ADVANCED PRACTICE NURSING

Essentials for Role Development

Third Edition

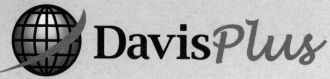

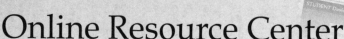

ADVANCED PRACTICE NURSING

Essentials for Role Development

Third Edition

Lucille A. Joel, EdD, APN, FAAN

Professor II
Rutgers, The State University of New Jersey
College of Nursing
Newark, New Jersey

F.A. Davis Company • Philadelphia

F. A. Davis Company
1915 Arch Street
Philadelphia, PA 19103
www.fadavis.com

Printed in the United States of America

Last digit indicates print number: 10 9 8 7 6 5 4 3 2

Publisher, Nursing: Joanne Patzek DaCunha, RN, MSN
Director of Content Development: Darlene D. Pedersen, MSN, APRN, BC
Project Editor: Victoria White
Electronic Project Manager: Tyler Baber
Design and Illustration Manager: Carolyn O'Brien

Library of Congress Cataloging-in-Publication Data

Advanced practice nursing : essentials for role development / [edited by]
Lucille A. Joel.—3rd ed.
p. ; cm.
Includes bibliographical references and index.
ISBN 978-0-8036-2785-7
I. Joel, Lucille A.
[DNLM: 1. Advanced Practice Nursing. 2. Nurse's Role. WY 128]

610.7306'92—dc23 2012037555

Preface

The content of this text was identified only after a careful review of the documents that shape both the advanced practice nursing role and the educational programs that prepare for practice. That review allowed some decisions about topics that were essential to all advanced practice nurses (APNs), whereas others were excluded because they are traditionally introduced during baccalaureate studies. This text is written for the graduate-level student in advanced practice and is intended to address the nonclinical aspects of the role.

Unit 1 explores *The Evolution of Advanced Practice* from the historical perspective of each of the specialties: the nurse-midwife, nurse anesthetist, clinical nurse specialist, and nurse practitioner. This historical background moves to a contemporary focus with the introduction of the many and varied hybrids of these roles that have appeared over time. These dramatic changes in practice have been a response to societal need. Adjustment to these changes is possible only from the kaleidoscopic view that theory allows. Skill acquisition, socialization, and adjustment to stress and strain are theoretical constructs and processes that will challenge the occupants of these roles many times over the course of a career, but coping can be taught and learned. Our accommodation to change is further challenged as we realize that advanced practice is neither unique to North America nor new on the global stage. Advanced practice roles, although accompanied by varied educational requirements and practice opportunities, are well embedded and highly respected in international culture. In the United States, education for advanced practice had become well stabilized at the master's-degree level. Such is no longer true, and the story of our recent transition to doctoral preparation is laid before us, with the subsequent issues this creates.

The Practice Environment, the topic of Unit 2, dramatically affects the care we give. With the addition of medical diagnosis and prescribing to the advanced practice repertoire, we became competitive with other disciplines, deserving the rights of reimbursement, prescriptive authority, clinical privileges, and participation as a member on health plan panels. There is the further responsibility to understand budgeting and material resource management, and the nature of different collaborative, responding, and reporting relationships. The APN often provides care within a mediated role, working through other professionals, including nurses, to improve the human condition.

Competency in Advanced Practice, the topic of Unit 3, demands an incisive mind capable of the highest order of critical thinking. This cognitive skill becomes refined as the subroles for practice emerge. The APN is ultimately a direct caregiver, client advocate, teacher, consultant, researcher, and case manager. The APN's forte is to coach individuals and populations so that they may take control of their own health in their own way, ideally even seeing chronic disease as a new trajectory of wellness. The APN's clients are as diverse as the many ethnicities of the U.S. public, and the challenge is often to learn from them, taking care to do no harm. The APN's therapeutic modalities go beyond traditional Western medicine, reaching into the realm of complementary therapies and integrative healthcare practices that have become expected by many consumers. Any or all of these role competencies are potential areas for conflict, needing to be understood, managed, and resolved in the best interests of the client. The chapters in this section aim to introduce these competencies, not to provide closure on any one topic; the art of direct care in specialty practice is not broached.

When you have completed your course of studies, you will have many choices to make. There are opportunities to pursue your practice as an employee, an employer, or an independent contractor. Each holds different rights and responsibilities. Each demands *Ethical, Legal, and Business Acumen,* which is covered in Unit 4. Each requires you to prove the value you hold for your clients and for the systems in which you work. Cost efficiency and therapeutic effectiveness cannot be dismissed lightly today. The nuts and bolts of establishing a practice are detailed, and although these particulars apply directly to independent practice, they can be easily extrapolated to employee status. Finally, experts in the field discuss the legal and ethical dimensions of practice, and how they uniquely apply to the role of the APN to ensure protection for ourselves and our clients.

This text has been carefully crafted based on almost 40 years of experience teaching APNs. It substantially includes the nonclinical knowledge necessary to perform successfully in the APN role and raises the issues that still have to be resolved to leave this practice area better than we found it.

LUCILLE A. JOEL

Contributors

Judith Barberio, PhD, APNC
Assistant Clinical Professor
Rutgers, The State University of New Jersey
College of Nursing
Newark, New Jersey
jabphd83@aol.com

Deborah Becker, PhD, ACNP, BC, CCNS
Practice Assistant Professor of Nursing
Biobehavioral and Health Sciences Department
University of Pennsylvania School of Nursing
Philadelphia, Pennsylvania
debecker@nursing.upenn.edu

Suzanne M. Burns, MSN, RRT, ACNP, CCRN, FAAN, FCCM, FAANP
Professor of Nursing and APN 3
Director of PNSO Research Program, UVA Health System
University of Virginia
Charlottesville, Virginia
smb4h@virginia.edu

Edna Cadmus, RN, PhD, NEA-BC
Clinical Professor, Specialty Director—Graduate Leadership Tracks
Rutgers, The State University of New Jersey
College of Nursing
Newark, New Jersey
ednacadm@rutgers.edu

Ann H. Cary, RN, MPH, PhD
Director and Professor
Robert Wood Johnson Executive Nurse Fellow
Loyola University
School of Nursing
New Orleans, Louisiana
ahcary@loyno.edu

Caroline Doherty, MSN, CRNP, ACNP-BC, AACC
Senior Lecturer
Associate Program Director
Adult Gerontology Acute Care Nurse Practitioner, Clinical Nurse Specialist, and
Adult Oncology Specialty Minor/Post Master's Certificate Program
University of Pennsylvania
School of Nursing
Interventional Cardiology Nurse Practitioner
Hospital of the University of Pennsylvania
Philadelphia, Pennsylvania
ctl@nursing.upenn.edu

H. Michael Dreher, RN, PhD, FAAN
Associate Professor
Advanced Nursing Role Department
College of Nursing and Health Professions
Drexel University
Philadelphia, Pennsylvania
Hd26@drexel.edu

Lynne M. Dunphy, PhD, APRN, BC, FAAN
Routhier Chair of Practice
Professor of Nursing, Family Nurse Practitioner
College of Nursing
University of Rhode Island
Kingston, Rhode Island
ldunphy@mail.uri.edu

Mary Lou S. Etheredge, CNS, BC
Director, Nursing Practice Development
Brigham and Women's Hospital
Boston, Massachusetts
Mlse2222@aol.com

Denise Fessler, RN, MSN, CMAC
Vice President, Clinical Services
Capital BlueCross
Harrisburg, Pennsylvania
Denise.Fessler@CapBlueCross.com

Eileen Flaherty, RN, MBA, MPH
Staff Specialist
Massachusetts General Hospital
Boston, Massachusetts
edflaherty@partners.com

Jane M. Flanagan, PhD, ANP-BC
Associate Professor
Boston College
Connell School of Nursing
Boston, Massachusetts
jane.flanagan@bc.edu

Donna A. Gaffney, DNSc, PMHCNS-BC, FAAN
Advisor for Education and Research
Project Rebirth
New York, New York
donnaagaffney@gmail.com

Rita Munley Gallagher, RN, PhD
Nursing and Healthcare Consultant
Washington, District of Columbia
drritamunleygallagher@att.net

Mary M. Germain, EdD, ANP-BC, FNAP
Professor Emeritus
SUNY-Downstate Medical Center
College of Nursing
Brooklyn, New York
mary.germain@downstate.edu

Kathleen M. Gialanella, JD, LLM, RN
Law Offices
Westfield, New Jersey
Associate Adjunct Professor
Teachers College, Columbia University
New York, New York
kgialanella@verizon.net

Shirley Girouard, RN, PhD, FAAN
Dean, School of Nursing
Long Island University
Brooklyn Campus
Brooklyn, New York
sgirouard@aol.com

Allyssa L. Harris, RN, PhD, WHNP-BC
Assistant Professor
William F. Connell School of Nursing
Boston College
Boston, Massachusetts
allyssa.harris@bc.edu

Patricia M. Haynor, RN, PhD
Associate Professor
Coordinator
BSN/MSN Gateway Program for RNs
Villanova University
College of Nursing
Villanova, Pennsylvania
patricia.haynor@villanova.edu

Gladys L. Husted, RN, PhD
Professor Emeritus
Duquesne University
School of Nursing
Pittsburgh, Pennsylvania
husted@duq.edu

James H. Husted
Independent Scholar
Pittsburgh, Pennsylvania

Lucille A. Joel, EdD, APN, FAAN
Professor
Rutgers, The State University of New Jersey
College of Nursing
Newark, New Jersey
ljoel@rutgers.edu

Dorothy A. Jones, RN, EdD, FAAN
Professor, Boston College
Director, Yvonne L. Munn Center for Nursing Research
Massachusetts General Hospital
Boston, Massachusetts
dorothy.jones@bc.edu

David M. Keepnews, RN, PhD, JD, NEA-BC, FAAN
Associate Professor
Hunter-Bellevue School of Nursing
Hunter College
City University of New York Graduate Center
New York, New York
dkeepnew@hunter.cuny.edu

Phyllis Beck Kritek, RN, PhD, FAAN
Conflict Engagement Consultant, Trainer, Facilitator, and Coach
Self-employed
Half Moon Bay, California
pbkritek@msn.com

Alice F. Kuehn, RN, PhD, BC-FNP/GNP
Associate Professor Emeritus
University of Missouri–Columbia School of Nursing
Columbia, Missouri
External Evaluator, North American Mobility Project
University of Minnesota
Minneapolis, Minnesota
kuehna@socket.net

Irene McEachen, RN, MSN, EdD
Associate Professor
Saint Peter's College
Division of Nursing
Jersey City, New Jersey
imceachen@spc.edu

Deborah C. Messecar, RN, MPH, PhD, GCNS-BC
Associate Professor
Director, Master of Nursing Education and Master of Public Health
Oregon Health and Science University
School of Nursing
Portland, Oregon
messecar@ohsu.edu

Kammie Monarch, RN, MSN, JD
Chief Operating Officer
Nurse-Family Partnership
Denver, Colorado
Founder, NursingLaw USA
Kammie.Monarch@nursefamilypartnership.org

Marilyn H. Oermann, RN, PhD, FAAN, ANEF
Frances Hill Fox Term Distinguished Professor
Chair, Adult/Geriatric Health, School of Nursing
University of North Carolina at Chapel Hill
Chapel Hill, North Carolina
moermann@email.unc.edu

Karen Piren, MS, PMHNP-BC
Chief Nursing Officer
State of New Jersey, Division of Mental Health and Addiction Services
Trenton, New Jersey
Karen.piren@dhs.state.nj.us

Beth Quatrara, RN, DNP, ACNS-BC
Clinical Nurse Specialist and Clinical Instructor
Assistant Director of the PNSO Research Program
University of Virginia Health System
Charlottesville, Virginia
BAD3E@hscmail.mcc.virginia.edu

Karen R. Robinson, RN, PhD, FAAN
Research Consultant and Clinical Quality Analyst
Fargo, North Dakota
robinson.karen6@gmail.com

Al Rundio, RN, DNP, PhD, APRN, NEA-BC
Clinical Professor of Nursing
Assistant Dean for Advanced Practice
Chair, Doctor of Nursing Practice Program
Drexel University
College of Nursing and Health Professions
Philadelphia, Pennsylvania
aar27@drexel.edu

Mary E. Samost, RN, MSN, DNP
Associate Chief Nursing Officer
Professional Development and Academic Integration
Cambridge Health Alliance
Cambridge, Massachusetts
MSamost@challiance.org

Madrean Schober, RN, MSN, FAANP
Visiting Senior Fellow
National University of Singapore
madreans@yahoo.com

Carrie Scotto, RN, PhD
Assistant Professor, College of Nursing
University of Akron
Akron, Ohio
cscotto@uakron.edu

Thomas D. Smith, RN, DNP, NEA-BC
Senior Vice President and Chief Nursing Officer
Maimonides Medical Center
Brooklyn, New York
TSmith@maimonidesmed.org

Mary C. Smolenski, MS, EdD, FNP, FAANP, CAE
Independent Consultant
Washington, District of Columbia
marysmo@verizon.net

Christine A. Tanner, RN, PhD, FAAN
A.B. Youmans Spaulding Distinguished Professor
Oregon Health and Science University
School of Nursing
Portland, Oregon
tannerc@ohsu.edu

Carolyn T. Torre, RN, MA, APN, PNP-BC
Nursing Policy Consultant
Formerly, Director, Regulatory Affairs, New Jersey State Nurses Association
Trenton, New Jersey
ctorre46@yahoo.com

Jan Towers, PhD, NP-C, CRNP (FNP), FAANP
Director of Health Policy
American Academy of Nurse Practitioners
Washington, District of Columbia
jtowers@AANP.org

Maria L. Vezina, RN, EdD, NEA-BC
Senior Director, Nursing Education and Professional Practice
The Mount Sinai Hospital
New York City, New York
maria.vezina@mountsinai.org

Marylou Yam, RN, PhD
Provost and Vice President of Academic Affairs
Saint Peter's College
Jersey City, New Jersey
mayam@spc.edu

Rothlyn P. Zahourek, PhD, PMHCNS-BC, AHN-BC
Adjunct Faculty, University of Massachusetts
Amherst, Massachusetts
American Holistic Nurses Association, Coordinator for Research
Retired, Private Practice and Consultation CNS in Mental Health Nursing
RorryZ@aol.com

Reviewers

Nancy Bittner, RN, PhD
Associate Dean
School of Nursing Science and Health Professions
Regis College
Weston, Massachusetts

Cynthia Bostick, PMHCNS-BC, PhD
Lecturer
California State University
Carson, California

Susan S. Fairchild, EdD, APRN
Dean, School of Nursing
Grantham University
Kansas City, Missouri

Cris Finn, RN, PhD, FNP
Assistant Professor
Regis University
Denver, Colorado

Susan C. Fox, RN, PhD, CNS-BC
Associate Professor
College of Nursing
University of New Mexico
Albuquerque, New Mexico

Eileen P. Geraci, PhD candidate, MA, ANP-BC
Professor of Nursing
Western Connecticut State University
Danbury, Connecticut

Elsabeth Jensen, RN, PhD
Associate Professor
School of Nursing
York University
Toronto, Ontario
Canada

Linda U. Krebs, RN, PhD, AOCN, FAAN
Associate Professor
University of Colorado
Anschutz Medical Campus, College of Nursing
Aurora, Colorado

Sandra Nadelson, RN, MS Ed, PhD
Associate Professor
Boise State University
Boise, Idaho

Geri B. Neuberger, RN, MN, EdD, ARNP-CS
Professor
University of Kansas School of Nursing
Kansas City, Kansas

Julie Ponto, RN, PhD, ACNS-BC, AOCN
Professor
Winona State University–Rochester
Rochester, Minnesota

Susan D. Schaffer, PhD, ARNP, FNP-BC
Chair, Department of Women's, Children's and Family Nursing
FNP Track Coordinator
University of Florida College of Nursing
Gainesville, Florida

Lynn Wimett, EdD, APRN-C
Professor
Regis University
Denver, Colorado

Acknowledgments

This book belongs to its authors. I am proud to be one among them. Beyond that, I have been the instrument to make these written contributions accessible to today's students and faculty. I thank each author for the products of his or her intellect, experience, and commitment to advanced practice.

Contents

UNIT 1

The Evolution of Advanced Practice

1

Advanced Practice Nursing: Doing What Has to Be Done—Radicals, Renegades, and Rebels

Lynne M. Dunphy

"I don't want less chaos ever, because chaos is opportunity. The nurse practitioner is not the end, it's the beginning."

Loretta Ford, quoted in "The Nurse Practitioner Question" in the American Journal of Nursing,*1974(12), 2191.*

On October 2, 2011, the *New York Times* ran an article with the headline "Calling More Nurses Doctor—A Title Physicians Begrudge." The article, taken from an earlier version written by Gardiner Harris and published on October 1, 2011, in Nashville, outlines the broader issue: that of someone not a physician using the title of doctor. There are already laws in effect in Arizona, Delaware, and other states that forbid nurses, pharmacists, and others to use the title "doctor" unless they immediately identify their profession, with other state and even federal legislation pending. Despite a new appreciation of the term *teamwork* in health care, physicians are unwilling to surrender their roles as leaders of the health-care team. Holding onto the mantra of years of specialized training and education, alleged to be far more than the approximately 8 years required to achieve the professional doctorate for pharmacists, physical therapists, and doctorates of nursing practice (DNP), it is medical practitioners alone who should diagnose illness and institute treatment. Advanced practice nurses respond *en masse*, making the case that they are more than capable of recognizing the vast majority of patients' problems. They cite their advanced education often *after* many years of basic nursing practice, seeing multiple clinical situations, their humility—and common sense—to refer appropriately as warranted, and an increasing mountain of evidence to back up their effectiveness. But some advanced practice nurses themselves remain ambivalent about the need for a "doctorate" of nursing practice (Cronenwett et al., 2011), a new rendition of organized nursing's ongoing push for full professionalization and a bigger slice of the health-care pie. What we have now is a time of potentially creative chaos, which, as noted by Loretta Ford, is a time of opportunity.

Loretta Ford, acknowledged creator of the nurse practitioner (NP) role, noted in 1991 that "the movement thrived because the foundation of the nurse practitioner was deeply rooted in the enduring values and goals of professional nursing" (Ford, 1991, p. 287). This chapter makes the case that, far from being a new creation, advanced practice nurses (APNs) actually predate the founding of modern professional nursing. A look back into our past reveals legendary figures always responding to the challenges of human need, changing the landscape of health care, and improving the health of the populace. The titles may change—such as a doctor of nursing practice—but the essence remains the same.

Advanced practice is a contemporary term that has evolved to label an old phenomenon: nurses/women providing care to those in need in their surrounding communities. As Barbara Ehrenreich and Deidre English (1973) note, "Women have always been healers. They were the unlicensed doctors and anatomists of western history . . . they were pharmacists, cultivating herbs and exchanging the secrets of their uses. They were midwives, travelling from home to home and village to village" (p. 3). Today, with health care dominated by a male-oriented medical profession, APNs (especially those cheeky enough to call themselves "doctor" even while clarifying their nursing role and background) are viewed as nurses "pushing the envelope"—the envelope of regulated, standardized nursing practice. The reality is that the boundaries of professional nursing practice have always been fluid, with changes in the practice setting speeding ahead of the educational and regulatory environments. It has always been those nurses caring for persons and families who see a need and respond—at times in concert with the medical profession, and at times, at odds—who are the true trailblazers of contemporary advanced practice nursing.

PRECURSORS AND ANTECEDENTS

There is a long and rich history of female lay healing with roots in both European and African cultures. Well into the 19th century, it was the female lay healer who was the primary health-care provider for most of the population. The sharing of skills and knowledge was seen as one's obligation as a member of a community. These skills were broad based and might include midwifery, the use of herbal remedies, and even bone setting (Ehrenreich, 2000, p. xxxiii). Laurel Ulrich, in *A Midwife's Tale* (1990), notes that when the diary of the midwife Martha Ballard opens in 1785, ". . . she knew how to manufacture salves, syrups, pills, teas, ointments, how to prepare an oil emulsion, how to poultice wounds, dress burns, treat dysentery, sore throat, frost bite, measles, colic, 'whooping cough,' 'chin cough,' . . . and 'the itch,' how to cut an infant's tongue, administer a 'clister' (enema), lance an abscessed breast . . . induce vomiting, assuage bleeding, reduce swelling and relieve a toothache, as well as deliver babies" (p. 11).

Ulrich notes the tiny headstones marking the graves of midwife Ballard's deceased babies and children as further evidence of her ability to provide compassionate, knowledgeable care; she was able to understand the pain and suffering of others. The emergence of a male medical establishment in the 19th century marked the beginning of the end of the era of female lay healers, including midwives. The lay healers saw their role as intertwined with one's obligations to the community, whereas the emerging medical class saw healing as a commodity to be bought and sold (Ehrenreich & English, 1978). Has this really changed? Are not our current struggles still bound up with issues of gender, class, social position, and money? Have we not entered a phase of more radical than ever splits between the haves and have–nots, with grave consequences to our social fabric?

Nursing histories (O'Brien, 1987) have documented the emergence of professional nursing in the 19th century from women's domestic duties and roles, extensions of the things that women and/or servants had always done for their families. Modern nursing is usually pinpointed as beginning in 1873, the year of the opening of the first three U.S. training schools for nurses, "as an effort on the part of women reformers to help clean up the mess the male doctors were making" (Ehrenreich, 2000, p. xxxiv). The incoming nurses, for example, are credited with introducing the first bar of soap into Bellevue Hospital in the dark days when the medical profession was still resisting the germ theory of disease and aseptic techniques.

The emergence of a strong public health movement in the 19th century, coupled with the Settlement House Movement, created a new vista for independent and autonomous nursing practice. The Henry Street Settlement, a brainchild of a recently graduated trained nurse named Lillian Wald, was a unique community-based nursing practice on the lower east side of New York City. Wald described these nurses who flocked to work with her at Henry Street Settlement as women of above average "intellectual equipment," of "exceptional character, mentality and scholarship" (Daniels, 1989, p. 24). These nurses, as has been well documented, enjoyed an exceptional degree of independence and autonomy in their nursing practice, caring for the poor, often recent immigrants.

In 1893, Wald described a typical day. First, she visited the Goldberg baby and then Hattie Isaacs, a patient with consumption to whom she brought flowers. Wald spent 2 hours bathing her ("the poor girl had been without this attention for so long that it took me nearly two hours to get her skin clean"). Next, she inspected some houses on Hester Street, where she found water closets that needed "chloride of lime" and notified the appropriate authorities. In the next house she found a child with "running ears," which she "syringed," showing the mother how to do it at the same time. In another room there was a child with a "summer complaint"; Wald gave the child bismuth and tickets for a seaside excursion. After lunch she saw the O'Briens and took the "little one, with whooping cough" to play in the back of the Settlement House yard. On the next floor of that tenement, she found the Costria baby, who had a sore mouth. Wald "gave the mother honey and borax and little cloths to keep it clean" (Coss, 1989, pp. 43–44). This was all before 2 p.m.! Far from being some new invention, midwives, nurse anesthetists, clinical nurse specialists (CNSs), and NPs are merely new permutations of these long-standing nursing commitments and roles.

NURSE-MIDWIVES

Throughout the 20th century, nurse-midwifery remained an anomaly in the U.S. health-care system. Nurse-midwives attend only a small percentage of all U.S. births. Since the early decades of that century, physicians laid claim to being the sole legitimate birth attendants in the United States (Dye, 1984). This is in contrast to Great Britain and many other European countries, where trained midwives attend a significant percentage of births. In Europe, homes remain an accepted place to give birth, whereas hospital births reign supreme in the United States. In contrast to Europe, the United States has little in the way of a tradition of professional midwifery.

As late as 1910, 50% of all births in the United States were reportedly delivered by midwives, and the percentage in large cities was often higher. However, the health status of the U.S. population, particularly in regard to perinatal health indicators, was poor (Bigbee & Amidi-Nouri, 2000). Midwives—unregulated and, by most accounts, unprofessional—were easy scapegoats on which to blame the problem of poor maternal and infant outcomes. New York City's Department of Health commissioned a study that claimed that the New York midwife was essentially "medieval." According to this report, fully 90% were "hopelessly dirty, ignorant, and incompetent" (Edgar, 1911, p. 882). There was a concerted movement away from home births. This was all part of a mass assault on midwifery by an increasingly powerful medical elite of obstetricians determined to control the birthing process.

These revelations resulted in the tightening of existing laws and the creation of new legislation for the licensing and supervision of midwives (Kobrin, 1984). Several states passed laws granting legal recognition and regulation of midwives, resulting in the establishment of schools of midwifery. One example, the Bellevue School for Midwives in New York City, lasted until 1935, when the diminishing need for midwives made it difficult to justify its existence (Komnenich, 1998). Obstetrical care continued the move into hospitals in urban areas that did not provide midwifery. For the most part, the advance of nurse-midwifery has been a slow and arduous struggle, often at odds with mainstream nursing. For example, Lavinia Dock (1901) wrote that all births must be attended by physicians. Public health nurses, committed to the professionalizing of nursing and adherence to scientific standards, chose to distance themselves from lay midwives. The heritage of the unprofessional image of the lay midwife would linger for many years.

A more successful example of midwifery was the founding of the Frontier Nursing Service (FNS) in 1925 by Myra Breckinridge in Kentucky. Breckinridge pursued a vision of autonomous nurse-midwifery practice, having been educated as a public health nurse and traveling to Great Britain to become a certified nurse-midwife (CNM). She aimed to implement the British system in the United States (always a daunting enterprise on any front). In rural settings, where doctors were scarce and hospitals virtually nonexistent, midwifery found more fertile soil. However, even in these settings, professional nurse-midwifery had to struggle to bloom.

Breckinridge founded the FNS at a time when the national maternal death rate stood at 6.7 per 1000 live births, one of the poorest rates in the Western world. More than 250,000 infants, nearly 1 in 10, died before they reached their first birthday (U.S. Department of Labor, 1920). The Sheppard-Towner Maternity and Infancy Act, enacted to provide public funds for maternal and child health programs, was the first federal legislation passed for specifically this purpose. Part of the intention of this act was to provide money to the states to train public health nurses in midwifery; however, this proved short-lived. By 1929, the bill lapsed; this was attributed by some to major opposition by the American Medical Association (AMA), which advocated the establishment of a "single standard" of obstetrical care, that is, provided by doctors in hospital settings (Kobrin, 1984).

Breckinridge saw nurse-midwives working as independent practitioners and continued to advocate home births. And even more radically, FNS saw nurse-midwives as offering complete care to women with normal pregnancies and deliveries. However, even Breckinridge and her supporters did not advocate the FNS model for cities where doctors were plentiful and middle-class women could afford medical care. She stressed that the FNS was designed for impoverished "remotely rural areas" without physicians (Dye, 1984).

The American Association of Nurse-Midwives (AANM) was founded in 1928, originally as the Kentucky State Association of Midwives, which was an outgrowth of FNS. First organized as a section of the National Organization of Public Health Nurses (NOPHN), the American College of Nurse-Midwives (ACNM) was incorporated in 1955 as an independent specialty nursing organization when the NOPHN was subsumed within the National League for Nursing (NLN). In 1956, the AANM merged with the college, forming the ACNM as it continues today. The ACNM sponsored the *Journal of Nurse-Midwifery,* implemented an accreditation process of programs in 1962, and established a certification examination and process in 1971. This body also currently certifies non-nurses as midwives and maintains alliances with professional midwives who are not nurses. As noted by Bigbee and Amidi-Nouri (2000), CNMs are distinct from other APNs in that "they conceptualize their role as the combination of two disciplines, nursing and midwifery" (p. 12).

Currently, the ACNM remains skeptical of the move toward the doctorate of nursing practice, although as of this writing, one midwifery program leading to the DNP does exist. At their core, midwives as a group remain focused on their primary commitment: care of mothers and babies, regardless of setting and ability to pay.

NURSE ANESTHETISTS

Nursing made medicine look good. — *Baer, 1982*

Sister Mary Bernard is recognized as the first nurse anesthetist to practice in the United States (Thatcher, 1953). Church records of 1877 identify her as being called on to function as an anesthetist while enrolled as a student in St. Vincent's Hospital in Erie, Pennsylvania.

Surgical anesthesia was born in the United States in the mid-19th century. Immediately there were rival claimants to its "discovery" (Bankert, 1989). In 1846, at Massachusetts General Hospital, William T. G. Morton first successfully demonstrated surgical anesthesia. Nitrous oxide was the first agent used and adopted by U.S. dentists. Ether and chloroform followed shortly as agents for use in anesthetizing a patient. One barrier to surgery had been removed. However, it would take infection control and consistent, careful techniques in the administration of the various anesthetic agents for surgery to enter its "Golden Age." It was only then that "surgery was transformed from an act of desperation to a scientific method of dealing with illness" (Rothstein, 1958, p. 258). For surgeons to advance their specialty, they needed someone to administer anesthesia with care. However, anesthesiology lacked medical status; the surgeon collected the fee. No incentive existed for anyone with a medical degree to take up the work. Who would administer the anesthesia? And who would administer it reliably, carefully? There was only one answer: nurses.

Marianne Bankert, in her landmark book *Watchful Care: A History of America's Nurse Anesthetists* (1989), explains how economics changed anesthesia practice. Physician-anesthetists "needed to establish their 'claim' to a field of practice they had earlier rejected" (p. 16), and to do this, it became necessary to deny, ignore, or denigrate the achievements of their nurse colleagues. The most intriguing part of her study, she says, was "the process by which a rival—and less moneyed—group (in this case, nurses) is rendered historically 'invisible'" (p. 16).

St. Mary's Hospital, later to become known as the Mayo Clinic, played an important role in the development of anesthesia. It was here that Alice Magaw, sometimes referred to as the "Mother of Anesthesia," practiced from 1860 to 1928. In 1899 she published a paper titled "Observations in Anesthesia" in *Northwestern Lancet* in which she reported giving anesthesia in more than 3000 cases (Magaw, 1899). In 1906 she published another review of more than 14,000 successful anesthesia cases (Magaw, 1906). Bigbee and Amidi-Nouri (2000) note, "She stressed individual attention for all patients and identified the experience of anesthetists as critical elements in quickly responding to the patient" (p. 21). She also paid special attention to her patients' psyches: She believed that "suggestion" was a great help "in producing a comfortable narcosis" (Bankert, 1989, p. 32). She noted that the anesthetist "must be able to inspire confidence in the patient" and that much of this depends on the approach (Bankert, 1989, p. 32). She stressed preparing the patient for each phase of the experience and of the need to "'talk him to sleep' with the addition of as little ether as possible" (p. 33). Magaw contended that hospital-based anesthesia services, as a specialized field, should remain separate from nursing service administrative structures (Bigbee & Amidi-Nouri, 2000). This presaged the estrangement that has historically existed between nurse anesthetists and "regular" nursing; again we see a nursing specialty with expanded clinical responsibilities developing outside of mainstream nursing.

It was around the turn of the century that the medical specialty of anesthesiology began to gain a foothold, led largely by women physicians. However, these physicians were unsympathetic to the role of the nurse anesthetists; they wanted/needed to replace them to establish their own controls. Different variants of this old power struggle echo today in legislative battles over the need for on-site oversight by an anesthesiologist.

The American Association of Nurse Anesthetists (AANA) was founded in 1931 by Hodgins and originally named the National Association for Nurse Anesthetists. This group voted to affiliate with the American Nurses Association (ANA), only to be turned away. As early as 1909, Florence Henderson, a successor of Magaw's, was invited to present a paper at the ANA convention, with no subsequent extension of an invitation to become a member of the organization (Komnenich, 1998). Thatcher (1953) speculates that organized nursing was fearful that nurse anesthetists could be charged with practicing medicine, a theme we will see repeated when we examine the history of the development of the nurse practitioner role. This rejection led AANA to affiliate with the American Hospital Association. The relationship between nurse anesthetists and anesthesiologists has always been, and continues to be, contentious. Despite a brief period of relative harmony, from 1972 to 1976, when its respective professional organizations issued the "Joint Statement on Anesthesia Practice," their partnership ended when the board of directors of the American Society of Anesthesiologists withdrew their support of this statement, returning to a model that maintained physician control (Bankert, 1989, pp. 140–150).

At present, there are approximately 44,000 (AANA, 2011) certified registered nurse anesthetists (CRNAs),* 41% of whom are males (compared to the approximately 13% male population in nursing overall, a figure that has held steady for some time).

Interestingly, the inclusion of large numbers of males in its ranks has not eased the advance of this venerable nursing specialty; turf wars between practicing anesthesiologists and nurse anesthetists remain intensely active as of this writing, further aggravated by the incursion of "doctor-nurses" or "nurse-doctors." Nonetheless, nurse anesthetists continue to thrive and have situated themselves in the mainstream of graduate-level nursing education, including a large portion of programs adapting curriculums leading to the Doctorate of Nursing Practice (DNP). Their inclusion in the spectrum of advanced practice nursing continues to be invigorating for us.

THE CLINICAL NURSE SPECIALIST

The role of the CNS is the one strand of advanced practice nursing that arose and was nurtured by mainstream nursing education and nursing organizations. Indeed, one could say it arose from the very bosom of traditional nursing practice. As early as 1900, in the *American Journal of Nursing,* Katherine DeWitt wrote that the development of nursing specialties, in her view, responded to a "need for perfection within a limited domain" (Sparacino, 1986, p. 1). According to DeWitt, nursing specialties were a response to "present civilization and modern science [that] demand a perfection along each line of work formerly unknown" (idem). She argued that "the new nurse is more useful, at least to the patient himself, and ultimately to the family and community. Her sphere is more limited, but her patient receives better care" (idem).

Nurses were trained and worked in hospitals that were structured for the convenience of the doctors around specific populations of patients. Early on, nurses initiated guidelines for the care of unique populations and often garnered a hands-on kind of intimacy, an expertise in the care of certain patients that was not to be denied. Caring day-in and day-out for patients suffering from similar conditions enabled nurses to develop specialized and advanced skills, not practiced by other nurses. Think of the nurses who cared exclusively for patients with tuberculosis, syphilis, and polio. Because these conditions are no longer common, any nursing expertise that might have been developed has been lost.

*In some states, the title CRNA has been changed to APN-Anesthesia.

In a 1943 speech, Frances Reiter first used the term *nurse-clinician.* She believed that "practice is the absolute primary function of our profession" and "that means the direct care of patients" (Reiter, 1966). The nurse-clinician, as Reiter conceived the role, consisted of three spheres. Clinical competence, the first sphere, included three additional dimensions of function, which she termed *care, cure,* and *counseling.* The nurse-clinician was labeled "the Mother Role," in which the nurse protects, teaches, comforts, and encourages the patient. The second sphere, as envisioned by Reiter, involved clinical expertise in the coordination and continuity of the patient's care. Last, she believed in what she called "professional maturity," wherein the physician and nurse "share a mutual responsibility for the welfare of patients" (Reiter, 1966, p. 277). It was only through such working together that the patient could best be served and nursing achieve "its greatest potential" (Reiter, 1966). Although Reiter believed that the nurse-clinician should have advanced clinical competence, she did not specify that the nurse-clinician should be prepared at the master's level.

In 1943, the National League for Nursing Education advocated a plan to develop these *nurse-clinicians,* enlisting universities to educate them (Menard, 1987). Traditionally, advanced education in nursing had focused on "functional" areas: that is, nursing education and nursing administration. Esther Lucile Brown, in her 1948 report *Nursing for the Future,* promoted developing clinical specialties in nursing as a way of strengthening and advancing the profession. The GI Bill was also available. Nurses in the Armed Services were eligible to receive funds for their education.

It took the entrance of another strong nurse leader, Hildegard Peplau, to move these ideas forward to fruition. In 1953, she had both a vision and a plan: She wanted to prepare psychiatric nurse clinicians at the graduate level who could offer direct care to psychiatric patients, thus helping to close the gap between psychiatric theory and nursing practice (Callaway, 2002). In addition, as always, there was a great need for health-care providers of all stripes in psychiatric settings. In her first 2 years at Rutgers University in New Jersey, Peplau developed a 19-month master's program that prepared only CNSs in psychiatric nursing. In contrast, existing programs, for example at Teachers College in New York City, attempted to prepare nurses for teaching and supervision in a 10-month program.

The field of psychiatric nursing was in the process of inventing itself. Before the passage of the National Mental Health Act in 1946, there was no such field as psychiatric nursing. It was the availability of National Institute of Mental Health funds to "seed" such programs as Peplau's that allowed psychiatric nursing to begin and eventually to flourish.

In retrospect, Peplau would note that no encouragement was received from the two major nursing organizations of the day, the NLN and the ANA. She stated, "We were highly stigmatized. Any nurse who worked in [the field of mental health] was considered almost certifiable. . . . We were thoroughly unpopular, we were considered queer enough to be avoided" (Callaway, 2002, p. 229). It should be emphasized that at this point in nursing history it was inconceivable that any nurse, under any circumstances, could become a specialist.

The "received wisdom" of the day was the axiom, followed by the vast majority of nurses, that "a nurse is a nurse is a nurse," opposing any differentiation between who was doing what among them. Peplau's rigorous curriculum and clinical and academic program requirements expected that faculty would continue their own clinical practice, do clinical research, and publish the results (Calloway, 2002). This was a radical model for nursing faculty, few of whom were doctorally prepared in the 1950s. In 1956, only 2 years following the initiation of the first clinically focused graduate program, a national working conference on graduate education in psychiatric nursing formally developed the role of the psychiatric clinical specialist.

Most hospital training schools remained embedded in a functional method of nursing well into the 1960s. As originally conceptualized by Isabel Stewart in the 1930s, "nurses were trained and much of nursing practice was rule-based and activity-oriented" (Fairman, 1999, p. 42), relying heavily on repetition of skills and procedures. There was little, if any, scientific understanding of the principles underlying care. There was little, if any, intellectual content to be found in nursing care. With the advent of antibiotics in the 1940s and the resulting decline of infectious diseases, nurses were confronted with patients with acute, often rapidly changing exacerbations of chronic conditions. Leaders like Peplau, along with others such as Virginia Henderson, Frances Reiter, and later Dorothy Smith, began developing a theoretical orientation for practice. Students were being taught to assess patient responses to their illnesses and to make analytical decisions. Smith experimented with the idea of a nurse-clinician who had 24-hour responsibility for a patient area and who was on call. Laura Simms at Cornell University–New York Hospital School of Nursing developed a CNS role to provide consultation to more generalist nurses. As opposed to the nurse who might have been expert in procedures, these new clinicians were experts in clinical care for a certain population of patients. This development occurred across specialties and was seen in oncology, nephrology, psychiatry, and intensive care units (Sills, 1983).

Role expansion of the CNS grew rapidly during the 1960s because of several factors. Advances in medical technology and medical specialization increased the need for nurses who were competent to care for patients with complex health needs. Nurses returning from the battlefields of Vietnam sought to increase their knowledge and skills, continuing to practice in advanced roles and nontraditional areas (such as trauma or anesthesia). Role definitions for women loosened and expanded. There was a shortage of physicians. The Nurse Training Act of 1964 allocated necessary federal funds for additional graduate nursing education programs in several different clinical specialties (Mirr & Snyder, 1995).

The terms *nurse-clinician, clinical nurse specialist,* and *nurse specialist,* among others, were used extensively by nurses with experience or advanced knowledge who had developed an expertise within a given area of patient care. There were no standards in regard to educational requirements or experience. In 1965, the ANA developed a position statement declaring that only those nurses with a master's degree or higher in nursing should claim the role of CNS (ANA, 1965). These trends continued into the 1970s. The number of academic programs providing master's preparation in a variety of practice areas increased. Federal grants including those from the Department of Health, Education, and Welfare continued to provide funding for nursing education at the master's and doctoral levels.

In 1976, during the ANA's Congress on Nursing Practice, a position statement on the role of the CNS was issued. The ANA position statement read as follows (ANA Congress for Nursing Practice, 1976):

> *The clinical nurse specialist (CNS) is a practitioner holding a master's degree with a concentration in specific areas of clinical nursing. The role of the CNS is defined by the needs of a select client population, the expectation of the larger society and the clinical expertise of the nurse.*

The statement went on to elaborate that "by exercising leadership ability and judgment," the CNS is able to both affect client care on the individual, direct-care provider level and affect change within the broader health-care system (ANA Congress for Nursing Practice, 1976).

The 1970s were a time of growth in academic CNS programs; the 1980s were years in which refinements occurred. In 1980, the ANA revised its earlier policy statement of 1976 to define the CNS as "a registered nurse who, through study and supervised clinical practice at the graduate level (master's or doctorate) has become an expert in a defined area of knowledge and practice in a selected clinical area of nursing" (ANA, 1980, p. 23). This statement was significant because it was the first time that education at the master's level had been dictated as a mandatory criterion for entry into expert practice.

The CNS role, more than any other advanced nursing role, was situated in the mainstream of graduate nursing education, with the first master's degree in psychiatric/mental health nursing conferred by Rutgers University in 1955. The inclusion of clinical content in master's degree education was an essential step forward for nursing's advancement. But the implementation and use of the CNS evaded easy categorization and their efficacy was elusive.

In February 1983, the ANA Council of Clinical Nurse Specialists met for the first time (Sparacino, 1990). The Council grew rapidly throughout the following years, supporting and providing educational conferences for the increasing numbers of CNSs. In 1986, the Council published the Clinical Nurse Specialist's role statement. This statement identified the roles of the CNS as specialist in clinical practice and as educator, consultant, researcher, and administrator. This role statement by the Council depicted the changing role of the CNS, notably delegating and overseeing practice, as its primary focus (Fulton, 2002). The year 1986 was also notable for the publication of the journal *Clinical Nurse Specialist: The Journal for Advanced Nursing.*

In 1986, the ANA's Council of Clinical Nurse Specialists and the Council of Primary Health Care Providers published an editorial comparing the similarities of the CNS and NP roles. Discussion surrounding the commonalities of both specialties occurred throughout the decade. In 1989, during the annual meeting of the National Organization of Nurse Practitioner Faculty (NONPF), the 10-year-old debate regarding the merger of the two roles reached a crescendo without resolution (Lincoln, 2000). It remains an issue of contention to the present day. Despite this, the two ANA councils did merge in 1990, becoming the Council of Nurses in Advanced Practice (Busen & Engleman, 1996; Lincoln, 2000). Following the merger of the councils, several studies were published comparing CNS and NP roles, finding the education for practice generally comparable (Joel, 2003). The 1990s was an era of health-care "reform." Health-care costs were skyrocketing; hospital stays were shorter, with acutely ill patients being discharged quicker and sicker. As a result of fiscal mandates, hospitals were downsizing the number of beds and personnel. The historically hospital-based CNS was considered too expensive and unproven, and the focus of health care shifted from hospital to ambulatory care within the community and home. CNSs all over were losing positions.

In 1993, the American Association of Colleges of Nursing (AACN) met to discuss educational needs and requirements for the 21st century. In December 1994, at the AACN's annual conference, members voted to support the merging of the CNS/NP roles in the curricula of graduate education in nursing. Although the structure of the curricula suggested in the "Essentials of Graduate Education" (AACN, 1995) has been widely adopted, the lived reality of role adaptation and its implementation in the marketplace has been less uniform and more divisive. Sparacino (1990) defined the scope of the CNS as "client-centered practice, utilizing an in-depth assessment, practiced within the domain of secondary and tertiary care settings" (p. 8). The NP role is defined by Sparacino (1986) as being responsible for providing a full range of primary health-care services, using the appropriate knowledge base and practicing in multiple settings outside of secondary and tertiary settings. The "other side" of this story of advanced practice nursing—nurse practitioner evolution—is addressed in the next section of this chapter. The futures of these various roles remain on some level intertwined and are further complicated by the emergence of a new role and title: the doctor of nursing practice (DNP).

In an effort to bring some clarity to, and standardization of, advanced practice nursing roles, in 2008 the APRN Consensus Model, also referred to as a regulatory model, was published by the APRN Consensus Work Group and the National Council of State Boards of Nursing (NCSBN) APRN Advisory Committee with extensive input from a larger APRN stakeholder community. The nomenclature *APRN (Advanced Practice Registered Nurse)* was adopted, and four APRN roles were defined in the document: certified nurse-midwives (CNMs), certified registered nurse anesthetists

(CRNAs), clinical nurse specialists (CNSs), and certified nurse practitioners (CNPs). An APRN is further defined as a registered nurse who has completed a graduate degree or postgraduate program that has prepared him or her to practice in one of these four roles. The acronym LACE—standing for "licensure, accreditation, certification, and education"—demonstrates alliances across these spheres for implementation of the APRN Consensus Model, thus promoting uniformity and standardization of the APRN role for the safety of the consumer of health care. The target date for model implementation is 2015, with an alignment of current certifying exams with educational program offerings and subsequent licensure.

THE EVOLUTION OF THE NURSE PRACTITIONER ROLE: "A DISRUPTIVE INNOVATION"

The history of the NP "movement" has been well documented (Brush & Capezuti, 1996; Fairman, 1999, 2008; Jacox, 2002). A lesser known story involves Dr. Eugene A. Stead, Jr., of Duke University, who in 1957 conceived of an advanced role for nurses, somewhere between the role of the nurse and the doctor. Thelma Ingles, a nursing faculty member on a sabbatical, worked with Stead, rounding with the interns and residents, seeing patients, and managing increasingly ill patients with acumen and sensitivity. Ingles shared Stead's ideas and returned to the Duke Nursing School to create a master of science in nursing program modeled on her experience with Stead. Stead was gratified and anxious to impart this expanded role to other nursing faculty, envisioning a new role for nurses, with, in his view, expanded autonomy. He was shocked at the "lukewarm" response of the dean of nursing at Duke and the nonsupportive stance of a number of prominent nurses at the university. On top of that, the NLN, the school's accrediting body, did not approve of Ingles's new program for nurse clinical specialization and withheld the program's accreditation. They found the program "unstructured" and criticized the use of physicians as instructors to teach courses for nurses in a nursing program. They disavowed the study of the esteemed discipline of medicine that Stead was so anxious to impart (Holt, 1998). Instead, they wanted the students to study "nursing." Stead could not understand this. What was there in nursing to study? Rejected and disheartened, Stead eventually turned to military corpsmen to actualize this new role, which he named *physician assistant.* He insisted that they be male. In his view, nurse leaders were very antagonistic to innovation and change (Christman, 1998). In the view of some, this was a missed opportunity for organized nursing, but one governed by historical circumstances when viewed on the broader stage of history. Fairman (2008) in an extensive study of Stead's papers offers the appraisement that "Stead's difficulties went beyond his experiences with organized and academic nursing. They reflected his perceptions of the kind of help his physician colleagues needed" (Fairman, 2008, p. 98).

Stead's original proposal was quite prescient. Gender roles were loosening, as were hierarchical structures in general; nurses were better educated and well able to assume the role responsibilities that Stead envisioned. Yet it came at a time when nursing was merely a fledgling discipline, new to the university, new to development as an academic discipline, and new to doctoral education. Academic nursing was fixated on defining its own knowledge base and developing its own unique science. Along with expanded opportunities for women came ideas of an autonomous nursing role, separate and distinct from medicine. Stead's deeply rooted gender-role stereotyping no doubt further inflamed nursing resistance to "his" new role. Other settings—such as the University of Colorado, where Henry Silver, pediatrician, and Loretta Ford, a master's prepared public health nurse, founded a partnership rooted in collaboration—provided more fruitful results. All these factors were in play when the first NPs emerged in the 1960s.

However, the NP was not really a new role for nurses. Examining our history, it is apparent that nurses functioned independently and autonomously before the rise of organized medicine. If medicine was ambivalent about the emergence of this new role, nursing itself was no less conflicted.

In 1978 the following statement appeared in the *American Journal of Nursing* (Roy & Obloy, 1978, p. 1698):

> *The nurse practitioner movement has become an issue in nursing, a topic on which there is no consensus. One question about the movement is whether the development of the nurse practitioner role adds to, or detracts from, the development of nursing as a distinct scientific discipline.*

This statement was issued more than 13 years after the initiation of the first NP program at the University of Colorado. If, as Sparacino (1990) spells out, the domain of the CNS is situated in the secondary and tertiary setting, the domain of the NP originally arose as a role situated in primary care.

Loretta Ford and Dr. Henry Silver designed a graduate curriculum for pediatric nurses to provide ambulatory care to poor rural Colorado children. The goal of this program was to bridge the gap between the health-care needs of children and the family's ability to access and afford primary health care (Ford & Silver, 1967; Silver, Ford, & Stearly, 1967). This program was situated in graduate education and included courses such as pathophysiology, health promotion, and growth and development, with the intent of the student understanding the principles of healthy child care and patient education. Nurses would then be able to provide preventive nursing services outside of the hospital setting in collaboration with physicians. Students had to have a baccalaureate degree and public health nursing experience to be admitted to the program.

Ford states the following in an interview: "We looked at the nurse practitioner preparation not as a separate program but as integrated into a role that had already been designed at the graduate level" (Jacox, 2002, p. 155). Ford notes that the lack of organizational leadership in the profession coupled with a lack of responsiveness in academic settings caused a "bastardization of the model" (Jacox, 2002, p. 157). She had envisioned that our professional organization, as in other professions, would identify, credential, and make public advanced nurse practitioners. However, Ford was to discover that the "ANA in those early years was reluctant to stick its neck out and give some leadership to the nurse practitioner groups that were growing rapidly," and that the lack of leadership in nursing education created "a patchwork quilt" of differently prepared NPs (Jacox, 2002, p. 157). Although clinically based programs were growing, there remained resistance to the NP model. Ford (Jacox, 2002, p. 155) says,

> *I understood that faculty members were supposed to be doing just that—push the borders of knowledge and publish their work. In my naiveté of faculty politics, I expected that since the NP model grew out of professional nursing and public health nursing—including primary, secondary, and tertiary prevention and community-based services—it was a perfectly legitimate investigation. Instead, it became a battleground, and even recently was labeled in the Harvard Business Review as a "Disruptive Innovation." What a compliment!*

The collaboration between NP and physician has been analyzed and debated since the advent of the NP role, including the relationship between Ford and Silver (Fairman, 2002, 2008). The sticking point of collaboration is that it has included the heavy implication of supervision and thus control. In truth, in the early 1970s both NPs and physicians had to give up their traditional roles, tasks, and knowledge to establish this new provider role, often in the face of organizational and societal opposition. Jan Towers describes the growth of her own NP practice as follows: "The area that I perhaps most feared turned out to be the least troublesome, after some initial adjustments between the physician with whom I was working and me were made" (Towers, 1995, p. 269). What would often be impossible on an organizational level was more easily resolvable among professionals with a shared interest and commitment: the good of the patient.

Prescriptive authority was a major issue, and it was either delegated from the medical practice act and carried out under physicians' standing orders or protocols, or it came directly from the nursing practice acts. Nurse historian Arlene Keeling has argued that far from being a new realm of nursing practice, the "prescribing"—or use—of a variety of techniques/substances for therapeutic effect has always been a dimension of nursing practice (Keeling, 2007). The states of Oregon and Washington allowed nurses the freedom to prescribe independently in 1983 (Kalisch & Kalisch, 1986). Some of the fiercest turf battles have heated up over prescriptive privileges. By 1984, nurses were accused of practicing medicine, although they were practicing well within the scope of their expanded role. Physicians remained ambivalent. They pushed NPs to function broadly but did not usually support legislation that authorized an increased scope of practice, especially in the area of prescriptive privileges. Joan Lynaugh, nurse historian, describes nurse practitioners as looking for an "exam room of their own"—essentially a clinical space in which to provide nursing care (Fairman, 2008, p. 7). This space is indeed a crowded one (Fairman, 2008, p. 200, note 9).

The Great Society entitlement programs significantly influenced the need for NPs to care for people who were covered under Medicare and Medicaid. Predominant social movements—women's rights, civil rights, antiwar protest, consumerism—had a profound impact on the need for groups to assert their place in the society of the 1960s and early 1970s. Nurses were not immune to the forces unleashed in these years and took advantage of the opportunities to work with physicians "in relationships that were entrepreneurial and groundbreaking, and to engage in a kind of dialogue that supported new models of care" (Fairman, 2002, p. 165). These nurses were pioneers, rebels, and renegades treading on uncertain ground.

The National Advisory Commission on Health Manpower supported the NP movement (Moxley, 1968). The Committee to Study Extended Roles for Nurses in the early 1970s recommended that the expanded role for nurses was necessary to provide the consumer with access to health care and proposed the inclusion of highly developed health assessment skills (Kalisch & Kalisch, 1986; Leininger, Little, & Carnevali, 1972; Marchione & Garland, 1997). Although the committee did stop short of providing a definitive scope of practice statement, it recommended support for licensure and certification for advanced practice, recognition in the nursing practice act, further cost-benefit research, and surveys on role impact. Government and private groups rapidly developed funding support for educational programs (Hamric, Spross, & Hanson, 1996). According to Marchione and Garland (1997), "The traditional role of humanistic caring, comforting, nurturing and supporting was to be maintained and improved by the addition" of new primary care functions that the Department of Health, Education, and Welfare approved: total patient assessment, monitoring, health promotion, and a focus that encompassed not only disease prevention but health promotion and maintenance, treatment, and continuity of care.

The Division of Nursing of the Department of Health, Education, and Welfare tracked the development of the NP role from 1974 to 1977, during which time the number of NP programs rose from 86 to 178 across the country, with significant governmental support through the Nurse Training Act to advanced practice nursing education programs of all types. Although nurse educators by this time wanted NP education standardized, in 1977 most NP programs awarded a certificate with some still using continuing education models and accepting less than a baccalaureate degree for entry. However, the number of NP graduates of master's programs did increase from 20% in 1975 to 26% in 1977, again largely encouraged by the availability of federal funds for support. The education of nurse practitioners was the rallying cry for the formation of the NONPF in 1980, dedicated to defining curriculum and evaluation standards, as well as pioneering research and development related to nurse practitioner practice and teaching-learning methodologies. The political voice for NPs was enhanced with the formation of the American Academy of Nurse Practitioners (AANP) in 1985 and the American College of Nurse Practitioners in 2003.

The Nurse Training Acts of 1971 and 1975 were critical in providing federal funding to support NP programs. By 1979, more than 133 programs and tracks existed, and approximately 15,000 NPs were in practice. By 1983 and 1984, NP graduates numbered approximately 20,000 to 24,000; they were primarily employed in sites that served those in greatest need: public health departments, community health centers, outpatient and rural clinics, health maintenance organizations, school-based clinics, and occupational health clinics (Hamric et al., 1996; Kalisch & Kalisch, 1986; Pulcini & Wagner, 2001). NPs were typically providing care for health promotion, disease prevention, minor acute problems, chronic stabilized illness, and the full range of teaching and coaching that nurses have always provided for patients and families. A hindrance to practice in rural areas was finding appropriate physician backup. By 1987, the federal government had spent $100 million to promote NP education, primarily through the U.S. Public Health Service Division of Nursing (Pulcini & Wagner, 2001). By the 1980s, the master's degree was viewed broadly as the educational standard for advanced practice (Geolot, 1987; Sultz et al., 1983), and by 1989, 90% of programs were master's and post master's level (Pulcini & Wagner, 2001). NONPF thrived in the 1980s, developing curriculum guidelines and competencies, surveying faculties, and studying role components.

An interorganizational task force to identify criteria for quality NP educational programs occurred as an outgrowth of the work to unify certification. This work, begun in 1995 by NONPF and the NLN, was the beginning of the development of a model curriculum for NP education that would be used nationally and provide the basis for certification eligibility (Hamric et al., 1996). At that time, the NLN was the only accrediting body for nursing graduate programs, and program standards, curriculum guides, and domains and competencies for NP education from NONPF were often used by the NLN in the accreditation process. In 1998, the Commission on Collegiate Nursing Education, an accreditation arm of the American Association of Colleges of Nursing (AACN), was formed to provide an alternative to the NLN as a source of accreditation to schools offering baccalaureate and higher degrees in nursing. The thrust of the 2001 meeting of the NP task force when it reconvened was for accrediting bodies to move toward the approval of NONPF guidelines and standards as the reigning accepted standards for accreditation of programs preparing NPs (Edwards et al., 2003). In addition, the APRN Consensus Model spells out specific criteria for preapproval and accreditation of APRN education.

There is a cautionary note to this perception of progress. Despite clear statutes in some states, credentialing by insurers for nurse practitioners may still lag behind, providing additional barriers to care. Scope of practice, a primary focus of the 2010 Institute of Medicine *Future of Nursing* recommendations, remains a contested battleground for control of professional practice and reimbursement.

In 2008, the adoption of the Consensus Model for Advanced Practice Registered Nurse (APRN) Regulation by the National Council of State Boards of Nursing gave direction for gains in legal authority, prescriptive privilege, and reimbursement mechanisms across the 50 states and the District of Columbia. Current NPs have achieved a higher degree of autonomy in practice and associated prestige (Phillips, 2011) with the mandate for continued advancement contained in the IOM report, *The Future of Nursing* (2010). More victories than failures provide evidence of success, but, as in the late 1970s, today's NP is still battling for autonomy and consumer recognition in practice, especially in states with many physicians. As early as 1985, Hayes stated, "No role in nursing, or for that matter, in any field has been so debated in the literature, and possibly no other nursing function has ever been so obsessed about by those performing it as has been the NP role" (Hayes, 1985, p. 145). Yet, as Hayes asserts, there has been an avalanche of support from satisfied consumers of NP services.

YET ANOTHER "DISRUPTIVE INNOVATION": THE DOCTOR OF NURSING PRACTICE

However, the future contains clouds on the horizon as well as sunshine. Fairman (1999) cautions that although local negotiations between individual physicians and nurses may have been, in some cases, easily traversed in the interest of the good of the patient, on the professional level hierarchical relationships and power are at stake. As noted at the start of this chapter, within this hotly competitive health-care environment, with massive looming health-care reform legislation, as well as ever-increasing numbers of uninsured patients, all health-care professional groups face hurdles, challenges, and assaults.

In October 2004, the members of the AACN endorsed the *Position Statement on the Practice Doctorate in Nursing*, which called for the movement of educational preparation for advanced practice nursing roles from the master's degree to the doctoral level by 2015. This "new" doctorate would be a "practice" doctorate in contrast to the doctor of philosophy (PhD)—the traditional research degree—and is not intended to "replace" the PhD. There are many reasons for this development. Some master's programs for APNs had become very lengthy, without any change in the credential awarded at the completion of studies. The numbers of credits, in many cases, approaches what is required for a doctoral degree. And many educators believe this is necessary to ensure clinical competency. Furthermore, other practice disciplines such as pharmacy, physiotherapy, and occupational therapy have moved on to doctoral-level preparation. The debate continues.

The case can also be made that APNs across the country have been expanding their skills, both formally and informally. One example is the role of "intensivist" in the hospital, which is being assumed by many NPs and CNSs (Mundinger, 2005). This is consistent with nursing's lengthy history of moving where the need in health care surfaces. The aging of the population, the increased acuity and complexity of care, the continuation of a dwindling number of primary care physicians, and the decreased hours for residents in the hospital due to legislative and accreditation criteria have fostered the need for these nurses to move well beyond the primary care arena. For example, when Columbia University School of Nursing was asked by Presbyterian Hospital to establish two new ambulatory care clinics to meet the growing demand for primary care among the underserved immigrant populations, the faculty accepted. They also proposed conducting a randomized trial comparing independent NPs and primary care physicians. To reduce the variability among roles and strengthen the study, the faculty requested that the hospital's medical board grant the faculty NPs admitting privileges. Mundinger (2005) describes this evolution at Columbia: "Several physician(s) . . . provided additional training for our faculty nurse practitioners in dermatology, radiology, and cardiology and helped mentor them through the process of admitting, and co-managing patients and conducting emergency room evaluation" (p. 175).

The results of the randomized trials, with excellent patient care outcomes achieved by NPs, on a par with primary care physicians, were published in the *Journal of the American Medical Association* (Mundinger et al., 2000). This contributed to a change in hospital bylaws, granting faculty NPs hospital admitting privileges. Mundinger sees the level of service delivered by these faculty NPs as beyond that achieved by colleagues with the traditional master's degree preparation for practice. Based on these observations comes the call for a formal and standardized curriculum leading to a doctoral degree consistent with the practice needs for advanced competencies and increased knowledge. Mundinger

(2005) states, "We know that thousands of nurses aspire to this level of education and schools are responding by developing the new degree. We know that the research degree is asynchronous with these goals, and we know from every other profession that when you reach the competency associated with doctoral achievement, one should receive a doctorate not another MS degree" (p. 175).

As part of the APRN Consensus Model, 2015 was targeted as the year anyone seeking to sit for certification as an APRN would need a doctorate of nursing practice. Although the DNP degree has spread and prospered since 2008, there have always been vocal detractors. Recently, opposition to this mandate was voiced by a significant cohort of national nursing leaders in a paper titled "The Doctor of Nursing Practice: A National Workforce Perspective" (Cronenwett et al., 2011), making the case that the need for care providers should take precedence over a professionalizing agenda. Significant retrenchment of the 2015 mandate has occurred, with moves to preserve existing master's programs producing APRNs. See Chapter 4 for more discussion on this issue.

THE INSTITUTE OF MEDICINE ISSUES ITS 2010 REPORT: *THE FUTURE OF NURSING: LEADING CHANGE, ADVANCING HEALTH*

This dramatic, evidence-based report presents the results of 2 years of study by the Committee on the Robert Wood Johnson Foundation Initiative on the Future of Nursing at the Institute of Medicine (IOM). This committee was chaired by long-time nurse advocate, former head of the U.S. Department of Health and Human Services (1992–2000), now University of Miami President, Donna Shalala, PhD, FAAN, in concert with Nursing Vice Chair, Linda Burnes Bolton, RN, DrPH, FAAN. This report was presented in November 2010. Now, the far-reaching impact of the report's recommendations are just beginning to be fully absorbed. Key recommendations begin with the assumption that "nursing can fill ... new and expanded roles in a redesigned healthcare system" (IOM, 2010, p. xi). We will need our renegades, rebels, and trailblazers more than ever.

CONCLUSION

The boundaries of practice are always malleable. They are always subject to myriad external forces—political, economic, social, and cultural—and are interpreted in different ways by different practitioners. APNs are a mixed breed; each trajectory under the umbrella of advanced nursing practice has evolved differently and under variable circumstances. This leads to vigor, strength, and diversity. The struggles documented within this chapter have aimed to strengthen each variant of the nursing advanced practice role. The struggles are not over; in many ways they are just beginning. It is our hope that nursing will continue to produce rebels, renegades, and trailblazers, motivated by concern for patients, concern for community, and concern for humanity. We have no doubt that we will continue to take on new and challenging roles, using creative and diverse strategies. Nursing continues to lurch forward; progress is sometimes slow, sometimes variable, sometimes unsteady—but as always, continuing to find opportunity in chaos, motivated, as ever, by commitment to patients, families, and communities, to human need and suffering.

REFERENCES

American Association of Colleges of Nursing. (1995/2010). *Essentials of master's education.* Washington, DC: American Association of Colleges of Nursing.

American Association of Nurse Anesthetists. (2011). *Credential verification.* Retrieved November 12, 2011, from http://www.aana.com.

American College of Nurse-Midwives. (2011). *Basic facts about certified nurse midwives.* Retrieved November 11, 2011, from http://www.midwife.org.

American Nurses Association. (1965). *Educational preparation for nurse practitioners and assistants to nurses: A position paper.* New York: American Nurses Association.

American Nurses Association. (1980). *Nursing: A social policy statement.* Kansas City, MO: American Nurses Association.

American Nurses Association. (1993). Nursing facts from the American Nurses Association. In *Primary health care: The nurses' solution.* New York: American Nurses Association.

American Nurses Association Congress for Nursing Practice. (1976). *Definition: Nurse practitioner, nurse clinician, and clinical nurse specialist.* Kansas City, MO: Author.

Baer, E. (1982). The conflictive social ideology of American nursing, 1893: A microcosm. Unpublished dissertation, New York University, School of Education.

Bankert, M. (1989). *Watchful care: A history of America's nurse anesthetists.* New York: Continuum.

Bigbee, J. L., & Amidi-Nouri, A. (2000). History and evolution of advanced nursing practice. In A. B. Hamric, J. A. Spross, & C. M. Hanson (Eds.), *Advanced nursing practice: An integrative approach* (2nd ed., pp. 4–32). Philadelphia: WB Saunders.

Brush, B., & Capezuti, E. A. (1996). Revisiting "A Nurse for All Settings": The nurse practitioner movement, 1965–1995. *Journal of the American Academy of Nurse Practitioners, 8*(1), 5–11.

Busen, N., & Engleman, S. (1996). The CNS practitioner preparation: An emerging role in advanced practice nursing. *Clinical Nurse Specialist: The Journal of Advanced Nursing, 10*(3), 145–150.

Callaway, B. J. (2002). *Hildegard Peplau: Psychiatric nurse of the century.* New York: Springer Publishing Company.

Christman, L. (1998). Advanced practice nursing: Is the physician's assistant an accident of history or a failure to act? *Nursing Outlook, 46*(2), 56–59.

Coss, C. (Ed). (1989). *Lillian D. Wald: Progressive activist.* New York: The Feminist Press.

Cronenwett, L., Dracup, K., Grey, M., McCauley, L., Meleis, A., & Salmon, M. (2011). The doctor of nursing practice: A national workforce perspective. *Nursing Outlook, 59,* 9–17.

Daniels, D. G. (1989). *Always a sister: The feminism of Lillian D. Wald.* New York: The Feminist Press.

DeWitt, K. (1900). Specialties in nursing. *American Journal of Nursing, 1*(1), 14–17.

Dock, L. L. (1901). In I. A. Robb, L. L. Dock, & M. Banfield (Eds.), *The Transactions of the Third International Congress of Nurses with the Reports of the International Council of Nurses* (p. 15). Cleveland, OH.

Dye, N. S. (1984). Mary Breckenridge, the frontier nursing service, and the introduction of nurse-midwifery in the United States. In J. Leavitt & R. L. Numbers (Eds.), *Women and health* (pp. 336–337). Madison: University of Wisconsin.

Edgar, C. J. (1911). The remedy for the midwife problem. *American Journal of Obstetrics and Gynecology, 63,* 882.

Edwards, J., Oppewal, S., & Logan, C. (2003). Nurse-managed primary care: Outcomes of a faculty practice network. *Journal of American Academy of Nurse Practitioners, 15*(12), 563–569.

Ehrenreich, B. (2000). Introduction: Emergence of nursing as a political force. In D. Mason, J. Leavitt, & M. Chafee (Eds.), *Policy and politics in nursing and health care* (4th ed., pp. xxxiii–xxxvii). Philadelphia: Saunders.

Ehrenreich, B., & English, D. (1973). *Witches, midwives, and nurses: A history of women healers.* New York: The Feminist Press.

Ehrenreich, B., & English, D. (1978). *For her own good—150 years of expert advice to women.* New York: Anchor Books.

Fairman, J. (1999). Delegated by default or negotiated by need? Physicians, nurse practitioners, and the process of clinical thinking. *Medical Humanities Review, 13*(1), 38–58.

Fairman, J. (2002). The roots of collaborative practice: Nurse practitioner pioneers' stories. *Nursing History Review, 10,* 159–174.

Fairman, J. (2008). *Making room in the clinic: Nurse practitioners and the evolution of modern healthcare.* New Brunswick, NJ: Rutgers University Press.

Ford, L. C. (1991). Advanced nursing practice: Future of the nurse practitioner. In L. H. Aikein & C. M. Fagin (Eds.), *Charting nursing's future: Agenda for the 1990s* (pp. 287–299). New York: JB Lippincott.

Ford, L. C., & Silver, H. K. (1967). The expanded role of the nurse in child care. *Nursing Outlook, 15,* 43–45.

Fulton, J. (2002). Defining our practice. *Clinical Nurse Specialist: The Journal for Advanced Nursing, 16*(4), 1–3.

Geolot, D. (1987). Nurse practitioner education: Observations from a national perspective. *Nursing Outlook, 35,* 132–135.

Hamric, A. B., Spross, J. A., & Hanson, C. M. (1996). *Advanced nursing practice: An integrative approach.* Philadelphia: WB Saunders.

Hayes, E. (1985). The nurse practitioner: History, current conflicts, and future survival. *Journal of Community Health, 34,* 144–147.

Holt, N. (1998). Confusion's masterpiece: The development of the physician assistant profession. *Bulletin of the History of Medicine, 72,* 246–278.

Institute of Medicine. (2010). *The future of nursing: Leading change, advancing health. A report of the Committee on the Robert Wood Johnson Foundation Initiative on the Future of Nursing at the Institute of Medicine.* Washington, DC: The National Academies Press.

Jacox, A. K. (2002). Dr. Loretta Ford's observations on nursing's past and future. *Nursing and Health Policy Review, 1*(2), 153–164.

Joel, L. A. (2003). *Dimensions of professional nursing* (9th ed.). New York: McGraw-Hill.

Kalisch, P. A., & Kalisch, B. J. (1986). *The advance of American nursing* (2nd ed.). Boston: Little, Brown.

Keeling, A. (2007). *Nursing and the privilege of prescription.* Columbus, OH: The Ohio State University Press.

Kobrin, F. E. (1984). The American midwife controversy: A crisis of professionalization. In J. Leavitt & R. L. Numbers (Eds.), *Women and health* (pp. 318–326). Madison: University of Wisconsin.

Komnenich, P. (1998). The evolution of advanced practice in nursing. In C. M. Sheehy & M. McCarthy (Eds.), *Advanced practice nursing: Emphasizing common roles* (pp. 9–41). Philadelphia: FA Davis.

Leininger, M., Little, D. E., & Carnevali, D. (1972). Primex. *American Journal of Nursing, 72*(7), 1274–1277.

Lincoln, P. (2000). Comparing CNS and NP role activities: A replication. *Clinical Nurse Specialist: The Journal of Advanced Nursing, 14*(6), 1–4.

Magaw, A. (1906). A review of over fourteen thousand surgical anesthesias. *Bulletin of the American Association of Nurse Anesthetists 7,* 62.

Magaw, A. (1899). Observations in anesthesia. *Northwestern Lancet, 19,* 207.

Marchione, J., & Garland, T. N. (1997). An emerging profession? The case of the nurse practitioner. *Image: The Journal of Nursing Scholarship, 29*(4), 335–337.

Menard, S. (1987). The CNS: Historical perspectives. In S. Menard (Ed.), *The clinical nurse specialist: Perspectives on practice* (pp. 2–3). New York: John Wiley & Sons.

Mirr, M. P., & Snyder, M. (1995). Evolution of the advanced practice nursing role. In M. P. Mirr & M. Snyder (Eds.), *Advanced practice nursing* (pp. 13–21). New York: Springer.

Moxley, J. H., 3rd. (1968). The predicament in health manpower. *American Journal of Nursing, 68*(7), 1486–1490.

Mundinger, M. O. (2005). Who's who in nursing: Bringing clarity to the doctor of nursing practice. *Nursing Outlook, 53*(4), 173–176.

Mundinger, M. O., Kane, R. I., Lenz, E. R., Totten, A. M, Tsai, W., & Cleary, P. D. (2000). Primary care outcomes in patients treated by nurse practitioners or physicians: A randomized trial. *JAMA, 283*(1), 59–68.

O'Brien, P. (1987). "All a woman's life can bring": The domestic roots of nursing in Philadelphia, 1830–1885. *Nursing Research, 36*(1), 12–17.

Phillips, S. J. (2011). 23rd annual legislative update: As healthcare reforms, NPs continue to evolve. *Nurse Practitioners, 36*(1), 30–52.

Pulcini, J., & Wagner, M. (2001). Perspectives on education and practice issues for nurse practitioners and advanced practice nursing. In *Nurse Practitioner/Advanced Practice Nursing Roles in the United States.* Education/Practice Subgroup of the International Nurse Practitioner/Advanced Practice Nursing Network. Geneva: ICN.

Reiter, F. (1966). The nurse clinician. *American Journal of Nursing, 66*(2), 274–279.

Rothstein, W. G. (1958). *American physicians in the nineteenth century: From sect to science.* Baltimore: Johns Hopkins Press.

Roy, C., & Obloy, M. (1978). The practitioner movement—toward a science of nursing. *American Journal of Nursing, 78*(10), 1698–1702.

Sills, G. (1983). The role and function of the clinical nurse specialist. In N. L. Chaska (Ed.), *The nursing profession: A time to speak up.* New York: McGraw-Hill.

Silver, H. K., Ford, L. C., & Stearly, S. G. (1967). A program to increase health care for children: The pediatric nurse practitioner program. *Pediatrics, 39*(5), 756–768.

Sparacino, P. S. A. (1986). The clinical nurse specialist. *Nursing Practice 1*(4), 215–228.

Sparacino, P. S. A. (1990). A historical perspective on the development of the clinical nurse specialist role. In P. S. A. Sparacino, D. M. Cooper, & P. A. Manarik (Eds.), *The clinical nurse specialist: Implementation and impact* (pp. 3–9). Norwalk, CT: Appleton & Lange.

Stone, S. (1990). A complete practice of midwifery. In L. T. Ulrich (Ed.), *A midwife's tale: The life of Martha Ballard* (pp. 12–40). New York: Alfred Knopf.

Sultz, H. A., Henry, O., Kinyon, J., Buck, G., & Bullough, B. (1983). Nurse practitioners: A decade of change. *Nursing Outlook, 31,* 137–141.

Thatcher, V. S. (1953). *History of anesthesia with emphasis on the nurse specialist.* Philadelphia: Lippincott.

Towers, J. (1995). Celebrating our 30th anniversary as nurse practitioners and our 10th anniversary as an academy. *Journal of the American Academy of Nurse Practitioners, 7*(6), 267–270.

Ulrich, L. T. (1990). *A midwife's tale: The life of Martha Ballard, based on her diary, 1785–1812.* New York: Alfred A. Knopf.

U.S. Department of Labor. (1920). *Children's Bureau publication no. 61.* Washington, DC: U.S. Government Printing Office.

2

Emerging Roles of the Advanced Practice Nurse

Deborah Becker
Caroline Doherty

EMERGING ROLES OF THE ADVANCED PRACTICE NURSE

Advanced practice nursing has evolved to meet the changing needs of patients, communities, and society as a whole. Advanced practice registered nurses (APRNs)* have successfully adapted their roles to meet these ever-changing needs and the expectations that go along with them. The growth occurring now can be attributed to a number of elements, such as health-care reform and the Affordable Care Act, a national emphasis on the provision of safe and high-quality care, pay-for-performance initiatives, and the call by the Institute of Medicine's *Future of Nursing* (2010) report for APRNs to work to the fullest extent of their scopes of practice without restrictions or barriers. These initiatives foster new opportunities for the development of advanced practice nursing roles.

Several factors have influenced the emergence and acceptability of advanced practice roles. These factors include the growing numbers of elderly patients as baby boomers reach retirement age, increased complexity and severity of illness in hospitalized patients, further reduction in medical residents' clinical work hours, a call for greater access to care for all citizens, and a varying degree of nursing shortages, depending on geographical region. These and other factors will continue to influence the emergence of the APRN role in the coming decades.

Currently, there are four major groups of APRNs in the United States: certified registered nurse anesthetists (CRNAs), certified nurse-midwives (CNMs), clinical nurse specialists (CNSs), and nurse practitioners (NPs). The range of current advanced practice roles and the numbers of nurses in these roles demonstrate the continued success and acceptance of APRNs. See **Table 2-1.** Studies evaluating clinical outcomes of care delivered by APRNs are overwhelmingly positive, as are surveys of patient satisfaction with the delivery of care by APRNs. Recently, a systematic review of outcomes studies conducted between 1990 and 2008 was published (Newhouse et al., 2011). The aim of the study was to compare patient outcomes between physician-and APRN-directed teams. The review found that patient outcomes of care provided by NPs and CNMs (in collaboration with physicians as required by state regulations) were similar to and in some ways better than care provided by physicians alone for the populations and in the settings included (Newhouse et al.). The review found that CNSs working in acute care settings can reduce length of stay and cost of care for hospitalized patients. Although no specific conclusions regarding CRNA patient outcomes were provided by this review, a few studies show CRNA patient outcomes to be comparable to those of anesthesiologists (Newhouse et al.).

*APRN is the title preferred by the American Nurses Association and used in most state practice acts. Throughout this chapter various acronyms will be presented to distinguish between specialty preparations, but the generic title for all of these practice roles is APRN.

TABLE 2-1

Numbers of Advanced Practice Nurses

Clinical nurse specialists	12,543
Certified registered nurse anesthetists	40,792
Certified nurse-midwives	7,383
Nurse practitioners	147,605

Source: Phillips, S. J. (2011). 23rd annual legislative update. *Nurse Practitioner, 36*(1), 30–52.

By accepting the responsibilities of the advanced practice role, APRNs have understood the need to expand legislative recognition of their professional status, including prescriptive authority and reimbursement for care delivered. Recognition of APRNs in the United States varies, with most states providing some level of legal recognition and prescriptive authority.

SCOPE OF PRACTICE

Professional nursing organizations and state boards of nursing understand the need to describe and interpret the responsibilities of advanced practitioners in their areas of specialization. Underlying the recognition of this need is the obligation to ensure public safety, to identify the essential characteristics of advanced practice, and to interpret for the practitioner the components of competent care (American Association of Critical Care Nurses & American Nurses Association, 1995). The scope of practice may be described by the functions performed by the APRN and the minimal competencies needed to perform those functions. These descriptions and guidelines direct APRNs in the implementation and conceptualization of their roles and responsibilities.

In addition, each state has a legislative/regulatory stance on issues affecting advanced practice within its jurisdiction (Phillips, 2011). The legal scope of practice, including prerogatives for diagnosing, prescriptive authority, and reimbursement, is described within these regulations. Scope and standards of practice are defined by the professional organization and enacted into law at the state level. The actual role is further delineated through credentialing of practice responsibilities at the institutional or employment level. Hospitals and other health-care organizations typically define role responsibilities and prerogatives through a review by other practitioners, and this is generally expressed through a contract identifying responsibilities, prerogatives, and limitations of the role. This review results in the granting of institutional or organizationally based practice privileges for the APRN. A specific example of this is a cardiac catheterization lab in New York State where, due to high volume and a shortage of fellows, nurse practitioners are trained to obtain arterial access and to cross uncomplicated coronary lesions (Stuppy, 2004).

Although scope of practice guidelines are important philosophically, and may even have the weight of law, they do not imply that the roles of APRNs are unchanging. When knowledge evolves and different care delivery models emerge, roles also evolve. More commonly, roles change as different practice settings become available and opportunities for improved patient access to care appear. The nature of advanced practice is broader than individual roles or functions.

Regulation of the Advanced Practice Registered Nurse

Regulation of APRNs occurs at the state level, but there are both educational and certification prerequisites. Graduate-level educational preparation of APRNs is guided by educators and members of professional organizations who identify essential curricular goals, content, and competencies expected of APN graduates. Recently a call for doctoral-level preparation for APRNs was made by the American Association of Colleges of Nursing (AACN). While many schools of nursing moved their APRN education to the doctoral level, most offering the doctorate of nursing practice (DNP) degree, only one APRN group has mandated doctoral education. The American Association of Nurse Anesthetists (AANA) has mandated that as of 2025 all graduates of educational programs must be prepared at the doctoral level for entry into practice (AANA, 2010).

Content and competencies core to all APRNs and those specific to a particular role must be provided in all APRN educational programs. **Table 2-2** lists major APRN organizations developing the educational and certification prerequisites and the APRN essential content and competency documents developed by the professional organizations and directing the preparation of APRNs for entry into practice. On completion of an accredited master's-level program, graduates generally must pass a national certification examination in the area of intended practice before applying for licensure at the state level.

APRNs may be recognized and licensed at the state level in one of the four aforementioned roles. However, many issues have been identified with the current regulatory process, particularly the ability of APRNs to move across states and remain eligible to be licensed and to practice. In response to this need to develop more consistent standards for APRN recognition across states, the APRN Consensus Work Group and the National Council of State Boards of Nursing have developed the Consensus Model for APRN Regulation: Licensure, Accreditation, Certification and Education (Consensus Model, 2008). This document has been accepted by numerous nursing organizations and stakeholder groups. The regulatory model acknowledges the four APRN roles and argues that advanced practice nursing must be regulated in one of the four roles and in at least one of six population

TABLE 2-2

Professional Organizations and Essential Educational Content

American Association of Colleges of Nursing	*The essentials of master's education in nursing.* Washington, DC: Author, 2011.
American Association of Colleges of Nursing	*The essentials of doctoral education for advanced nursing practice.* Washington, DC: Author, 2006.
American College of Nurse-Midwives	*Core competencies for basic midwifery practice.* Retrieved October 5, 2011, from http://www.midwife.org—standard setting documents.
American Association of Women's Health, Obstetric and Neonatal Nurses and National Association of Nurse Practitioners Women's Health	*The women's health nurse practitioner: guidelines for practice and education* (6th ed.). Washington, DC: Author, 2008.
Council on Accreditation of Nurse Anesthesia Educational Programs	*Standards for accreditation of nurse anesthesia educational programs.* Chicago: Author, 2004.
National Association of Clinical Nurse Specialists	*Statement on clinical nurse specialist practice and education* (2nd ed.). Harrisburg, PA: Author, 2004.
National Organization of Nurse Practitioner Faculties	*Domains and Core Competencies of Nurse Practitioner Practice.* Washington, DC: Author, 2006.
National Panel for Psychiatric–Mental Health Nurse Practitioner Competencies	*Psychiatric–mental health nurse practitioner competencies.* Washington, DC: National Organization of Public Health Nurses, 2002.

foci: psychiatric/mental health, women's health/gender specific, adult-gerontology, pediatrics, neonatal, and individual families across the life span. The adult-gerontology and pediatrics populations are further distinguished by either an acute care or a primary care focus. Of note is that clinical nurse specialist practice is described to occur across primary and acute care settings and as such must be reflected in their education.

Requirements for the consistent educational preparation across all APRN roles have provided greater uniformity. Content for all APRNs must include graduate-level courses in advanced pathophysiology, advanced physical assessment, and advanced pharmacology, called the *APRN core* (Consensus Model, 2008). In addition, content related to the population served, role development, and clinical experience in the specific role is required. The recommendations of the Consensus Model have and will continue to influence the licensure, accreditation, certification, and educational preparation of all future APRNs, and can be found in **Table 2-3**.

Clinical Nurse Specialist

CNSs are nurses with master's-or doctorate-level education in a defined area of knowledge and practice. They typically work in unit-based or population-based settings; in hospitals, offices, or clinic outpatient settings; and in community practice. Even with evidence of their favorable impact, hospital-based CNSs have been particularly vulnerable to administrative attempts to decrease health-care costs. Multiple studies have demonstrated the positive contributions of CNSs to patient care outcomes and patient satisfaction, but fewer studies have evaluated their economic impact and their ability to generate income and save costs. Cost-saving measures have been demonstrated, such as CNS impact on early discharge, product evaluation, and nursing practice changes (Scott, 1999). These savings are real, but they may not be returned to the CNS's home (usually nursing) department. Because of this,

TABLE 2-3

Essential Characteristics of the Advanced Practice Registered Nurse*

1. Completion of an accredited graduate-level program in one of the four areas: nurse-midwifery, nurse anesthesia, nurse practitioner, or clinical nurse specialist
2. Successful completion of a national certification examination measuring APRN role and population of focus competencies and maintains competence through recertification
3. Possession of advanced clinical knowledge and skills needed for direct patient care and a significant component of education and practice focuses on direct care of individuals
4. Practice builds on RN competencies and demonstrates depth and breadth of knowledge, data synthesis, complex skills, intervention, and role autonomy
5. Educational preparation for health promotion and maintenance, assessment, diagnosis, and management of patient problems including use and prescription of pharmacological and nonpharmacological interventions
6. Possesses depth and breadth of clinical experience reflecting intended area of practice
7. Possesses license to practice as APRN as CRNA, CNM, CNS, or CNP

APRN, advanced practice registered nurse; *CNM,* certified nurse-midwife; *CNP,* certified nurse practitioner; *CNS,* clinical nurse specialist; *CRNA,* certified registered nurse anesthetist; *RN,* registered nurse.

*Adapted from Consensus Model for APRN Regulation: Licensure, Accreditation, Certification and Education. (2008). Completed through the work of the APRN Consensus Work Group and the National Council of State Boards of Nursing APRN Advisory Committee.

the immediate supervisors of CNSs may not appreciate the benefits of expert CNS practice. This reality is compounded by the inability of CNSs to bill directly for services if they are salaried employees. Hospital-based employees cannot bill third-party payers for services delivered such as consultations, teaching programs, pain management, or wound-care activities. Skilled advanced practice nursing care is not directly reimbursed and remains bundled in the hospital's room, food, laundry, and supplies bill. More creative and appropriate financial models that could remedy the situation are needed. This limitation on role functioning is usually not faced by self-employed or practice-based CNSs, who likely are not institutional employees and generally work in outpatient or community settings.

The CNS shifts functions depending on the needs of the situation and participates in a mix of direct and indirect patient care activities. Still, the traditional roles of CNS practice remain, including those of expert practitioner, educator, consultant, manager, and researcher.

In an evaluation of CNS practice roles, Scott (1999) reported that CNSs nationwide were involved in clinical practice activities 29% to 91% of the time; in educational activities 24% to 89% of the time; as consultants 18% to 96% of the time; and in research activities 15% to 93% of the time. Scott also reported that CNSs were commonly found in community-based practice (32% of the sample). Community practice included such settings as clinics, private practice, school systems, nursing homes, corporations, and prisons.

In an analysis of acute care advanced practice nurses, performed by the American Association of Critical Care Nurses (Becker et al., 2006), CNSs were asked to rate activities they perform that are most critical to their practices. Activities selected include the following: synthesizes, interprets, makes decisions and recommendations, and evaluates responses on the basis of complex, sometimes conflicting, sources of data; identifies and prioritizes clinical problems on the basis of education, research, and experiential knowledge; facilitates development of clinical judgment in health-care team members (e.g., nursing staff, medical staff, other health-care providers) through serving as a role model, teaching, coaching, and/or mentoring; promotes a caring and supportive environment; promotes the value of lifelong learning and evidence-based practice while continually acquiring knowledge and skills needed to address questions arising in practice to improve patients' care; evaluates current and innovative practices in patients' care on the basis of evidence-based practice, research, and experiential knowledge; and incorporates evidence-based practice guidelines, research, and experiential knowledge to formulate, evaluate, and/or revise policies, procedures, and protocols. These results demonstrated the performance of activities that at one time were performed solely by physicians and currently also overlap those performed by acute care nurse practitioners.

An important concern was that only 6% of the nurses in this survey could identify ways in which they generated income. As Scott (1999) suggests, CNSs must have preparation in health-care economics if they are to have the requisite skills needed to flourish as independent advanced practice health-care providers. See **Boxes 2-1** and **2-2.**

Ambiguity and the Clinical Nurse Specialist Role

The observation that CNS practice reflects role ambiguity undoubtedly grows out of the ability of the CNS to adapt to changing patient, family, and nursing staff needs, supported by a broad clinical repertoire of skills and knowledge. There have been several responses to the problem of role ambiguity with in-hospital CNS roles. One has been the development of AACN's Scope and Standards for Acute and Critical Care Clinical Nurse Specialists (Bell & McNamara, 2010). This document provides guidelines for competent and professional care for acutely and critically ill patients. It also reflects the three spheres of CNS influence: patient/family; nursing personnel and other health-care providers;

BOX 2-1
The Psychiatric Clinical Nurse Specialist Profile

Jane is a psychiatric clinical nurse specialist (CNS) who is prepared at the master's level and for the past 25 years has worked in a private practice supporting clients with multiple psychological problems. Her clients include children over 10 years of age in the context of their families or support systems. She is certified as a marriage and family therapist, as an adolescent therapist, and in eye movement desensitization reprogramming (EMDR), a technique used in the treatment of clients with post-traumatic stress disorder (PTSD).

Jane describes her practice as taking place in an exciting time, with new information and research providing her with a broad repertoire of approaches and skills for her clients. She prefers to work as a solo practitioner without supervisory reporting requirements. She is able to set her own working schedule and see clients for as long as she judges appropriate. She bills directly and is not a member of managed care billing panels. She depends on referrals from physicians, other health-care workers, and school principals for her clients and does not advertise. Jane cannot prescribe medications in her state and relies on cooperation with physician colleagues if medications are necessary. Jane loves the work she is doing and plans to stay in the role as long as she can.

BOX 2-2
Population-Based Clinical Nurse Specialist Profile

Alicia is a nurse who has master's-level training and has been a clinical nurse specialist (CNS) for the past 12 years in a major teaching hospital. For the first 6 years she was a unit-based specialist providing direct care to seriously ill surgical patients and supervising and directing the care provided by unit-based staff nurses. For the past 6 years she has worked as a CNS in ostomy and wound care. In this capacity she serves as an educator and consultant for patients with ostomies (70%) and problems with wound healing (30%). These responsibilities require her to work directly with patients and their families and also with the nursing and medical staff. Alicia also has responsibility for ongoing in-service educational programs and for orientation for new surgical nurses. She reports to the nurse manager of a surgical nursing unit.

Alicia loves her position because she realizes that she is able to direct and coordinate the needs of these complex patients as she works with physicians, staff nurses, discharge planners, and health insurance representatives. Although her role is hospital based, the ongoing post-discharge needs of these patients require that she provide extended supervision and direction to patients struggling to assume responsibility for the complicated care of their ostomies or problem wounds. This follow-up care includes telephone and in-person evaluations, wound and ostomy product adjustments, education, and counseling.

In her role Alicia faces problems related to her inability to prescribe medications, supplies, and devices commonly required by her patients. Written prescriptions for medications, devices, and supplies are necessary, even if they are available over the counter, if patients are to receive insurance reimbursement. Because CNSs cannot prescribe in her state, Alicia directs residents, house staff, or nurse practitioners to write the necessary prescriptions. Similarly, Alicia cannot bill for the care she provides to her patients, even when provided postdischarge. These problems result from lack of title recognition at the state level (CNSs are not recognized as advanced practice nurses [APNs] in her state and therefore cannot become eligible for prescriptive privileges), from the lack of credentialing at the institutional level, and from a need to reconceptualize her role responsibilities to include postdischarge care. Alicia's responsibilities cross inpatient and outpatient settings, but her reporting lines are limited to a specific inpatient setting.

and the organizational system for care delivery in different settings (Bell & McNamara). Within this framework the CNS is expected to provide continuous and comprehensive care to improve outcomes for acutely and critically ill patients. This is done in a collaborative model that includes patients, families, significant others, nurses, and other providers and administrators (Bell & McNamara).

A contribution of this document is that it sets goals and standards for CNS practice and contributes to further role clarification for hospital-based CNSs. The values identified in this document for continuous and comprehensive care for acutely and critically ill patients suggest that the scope of the critical care CNS's responsibilities are not limited to acute or special care units. Seriously ill patients are found in most hospital units, and their continuing specialized care needs are now frequently required in nonhospital or outpatient settings. It is likely that postdischarge role functions will become more common for the acute or critical care CNS.

The publishing of CNS Core Competencies by the National CNS Competency Task Force (Clinical Nurse Specialist Core Competencies, 2010) also attempts to reduce role ambiguity for the CNS. This task force identified the various roles and activities of CNSs in a number of practice settings and validated them by surveying over 2000 CNSs. The range of agreement was 90% to 98%. These competencies will aid educators, employers, and new CNSs in understanding their role and responsibilities as well as their contributions to patient care outcomes.

CNS involvement in quality initiatives and their contributions to improved patient outcomes most recently has been recognized as agencies apply for Magnet Recognition. The Magnet Recognition Program® offered by the American Nurses Credentialing Center (ANCC) recognizes health-care organizations for quality patient care, nursing excellence, and innovations in professional nursing practice (ANCC, 2011). The CNS role is essential to implementing innovation and sustaining improved patient outcomes, integral components of the Magnet Recognition Program (Muller, Hujcs, Dubendorf, & Harrington, 2010). The CNS role broadly and specifically supports the process by which care is delineated, changes made, and improvements noted. CNS participation in the attainment of these goals and the movement of organizations toward achieving Magnet status will provide new and expanded opportunities for the CNS.

Nurse Practitioner

The educational preparation of NPs has moved from continuing education programs offering certification on completion to university-based graduate programs granting a master's degree in nursing. Today NPs are the largest group of APRNs and have prescriptive authority in all 50 states and the District of Columbia (Phillips, 2011). These APRNs assess and manage both medical and nursing problems, and serve as both primary and acute care providers.

Changing Roles for the Primary Care Nurse Practitioner

Initially, patient populations cared for by NPs were often uninsured immigrants or low-income individuals who were Medicaid recipients. However, NPs since have sought to meet the needs of larger groups of patients and have expanded their practice to include clients from suburban and urban outpatient settings and clinics. This shift to highly populated, high-income areas where physicians are also readily available has been supported by the decision of health insurance plans to add NPs to their direct provider lists and to reimburse them on par with physicians (Grandinetti, 1999). This move has supported the delivery of holistic primary care to larger groups of patients in community settings but sometimes has resulted in competition as primary care NPs and physicians attempt to serve similar populations. It has also resulted in NPs working for practices under umbrella corporations that contract with NPs to see a certain number of patients per day (perhaps every 15 minutes) and then build incentives for NPs to see more patients than their contract designates. The effect of this advancement is yet to be determined.

The development of the walk-in "retail clinic" has produced broad recognition of the NP role, has led to their "discovery" by the public, and has been described as "a significant move to reform U.S. health care by business and other groups outside the traditional medical industry" (Pearson, 2008, p. 10). Recognizing this development, the American Academy of Nurse Practitioners (AANP) has published *Standards for Nurse Practitioner Practice in Retail-based Clinics* (AANP, 2007).

A newer role for the primary care APN is that of concierge nurse practitioner. This role is in its development stages. As it is envisioned, the NP will directly contract with the patient for his or her services. The NP will provide health promotion and preventive services. When necessary, the patient receives priority care. The concierge NP will meet the patient at a convenient place, such as the patient's home or place of business; will provide on-the-spot care; and, if the patient's needs exceed the capabilities of outpatient care, the NP will accompany and/or facilitate the admission of the patient to an inpatient setting and coordinate care with the other providers. As the demand for this level of personalized care expands, so will this role.

Nurse Practitioners in the Community

Primary care NPs have established unique community-centered practice models. In an effort to develop an independent NP service model and to study the ways health care is delivered to various populations in the United States, many schools of nursing have opened Academic Community Nursing Centers (Grandinetti, 1999; Zachariah & Lundeen, 1997). These centers are used as settings in which to study how health care is provided to vulnerable populations with limited access to care, who face inefficiencies and a lack of coordination in health-care delivery; to determine the specific needs of the community in which the center is located; and to provide a means of improving the quality of the care delivered (Zachariah & Lundeen, 1997).

Building on the concept of nurse-run clinics, the National Committee for Quality Assurance (NCQA), a prominent health-care quality organization, reports that it will recognize "nurse-led" primary care practices as patient-centered medical homes under the Physician Practice Connections®–Patient-Centered Medical Home recognition program. In this program practices are being encouraged to add names of eligible nurse practitioners to their practice information. The "medical home" concept was developed to reward providers for the coordination and management of patient-centered care of individuals with complex and multiple chronic illnesses, and initially did not include APNs at all (Schram, 2010). Through the efforts of the American Nurses Association, the American Academy of Nurse Practitioners, and the American College of Nurse Practitioners, NPs are now included in the language of this initiative (Schram). The movement to more neutral language such as the primary care home model reflects the widespread recognition and acceptance of the critical role that NPs can play in increasing access to high-quality primary care (Summers, 2011).

Nurse Practitioners in Transitional Care Settings

Hospital-based nurses have traditionally focused their interventions on preparing patients for discharge from the hospital. Because of the success and effectiveness that nurses have demonstrated in coordinating care, in anticipating postdischarge concerns or potential complications, and in developing a means to manage these issues, various roles for NPs in home health-care settings have emerged. The need for APNs who can provide transitional care from hospital to community is particularly evident.

Until recently, home health nurses have identified problems and concerns regarding the health of their patients and have had to contact the patient's physician to determine the next course of action, a step that often caused a delay in treatment. The development of APRN roles that bridge the acute care and community setting for complex, chronically ill patients or those requiring support in making the transition from the acute care setting to home has promoted favorable patient care outcomes and decreased hospital readmission rates. These APRNs can recognize subtle changes in their patients' status and provide prompt care, potentially averting a more serious result (Craven & Keene, 2000; Naylor, Bowles, & Brooten, 2000). APRNs in home care settings engage in such activities as diagnosis and treatment of acute and chronic conditions, including consulting the physician when necessary; education of patients, families, and home care nurses; provision of cost-efficient and cost-effective care; and coordination of complex health-care services (Craven & Keene, 2000).

Several viable models of APRNs in transitional roles have been demonstrated through research efforts (Blewett et al., 2010; Brooten et al., 1989; Naylor et al., 2000). The clearly demonstrated, favorable patient-centered outcomes of Naylor's Transitional Care Model (2000) has gained significant recognition to the point of being named in the Affordable Care Act as an example of a program showing substantial contributions to reducing health-care costs. However, there is still a need to further develop reimbursement systems for the services of APRNs.

The NP as consultant in community health settings is another emerging advanced practice role. Long-term care facilities, nursing homes, and rehabilitation centers are settings that have few APRNs or professional nurses. However, these settings often have residents with chronic health needs that go untreated or unnoticed until they become serious. In response, some administrators have developed roles for APRNs to address health issues more quickly (Neal, 1999). These community-based APRNs assess problems and develop plans of care in an attempt to prevent further progression of symptoms or needless suffering. Because the NP consultant role in the community is a new and emerging role, many states continue to require that these NPs work in collaboration with, or under the supervision of, a physician. This restriction may limit the ability of these APRNs to function independently or may limit the range of services they can provide. In addition, there are restrictions on the type of services for which APRNs can bill directly. However, as changes in health-care reimbursement policies continue to occur, the consultant role in the community will grow more popular.

The Psychiatric/Mental Health Nurse Practitioner

Since the 1950s the APRN role of the psychiatric/mental health nurse has been conceptualized as a CNS role. With recent developments in the science underpinning mental health and psychiatric illnesses, a shifting emphasis is evolving from a traditional psychosocial approach to care to a biopsychosocial paradigm. In the latter model, psychopharmacology has assumed a prominent place in the treatment inventory (Moller & Haber, 1997). Acceptance of this movement is demonstrated by development of national certification examinations for the adult psychiatric and mental health NP, and the family and psychiatric mental health NP (American Nurses Credentialing Center [ANCC], 2008a, 2008b). With the adoption of the Consensus Model (2008), the psychiatric/mental health APRN will focus on the individual across the life span. With the increase in access to primary care providers, the psychiatric/mental health practitioner needs title protection, prescriptive authority, and the ability to have direct care billing of CPT codes (American Psychiatric Nurses Association, 2010). Currently this occurs in 37 states for both CNSs and NPs. Nurse practitioners have prescriptive authority across all 50 states; hence the psychiatric/mental health nurse practitioner may be the more feasible preparation for the mental health provider for these APRNs to effectively care for patients.

Women's Health Nurse Practitioners

The women's health NP role grew out of identification of the unique needs of women and initially focused on family planning, gynecological care, perimenopausal issues, and the diagnosis and treatment of sexually transmitted infections (STIs) throughout the life span. Due to low income and the lack of resources available to many women, the role expanded to include well-woman health with a focus on holistic care, prevention and healthy lifestyles, mental health issues, and identification of issues such as partner violence. The women's health NP also focuses on common urological problems such as incontinence and cystitis, and performs procedures such as cystoscopy, circumcision, intrauterine device (IUD) insertion, endometrial biopsy, and obstetrical ultrasonography.

Over the years, these experts recognized a need for providers to address men's sexual and reproductive health needs. Thus, the education and role of the women's health NP has expanded to include the diagnosis of, screening for, and evaluation and management of men's issues such as STIs and fertility issues. In recognition of the effectiveness of these women's health practitioners, the Consensus Model (2008) calls for women's health practitioners to expand their population focus. The formal recognition of care to men will undoubtedly provide for future expansion of the role.

Acute Care Nurse Practitioner

NPs are found not only in primary care but also in specialized settings such as neonatal, pediatric, geriatric, women's health, and acute and critical care settings. The term *acute* has always been associated with the type of facility in which patient care is provided, but it is also used to describe the patient who is experiencing either a new onset or an exacerbation between an existing illness and those patients who have complex chronic illnesses that teeter on the edge of wellness and illness (Bell, 2006). Thus, acute care nurse practitioners are no longer defined by the geographical setting in which they provide care but by the patient population they serve. Acute care nurse practitioners provide care in a variety of settings such as hospitals, intensive care units, long-term acute care hospitals, outpatient and inpatient hospices, specialty offices, and operating rooms. They may be practice based, such as those working on a cardiothoracic service, or may be unit based, such as those working in a medical intensive care unit or cardiac step-down unit. They may also be on teams, that provide care across settings such as those in hospitalist positions or on consultative teams such as acute diabetes management services.

Several studies have examined the quality of outcomes of care delivered by neonatal NPs compared to that delivered by medical house staff. Results demonstrated that care delivered by NPs was as good as, or better than, that delivered by house staff, on measures of cost-effectiveness and quality. In addition, care delivered by neonatal NPs had greater continuity and consistency (Bissinger, Allred, Arford, & Bellig, 1997; Mitchell-DiCenso et al., 1996). Other studies have demonstrated similarly favorable outcomes of NP practice in pediatric, rehabilitative, and inpatient trauma care settings (Borgmeyer et al., 2008; Gracias et al., 2008; Hoffman et al., 2005; Lambing et al., 2004; Lenz et al., 2002; Silver, Murphy, & Gitterman, 1984; Spisso, O'Callaghan, McKinnon, & Holcroft, 1990; Weinberg, Liljestrand, & Moore, 1983).

Another issue faced by the ACNP is that of reimbursement for services delivered. If employed by a medical practice group, NPs can bill directly for their services. However, reimbursement is not equal to that received by physicians in the practice. NPs who bill directly receive only 85% of the amount a physician would receive for the same services. See **Box 2-3.** Because of this disparity, many NPs working in hospitals have not directly billed but instead allowed their collaborating physicians to bill at the 100% rate. Recently nursing departments have decided to bring greater visibility to the NP contributions to the organization by requiring them to bill for their services. While this will require the addition of

BOX 2-3
Acute Care Nurse Practitioner Profile

Jim works as an acute care nurse practitioner in an open-model surgical intensive care unit. His professional responsibilities include total care of these patients, including admission and transfer, ventilator management, and management of their chronic comorbidities. He also manages acute issues such as sepsis and acute respiratory distress syndrome. In addition, he is privileged through the hospital to independently place central lines, arterial lines, chest tubes, dialysis catheters, and PICC lines, and to perform therapeutic paracentesis. He works in collaboration with physicians, and is responsible for the minute-to-minute management of patients. He provides bedside and formal education to staff and encourages growth of the individual nurses and advancement of nursing in the unit as a whole. Surgeons have vocalized their appreciation for the continuity of care, the thoroughness, and the knowledge that the NPs contribute to the medical and nursing care of these critically ill patients.

support services as the APNs learn the processes for billing and reimbursement, it will provide increased recognition of NP contributions in economic terms, leading to greater job security and less invisibility.

The Acute Care Nurse Practitioner in Pediatric Settings

NPs have practiced in neonatal intensive care units (ICUs) since the early 1970s. Until recently though, the role of the pediatric NP had not reached into other acute areas of pediatric care. This was related to the strong role of the CNS in pediatric settings. Clinical nurse specialists have long practiced in all pediatric acute care settings in roles such as case management; developing clinical pathways; participating in research; providing consultation; educating care providers, patients, and families; and collaborating with various members of the health-care team in an attempt to provide cost-efficient and high-quality patient care (Teicher, Crawford, Williams, Nelson, & Andrews, 2001).

In pediatric settings the role of the ACNP has evolved into one that assists with managing patients who are acutely ill or who have exacerbations of chronic health problems (Teicher et al., 2001). Initially, this new role in pediatric care blended the roles of the CNS and the NP in an attempt to provide comprehensive services and direct patient care to pediatric patients and their families. Now, as nurse practitioner roles are recognized for their contributions to patient outcomes, the blended role is being phased out. With implementation of the Consensus Model (2008), CNSs and NPs must be certified distinctly in one of these roles based on their educational preparation and eligibility for licensure in the state they practice. The many responsibilities of the APN in pediatrics include such activities as performing health histories and physical examinations; evaluating clinical data; prescribing treatments; performing invasive procedures, such as tracheal intubation and insertion of arterial lines; educating and supporting patients and families; facilitating patient discharge; participating in interdisciplinary rounds; and providing consultative services regarding such issues as wound care and infant feeding problems (Delametter, 1999; Pelosi, 2000; Rossetto & Fair, 1998; Teicher et al., 2001).

The pediatric NP can be found on specific patient care units such as the medical-surgical floor or the ICU; function in the hospitalist role; or be a member of a specialty service such as cardiology, pulmonary, oncology, transplantation, gastrointestinal, and general surgery (Brown et al., 2008; Delametter, 1999; Hittle & Tilford, 2010; Okuhara et al., 2011; Pelosi, 2000; Teicher et al., 2001).

Pediatric ACNPs may also work outside the hospital setting in other areas in which acutely ill pediatric patients are found. Such areas include HIV clinics, centers for the management of mechanically ventilated patients, transport services, and home settings (Delametter, 1999; Dwyer, 2000; King, Foster, Woodward, & McCans, 2001; Teicher et al., 2001). The role that each NP assumes depends largely on the specific needs of the patients cared for. The focus of the role, regardless of the geographical location in which the pediatric ACNP works, is to provide cost-effective and high-quality patient care.

Adult Acute Care Nurse Practitioners

Like the roles of their pediatric counterparts, the roles of adult ACNPs are evolving and expanding in the acute care setting. Settings in which ACNPs deliver care include emergency rooms, ICUs, step-down or progressive care units, and medical-surgical floors. ACNPs also deliver care to patients outside the tertiary or quaternary care institutions in settings such as outpatient surgical centers, centers for the management of mechanically ventilated patients, long-term acute care hospitals, psychiatric evaluation centers, dialysis units, heart failure centers, and correctional facilities.

In the Kleinpell and Goolsby (2006) study of acute care nurse practitioner practice as part of the larger 2004 National Nurse Practitioner Survey, ACNP respondents continued to develop new roles to fulfill identified needs for APNs to manage aspects of patient care in a variety of settings. NPs were found to be practicing in specialty care areas such as the cardiology, pulmonary, and specialized neurology settings; hematology/oncology; specialty ear-nose-throat (ENT) services; a variety of surgery services; palliative care; pain management services; and others (Kleinpell & Goolsby, 2006; Kleinpell-Nowell, 1999). New areas of practice for ACNPs were hospitalist roles and as surgical first assistants. A new leadership role that has emerged is director of nurse practitioners. This role has improved the work environment for NPs who had previously reported to office managers or physicians. The director of NPs is in tune with issues regarding scope of practice, licensure, and certification. He or she can serve as an advocate as well as a mentor for professional development projects such as publications and presentations (D'Agostino & Halpern, 2010). These new practice areas demonstrate the diversity of practice opportunities available to meet the needs of acutely ill patients.

As of 2004, only a little over 50% of ACNPs continued to work in hospitals, and this change is projected to continue as the role of the ACNP expands into more specialty, rural, and nontraditional areas (Kleinpell & Goolsby, 2006). This evolution in practice setting parallels that of the CNS who was originally totally hospital based, but now one-third of practicing CNSs are found in community settings (Scott, 1999).

Acute Care Nurse Practitioners in Specialty Practices

In tertiary health-care centers, cyclic changing of medical residents from one service to another has contributed to fragmented care. The ACNP can provide much-needed stability and continuity known to produce positive patient outcomes. Complex settings, in which the continuous follow-up of patients is necessary, are ideal practice areas for the ACNP. ACNPs can make a positive impact on the health-care delivery system by providing a continuous and comprehensive approach to the management of their patients' needs.

Oncology is one of those specialty areas in which nurse practitioner expertise for continuous and comprehensive care is crucial. Oncology settings span the cancer trajectory from high-risk cancer clinics to hospice and palliative care (Vogel, 2010; Volker & Limerick, 2007). In 2007, the American Society of Clinical Oncology (ASCO) Workforce Study predicted a 48% increase in the demand for medical oncology services by the year 2020. This need far exceeds the number of medicine trainees that will be able to fill this need (Erikson et al., 2009). Perhaps more important, NPs in oncology bring a unique holistic perspective that enables them to provide expert care with issues such as pain management, symptom palliation, and sensitivity to the psychological aspects of a cancer diagnosis. NP roles in oncology are varied and can include outpatient roles in radiation therapy, chemotherapy, surgical clinics (preoperative and postoperative global care), palliative care, survivorship and prevention, and genetic counseling related to cancer risk. These NPs can also be found in intensive care units as well as medical/surgical oncology units. As a result of the Consensus Model, there are no longer stand-alone oncology NP programs. NPs must be prepared as either primary care or acute care nurse practitioners and then can complete additional training and obtain specialty certification in oncology.

Care of the Elderly

The aging population is projected to increase by over 70% between 2010 and 2030. Coinciding with this is a projected worsening of the shortage of critical care intensivists and nurses. These shortages provide considerable concern for those working in, or relying on, acute health-care services (Angus, Kelley, Schmitz, White, & Popovich, 2000). Undoubtedly, the ACNP working in the acute and critical care areas will be confronted with caring for more elderly patients who are subject to significant physiological, social, psychological, and developmental changes that affect their recovery from and survival after an acute illness (Miller, 2001).

In response to the need for more adequately prepared health-care professionals who can meet the growing needs of critically ill older patients, the Critical Care Workforce Partnership was formed. This partnership collectively represented more than 100,000 health-care professionals who specialize in critical care (Angus et al., 2000). Their goals were to help inform policy makers and other key audiences of the complex issues associated with shortages of critical care physicians, nurses, pharmacists, and respiratory therapists trained to care for the critically ill, and especially the critically ill aged; to educate health-care professionals in critical care; to promote effective and safe systems of patient care; and to ensure an adequate workforce of trained critical care professionals. Simultaneously, cooperatives between the Hartford Institute for Geriatric Nursing at New York University and the National Association of Clinical Nurse Specialists developed competencies for clinical nurse specialists caring for the adult-gerontology population (AACN, 2010).

These partnerships informed those involved in the development of the Consensus Model. As such, the adult population has been redefined to better reflect the growing demographic and is now the adult-gerontology population. All advanced practice nurses caring for the adult population must now be educationally prepared to manage the issues of the adult population across the adult continuum from young adulthood through older adulthood. Moreover, the National Organization of Nurse Practitioner Faculties (NONPF) has developed competencies for acute care nurse practitioners and primary care nurse practitioners specific to the adult-gerontology population that must be met before students graduate from their educational programs. Specific competencies regarding adult-gerontology patients have also been developed for those NPs whose primary focus is not adult-gerontology patients but who may encounter them in their practices. Thus, all nurse practitioner educational programs are recommended to include additional gerontology-specific content based on competencies developed by NONPF.

Nurse-Midwifery

Nurse-midwives are registered nurses who are primary health-care providers to women throughout the life span. They perform physical exams; prescribe medications, including contraceptive methods; order laboratory tests as needed; and provide prenatal care, gynecological care, and labor and birth care, as well as health education and counseling to women of all ages. Per the American College of Nurse-Midwives (ACNM) position statement, *Mandatory Degree Requirements for Entry into Midwifery*

Practice, a graduate degree is required for entry into midwifery practice (ACNM, 2009). All midwifery education programs provide the necessary education for graduates to be eligible to take the examination offered by the American Midwifery Certification Board (AMCB) and become certified nurse-midwives (CNMs). The Accreditation Commission for Midwifery Education (ACME) (formerly the ACNM Division of Accreditation [DOA]) assesses the quality and content of midwifery education programs and ensures that they reflect the ACNM core competencies.

Since the ACNM has mandated graduate-level education for entry into midwifery clinical practice, the multiple entry options into midwifery have dwindled. Graduate programs predominate in nurse-midwifery preparation (91% of nurse-midwifery programs) versus certificate programs (9% of programs).

Nurse-midwifery is recognized in all 50 states, although it is regulated by various agencies in the different states and has varying scopes of practice from state to state. Physician practices and hospitals are identified as the primary employers of nurse-midwives (Schuiling, Sipe, & Fullerton, 2010). For nurse-midwives practicing in hospital settings, clinical privileges may be granted through membership in the medical staff or through other privileging routes (Cooper, 1998). The purpose of requiring institutional credentialing and practice privileges is to ensure that nurse-midwives provide patient care within the parameters of professional practice (Cooper, 1998). Presently nurse-midwives practice in hospitals, physician-owned practices, educational institutions, midwife-owned practices, community health centers, nonprofit health agencies, military or federal government agencies, and birthing centers (Schuiling et al., 2010).

Primary Care Focus in Nurse-Midwifery

As nurse-midwives continued to provide obstetrical care to women throughout their childbearing years, they realized that many women did not have access to physician services. It became a natural progression for women to seek their primary health-care needs from the health-care provider they had trusted during their childbirths. As a result, nurse-midwives began to provide care to perimenopausal and postmenopausal women, a natural expansion of their scope of practice. As the aging of U.S. Americans evolves in the 21st century, the number of women approaching menopause is growing. Large numbers of women are expected to seek menopausal and postmenopausal care from nurse-midwives. In response to this change in demographics and the need for greater access to primary care providers, CNMs have expanded their scope of practice. Currently, CNMs' scope of practice includes provision of primary care to women across the life span from adolescence to beyond menopause, with a special emphasis on pregnancy, childbirth, and gynecological and reproductive health. Midwives perform comprehensive physical exams, prescribe medications (including contraceptive methods), order laboratory and other diagnostic tests, and provide health and wellness education and counseling. The scope of practice for CNMs also includes treatment of male partners for sexually transmitted infections and reproductive health, and care of the normal newborn during the first 28 days of life (ACNM, 2011a). Interestingly, this scope of practice reflects the changes in the Consensus Model: the population focus of midwives from women's health to women's health–gender-related care. CNMs continue to focus on midwifery so as to not lose the essence of nurse-midwifery practice, while acknowledging those aspects of primary care that are part of the services offered to patients and their families.

Issues Related to Primary Care Practice

CNMs provide primary and preventive care in clinics and other outpatient settings. The ACNM calls for care delivered by CNMs to include all essential factors of primary care and case management.

This focus on the ambulatory care of women and newborns emphasizes health promotion, education, and disease prevention, and identifies women as central in providing this care (ACNM, 1997). CNMs have also focused on the care of adolescent women, noting that they are largely a medically underserved group.

Nurse-Midwife as First Assistant for Cesarean Section

Another role of the CNM in birthing emergencies has developed out of necessity, that of the surgical first assistant. As a result of obstetrical residency programs across the nation closing and cost containment resulting in fewer physicians available to serve as first assistants, CNMs have expanded their roles to fill the gap (Moes & Thatcher, 2001). Because in many cases the CNM was already present at the time of an emergency, the delivery could progress without interruption, resulting in better outcomes for both the mother and the newborn, if the CNM was prepared as a surgical first assistant.

Not unexpectedly, there is opposition to this expansion of the CNM role. The Association for Perioperative Registered Nurses (AORN) and some surgeons are not convinced that CNMs possess adequate knowledge to perform the first assistant role safely. In response to this criticism, the ACNM (1998) has set guidelines for those CNMs who wish to serve as a first assistant and defined the role of the first assistant in Cesarean sections as a frequently performed advanced midwifery skill requiring training and supervision in patient assessment, anatomy and physiology, principles of wound repair, and the development of basic surgical skills such as aseptic technique and suturing. At present, each state is addressing the requirements for CNMs who practice as first assistants. Although the number of CNM–first assistants is still small, this may change as appropriate content and supervision are provided in curricula that prepare CNMs.

More recently, midwives have added the use of obstetrical ultrasound examinations to their repertoire of skills (ACNM, 2011b). Ultrasound examinations may be performed in all trimesters of pregnancy to obtain specific information: determining gestational age, assessing fetal well-being, monitoring interval fetal growth, and measuring maternal cervical length. ACNM (2010) recognizes the need for additional educational content, credentialing, and privileging for midwives who choose to incorporate this into their practices. ACNM is not mandating this as a required skill for all midwives but recognizes that ultrasound examinations may be a necessary tool in meeting the needs of one's patients.

As the needs of childbearing women have changed over the years, the practice and skills of the nurse-midwife have expanded to meet them. This trend will continue as additional needs are identified. See **Box 2-4.**

Nurse Anesthetist

CRNAs* are APRNs who are anesthesia specialists with authority to practice in all 50 states and the District of Columbia. They administer all types of anesthesia and provide anesthesia-related care in the following categories: preanesthetic preparations and evaluation; anesthesia induction, maintenance, and emergence; postanesthesia care; and perianesthetic and clinical support functions (Department of Health and Human Services [DHHS], Public Health Service [PHS] Division of Acquisition Management, 1995).

---

*In the state of New Jersey, the title APN has been substituted for the CRNA title, providing consistency among all advanced practice nurses.

BOX 2-4
Nurse-Midwife Clinical Profile

Carol is the practice director of a busy obstetrical, gynecological, and midwifery care program that includes nine midwives and five physicians. She is responsible for the recruitment and evaluation of staff members and serves as liaison to hospital administrators and to the professional and lay community.

As she has progressed in her role, she has assumed more administrative responsibilities, especially those dealing with the need to break even financially. The high costs of health care have forced her to learn the business end of the practice. She completed a midwifery business institute course to learn the intricacies of reimbursement because her practice accepts numerous health-care plans, and she acknowledges a steep learning curve.

Billing is done through the clinical care association (CCA) that employs her. Nurse-midwives in her practice were offered an incentive-based contract with the CCA but refused this opportunity, choosing instead a guaranteed base salary with bonuses.

Nurse anesthetists provide a significant amount of the anesthesia given for surgical procedures in the United States, including that delivered in federal agencies and military installations (Fehder, 2003). These APRNs work in urban and rural settings, and provide more than 50% of the anesthesia administered in rural areas (RAND Corporation, 2010). In contrast to the high numbers of women in the other APRN categories, 41% of CRNAs are men (American Association of Nurse Anesthetists [AANA], 2011).

Employment patterns for CRNAs have evolved in recent years as a result of their achievement of independent billing rights under Medicare, decreases in anesthesia reimbursement rates, efforts to reduce hospital-based costs, and the growth of nonhospital-based surgical settings in which anesthesia is administered. As of 2007, 44% of CRNAs were employed in urban areas compared to 56% in rural areas. Further geographical analysis by U.S. region shows the majority of CRNAs providing anesthesia services in the South (36%), then the Midwest (25%), then the Northeast (12%), followed by 10% working in the West (RAND Corporation, 2010). Nearly 80% of CRNAs report their primary employment to be within one facility or one group, whereas anesthesiologists were noted to work for one group, but usually in multiple facilities (RAND Corporation).

The American Association of Nurse Anesthetists (AANA) serves as the guiding professional organization for CRNAs, setting the educational and certification standards and promulgating a code of ethics for CRNAs (AANA, 2005), along with scope and standards for nurse anesthesia practice (AANA, 2006) and standards for office-based practice (AANA, 2009). Nurse anesthetist students must enroll in schools accredited by the AANA, and upon graduation they must successfully complete a certification examination. They must also participate in mandatory biennial recertification through the National Board on Certification and Recertification of Nurse Anesthetists (NBCRNA) that includes 40 hours of accredited continuing education (NBCRNA, 2011).

In 1998, master's-degree preparation was required for beginning nurse anesthesia practice. Although the required master's degree does not have to be in nursing, about 50% of graduate CRNA programs are located within schools of nursing (McCarthy et al., 2000). By 2025 the entry-into-practice educational requirement will be at the doctoral level.

CRNAs face significant ongoing difficulties in establishing their practice prerogatives. They face considerable pressures from anesthesiologists who have attempted to limit their scope of practice by conceptualizing the administration of anesthesia as the practice of medicine (Shumway & Del Risco,

2000). In 1982, the American Society of Anesthesiologists (ASA) introduced the concept of an anesthesia care team (ACT), a practice model requiring that all anesthetics be given under the direction and supervision of an anesthesiologist (Shumway & Del Risco, 2000).

These restrictive efforts were inadvertently fostered with the introduction of an insurance reimbursement regulation policy by Medicare in 1982. This policy attempted to reduce charges of fraud for anesthesia care by establishing specific conditions that held anesthesiologists accountable for services they claimed to perform when working with or employing CRNAs (Fehder, 2003; Shumway & Del Risco, 2002). The Tax Equity and Fiscal Responsibility Act (TEFRA) regulations set specific conditions for reimbursable services that seemed to require physician leadership for the delivery of anesthesia as a standard of care. Later attempts to eliminate the necessity for anesthesiologist supervision for Medicare reimbursement of CRNA services have resulted in an "opt out" option for states. If the governor of a state completes three criteria (consults the state boards of medicine and nursing about issues related to access to and the quality of anesthesia services in the state, determines that opting out is consistent with state law, and determines that opting out is in the best interest of the state's citizens), he or she can "opt out," resulting in CRNAs being permitted to provide anesthesia without physician supervision (AANA, 2011). As of 2011, 16 states have chosen to do this.

One result of the struggle for CRNA practice prerogatives and leadership has been the establishment of the ACT as the predominant practice model. To clarify whether differences exist between CRNAs who work in ACTs and those who do not, Shumway and Del Risco (2000) evaluated personal and professional characteristics, scope of practice, workload, income, and employment arrangements in a sample of over 400 CRNAs. They found that CRNAs who practiced in ACTs were more likely to be women, have less experience, be younger, have a master's degree, and practice in larger cities. ACT-based CRNAs also had a broader scope of practice and used more airways, regional anesthesia, and monitoring techniques, and performed more varied cases and services. They used more laryngeal mask airways and arterial catheters, and provided more anesthesia for cardiopulmonary bypass, pediatric, intracranial, and trauma cases than non-ACT anesthetists. However, they were less likely to be involved with the placement of epidural and central venous catheters and to participate in pain management and critical care services (Shumway & Del Risco, 2000).

Non-ACT-based anesthetists worked more hours per week and were reimbursed $40,000 more per year. Finally, 91% of ACT-based anesthetists in this sample were employees compared to 4% who were self-employed, whereas 49% of non-ACT-based anesthetists were employees compared to 43% who were self-employed (Shumway & Del Risco, 2002). See **Box 2-5.**

FUTURE DIRECTIONS FOR ADVANCED PRACTICE NURSES

APRNs are thriving, as shown in the increased numbers of practitioners; in the expansion of practice roles and settings; in the opportunity for reimbursement for services; and in the numerous studies demonstrating favorable patient outcomes related to APRN delivery of care. The growth and expansion of these roles will undoubtedly continue.

APRN roles present exciting challenges and enormous diversity, satisfaction, and rewards. But they also present challenges that reflect those found in the larger health-care arena, including those related to the high cost of health care, reimbursement limitations, and the need for greater access to care. They also have problems unique to those found in a predominantly female profession, including the need to recruit an outstanding new generation of APRNs in a climate that offers many role opportunities to women and men.

BOX 2-5
Nurse Anesthetist Clinical Profile

Marcy is a certified registered nurse anesthetist (CRNA) who has master's-level training and works as a member of an anesthesia care team (ACT) in a university-related urban medical center. She has been a clinical coordinator for the team for the past 2 years and before that was a team member for 2 years. Her clinical responsibilities involve providing anesthesia for patients requiring ear-nose-throat (ENT), plastic, neurosurgical, thoracic, cardiac, and orthopedic surgery.

Marcy works in a busy practice setting with 24 operating rooms and plans to expand the practice to two other sites. She typically works four 10-hour days. Three are spent in the operating room and one involves administrative duties. She regularly supervises anesthesia students in the operating rooms and teaches and co-directs an accredited educational program for nurse anesthetists.

Marcy's responsibilities include the provision of general, regional, and local anesthesia and conscious sedation. She likes the autonomy and independence of her job, and the opportunity it presents to integrate her skill and knowledge in the clinical setting.

Marcy is an employee of the ACT and does not bill directly for her services. Billing is done through the supervising anesthesiologist to maximize full billing potential. Although she cannot prescribe medications in her state, she uses the unit-supplied medications for her patients. Her choices are guided by the patient's history and needs, the surgeon's preference, the surgical procedure, and the patient's preference when possible.

The future for APRNs, although promising, will continue to be affected by knowledge development in the biological and social sciences and in the evolving political and social climate. The call for a practice doctorate in nursing, as a proposed terminal degree for APRNs (AACN, 2004), will provide stimuli for role expansion or contraction and for possible changes in educational programs preparing future APRNs. APRN organizations have varied in their response to the call for a practice doctorate for APRNs by 2015: the American Association of Nurse Practitioners (AANP) has endorsed this call; the AANA has endorsed both the PhD and the DNP by 2025, whereas the ACNM and the National Association of Clinical Nurse Specialists (NACNS) have not endorsed this requirement. In addition, as the Consensus Model (2008) recommendations are implemented, the licensure, accreditation, certification, and education of APRNs will continue to evolve. What effect this will have on APRN practice is yet to be seen.

REFERENCES

American Academy of Nurse Practitioners. (2007). *Standards for nurse practitioner practice in retail-based clinics.* Austin, TX: Author.

American Association of Colleges of Nursing. (2004). *Position statement on the practice doctorate in nursing.* Washington, DC. Retrieved May 10, 2008, from www.aacn.nche.edu/DNP/DNPPositionStatement.htm.

American Association of Colleges of Nursing. (2010). *Adult-gerontology clinical nurse specialist competencies.* Developed in collaboration with the Hartford Institute for Geriatric Nursing at New York University and the National Association of Clinical Nurse Specialists. Washington, DC: Author.

American Association of Critical Care Nurses & American Nurses Association. (1995). *Standards of clinical practice and scope of practice for the acute care nurse practitioner.* Washington, DC: American Nurses Publishing.

American Association of Nurse Anesthetists. (2005). *Code of ethics for the certified registered nurse anesthetist.* Park Ridge, IL: Author.

American Association of Nurse Anesthetists. (2006). *Scope and standards for nurse anesthesia practice.* Park Ridge, IL: Author.

American Association of Nurse Anesthetists. (2009). *Standards for office based anesthesia practice.* Park Ridge, IL: Author.

American Association of Nurse Anesthetists. (2010). *Nurse anesthesia education.* Park Ridge, IL: Author. American Association of Nurse Anesthetists. (2011). *Certified registered nurse anesthetists (CRNAs) at a glance.* Retrieved September 28, 2011, from http://www.aana.com/ataglance.aspx.

American College of Nurse-Midwives. (1997). *Position statement. Certified nurse-midwives and certified midwives as primary care providers/case managers.* Retrieved May 10, 2008, from www.midwife.org.

American College of Nurse-Midwives. (1998). *ACNM clinical practice statement: The certified nurse-midwife/certified midwife as first assistant in surgery.* Washington, DC: Author.

American College of Nurse-Midwives. (2009). *Position statement. Mandatory requirements for entry into midwifery practice.* Retrieved September 12, 2011, from www.midewife.org.

American College of Nurse-Midwives. (2010). *Essential facts about midwives: Midwives and birth in the United States.* Retrieved September 12, 2011, from www.midwife.org/essential-facts-about-midwives.

American College of Nurse-Midwives. (2011a). *Scope of practice.* Retrieved September 22, 2011, from http://www.midwife.org/Our-Scope-of-Practice.

American College of Nurse-Midwives. (2011b). *Position statement. Midwive's performance of ultrasound in clinical care.* Retrieved October 5, 2011, from www.midwife.org.

American Nurses Credentialing Center. (2011). *Magnet Recognition.* Retrieved September 29, 2011, from http://www.nursecredentialing.org/Magnet.aspx.

American Nurses Credentialing Center. (2008a). *Adult psychiatric and mental health nurse practitioner certification. Description of practice.* Retrieved April 23, 2008, from www.nursecredentialing.org/cert/eligibility/apmhnp.htlm.

American Nurses Credentialing Center. (2008b). *Family psychiatric and mental health nurse practitioner certification. Description of practice.* Retrieved April 23, 2008, from www.nursecredentialing.org/cert/eligibility/fpmhnp.htlm.

American Psychiatric Nurses Association. (2010). *Position statement: Psychiatric mental health advanced practice nurses.* Retrieved September 3, 2011, from http://www.apna.org/files/public/PMH_Advanced_Practice_Nurses_Position_Statement.pdf.

Angus, D. C., Kelley, M. A., Schmitz, R. J., White, A., & Popovich, J. (2000). Current and projected workforce requirements for care of the critically ill and patients with pulmonary disease: Can we meet the requirements of an aging population? *Journal of the American Medical Association, 284*(21), 2762–2770.

Becker, D., Kaplow, R., Muenzen, P., & Hartigan, C. (2006). Activities performed by acute and critical care advanced practice nurses: American Association of Critical Care nurses study of practice. *American Journal of Critical Care, 15*(2), 130–148. PMID: 16501133.

Bell, L. J. (2006). *Scope and standards of practice for the acute care nurse practitioner.* Aliso Viejo, CA: American Association of Critical Care Nurses.

Bell, L. J., & McNamara, L. J. (Eds.). (2010). *AACN scope and standards for acute and critical care clinical nurse specialist practice.* Aliso Viejo, CA: American Association of Critical-Care Nurses.

Bissinger, R. L., Allred, C. A., Arford, P. H., & Bellig, L. L. (1997). A cost-effectiveness analysis of neonatal nurse practitioners. *Nursing Economics, 15*(2), 92–99.

Blewett, L. A., Johnson, K., McCarthy, T., Lackner, T., & Brandt, B. (2010). Improving geriatric transitional care through inter-professional care teams. *Journal of Evaluation in Clinical Practice, 16*(1), 57–63.

Borgmeyer, A., Gyr, P. M., Jamerson, P. A., & Henry, L. D. (2008). Evaluation of the role of the pediatric nurse practitioner in an inpatient asthma program. *Journal of Pediatric Health Care, 22*(5), 273–281.

Brooten, D., Gennaro, S., Knapp, H., Brown, L., & York, R. (1989). Clinical specialist pre and postdischarge teaching of parents of very low birthweight infants. *Journal of Obstetrical, Gynecological, and Neonatal Nursing, 18*(4), 316–322.

Brown, A. M., Besunder, J., & Bachman, M. (2008). Development of a pediatric intensive care unit nurse practitioner program. *Journal of Nursing Administration, 38*(7-8), 355–359.

Clinical Nurse Specialist Core Competencies Executive Summary 2006–2008. (2010). The National CNS Competency Task Force. Retrieved August 10, 2012, from http://www.aacn.org.

Consensus Model for APRN Regulation: Licensure, Accreditation, Certification and Education. (2008). Completed through the work of the APRN consensus work group and the National Council of State Boards of Nursing APRN Advisory Committee. Retrieved October 5, 2011, from http://www.aacn.nche.edu/Education/pdf/APRNReport.pdf.

Cooper, E. (1998). Credentialing and privileging nurse-midwives. *Journal* of *Nursing Care Quality, 12*(4), 30–35.

Craven, R. F., & Keene, T. L. (2000). The advanced practice nurse and home care. *CARING Magazine, 19*(11), 38–40.

D'Agostino, R., & Halpern, N. (2010). Acute care nurse practitioners in oncologic care: The Sloan Kettering Memorial experience, *Critical Care Clinics, 26,* 207–217.

Delametter, G. L. (1999). Advanced practice nursing and the role of the pediatric critical care nurse practitioner. *Critical Care Nursing Quarterly, 21*(4), 16–21.

Department of Health and Human Services, Public Health Service Division of Acquisition Management. (1995). *Expanding the capacity of advanced practice nursing education. Final report* [data file]. Retrieved May 10, 2008, from http://bhpr.hrsa.gov/nursing/lewin95.html.

Dwyer, M. L. (2000). Advanced practice nursing for children with HIV infection. *Nursing Clinics of North America, 35*(1), 115–123.

Erikson, C., Schulman, S., Kosty, M., & Hanley, A. (2009). Oncology workforce: Results of the ASCO 2007 program directors survey. *Journal of Oncology Practice, 5*(2), 62–65.

Fehder, W. (2003). Nurse anesthetists: Evolution from critical care practitioners to anesthesia providers. In D. O. McGivern, E. M. Sullivan-Marx, & S. A. Greenberg (Eds.), *Nurse practitioners: Evolution of advanced practice* (4th ed., pp. 269–283). New York: Springer.

Gracias, V. H., Sicoutris, C. P., Stawicki, S. P., Meredith, D. M., Horan, A. D., Gupta, R., et al. (2008). Critical care nurse practitioners improve compliance with clinical practice guidelines in "semiclosed" surgical intensive care unit. *Journal of Nursing Care Quality, 23*(4), 338–344.

Grandinetti, D. (1999). NP progress report: How is this practice doing? *RN, 62*(7), 36–38.

Hittle, K., & Tilford, A. K. (2010). Pediatric nurse practitioners as hospitalists. *Journal of Pediatric Health Care, 24*(5), 347–350.

Hoffman, L. A., Tasota, F. J., Zullo, T. G., Scharfenberg, C., & Donahoe, M. P. (2005). Outcomes of care managed by an acute care nurse practitioner/attending physician team in a subacute medical intensive care unit. *American Journal of Critical Care, 14*(2), 121–130.

Institute of Medicine. 2010. *A summary of the October 2009 forum on the future of nursing: Acute care.* Washington, DC: The National Academies Press.

King, B. R., Foster, R. L., Woodward, G. A., & McCans, K. (2001). Procedures performed by pediatric transport nurses: How "advanced" is the practice? *Pediatric Emergency Care, 17*(6), 410–413.

Kleinpell, R., & Goolsby, M. J. (2006). 2004 American Academy of Nurse Practitioners national nurse practitioner sample survey: Focus on acute care. *Journal of the American Academy of Nurse Practitioners, 18,* 393–394.

Kleinpell-Nowell, R. (1999). Longitudinal survey of acute care nurse practitioner practice: Year 1. *AACN Clinical Issues, 10*(4), 510–520.

Lambing, A. Y., Adams, D. L., Fox, D. H., & Divine, G. (2004). Nurse practitioners' and physicians' care activities and clinical outcomes with an inpatient geriatric population. *Journal of the American Academy of Nurse Practitioners, 16*(8), 343–352.

Lenz, E. R., Mundinger, M. O., Kane, R. L., Hopkins, S. C., & Lin, S. X. (2004). Primary care outcomes in patients treated by nurse practitioners or physicians: Two-year follow-up. *Medical Care Research and Review, 61*(3), 332–351.

McCarthy, E. J., Pearson, J., McCall, W. G., Fault-Callahan, M., Lovell, S. L., & Sanders, B. D. (2000). Education of nurse anesthetists in the United States. *AANA Journal, 68*(2), 111–113.

Miller, S. K. (2001). Gerontology and geriatrics: Considerations for the acute care nurse practitioner. *Nurse Practitioner Forum, 12*(3), 155–160.

Mitchell-DiCenso, A., Guyatt, G., Marrin, M., Goeree, R., Willan, A., Southwell, D., et al. (1996). A controlled trial of nurse practitioners in neonatal intensive care. *Pediatrics, 98*(6), 1143–1148.

Moes, C. B., & Thacher, F. (2001). The midwife as first assistant for Cesarean section. *Journal of Midwifery and Women's Health, 46*(5), 305–312.

Moller, M. D., & Haber, J. (1997). Advanced practice psychiatric nursing: The need for a blended role. *Online Journal of Issues in Nursing, 2*(1). Retrieved May 10, 2008, from www.nursingworld.org/ojin.

Muller, A. C., Hujcs, M., Dubendorf, P., & Harrington, P. T. (2010). Clinical nurse specialist practice and Magnet designation. *Clinical Nurse Specialist, 24*(5), 252–259.

National Board on Certification and Recertification of Nurse Anesthetists. (2011). *Criteria for recertification.* Park Ridge, IL: Author.

Naylor, M. D., Bowles, K. H., & Brooten, D. (2000). Patient problems and advanced practice nurse interventions during transitional care. *Public Health Nursing, 17*(2), 94–102.

Neal, L. J. (1999). Role of the advanced practical nurse. *Home Healthcare Nurse, 17*(5), 323–325.

Newhouse, R. P., Stanik-Hutt, J., White, K. M., Johantgen, M., Bass, E. B., Zangaro, G., et al. (2011). Advanced practice nurse outcomes 1990–2008: A systematic review. *Nursing Economics, 29*(5), 1–21.

Okuhara, C. A., Faire, P. M., & Pike, N. A. (2011). Acute care pediatric nurse practitioner: A vital role in pediatric cardiothoracic surgery. *Journal of Pediatric Nursing, 26*(2), 137–142.

Pearson, L. J. (2008). The Pearson report. *American Journal for Nurse Practitioners, 12*(2), 9–10.

Pelosi, L. (2000). The role of the advanced practice nurse in pediatric general surgery. *Pediatric Advanced Practice Nursing, 35*(1), 159–171.

Phillips, S. J. (2011). 23rd annual legislative update. *Nurse Practitioner, 36*(1), 30–52.

RAND Corporation. (2010). An analysis of the labor markets for anesthesiology. Retrieved September 6, 2011, from http://www.rand.org/pubs/technical_reports/2010/RAND_TR688.pdf.

Rossetto, C. L., & Fair, J. (1998). Assessing competencies for medical procedures as an advanced practice nurse. *Journal of Pediatric Health Care, 12*(2), 102–104.

Schram, A. (2010). Medical home and the nurse practitioner: A policy analysis. *Nurse Practitioner, 6*(2), 132–139.

Schuiling, K. D., Sipe, T. A., & Fullerton, J. (2010). Findings from the analysis of the American College of Nurse-Midwives' membership surveys: 2006–2008. *Journal of Midwifery and Women's Health, 55*(4), 299–307.

Scott, R. A. (1999). A description of the roles, activities, and skills of clinical nurse specialists in the United States. *Clinical Nurse Specialist, 13*(4), 183–190.

Shumway, S. H., & Del Risco, J. (2000). A comparison of nurse anesthesia practice types. *AANA Journal, 68*(5), 452–462.

Silver, H. R., Murphy, M. A., & Gitterman, B. A. (1984). The hospital nurse practitioner in pediatrics: A new expanded role for staff nurses. *American Journal of Disease of Children, 138*(3), 237–239.

Spisso, J., O'Callaghan, C., McKennan, M., & Holcroft, J. (1990). Improved quality of care and reduction of house staff workload using trauma nurse practitioners. *Journal of Trauma, 30*(6), 660–664.

Stuppy, M. (2004). The role of the nurse practitioner in the cardiac cath lab. *Cath Lab Digest, 12*(7), 1, 6–12.

Summers, L. (2011). Developments in primary care affect APRNs. *American Nurse,* Jan/Feb, 12. Retrieved September 15, 2011, from http://www.nursingworld.org/MainMenuCategories/ANAMarketplace/ANAPeriodicals/TAN/2011-TAN/TAN-JanFeb11.aspx.

Teicher, S., Crawford, K., Williams, B., Nelson, B., & Andrews, C. (2001). Emerging role of the pediatric nurse practitioner in acute care. *Pediatric Nursing, 27*(4), 387–390.

Vogel, W. (2010). Advanced practitioners in oncology: Meeting the challenges. *AdvancedPractioner.com 1*(1), 13–18.

Volker, D. L., & Limerick, M. (2007). What constitutes a dignified death? The voice of oncology advanced practice nurses. *Clinical Nurse Specialist, 21,* 241–247.

Weinberg, R. M., Liljestrand, J. S., & Moore, S. (1983). Inpatient management by a nurse practitioner: Effectiveness in a rehabilitation setting. *Archives of Physical Medicine and Rehabilitation, 64*(12), 588–590.

Zachariah, R., & Lundeen, S. P. (1997). Research and practice in an academic community nursing center. *Image: Journal of Nursing Scholarship, 23*(3), 255–260.

3 Role Development: A Theoretical Perspective

Lucille A. Joel

There is a role only for the moment, not any role that will serve for the entire life of a career. Role modifications depend on a theoretical body of knowledge, more of it hypothetical than empirical research. These concepts and relationships allow a comfortable paradigm shift as necessary, with an awareness of the elements of continuity from here to there.

A THEORETICAL PERSPECTIVE ON ROLE: AN OVERVIEW

There are two diametrically opposed theoretical perspectives in the behavioral sciences that provide a context for the study of role performance: structural-functionalist theory and symbolic-interactionist theory. The former is based on the assumption that roles are more or less fixed within the society to which they are attached and that opportunities for individuals to alter patterns of social interaction are limited. This is in contrast to the latter, which proposes the more individualistic perspective, that people do not merely learn responses but organize and interpret cues in the environment and choose those to which they wish to react.

Structural-functionalist theory subordinates the individual to the society; it is deductive in its analysis of role. All situations that arise within a society do so because they fill a social need. One such example is the division of labor. The more complex a society, the more differentiated its labor source will become, readjusting and reconstructing over time. Specialization becomes guaranteed, and associates and assistants are created to share in a domain of the work. This concept is dramatically displayed by the division of labor and reordered roles within the health-care delivery system, each role creating its own cadre of technologists, technicians, associates, and assistants. Why should nursing be different?

Altruism also plays a major part here because individuals subordinate their will to the social order. The social forces in a given society validate the roles and the associated behaviors of the individual. Consensual validation is the vehicle for both the maintenance and change of these norms. In many instances, norms are codified by government; in others, they continue to exist in veritable limbo, changing or resisting change according to time and place. A continuing debate exists about the relationship between the fixed norms of a society and the individual's perception of those norms. Often there is no route to interpretation of the social norm except cues offered by others in the situation, and often those cues may be misleading. From another perspective, where may nonconformity be tolerated, to what degree, and in what areas of social participation? Examples abound both professionally and in life. Consider for a moment the immigrant family whose children are schooled in the United States and socialized to the prevailing culture in this country. Are their new ways accepted at home and to what extent? Must they change like a chameleon from place to place or jeopardize belonging or perhaps even sustenance? To what extent can advanced practice nurses

(APNs) feel confident in establishing their personally preferred values, attitudes, and behaviors in a new role or employment situation? See **Box 3-1** for cues that may predict limits on flexibility in defining role behaviors.

In contrast, the symbolic-interactionist view emphasizes the meaning that symbols hold for actors in the process of role development, rather than the constraints presumed to be exerted by the social structure. The interactionist sees the formation of role identity as inductive and complex. The role is a creative adaptation to the social environment and the result of the reciprocal interaction of individuals. It is the product of self-conception and the perspective of generalized others. To facilitate communication toward these ends, symbols are essential, and they must be social and hold the same meaning for each actor in the process. In other words, self-identity is shaped by the reflected appraisals of others, and it is desirable that individuals' self-perception should be highly congruent with the way they are perceived by others and the way they see themselves as being perceived by others. Should these pieces show a poor fit, an individual could waste a lifetime of effort creating evidence that justifies his or her personal view of self.

Many have rejected the structuralist approach because it seems limited in accounting for the wide variation in roles and behaviors that we see today. Yet, it is impossible to ignore the effect that the culture and the "collective conscience" have on our development of identity and role behaviors. There is recent interest in building conceptual frameworks that are inclusive of both the interactionist and structural perspectives, and promise a greatly enlarged understanding of role development. This eclecticism characterizes this chapter's discussion.

ROLE DEVELOPMENT

The concept of reference groups and the process of socialization are central to role development. Reference groups are the frame of reference for the process of socialization. Through socialization, individual behavior is shaped to conform to the standard of the group in which one chooses to seek membership.

BOX 3-1
Cues That May Predict Limits on Flexibility in Defining Role Behaviors

Highly precise and detailed job descriptions
Management by memorandum in situations in which personal communication would have sufficed
Guarded interdisciplinary boundaries that hamper smooth operation
A hierarchy that is an obstacle to work rather than a facilitator
Policies, procedures, and documentation systems that are cumbersome and even inconsistent with current practice
Absence of staff nurse autonomy in caring for patients
Organizational relationships designed for supervision, as opposed to reporting
Absence of inventiveness and creativity
Verbalized discontent from staff, but no evidence of any attempt to change things
High turnover rate among employees
Maintenance of a "screen" for attitudes, values, and behaviors not supported by historic antecedents

Reference Groups

Reference groups convey a standard of normative behavior in terms of values, attitudes, knowledge, and skills. For an individual, this may be a group to which he or she belongs or aspires. In moving toward a standard that is either consciously or unconsciously desired, discussion of several reference groups is in order, including normative groups, comparison groups, and audience groups. The normative group sets explicit standards and expects compliance, and it rewards or punishes relative to that degree of compliance. The church, community, and family are good examples of normative groups. The behaviors that are expected may have wide or narrow latitude, but somewhere there is a "bottom line." The comparison group sets its own standards and becomes a comparison group only when an individual accepts it as such. The nursing staff of a magnet facility may be a comparison group, demonstrating longevity in employment and satisfaction with work, seeking upward mobility through education, and so on. The nursing staff and their leadership in other facilities may aspire to these qualities, making it a comparison group for them. The audience group is a collective group whose attention an individual wishes to attract. The audience group holds certain values but does not demand compliance from the person for whom they serve as a referent (Lum, 1988). In fact, the audience group may not even be aware of this individual. To be recognized, the individual takes note of the group's values and plays to that audience for attention. Staff nurses may observe that physicians value being able to proceed with the treatment of their patients unencumbered by the bureaucratic constraints of health care. Administrators are overwhelmed by the cost factors in health care. Nurses are best positioned if they are aware of these values and attitudes, and try to minimize the obstacles they represent to these groups. In other words, they play to the audience through either word or deed.

Socialization

Socialization refers to the learning of the values, attitudes, knowledge, and skills that enable the behavior prescribed for a specific social position or role. The fact that these components are society specific indicates that there are social norms involved. Values are ideas held in common by members of a social structure that prioritizes goals and objectives (Scott, 1970). Values are generally the abstract but relatively stable aspects of a person's belief system. Attitude is the tendency to respond to social objects or events in a favorable or unfavorable way. Opinion is defined as expressed attitude (Katz, 1960). Behaviors are observable social acts performed by an individual. Attitudes guide judgment and subsequently behavior, but this assumption of a relationship between attitude and behavior is controversial.

Operationally, the concept of socialization refers to individuals acquiring the necessary knowledge and skills, as well as internalizing and shaping the values and attitudes of a particular social system, in preparation for fulfilling a specific role in that system (Lum, 1988). This process is no less true for the roles of nurse and APN than it is for the role of mother, father, husband, or wife. Further, whereas some roles or statuses have highly specific role prescriptions, others are extremely vague and open to wide variation of interpretation. This latitude may be observed in the setting in which the role is played out, the society in which it is placed, or both. Harmony among these systems enhances role execution. There is often significant discrepancy between the public, professional, legal, and institutional definitions of the role of the nurse. Even if the society and role occupant are bound by the legal role as defined, discrepancies among the other definitions cause problems in recruitment, retention, job satisfaction, and more.

Socialization is a continuous and cumulative process that evolves over time through role-taking and role-making, both of which are techniques of role bargaining. Social behavior is not simply a learned response. It depends on the processes of interaction and communication. To be successful, role-taking requires skill in empathic communication. There is a requirement to project oneself into the circumstances of another and then step back to imagine how one would feel in the other's situation. If there is accurate determination of the motives and feelings of the other, the actor can modify his or her own behavior to sustain or alter the other's response (Hardy & Hardy, 1988a). The process here is unidirectional. The APN "reads" his or her peers and supervisor as seeing staff development as the major focus of the APN role, although she or he may have preferred to carry a significant personal case load of the most complex patients. Staff development is accepted as the priority, but the APN takes on cases as vehicles for teaching at every opportunity.

Put in another way, the less desirable activities are accommodated (first-order change) and even eventually assimilated (second-order change), becoming an integral part of the role. First-order changes are *behavioral shifts* that do not permanently achieve a desired result. Old preferences keep returning like antagonists because we shift our behaviors, but not the core values or attitudes causing the behaviors. Second-order changes are *permanent attitude shifts that cause new behaviors.* The "old ways" stay gone and are not replaced by a new version (like giving up alcohol and starting a nicotine or work addiction).

In contrast, role-making is bidirectional and interactive, with both actors presenting behaviors that are interpreted reciprocally for the purpose of creating and modifying their own roles. This process is analogous to a dance, each partner seeking to complement the other while maintaining his or her own uniqueness. The APN notices surprise from the physician when she or he suggests a modification in treatment for a patient. The APN supplies cogent and sophisticated reasoning, and the physician agrees, although skeptical of this behavior. Over time, the physician becomes comfortable with the APN's prescriptions and actually looks for the clinical input. Both role-taking and role-making depend on success in reading role partners correctly. This skill is enhanced by broad social experience, rehearsal of the role anticipated, the recentness of those experiences, attentiveness to role behaviors, and good memory skills. These skills can be developed and honed during the educational experience.

As challenging as internalizing role behaviors is the movement from one role or subrole to another. This process is described in **Box 3-2.** Not only must one learn new behaviors, but one must break from old ones. Inadequate socialization predicts marginalization or the inability to either remain in a previous role or move on to another. A case in point is the nurse who hangs on to the periphery of a system, never quite becoming part of it or bothering to know the personalities involved and refusing to assimilate nursing with the other aspects of life. This is particularly common in people who try to juggle multiple aspects of life, keeping each separate—obligations everywhere, multiple lists of things to do, each with a first-place priority, a comprehensive plan nowhere. The wiser strategy is to integrate the dimensions of life, with professional colleagues becoming personal friends, family participating in workplace and professional events, and so on (one list with one rank ordering of priorities).

Role Acquisition

Knowledge and skill acquisition are important aspects of role implementation in nursing, both for the entry-level registered nurse and the APN. This is not to ignore the essential part played by attitudes and values (the belief system), but to acknowledge that knowledge and skill are expected of professionals by the public (audience group), leadership in the field (comparative group), and peers (normative group). The skill acquisition model, developed by Dreyfus and Dreyfus (1977) and later applied to nursing by Benner (1984), tells us that even experts perform as novices when they enter new roles or subroles, although they proceed to acquisition at a quicker pace. This pattern is verified by several

BOX 3-2
Socialization as Continuous

Break from Previous Roles
Minimize previous advantage.
Break previous peer relationships.
Convert previous peer relationships into friendship relationships.
Maintain a portfolio or clinical log reflecting on your evolving practice, values, and attitudes.

Establish a New Peer Group
Clarify new responsibilities that accompany changed status.
Consider the values, attitudes, knowledge, and skills that will contribute to success.
Develop new peer group associations.

Movement to the New Role Prescription (Accommodation)
Provide role rehearsal opportunities.
Review benefits of mastery.
Consider a mentor.
Identify support systems among role partners.*

Assimilation of Role Behaviors
Be aware of change of self-concept.
Recognize the rites of passage as more than symbolic.
Create opportunities for success.
Treat failure as a learning experience.
Move on to process and outcome evaluation once the role is established, although not matured.

*A role partner may hold the same role or a role that is reciprocal but definitely has role expectations of the primary role occupant.

authorities, including Brykczynski (2000) and Roberts, Tabloski, and Bova (1997). In observing APN students, they report periods of regression, anxiety, and conflict before the incorporation of new role behaviors. This is not unexpected, and an analogy can be drawn from work with groups. It is common that in the beginning of a group or when a new member is introduced into an established group, there is a loss of confidence among individual members. The introduction of a person into a milieu with new role expectations is a temporary setback, even when some of the behaviors have been well established in a previous role. The regression and loss of confidence are often followed by anger directed toward faculty and preceptors whom they see as guilty of not giving them enough knowledge or skill. In many ways, they are grieving the role they had previously mastered and responding to the anxiety over moving on.

Anticipatory socialization should be a planned goal during the student period and not left to chance. Ample opportunity should be provided for students to get to know APNs who may just be beginning their careers (peer group) and to participate in discussions with seasoned APNs regarding practice issues (accommodation). Both of these goals may be accomplished through the state nurses association, especially if there is a forum or division on advanced practice. Other experiences should be incorporated in the educational program, such as the opportunity to dialogue with employers and

BOX 3-3
Questions to Guide Advanced Practice Nurse Participation in a Panel on Advanced Practice

How did you find your first position after graduation?
What job-seeking strategies would you advise new graduates to use in today's market?
How do any or all of the following fit into your specific position?
What is your prescriptive authority?
What kind of practice privileges (i.e., admitting, treating, consulting, and discharging) do you have?
What system do you have for reimbursement?
Do you participate in a managed-care panel?
How have your functions or role changed over the years, and were those changes the result of the evolution of the profession, your choices, your advocacy, or the expectations of an employer?
Have you been an active participant in developing your role? How so?
What are the major stresses and strains in your practice? How do you handle them?
Describe your collaborative arrangement with a physician.
How do you show outcomes or document the value of your contribution to the practice? (Or to your employer?)
How do you maintain your practice credibility?
Do you plan to further develop your own role or skill set? If so, how?
What were the most valuable aspects of your graduate educational preparation for advanced practice? The least valuable?
What do you know now that you wish you had known earlier in your career?
What is your experience with mentoring, either as mentor or protégé?
How important to your professional development was this mentor(ed) experience?

practicing APNs about their expectations of the role. **Box 3-3** contains a format for the participation of APNs on a panel describing their practice and role development for students. These anticipatory experiences should facilitate the period of resocialization as a graduate.

It would be remiss not to mention the clinical competency of faculty. Clinically competent faculty are necessary to give credibility to the program and to narrow the gap "between education and practice" (Brykczynski, 2000, p. 121). The best of all worlds would be for faculty to teach using their own panel of patients. This being impossible much of the time, it is still necessary for faculty to have clinical skill to be able to critique practice and provide the proper oversight for preceptors.

Benner (1984) describes five levels of skill acquisition: novice, advanced beginner, competent, proficient, and expert. As one proceeds along this continuum, one becomes more involved in the process of caring, until at the expert stage, situations are recognized in terms of their holistic patterns rather than a cluster of component parts, and the context becomes somewhat irrelevant. In the early stages, new behaviors are accommodated, and they later become assimilated in the practice repertoire, until at the highest level they appear intuitive. Movement from accommodation to assimilation or from novice to expert with its intermediate steps is best accomplished through accruing experience with the opportunity to apply both practical and theoretical knowledge, and providing situations in which failure is allowed and treated as a learning experience (Roberts et al., 1997). It should be noted that Benner's model is experiential and does not consider education as a variable in distinguishing these skill levels. However, you cannot apply what you do not know. It would be interesting to use Benner's model to compare an APN and a non–master's-prepared registered nurse, both with similar experience.

It is helpful for APN students to consciously approach the socialization process knowing their normative, comparative, and audience groups, and being aware of the changes that are expected to take place in their own behaviors, values, and attitudes. Socializing experiences, provided during the course of studies, are presented in **Box 3-4.**

Socialization Deficits

One of the most compelling challenges in professional education is to provide adequate socialization. Socialization deficits are guaranteed to inhibit role performance, introducing additional stress into roles that are already by nature stressful.

APNs are increasingly prepared in programs of part-time study. In addition, the movement into the community college and university settings for entry-level education has, to some degree, diluted the intensity of the socialization experience for nursing. Off-campus living arrangements, a cohort of students who depend on full-time or part-time employments or who have family obligations, courses of study that may be protracted over many years, and so on, all reduce the strength of the primary socialization into the profession. What is the result of an incomplete or weak primary socialization into nursing when moving on to the next role transition to advanced practice (Chen, Chen, Tsai, & Lo, 2007)? This remains a serious question yet to be answered. Further, even if the primary socialization is solid, what does incomplete anticipatory socialization as an APN mean for role acquisition? This

BOX 3-4

Role-Enhancing Experiences Planned During Your Education (Applicable to Either Entry-Level or Graduate Education)

A synthesis semester at the end of the educational program that incorporates, as far as legally possible, all the ingredients of full-time employment

Work-study programs that alternate semesters with work placements in your anticipated field

A curriculum that progresses toward more independence and personal accountability, with students and faculty moving to a collegial relationship as opposed to superiors and subordinates

Service-education partnerships, with faculty teaching students as they practice with their own patients

Opportunity for students to work with faculty on their personal research or in their practice

Summer externships and new graduate internships or residencies

Patient clinical areas with a primary commitment to the clinical learning needs of students (the designated teaching unit)

Participation in activities suited to advanced practice nurses (e.g., conferences, meetings, and peer review sessions)

Preceptor or "buddy" system involving agency staff

An experience with interdisciplinary (or at the least multidisciplinary) education (Joel, 2003)

could create a situation of "marginal man," in which a person is a member of one or more cultures but belongs to none. It also presents a strong case for externships and residency programs through which a concentrated exposure to the role is guaranteed (Santucci, 2004; Starr, 2006). Certification also promises to help role acquisition and role progression with its expectation of additional education and investment in practice.

STRESS AND STRAIN

Stress and strain are natural companions of advanced practice, given the chaotic health-care environment and the fact that these roles are evolving and growing in prominence. Hardy and Hardy (1988b) tell us that role stress is primarily located in the social structure, external to the individual, and owing to incompatible normative expectations. It may or may not generate role strain, the feeling of frustration and anxiety internal to the individual.

Antecedents of Stress and Strain

The situations that create stress and strain for the APN are abundant. They are apparent in the educational preparation in which we may overlook opportunities for anticipatory socialization and in a rapidly restructuring health-care delivery system that demands continuous minor or major modification in roles. Specialization and advances in technology make roles that have become well established over time obsolete and require the role occupants to face a new cycle of ambiguity and transition (Creakbaum, 2011). Beyond this, there is also the growing emphasis on cost efficiency, consumerism, and the demedicalization of health care. None of these trends are surprising to the reader, but the effect they have on role is often unexpected and unintended. The traditional hierarchy of the system is radically changed, and the primary care provider is as likely an APN or physician's assistant as a physician. Consumer is "king," and health-care organizations are competing to corner their market share of clients. Consumer satisfaction is a major outcome measure against which everyone is measured. In fact, consumers often enter the system with as much information about their condition as the professional who attends them. In the midst of this evolving system, we see the slow but decisive movement toward complementary therapies that have not been part of our nursing repertoire in the past, but that are demanded by the public.

To further complicate the situation, reality finds most nurses as employees in health-care systems. One should never lose sight of the fact that systems (whether large or small, simple or complex) exist to secure their goals and preserve their values. They accomplish this by responding to changing conditions, achieving solidarity among their parts, using a division of labor to accomplish work, controlling the environment, maintaining order, and using resources efficiently. Efficiency has caused a move to accomplish many things through "adhocracy"—systems established for a limited goal and then disbanded. Subcontracting in addition to internal departments allows greater flexibility to adjust to change. In like manner, the nursing role has been forced to readjust or jeopardize organizational stability (Ball, 2011), so resocialization becomes a continuing process, and stress and strain a constant by-product of this process.

Classifying Role Stress

After an exhaustive analysis of research on role stress as it existed in 1988, Hardy and Hardy developed the classification system presented in **Box 3-5** that was subsequently expanded by the work of Schumacher and Meleis (1994).

BOX 3-5
Classification of Role Stress

Role ambiguity—There is vagueness, lack of clarity of the role expectations.

Role conflict—Role expectations are incompatible.

Role incongruity—There is a poor fit between the persons' abilities and their expectations or the expectations of the systems with which they interface.

Role overload—There is too much expected in the time available.

Role underload—Role expectations are minimal and underuse the abilities of role occupant.

Role overqualification—Role occupant's motivation, skills, and knowledge far exceed those required.

Role underqualification (role incompetence)—Role occupant lacks the necessary resources (Hardy & Hardy, 1988b).

Role transition—Person moves to a new role.

Role supplementation—There is anticipatory socialization (Schumacher & Meleis, 1994).

Stress and strain are predictable in situations that include ambiguity, ambivalence, incongruity, conflict, and underload and overload, and in situations in which the role occupants see themselves as underqualified or overqualified or are moving into a new role or engaged in anticipatory socialization. An example of ambiguity is the new APN who accepts a position without an adequate job description in a setting where there has been little experience with advanced practice, and so there are no seasoned peers to provide direction or support. An example of incongruity is the nurse who has been prepared for primary care practice exclusively and accepts a position that requires extensive coaching and teaching of nursing staff in a specialty area. Role conflict may result when the staff nurse feels an obligation to provide quality care but then finds it impossible to achieve satisfactory outcomes within the limits of a predetermined length of stay or in a situation in which the nurse believes that his or her clinical judgment is superior to the client's own choices, but the client refuses to comply. Overload and underload often require a more objective opinion, and the self-assurance to revisit goals and objectives to make them more realistic. Being overqualified or underqualified moves into areas of competence. Some individuals may consider themselves overqualified because they never strain to see or are untrained to see the complexities of a situation. The same circumstances may give rise to feelings of underload. Peer discussion of such clinical situations is helpful to verify your opinion of yourself. Feelings of being underqualified must be talked through and validated, or they result in living the life of an "impostor" (Arena & Page, 1992).

The stress and strain that come with most of the service occupations are labeled *codependency* or *burnout* in the literature. These two terms are related but different. In codependency, a person controls a situation through the assurance that he or she is needed and works to keep things that way, whereas in burnout there is difficulty determining who owns a problem. The result is anger stemming from the moral imperative to make a difference, yet the inability to succeed. The natural impulse of nurses to feel for their patients and occasionally bring home their frustrations is played out with exaggeration and eventually rejected. With time, where once they felt too much, they now feel too little in defense of their ego. The result is poor judgment, insensitivity, and intolerance (Joel, 1994). This is the end result of burnout. The codependent personality is at particularly high risk for burnout, which eventually results in negativism and the severe loss of self-esteem as one's clinical competence is questioned.

Responding to Role Strain

Kramer (1974), in an extensive longitudinal study that is still relevant after almost 40 years, identified the problems of new graduates in establishing their roles in the midst of bureaucratic-professional conflict and has termed it *reality shock.* Kramer speaks of "the specific shock-like reactions of new workers when they find themselves in a work situation for which they have spent several years preparing and for which they thought they were going to be prepared, and then suddenly find that they are not" (p. vi). When the new nurse, who has been *in* the work setting but not *of* it, embarks on a first professional work experience, there is not an easy adaptation of previously learned values, attitudes, and behaviors, but the necessity of an entirely new socialization to practice and simultaneous resolution of conflict with the bureaucracy. This process of resocialization from student to graduate can be easily applied to the APN. Kramer (1974, pp. 155–162) describes the steps as follows:

> *Skills and routine mastery: The expectations are those of the employment setting. A major value is competent, efficient delivery of procedures and techniques to clients. New graduates immediately concentrate on skill and routine mastery.*
>
> *Social integration: [Social integration is] getting along with the group; being taught by them how to work and behave; the "backstage" reality behaviors. If individuals stay at stage one, they may not be perceived as competent peers; if they try to incorporate some of the professional concepts brought over from the educational setting and adhere to those values, the group may be alienated.*
>
> *Moral outrage: With the incongruence identified and labeled, new graduates feel angry and betrayed by both their teachers and employers. They weren't told how it would be and they aren't allowed to practice as they were taught.*
>
> *Conflict resolution: The graduates may and do change their behavior, but maintain their values, or change both values and behaviors to match the work setting; or change neither values nor behavior; or work out a relationship that allows them to keep their values, but begin to integrate them into the new setting.*

The individuals who make the first choice have selected what is called *behavioral capitulation.* They may be the group with potential for making change, but they simply slide into the bureaucratic mold, or more likely, they withdraw from nursing practice altogether. Those who choose bureaucracy *(value capitulation)* may either become "rutters" (staying in a rut), with an "it's a job" attitude, or they may eventually reject the values of both themselves and the system. Others become organization men and women, who move rapidly into the administrative ranks and totally absorb the bureaucratic values. Those who will change neither values nor behavior, what might be called "going it alone," either seek to practice where professional values are accepted or try the "academic lateral arabesque" (also used by the first group), going on to advanced education with the hope of new horizons or escape. The most desirable choice, says Kramer (1974, p. 162), is biculturalism:

> *In this approach the nurse has learned that she possesses a value orientation that is perhaps different from the dominant one in the work organization, but that she has the responsibility to listen to and seek out the ideas of others as resource material in effecting a viable integration of both value systems. She has learned that she is not just a target of influence and pressure from others, but that she is in a reciprocal relationship with others and has the right and responsibility to attempt to influence them and to direct their influence attempts. . . . she has learned a basic posture of interdependence with respect to the conflicting value systems.*

Even though complicated by the bureaucratic-professional conflict, our original paradigm for socialization is visible in biculturalism.

New graduates do indeed go though variations of this experience, including role-taking, role-making, and bargaining. That there was little change in the adjustment process for decades can be seen by reviewing journals in the interim and by the nomadic workplace patterns of nurses, which must reflect deep-seated job dissatisfaction. Turnover may be a response to boredom, lack of involvement, and apathy, and may trace its origin to incomplete or ineffective socialization, or more correctly, ignorance of the socialization process. Hardy and Hardy (1988a) propose that strain may be handled by redefining the role or its expectations, by bargaining among role partners to reestablish priorities, or by decreasing or increasing the degree of interaction.

Managing Role Strain

There is no one prescription for coming to terms with an unmanageable personal or professional life. The problems are relative to the personality of the afflicted, and solutions must be individualized. The ultimate goal is to establish control and identity that is driven by internal strength, rather than being captive to the volatility of the environment. Given that your best investment is in self-care, consider the following (Joel, 2003, p. 7):

> *Learn to use distance therapeutically. Allow people to fail and learn from their own mistakes. Find a comfortable and private place to which you can retreat when you are stressed. If you cannot physically distance yourself, try meditation techniques.*
>
> *Decide who owns a problem. If you don't own it, you have no obligation to fix it, especially if it requires self-sacrifice.*
>
> *Examine the quality of the peer support you give and get, and correct the situation if needed. Sometimes support systems become habits as opposed to helps.*
>
> *Invest in upgrading yourself. Expose yourself to new experiences; learn new skills. Plan your self-care as seriously as you plan your patient care.*
>
> *Consciously schedule routine tasks and those requiring physical exertion as a break from complex and stressful activities.*
>
> *Learn to trust your instincts. Every problem does not have a rational and logical solution.*
>
> *Sometimes think in terms of what could be the worst consequence, then anything short of that is a bonus.*
>
> *Identify one person willing to serve as your objective sounding board. This may be one way to find out how you come across to people.*
>
> *Make contact with your feelings about situations. Feelings are neither good nor bad; they just are.*
>
> *Create options for yourself. Identify those circumstances that you need to personally control, those that are just as well controlled for you, and those that you choose to wait out.*

CONCLUSION

Socialization into role is a major responsibility of the nursing profession, whether at the point of immersion into the student role and anticipatory socialization to the profession or later with transition to registered nurse and for some on to advanced practice. Socialization requires personalizing a role to your preferences while complying with norms established by the government, the profession, the public, and the institution that employs you. These are your normative, comparative, and audience groups, your major referents; there may be others. The norms held by these groups may be broadly or narrowly interpreted and are revealed through the process of role-taking or empathic communication. There is an opportunity to modify these expectations once you are sensitive to the degree of flexibility allowed by each referent system. This process involves skill in reading our role partners and the environment and reciprocally working to make the role to our liking. This skill can be learned.

Stress and strain are natural companions to nurses, given the environment in which we work, and the work we do. Role stress is located in the social structure, and role strain in the person. Not all stressful circumstances produce strain; this depends on the individual and his or her ability to cope, problem solve, and search for meaning in difficult situations. Success in dealing with stress and strain may be related to complete and effective socialization. This observation reinforces the obligation to both provide socialization experiences and to equip nurses with the resources for self-care.

REFERENCES

Arena, D. M., & Page, N. E. (1992). The impostor phenomena in the clinical nurse specialist role. *Image: The Journal of Nursing Scholarship, 24*(2), 121–125.

Ball, E. (2011). A social purpose model for nursing. *Nursing Forum, 46*(3), 152–156.

Benner, P. E. (1984). *From novice to expert: Excellence and power in clinical nursing practice.* Menlo Park, CA: Addison-Wesley.

Brykczynski, K. A. (2000). Role development of the advanced practice nurse. In A. B. Hamric, J. A. Spross, & C. M. Hanson (Eds.), *Advanced nursing practice* (2nd ed., pp. 107–134). Philadelphia: WB Saunders.

Chen, Y. M., Chen, S. H., Tsai, C. Y., & Lo, L. Y. (2007). Role stress and job satisfaction for nurse specialists. *Journal of Advanced Nursing, 59*(5), 497–509.

Creakbaum, E. L. (2011). Creating and implementing a nursing role for RN retention. *Journal for Nurses in Staff Development, 27*(1), 25–28.

Dreyfus, H. I., & Dreyfus, S. E. (1977). *Uses and abuses of multi-attribute and multi-aspect model of decision-making.* Unpublished manuscript. Department of Industrial Engineering and Operations Research. Berkeley: University of California.

Hardy, M. E., & Hardy, W. L. (1988a). Managing role strain. In M. E. Hardy & M. E. Conway (Eds.), *Role theory* (2nd ed., pp. 241–255). Norwalk, CT: Appleton & Lange.

Hardy, M. E., & Hardy, W. L. (1988b). Role stress and role strain. In M. E. Hardy & M. E. Conway (Eds.), *Role theory* (2nd ed., pp. 159–239). Norwalk, CT: Appleton & Lange.

Joel, L. A. (1994). Maybe a pot watcher but never an ostrich. *American Journal of Nursing, 94*(46), 7.

Joel, L. A. (2003). *Kelly's dimensions of professional nursing* (9th ed.). New York: McGraw-Hill.

Katz, D. (1960). The functional approach to the study of attitudes. *Public Opinion Quarterly, 24,* 163–204.

Kramer, M. (1974). *Reality shock.* St. Louis: Mosby.

Lum, J. L. J. (1988). Reference groups and professional socialization. In M. E. Hardy & M. E. Conway (Eds.), *Role theory* (2nd ed., pp. 257–272). Norwalk, CT: Appleton & Lange.

Roberts, S. J., Tabloski, P., & Bova, C. (1997). Epigenesis of the nurse practitioner role revisited. *Journal of Nursing Education, 36*(2), 67–73.

Santucci, J. (2004). Facilitating the transition into nursing practice. *Journal for Nurses in Staff Development, 20*(6), 274–286.

Schumacher, K. L., & Meleis, A. I. (1994). Transitions: A central concept in nursing. *Image: The Journal of Nursing Scholarship, 26*(2), 119–127.

Scott, W. R. (1970). *Social processes and social structure: An introduction to sociology.* New York: Holt, Rinehart & Winston.

Starr, K. (2006). Becoming a registered nurse: the nurse extern experience. *Journal of Continuing Education in Nursing, 37*(2), 86–92.

4

Education for Advanced Practice

The "Big Tent" for Educating Advanced Practice Nurses: Issues Surrounding MSN, DNP, and PhD Preparation

H. Michael Dreher
Al Rundio

BACKGROUND: MASTER'S PREPARATION FOR APRNS CONTINUES

The advanced practice nursing landscape continues to evolve. Some might even say that it is in upheaval. In 2011, the *New York Times* featured the article "When the Nurse Wants to Be Called 'Doctor'" (Harris, 2011) where a "doctor," who was wearing a white lab coat with a stethoscope in one pocket, introduced herself to a patient by saying, "Hi. I'm Dr. Patti McCarver, and I'm your nurse" (p. 1). A few years earlier, the *Wall Street Journal* featured an article called "Making Room for 'Dr. Nurse'" (Landro, 2008), and in 2005 *U.S. News & World Report* featured a cover reading "Who needs doctors? Your future physician might not even be an M.D.—and you might be better off" (Levine & Marek, 2005). The explosive growth in doctor of nursing practice (DNP) programs since 2005, preparing a new generation of advanced practice nurses, means there is now an emerging critical mass of DNP graduates who are challenging assumptions about who should be allowed to use the title "doctor" in health-care environments. And while not the purpose of this chapter, this issue of using the title "doctor" by doctoral advanced practice nurses, a new description of the DNP-prepared advanced practice nurse proposed by Dreher and Montgomery (2009), is thoroughly discussed with both pro and con arguments by Oldfield (a nurse practitioner), Montgomery (a physician), and Miller (an attorney) (Miller, 2011; Montgomery, 2011; Oldfield, 2011). But despite the enormous energy and attention being given to DNP-educated advanced practice nurses, the master's degree remains the most common preparation for nurse practitioners (NPs), certified nurse-midwives (CNMs), certified registered nurse anesthetists (CRNAs), and clinical nurse specialists (CNSs). The reality is that it has not been long that a master's degree is required for the advanced practice registered nurse (APRN). O'Sullivan, past president of the National Organization of Nurse Practitioner Faculty (NONPF), at the 2008 national convention reminded the audience that it has taken 40 years to move from the origins of the nurse practitioner certificate to the requirement of the master's degree for entry into advanced practice. And now comes the arrival of a new practice doctorate, giving prospective advanced practice nurses another degree option.

The rise of the DNP degree as an alternative to the MSN has also created confusion about whether current MSN-prepared APRNs will be required to obtain their DNP degrees by 2015 (which the American Association of Colleges of Nursing stated was a goal in 2004a) or whether they will be grandfathered. The issue of "grandfathering" has been of interest to APRNs for many years. In 1965, the certificate became the first advanced educational credential of the first generation of pediatric nurse practitioners (the first nurse practitioner role). There were intense concerns over grandfathering NPs with certificates when MSN degree preparation became the standard requirement (Ford, 1975). At present, there is no grandfathering clause remaining in any state that would allow any APRN (nurse-midwife, nurse anesthetist, clinical nurse specialist, or nurse practitioner) to *enter practice* without an advanced degree. However, since advanced practice nursing is regulated by state statute, older nurses with an advanced practice certificate have often been able to continue to practice so long as their status is recognized by the state and, in some situations, specialty-certifying bodies. There are 50 different nurse practice acts and state laws under which the advanced practice roles are regulated. For this reason, in 2008 the National Council of State Boards of Nursing (NCSBN) introduced the *Consensus Model for APRN Regulation: Licensure, Accreditation, Certification and Education,* designed to provide some common structural guidance for the preparation and practice of advanced practice nurses. However, it is widely but wrongly assumed that the Consensus Model document addresses DNP preparation. It does not.

The American Midwifery Certification Board (AMCB) and the American College of Nurse-Midwives (ACNM) recently eliminated all post-baccalaureate certificate options in midwifery, and the ACNM Board of Directors in July 2009 mandated that a graduate degree is required for entry into practice starting in 2010 (ACNM, 2009). Moreover, in 2009 the AMCB also moved (despite significant opposition by practicing midwives) to require recertification for CNMs certified before 1996 to ensure the highest quality of continuing nurse-midwifery care. In 1990, the Council on Accreditation of Nurse Anesthesia Educational Programs (2003, 2004) moved to require the master's degree for entry into nurse anesthesia practice. However, the master's degree is not mandated to be in nursing, as many nurse anesthesia programs do not reside in colleges or schools of nursing. The Council included a grandfather clause that allowed current CRNAs to continue to practice without obtaining a master's degree (Kinslow, 2005). In September 2007 the American Association of Nurse Anesthetists (AANA) announced support for doctorate entry into nurse anesthesia practice by 2025 (AANA, 2007). However, the requirement is for "any doctorate" that will prepare a CRNA, and the DNP degree was not specifically endorsed. For the clinical nurse specialist, in states where this status is recognized, the master's degree in nursing is required. Further, the National Association of Clinical Nurse Specialists (NACNS) in May 2011 proposed that the education of clinical nurse specialists continue to be at the master's, practice doctorate, or post–master's degree certificate level (NACNS, 2011).

Finally, the educational preparation of nurse practitioners was the driving force behind the October 2004 vote by the American Association of Colleges of Nursing (AACN, 2004a) membership (nursing deans only) to support the doctor of nursing practice degree (DNP) as the entry-level educational credential for advanced practice by 2015. The actual vote was 162 for, 101 opposed, and 13 abstentions. However, despite this vote, none of the major APRN organizations ever endorsed the 2015 goal. As of publication, no APRN organization has moved to DNP entry level only for APRN practice at some future date, aside from the AANA, which is endorsing doctoral degree entry level (not specifically the DNP) to practice by 2025. In 2010, the American Academy of Nurse Practitioners reaffirmed this (American Academy of Nurse Practitioners, 2010, p. 1).

> *It is clear that the course work currently required in NP master's programs is equivalent to that of other clinical doctoral programs. It is important however, that the transition to clinical doctoral preparation for NPs continue to be conducted so that master's prepared NPs will not be disenfranchised in any way.*

THE RISE OF THE DOCTOR OF NURSING PRACTICE AS AN ALTERNATIVE

Much of the controversy over whether the DNP degree is a good idea has subsided, but not all. From the previously cited 2011 *New York Times* article, the Dean of the University of Pennsylvania School of Nursing, Afaf Meleis (and she is not alone), stated "If it ain't broke [MSN preparation], why fix it?" The more contemporary argument has changed to whether the DNP degree ought to be ultimately required for entry into advanced practice and whether phasing out the MSN is in the best interest of the nursing discipline or not (Cronenwett et al., 2011). This important discussion will occur later in this chapter.

Impressively, the development of new DNP programs continues to surge. According to the AACN's *2011 Annual Report: Shaping the Future of Nursing Education* (AACN, 2011a), some 72% of schools with APRN programs (388 schools) are either offering (120) or planning (161) a DNP program. That leaves 38% of schools that are not doing either. Moreover, 33 new DNP programs have opened since that report, bringing the total to 153 programs.

As of 2008, there were over 270,000 U.S. advanced practice nurses—158, 348 NPs; 59,242 CNSs; 34,821 nurse anesthetists; and 18,492 nurse-midwives, with most overwhelmingly prepared with the minimum of a master's degree (American Nurses Association, 2011). However, the goal to migrate these 270,000 APNs to the doctorate (excluding those who already have the degree) is an ambitious undertaking. Some question whether this is a realistic goal. In reality, the movement to require the entry-level doctorate for advanced nursing practice will be a complex process as the AACN has no legal authority to enforce this on the various state nursing regulatory bodies nor on the respective advanced practice specialty organizations. Further, the two chief accrediting bodies in nursing, the Commission on Collegiate Nursing Education (CCNE) and the National League for Nursing Accrediting Commission (NLNAC), have taken different positions on the approval of doctor of nursing practice programs. The CCNE has elected to accredit only practice doctorate programs with the initials "DNP," whereas the NLNAC has stated: "As advanced practice nursing moves in new directions, NLNAC will accredit the nursing practice doctorates, whatever their title. We believe that the interests of nursing and health care are best served by focusing on competencies and curriculum content, rather than degree title, and learning outcomes rather than specific curriculum mandates" (2005, p. 1).

Traditionally, advanced practice nurses who pursued the doctorate pursued the PhD, although historically APNs also pursue the DNSc, DNS, DSN, EdD, or even sometimes doctorates in another field. Most of these various nursing doctoral degrees have converted to the PhD (Dreher, Fasolka, & Clark, 2008), leaving the PhD in Nursing or Nursing Science as the gold standard research doctoral degree in nursing. And so APNs enter a new conundrum with the emergence and surge of the doctor of nursing practice degree. The critical question is whether the DNP will become fully accepted by society and the health-care market, and whether it can overcome some of the recurring perceptions of the degree as "an easy doctorate," or "less rigorous than the PhD," or, as Beckstead (2010) wonders, does the "DNP = PhD-*light*?" Unlike the nursing doctorate (ND) degree model, which failed as an idea and lasted some 25 years but only had four schools ever adopt it, the DNP degree looks as though it has more staying power. Fink (2006) indicates that the professional (or practice) doctorate "should not be a watered down version of the PhD but offer a valid alternative in doctoral education" (p. 38). Dreher and Smith Glasgow (2011) write that at the First International Conference on Professional Doctorates (London, 2009) one of the primary themes at the conference was that a professional/practice doctorate *is* a doctorate like any other. Moreover, they state that "the degree should not be marginalized or even have less rigor than a PhD. Its aims, however, should be very different from a PhD" (p. 403).

The central focus of this chapter is whether the DNP can coexist with other degree options for advanced nursing practice, particularly the MSN and post–master's degree certificate (the "big tent" for advanced practice preparation), or whether the trajectory of the DNP should be aimed at eliminating the MSN. Moreover, where do PhD degree–prepared APNs fit into this picture? If all new APRNs were to obtain the DNP instead of the MSN (as originally envisioned by the AACN), there would be no PhD-prepared APRNs and no one adequately prepared to conduct nursing research.

Some propose the idea of dual DNP/PhD preparation, and such programs now exist at Barnes/Jewish College of Nursing, University of Tennessee Health Sciences Center, and Case Western Reserve University. And with few exceptions, most remain very skeptical of BSN-to-PhD programs except for the relatively experienced BSN-prepared RN. As nursing is a practice discipline, it is futile to graduate doctoral-prepared graduates who have had limited exposure to clinical practice. Highly educated but inexperienced clinicians are not who the nursing profession needs to help alleviate the nursing faculty shortage. In considering admission to any of these doctoral programs, when should we encourage the bachelor's-prepared RNs to matriculate? After two years of practice? Three years? More than three? And should they undertake full-time study? If that happens, there will be few takers. Programs that accommodate those who need to work full-time to support themselves need to be created, although full-time PhD study is preferred, so nurse scientists can be productive earlier in their careers. It is unlikely there will ever be a critical mass of DNP/PhD graduates, and suggesting that nurses obtain *two* doctorates in nursing is illogical (or maybe too idealistic) when there is such an enormous shortage of nurses with *one* doctorate.

There are serious implications for our profession with the rise of the DNP. Will the PhD diminish in importance? Will this new nonresearch, practice doctorate negatively affect the expansion of nursing knowledge and erode the major progress nursing has made as a scientific discipline over the past three decades (Dracup, Cronenwett, Meleis, & Benner, 2005; Dreher & Smith Glasgow, 2011)? If, in nursing's future, advanced practice nurses are required to pursue the DNP, will any of them ever accede to the PhD? And as mentioned previously, if few APNs obtain the PhD, who will be conducting research and contributing to the evidence base of advanced practice nursing? These are important issues, and many contemporary critics of the DNP believe the future of nursing as a science is at stake and that the sudden rise of the DNP has untold implications for our profession as it takes hold and proliferates (Beckstead, 2010; Florczak, 2010; Meleis & Dracup, 2005). Besides advocating for a "big tent" for advanced practice preparation, this chapter examines the tension between the PhD and the new DNP degree, and poses the question of whether they can coexist and flourish. And should these two degrees be the profession's only doctoral degree alternatives?

Our history began in 1932 with the EdD in Nursing Education at Teacher's College, and along the way our educational tradition has included several other doctoral degrees, sometimes for good reasons and at other times probably not (Oldfield, 2011). One basic question being considered is whether advanced practice nursing should abandon the MSN and move to the doctorate. We subscribe to the viewpoint that indeed "this train has left the station." There are just too many internal and external forces driving the new DNP degree (some good and some bad) to inhibit its current progression. But just because there is this sudden surge of growth does not guarantee that this degree is ultimately a good idea for advanced practice nursing. Further, the urgency to abandon the MSN has abated considerably, both because of the economic pressures of the current great recession that began after the 2004AACN vote for the DNP (AACN, 2004a) and because not even the recent 2010 Institute of Medicine's *The Future of Nursing: Leading Change, Advancing Health* report endorsed the DNP degree, saying more outcome data were necessary first. Will the DNP take hold in the marketplace and ultimately assuage concerns over health-care cost and quality?

THE PHD IN NURSING: THE FUTURE IS UNCERTAIN

Data from 1996–2010 indicate that enrollment in research-focused doctoral programs (largely PhD, but also DNS, DSN, DNSc, and EdD) remains largely in flux. For 1996–2006 (largely the period before the surge of DNP programs), **Figure 4-1** indicates that despite a significant increase in new PhD programs over that decade (59%), there was a trend toward flat enrollment (12%) and graduation numbers remained erratic (19%). However, in the following four years (2006–2010) there was a new trend that is difficult to interpret: PhD programs increased by 20% and enrollment by a modest 17.4%, but DNP programs increased in number by 665% and enrollment by 716% (AACN, 2005; AACN, 2011a). There is concern that the PhD may be overwhelmed by the DNP, and experience a shifting allocation of research-focused resources. Moreover, the Robert Wood Johnson Foundation (2007) indicates that a large percentage of senior nursing faculty will retire by 2012, and nearly half the current nursing faculty is likely to retire by 2016. Dreher and Smith Glasgow (2011) point out that many senior faculty members, as well as funded researchers are PhD-prepared and, express concerns that the pipeline for nurse scientists may be threatened, a concern shared by Potempa, Redman, and Anderson (2008). This trend also has implications for the future of advanced practice research, which may be threatened without a cadre of APRN nurse scientists who are adept clinical researchers and best poised to ask the right questions.

The AACN (2006) does not believe that DNP graduates are prepared for the full scope of the faculty role without additional education and supervision (McKenna, 2005; Wittmann-Price, Waite, &

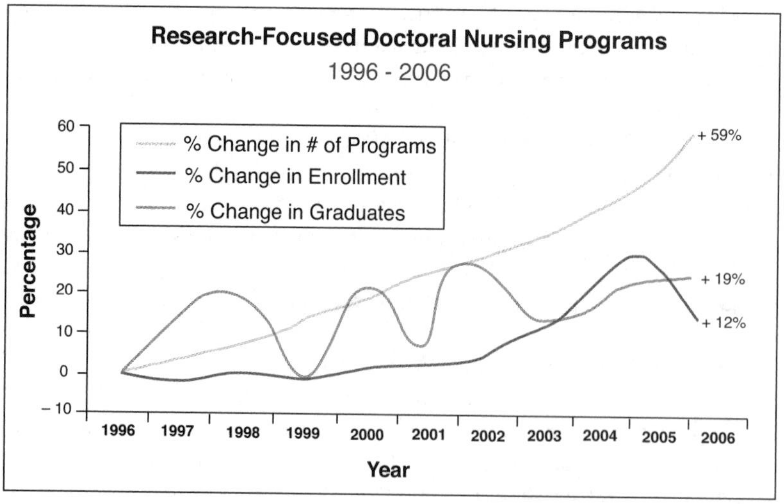

FIGURE 4-1 Research-focused doctoral nursing programs. *(Data from AACN 1996–2006. Analyzed by H. M. Dreher.)*

Woda, 2011). According to testimony by Valiga (2004), speaking for the National League for Nursing (NLN) at a congressional briefing on the nursing faculty shortage, it takes a registered nurse an average 8.3 years to complete the doctorate versus 6.8 years for other fields. When the endpoints are from the beginning of master's study to the awarding of the doctorate, a registered nurse takes an astounding 15.9 years versus 8.5 years for other disciplines. It is not surprising that a massive cadre of nurses are choosing to enter shorter DNP programs as opposed to taking much longer to complete a PhD program.

Although there has been a proliferation of new PhD in Nursing programs in the last 15 years, there has been limited support to properly socialize and mentor students in the nurse scientist role, leaving many unprepared for the rigors of conducting postdissertation research (Dreher & Smith Glasgow, 2011; Potempa et al., 2008). This is a criticism widely proffered by the University of Washington's project on *Re-envisioning the PhD* (Nyquist & Wilff, 2000). Similar commentary can be found in "How Business Schools Lost Their Way" from the *Harvard Business Review* (Bennis & O'Toole, 2005). The parallels between business education and nursing are striking. For almost a decade, professional business schools have come under intense criticism for failing to impart useful skills, instill norms for ethical business behavior, and even lead graduates to good corporate jobs. And the role of those graduates who occupied top corporate jobs during the Wall Street debacle and great recession of 2007–2009 is indicative of problems in graduate business education, particularly ethics. Part of the problem is that many graduate business schools measure their success by the rigor of scientific research of their faculty and hire and promote research-oriented professors who haven't spent much time working in industry. Many business school faculties seem more comfortable teaching methodology than competently providing experiential discourse on the messy, multidisciplinary issues that are at the very core of contemporary business management. To regain relevancy, Bennis and O'Toole (2005) say business schools must *rediscover the practice of business* and find a way to do both: educate the practitioner and create knowledge through research. Doesn't this argument sound very similar to the current discourse in the nursing discipline?

Like business, nursing finds itself trying to replicate the academic and scientific traditions of fields such as chemistry and psychology. Consequently, PhD nursing education is often divorced from contemporary nursing practice, a critique discussed at length in the chapter "Nursing as a Practice Discipline" (Dreher, 2011a) in *Philosophy of Science for Nursing Practice: Concepts and Application* (Dahnke & Dreher, 2011). This is particularly common when PhD faculty have often left clinical nursing practice perhaps decades earlier. The mission to educate the doctoral-prepared practitioner/scholar seems to have been lost or at least severely mismanaged in the rush to create the proper nurse scientist. Or perhaps that was never the early vision of doctoral nursing education (to prepare a practitioner/scholar), but instead to educate the nurse more in the mold of a typical bench scientist. This is unfortunate, since historically nursing probably shares more in common with another practice discipline, social work, than with, say, developmental biology—yet our PhD programs seem to operate more like we are preparing a developmental biologist (postdoc and all) rather than a scientist working in a practice and professionally oriented discipline. This is where both nursing and business share common challenges in graduate education. Thus, it should not be surprising that so many practicing APNs in particular are not that attracted to their own socially constructed vision of what a PhD-prepared nurse is and does. They do not want to forgo employment to attend full-time PhD study and thereby weaken their clinical skills. Consequently, the other downside to part-time PhD study is the excessive length it takes to complete the degree.

Nursing science that contributes critical, high-impact translational health research can distinguish the profession of nursing, raise our credibility, better position our discipline within the community of science, and move the science from "bench to bedside." However, nursing research at this point remains insufficiently visible and insufficiently supported. In 2005 Aaronson pointed out that the National Institute of Nursing Research (NINR) remained the lowest-funded institute at the National Institutes of Health (NIH) by far, with only $139 million requested for the fiscal year (FY) 2006 president's budget and remained just slightly more funded than the National Center for Complementary and Alternative Medicine (NIH, 2005). By 2010 the NINR's budget grew to only $146 million, representing only 0.47% of NIH's budget and only a 5% increase from the FY 2006 budget (AACN, 2010). In FY 2011, the NINR's funding level was $144.4 million, and the FY 2012 consolidated bill from the Senate and House allocates $144.77 million, again reflecting a poor economic environment (AACN, 2012). With such a low level of funding, unless more nurse scientists extend the boundaries of their research questions and submit successful proposals to the other NIH institutes (certainly in addition to the NINR), our discipline and science will suffer. Given the move by government to fund more interdisciplinary translational research, the need for well-trained nurse scientists is more apparent than ever (National Academy of Sciences, 2005). Further, nursing scientists and researchers should not confine their research efforts to those funded solely by the NIH and other governmental agencies, but use the private sector as well. Nursing needs more properly mentored PhD-prepared researchers who can move into faculty positions in research-intensive universities and quickly embark on research careers. However, given the nature of the discipline, it is clear that nurses who do not necessarily want full-time research careers need training to contribute to knowledge generation in the context of practice.

THE RAPID EMERGENCE OF THE DOCTOR OF NURSING PRACTICE DEGREE

The doctor of nursing practice (DNP or DrNP) is a still a relatively new degree (remember that the first EdD in Nursing Education was created in 1932 and the first PhD in 1934 at New York University). It was first offered by the College of Nursing at the University of Kentucky in 2001 with their first nine students graduating in 2005. It is confusing that some schools today claim to have had "practice doctorate graduates" in the 1980s or 1990s. This is a historical fallacy. These degree programs were either ND or DNSc programs that converted to the DNP in 2005 or later and then had their university board of trustees approve the conversion of the previously awarded degree to the new DNP. **Table 4-1** indicates the historical progression of the first doctor of nursing practice programs starting in 2001.

Where did this degree suddenly come from? It is probably historically accurate to describe the first doctor of nursing science (DNS) and doctor of science in nursing (DSN) programs as degrees originally designed to be *clinical* (or practice) *doctorates*. The original intent was that they would be different from the two research degrees in the profession, the PhD and the DNSc (also a doctor of nursing science degree, but a research doctorate unlike the DNS and DSN) (Apold, 2008). Other authors have previously identified that some of the early DNSc programs were not permitted to be founded as PhD programs, often because of prejudice by many university faculty in other disciplines who did not fully recognize nursing as a science, and thus were ineligible to award the PhD. Only recently have all the remaining DNSc degrees in the country (Yale, Columbia, and Widener) completed conversion to the PhD (Dreher, Fasolka, & Clark, 2008). But retrospectively, although the DNS and DSN were originally designed as clinical doctorates and an alternative to the research-focused PhD or DNSc, they ultimately became *de facto* research degrees and analogous to the PhD. Thus the first attempt in nursing education to create a true clinical doctorate was not successful. A couple

TABLE 4-1

Inaugural Doctor of Nursing Practice Programs

School	Year Program Founded	DNP or DrNP	Major	Final Scholarly Work Product
University of Kentucky	2001	DNP	**Then:** post–master's degree clinical leadership/executive management **Now:** BSN-DNP public health, management, NP, and CNS options; post–master's degree clinical leadership/executive management	Research utilization project
Case Western Reserve University (OH)	2005	DNP (converted from ND)	**Then:** post–master's degree educational leadership and clinical leadership tracks **Now:** BSN-DNP post–master's degree practice or educational leadership	**Then:** scholarly project—DNP thesis or applied research project **Now:** scholarly project (thesis or a manuscript suitable for publication)
Columbia University (NY)	2005	DNP (was DrNP 2005–2008)	Post–master's degree clinical doctorate for certified APRNs	Portfolio
Drexel University (PA)	2005	DrNP	Clinical research–oriented doctor of nursing practice Four tracks: practitioner, educator, clinical scientist, & clinical executive	Clinical dissertation
Rush University (IL)	2005	DNP (converted from ND)	**Then:** post–master's degree leadership and the business of health care **Now:** BSN-DNP in adult-gerontology, family, neonatal, pediatric, or psychiatric–mental health NP, CNS, CRNA, or advanced public health nursing (APHN); post–master's degree in systems leadership and APHN	Capstone project

Continued

TABLE 4-1

Inaugural Doctor of Nursing Practice Programs–cont'd

School	Year Program Founded	DNP or DrNP	Major	Final Scholarly Work Product
Tri-College University Concordia College, Minnesota State University; North Dakota State University Note: NDSU left the consortium in 2007 and the consortium disbanded in 2008.	2005	DNP	Family nurse practitioner/ generic DNP completion for APNs	None
University of Colorado at Denver	2005	DNP (converted from ND)	**Then:** generic post–master's degree **Now:** BSN-DNP in adult CNS, ANP, FNP, family psych MHNP, health-care informatics, midwifery, PNP, WHNP; post–master's degree for certified APRNs	**Then:** DNP capstone project **Now:** DNP capstone clinical project
University of South Carolina	2005	DNP (converted from ND)	**Then:** multiple primary and non–primary care options BSN-DNP and post–master's degree options **Now:** BSN-DNP FNP and ACNP; post–master's degree clinical and organizational leadership	Research utilization project
University of Tennessee Health Science Center	2005	DNP (converted from DNSc)	**Then:** BSN-DNP primary care; acute critical care, forensic nursing, gerontology, nursing administration, psychiatric/family nurse practitioner, and public health nursing and post–master's degree **Now:** BSN-DNP and post–master's degree options for primary care; acute critical care, forensic nursing, gerontology, psychiatric/family nurse practitioner, public health nursing, and CRNA	Residency project

For a complete list of current programs, see http://www.aacn.nche.edu/dnp/program-schools.

of DNS programs still exist (e.g., LSU Health Sciences University/New Orleans and CUNY Graduate Center).

The origin of today's doctor of nursing practice degree model can be traced to Dean Mundinger of Columbia University School of Nursing. In 2000, Mundinger and her colleagues published a clinical trial in the *Journal of the American Medical Association* titled "Primary Care Outcomes in Patients Treated by Nurse Practitioners or Physicians: A Randomized Trial." It was this seminal work on the nurse practitioner model at Columbia that ultimately led to development of the clinical doctorate or DrNP degree at that institution. Columbia's DrNP was finally approved in 2005. But even the Columbia DrNP model went through an evolution during which the faculty first described the degree as a "DrNP in Primary Care," later simply the "first clinical doctorate" (instead of a "practice doctorate" as the DNP is commonly referred to), and then in 2008 the degree was changed to the DNP to satisfy CCNE accreditors. It should be noted that despite the University of Kentucky initiating their DNP in 2001, the degree prepared clinical executives with a focus on leadership and management. It did not prepare nurses for advanced nursing practice as APRNs. So this author and perhaps others still wonder why the AACN in 2004 voted to endorse the DNP degree awarded through the University of Kentucky, which was not designed for MSN-prepared APRNs, while rejecting the DrNP model at Columbia University, which was.

Dean Donnelly of the Drexel University College of Nursing and Health Professions (personal communication, June 11, 2008) recalls that the AACN sponsored a speaker at the annual meeting some years ago to present pharmacy's movement toward the doctorate (PharmD) for entry into practice. The PharmD is a nonresearch doctorate. According to Donnelly, the membership thought there was a desire by the AACN leadership to move in this direction, but at that time there were no concrete proposals to move advanced practice nursing to the entry-level doctorate. In 2002, a task force was formed by the AACN to explore the practice doctorate (AACN, 2006). The history of the PharmD model and how it is not an ideal comparison to the DNP has been explored by Upvall and Ptachcinski (2007). Even today, the AACN Web site still presents the DNP as a practice doctorate analogous to doctorates in medicine (MD), dentistry (DDS), pharmacy (PharmD), psychology (PsyD), physical therapy (DPT), and audiology (AudD) (AACN, 2011b).

The reality is that the DNP is similar in some ways to these degrees and very different in other ways. The MD and DDS are professional practice degrees (nonresearch) like the DNP, but they are required entry-level degrees to practice medicine or dentistry. Although the BSN is preferred by the AACN for entry into professional nursing practice, even today there are alternate degree paths to RN licensure. The DPT and AuD are *options* for entry into physical therapy and speech/audiology practice, respectively, but are not required by these disciplines to practice. Further, the AuD and in particular the PsyD (Peterson, 1976, 1982) are not analogous to the DNP. The DNP was originally conceived as a nonresearch degree by the AACN, stating in their 2006 *Essentials of Doctoral Education for Advanced Nursing Practice* that "practice doctorates, requiring a dissertation or other original research is contrary to the intent of the DNP" (p. 20). But some AuD programs require an original research project (Boston University, 2004; University of Washington, 2008) and practically all PsyD programs require a clinical dissertation (Murray, 2000; Widener, 2004; Wheaton, 2004). In the literature, these practice doctorates that include some form of original research or dissertation are termed *hybrid doctorates* as differentiated from the pure research degree (PhD) and nonresearch professional doctorate (PharmD, DPT, or DNP) (Dreher, Donnelly, & Naremore, 2005; Smith Glasgow & Dreher, 2010). This is an important distinction. The question is whether the DNP as an alternative to the PhD in Nursing will result in a decrease in the expansion of nursing knowledge. Or should the DNP student and graduate become the leader in the development of practice-based evidence, as Dreher (2011b) has proposed? On this point there must be more discussion in the nursing discipline as the continuing maturation of our science is at stake. It seems unegalitarian to say that the PhD nursing graduate will generate new nursing knowledge and the DNP nursing graduate will translate and disseminate it.

COMPELLING ARGUMENTS FOR AND AGAINST THE DOCTOR OF NURSING PRACTICE DEGREE

Despite the plethora of DNP programs, it is likely that many students who use this text will be in both MSN and DNP programs. And further, despite a national movement toward more doctoral-prepared APRNs (particularly NPs), this chapter began by indicating that the MSN remains an acceptable degree for the preparation for advanced nursing practice, and it has historical outstanding outcomes. So this section is therefore more designed to weigh whether an individual MSN graduate should pursue the DNP. There are compelling reasons for why the AACN pushed for an entry-level doctorate for nursing. Three Institute of Medicine (IOM) reports (1999, 2001, and 2003) called for reform in health professions education mainly because of rising health-care errors and patient safety issues, failure of the health disciplines to work collaboratively and deliver optimal health outcomes, and a recognition that the education of students in the health professions, from medicine to nursing to occupational therapy and more, varies too considerably from discipline to discipline. The central arguments for why the AACN advocated that entry into advanced practice nursing should require the doctorate instead of the master's degree are as follows: (1) master's in nursing degrees, especially those preparing the nurse practitioner, nurse anesthetist, or midwife, often required as many credit hours as some clinical doctorate programs in other disciplines; (2) other disciplines such as physical therapy (DPT) and pharmacy (PharmD) had begun offering a clinical doctorate, and nursing (as the largest health-care profession) should not be any different; and (3) contemporary knowledge is growing exponentially and the master's degree can no longer fully encompass the breadth of coursework necessary for advanced practice (Apold, 2008).

As compelling as these arguments are, they are not all based on data, and this was one central reason the latest IOM report on *The Future of Nursing* (2010) did not endorse the degree, although acknowledging its rapid rise. Although the statement about the total number of credits appears to be a salient one, no one would agree that simply the accumulation of credits should merit the attainment of a doctoral degree. Alternatively, perhaps master's degree nursing credits ought to be used more selectively, rather than reflexively moving to a doctoral degree. Second, the issue of whether nursing ought to require an entry-level doctorate for advanced practice, merely because other health professions have moved to do so, is also not necessarily a strong point (Dracup & Brown, 2005). Bloch (2007), in a paper delivered at the first annual conference on the doctor of nursing practice degree in Annapolis, Maryland, argued that the cost and length of new DNP programs will decrease the number of women's health nurse practitioners and thus harm access to care for vulnerable populations. Indeed, what is still missing from the debate on the DNP versus the MSN is a cost/benefit analysis. What is the value of this degree to the health-care system?

The strongest argument against the DNP as the only future option for entry into advanced nursing practice is the decades of strong outcome data supporting the excellence of advanced practice nursing, particularly in comparison to primary medical care (Horrocks, Anderson, & Salisbury, 2002; Mundinger et al., 2000). Nurse-midwives, nurse anesthetists, clinical nurse specialists, and nurse practitioners are widely recognized by the public and supported in the literature as providing high-quality care. Therefore, the argument that a doctorate instead of a master's is needed to provide high-quality care is fallacious. Lending to the confusion, a National Research Council report of the National Academy of Sciences titled *Advancing the Nation's Health Needs: NIH Research Training Programs* reads as follows (National Academy of Sciences, 2005, p. 74):

The need for doctorally prepared practitioners and clinical faculty would be met if nursing could develop a new nonresearch clinical doctorate, similar to the M.D. and Pharm.D in medicine and pharmacy, respectively. The concept of a nonresearch clinical doctorate in nursing is controversial, but some programs of this type exist.

No one should be mistaken that the DNP degree has gained wide acceptance by the academic nursing community, but it is likely that having a practice doctorate may give an applicant an edge in hiring in some markets. The nursing community is challenged to prove that the extra cost, time, and resources necessary to produce such a doctoral graduate will improve health, not just improve the status of the practitioner.

TENSION BETWEEN THE DNP AND PhD: NECESSARY GROWING PAINS?

It is this new tension over the sudden rise of the DNP at the potential expense of the PhD that serves as a primary concern. New doctoral programs in any discipline are not created without additional resources or the reallocation of resources from other academic programs. Although some universities that offer both the DNP and PhD report no decline in their PhD enrollment, the first author is aware of many nursing schools (even the top ones) where faculty report a decline in the number of applicants for the PhD and a decline in the quality of the applicants. Further, the new data indicating an increase in PhD enrollment do not necessarily translate into more graduates, particularly when the time to the PhD averages 8.3 years as previously noted (AACN, 2011b; Valiga, 2004). Indeed, the trend lines to replace the flux of retirements from the nursing profession are worrisome. Further, we have only to look at the decline of nursing scholarship with the near extinction of the master's thesis to imagine that when given a doctoral option requiring a dissertation versus *not requiring a dissertation,* it is likely many or possibly most graduate students will take the path of least resistance and avoid the research degree. This first author anticipates a real risk of decreased expansion of nursing knowledge with the DNP as the primary alternative to the PhD and that other options for knowledge development must be explored, without assuming only PhD graduates will conduct original research. One option is the hybrid DrNP degree, now only at Drexel University, where advanced practice nurses are prepared for the conduct of relevant, practical clinical research culminating in a clinical dissertation (Dreher, Donnelly, & Naremore, 2005; Dreher & Smith Glasgow, 2011).

Another option is to reengineer the DNP, particularly at research-intensive and research-oriented universities, by emphasizing the conduct of research that leads to evidence-based practice. We are seeing some schools move toward this. The University of Connecticut has changed its DNP curriculum to emphasize research methods, and its DNP project has changed to a clinical practice dissertation (Bellini & Cusson, 2011). Fairfield University and Sacred Heart University (both in Connecticut) also require a practice dissertation in their DNP programs. What is unique about the clinical or practice dissertations is that students are less restricted in their mode of scholarly inquiry. The research need not be "original," as is the PhD criterion. DNP/DrNP students have more freedom to generate applied knowledge and use less traditional PhD formats, including pilot studies, replication studies, secondary analyses, and quality improvement or studies of evidence-based practice. We highly suggest that DNP programs use the "practice dissertation" format, and the faculty can decide what formats (likely multiple ones) are acceptable. Undergraduate students complete "projects." Doctoral-level scholarship needs the appropriate description and titling of the end-of-degree work product.

In summary, it is risky for the profession to rely solely on nursing PhD graduates to conduct original research. That clearly is not in the discipline's best interest. Of course, O'Sullivan and colleagues (2005) rightly raise the argument that many PhD graduates never conduct research past their dissertation and perhaps these students may have been better served by a practice doctorate option. We have repeatedly posed the following question: If *every* prospective APRN in 2015 were to obtain a DNP, what would nursing knowledge look like in the future? Is the combined DNP/PhD really the best option at double the credits (most universities have a policy on the minimum number of credits required for any baccalaureate student who is skipping the master's degree and pursuing a doctorate, e.g., BSN-to-PhD or BSN-to-DNP), double the cost, and double the time? And what if the student attends this program part-time? This strategy just does not seem realistic to create a critical mass of APRN nurse scientists. It is regrettable that the DSN/DNS became *de facto* PhD degrees. An opportunity to create a real clinical doctorate for the profession was lost. It is also unfortunate that university politics and, sometimes, elitist prejudice against nursing by other scientific disciplines prevented the timely conversion of many of these programs to the PhD until recently. The University of Alabama at Birmingham (2005) is a good example of a DSN program that converted to the PhD in 1999. Most nursing academicians would agree with Fitzpatrick (2003) that the PhD is the proper doctoral degree to prepare the nurse scientist. Therefore, as these other degree models have served their purpose historically, it is proper that most of them have now converted to the PhD.

The critical question remains: Who will be left to expand nursing knowledge if DNP graduates do not have clinical research skills? PhD candidates are overwhelmingly recruited from a pool of students who have their master's degree. What will happen when our students pursue entry into advanced practice directly from the BSN? This master's pool will thus diminish and there will likely be very few DNP graduates who will make the decision to return to school for yet another doctorate, the PhD. Yet, expert DNP practice must rely on *new* evidence. Can our scholarship be sustained with a research doctorate (PhD) and a nonresearch doctorate (DNP)? It is unfortunate that the profession has no viable clinical doctorate option that emphasizes the expansion of clinical nursing science, a middle path between the PhD and DNP degree, such as occupational and physical therapy have maintained (Smith Glasgow & Dreher, 2010). The Columbia and Drexel DrNP tried to fill this void but failed to proliferate largely because of nursing politics surrounding degree initials (DrNP versus DNP). The remaining DNS programs still look like PhD degrees, but it is unlikely this old degree could suddenly catch fire. Is innovation in doctoral nursing education over? Or is the better strategy to innovate *within* the current dominant paradigm of MSN, DNP, and PhD?

MSN, DNP, AND PhD PRACTICE: PERSPECTIVES FROM AN APRN WITH ALL THREE DEGREES

Thoughts on the MSN, PhD, and DNP

Al Rundio

As an APRN with two master's degrees (one outside of nursing and one in nursing administration), three post–master's degree certificates in nursing, a PhD in Educational Leadership with a concentration in Infection Control Education, and most recently a doctor of nursing practice, I am certainly a proponent of advanced education for all nurses. I think that Luther Christman (1915–2011) had it correct many years ago with his unification model for nursing, in which he proposed that all nurses have advanced education to practice. His unification model incorporated teams of physician and nurses practicing together. Education, practice, and research were apparent on every nursing unit at

Rush-Presbyterian Medical Center in Chicago, where he was Dean of the School of Nursing (Pittman, 2005). It was his belief that nursing would be equal to medicine and more respected if they had similar credentials, that is, the doctorate. Time has certainly changed things since Christman's original proposal, but certain elements remain. The health disciplines now realize that no one profession can be an island. The disciplines must work collaboratively to ensure the best patient outcomes, regardless of their educational level.

In lieu of the many forces driving health care at this time (i.e., many uninsured or under-insured Americans, a strained economy, lack of primary care providers, and the move from an intervention to a prevention health-care delivery system), I am in favor of maintaining the master's degree in nursing as the entry point for advanced practice. I believe that an articulation model would work best, much like the RN-to-BSN articulation model proposed by many states such as New Jersey and New York (Trossman, 2008). I believe that one must be a master at something before claiming the title of "doctor." Many of the DNP programs that I have surveyed collapse the MSN course content into the DNP program, so the credit allocation is similar to acquiring both degrees separately. I also believe that by maintaining the DNP as a separate entity, a more rigorous doctoral program can result. Some questions surrounding DNP education need to be addressed. First, are DNP programs doing a disservice to the doctoral-prepared nurse and the profession by not requiring a practice dissertation? Second, is it fair to require a doctorate for beginning advanced practice, when every future APRN may not be ready for the pursuit of what a rigorous doctoral program in nursing entails? Further, the Affordable Care Act passed by Congress in 2010 will create more access to health care for many Americans. APRNs have the potential to be the primary care providers of the nation as physicians are more intrigued by specialty practice. The DNP as entry for advanced practice nursing may limit the number of APNs available to the nation.

My New Role: Chairing a DrNP Program

The College of Nursing and Health Professions at Drexel University embarked on the implementation of a unique doctoral program in 2005. The doctor of nursing practice (DrNP) program at Drexel is currently the only DrNP program in the country, and students complete a clinical (or practice) dissertation. I have had the opportunity to chair this program since April 2011. The decision had been made before my taking the chair to convert the in-class program to an online program starting September 1, 2011. During this transition I contemplated whether our program should convert to a DNP like, the rest of the nation. After pondering this question for some time, I have concluded that Drexel's program is unique and rightfully so. Having interviewed 70 potential applicants to this program this past summer, it was apparent to me that these applicants sought out Drexel's program particularly because of the research component and the rigor of this particular degree. The course of studies includes a 3-day campus orientation and two 1-week residencies.

The program at Drexel also incorporates a mandatory 2-week global health experience in a foreign country. Our students have been in Ireland, England, and Scotland. This year they will spend 1 week in Florence, Italy, followed by a week in London, England. The students attend the annual International Conference on the Professional Doctorate (ICPD), and they submit abstracts independently and jointly with faculty. These students have also made podium presentations and conducted workshops and poster sessions. This experience has enabled them to develop as doctoral clinical scholars within a global context. Colleagues from other universities have used Drexel's DrNP program as an exemplar of a rigorous doctor of nursing practice experience. It is my belief that our accrediting agencies need to recognize that practice doctorates can be packaged in more than one box. One has to raise a very important question: How can an accrediting agency not support increased rigor in doctoral nursing education? One corollary is the Joint Commission. Would the Joint Commission not support more rigorous quality improvement and patient safety programs in a hospital with more ambition than typically exists?

In view of societal health-care needs, the nursing faculty shortage, and the change in APN education and practice, it is prudent that APNs should continue to be educated with a master's degree and then encouraged to pursue a doctoral degree as a post–master's degree option. This is what Cronenwett et al. (2011) have recently called for—an admonition that the nursing discipline revisit the AACN's mandate for APRNs to have the DNP for entry into advanced nursing practice by 2015. Retaining the MSN and allowing the DNP as an option definitely fits the call for an articulation model for nursing. It is the view of both authors of this chapter that this option is best for nursing and for the health care of the nation in the immediate future.

SUMMARY: THE FUTURE OF NURSING EDUCATION FOR ADVANCED PRACTICE, A NEW VISION

As advanced practice nursing specialty organizations and other interested parties consider the implications of the AACN 2015 mandate, we offer some suggestions for the future of nursing education for advanced practice. As aggressive as the AACN has been in promoting the dissolution of the master's degree for advanced nursing practice, it now appears that the mandate to require the DNP will fall short. Indeed, Cronenwett and colleagues (2011) and many others are now suggesting that this decision must be revisited and the MSN retained. Certainly, the AACN could not have foreseen the global recession, which has caused many nursing programs to reevaluate closing down MSN programs in favor of the DNP. The 2010 IOM report on *The Future of Nursing* did not believe there were enough data to support DNP entry for advanced practice at this time. Although the report called for a doubling of the percentage of nurses with a doctorate by 2020, they were referring to the PhD and nursing professor/nurse scientist role, not the DNP degree for clinical practice (Dreher, 2011c).

Although we respect the early developmental work that led to the original Columbia Model DrNP in Primary Care (Mundinger & Kane, 2000), the current DNP degree would have more value if it explicitly advanced practice knowledge and was not promoted as an exclusively nonresearch doctorate. Whether fair or not, if doctoral-prepared APNs want parity with physicians, their educational preparation must arm them with competencies that hold "extra value" *over* the MD. It can be said that this extra value is clinical research skill that physicians acquire only through the apprentice model or pursuit of the PhD. Further, O'Sullivan, during her presidency of the National Organization of Nurse Practitioner Faculty (NONPF), commented that "many clinicians and faculty have questions about what additional skills and knowledge a NP would have at the practice doctorate level" (2005, p. 12). One answer would be clinical research competencies gained from an emphasis on scholarly inquiry, and practical clinical research questions that MSN-prepared APRNs enrolled in doctoral study are perfectly poised to ask. And while it is not realistic to expect that other nursing schools will adopt the Drexel "hybrid" DrNP model since it is not accreditable by CCNE, it *is* realistic to imagine that some DNP programs will be reengineered to produce practice knowledge.

The hybrid model for nursing is the global model for the professional doctorate outside the United States. More discussion is needed about how best to prepare the APRN as a *practitioner/researcher* or *local or field scientist* (a term often used to describe the competencies and role of the PsyD graduate) who would apply research methods to specific problems identified in direct practice. Surely doctoral-prepared advanced practice nurses of the future would have the basic skills to conduct small-scale studies that would contribute to the evidence base of practice.

The discussion of preparation of the future advanced practice nurse must also include preparation of the advanced practice nursing educator. To prepare the nurse whose primary role is the didactic and clinical education of future advanced practice nurses, serious consideration should be given to establishing a PhD in nursing designed principally for the student who is inclined to conduct nursing education research. For clarity, the degree should be a separate PhD in Nursing (like the Villanova University program) from the PhD in Nursing Science degree, which is reserved for programs that prepare the nurse scientist. Despite intense focus on nursing practice, these authors still advocate for high-quality nursing education research.

In 2005 Broome identified two serious issues that nursing still faces today: an urgent need for more BSN-prepared nurses and a severe nursing faculty shortage that is only going to get worse in the next decade. With these two problems still perilously facing the nursing profession, only time will tell if the DNP degree is indeed a prudent move by leadership. In just 6 years there has been an explosion of DNP programs, and though the majority are post–master's degree options, many have moved to offer BSN-to-DNP programs while seriously considering dropping the MSN altogether. With concomitant fluctuations in PhD enrollments, real questions arise about whether there will be enough doctoral-prepared nurses conducting clinical research to provide the evidence for nursing practice.

Discussion of the DNP for advanced practice students cannot be separated from a discussion about what type of academic is best to teach them. Mundinger (2005), of Columbia University, has described the ways in which the doctoral role of advanced practice differs from MS-level practice. She emphasizes that the doctor of nursing practice graduate shows "a greater depth and breadth of knowledge and practice (and) significant additional science education is provided by courses in genetics, advanced pathophysiology, pharmacology, differential diagnoses, chronic illness, bioinformatics, research methods, and identification and use of medical evidence" (p. 173). How do new DNP programs *really change* their curricula beyond the scope of the MSN? This author has served as a consultant to several DNP programs and sees very uneven attention to skills, knowledge, and competencies beyond the MSN. As the IOM report illustrates, the practice doctorate in nursing is still so new that there are *practically no data* on the productivity of its graduates. It is currently impossible to attribute direct outcomes to their practice. Indeed, the DNP was a bold move, and yet the unfolding of its true impact on the nursing profession and the health of a nation is yet to be seen. It is likely that MSN preparation will continue unabated for some time and how multiple preparations for advanced practice play out in the future will be revealed in time. We conclude by asking, do you favor this "big tent strategy" for advanced nursing practice preparation or not?

REFERENCES

Aaronson, L. (2005, January). *The road to interdisciplinary research: NINR and the NIH roadmap.* Paper presented at the 2005 AACN Doctoral Education Conference, Coronado, California.

American Academy of Nurse Practitioners. (2010). *Discussion paper: Doctor of nursing practice.* Austin, Texas: Author.

American Association of Colleges of Nursing. (2004a). *AACN position statement on the practice doctorate in nursing.* Retrieved June 8, 2005, from http://www.aacn.nche.edu/DNP/pdf/DNP.pdf.

American Association of Colleges of Nursing. (2004b). *2004 annual state of the schools.* Washington, DC: Author.

American Association of Colleges of Nursing. (2005). *Institutions offering doctoral programs in nursing and degrees conferred.* Retrieved March 18, 2005, from http://www.aacn.nche.edu/Education/pdf/DoctoralPrograms05.pdf.

American Association of Colleges of Nursing. (2006). *Essentials of doctoral education for advanced nursing practice.* Retrieved November 13, 2011, from http://www.aacn.nche.edu/publications/position/DNPEssentials.pdf.

American Association of Colleges of Nursing. (2010). *National Institute of Nursing Research: Promoting America's health through nursing science.* Retrieved November 13, 2011, from http://www.aacn.nche.edu/government-affairs/AACN_NR.pdf.

American Association of Colleges of Nursing. (2011a). *2011 annual report: Shaping the future of nursing education.* Retrieved November 12, 2011, from http://www.aacn.nche.edu/aacn-publications/annual-reports/AR2011.pdf.

American Association of Colleges of Nursing. (2011b). *Talking points.* Retrieved November 13, 2011, from http://www.aacn.nche.edu/dnp/talking-points.

American Association of Colleges of Nursing. (2012). *FY 2012 appropriations.* Retrieved January 13, 2012, from http://www.aacn.nche.edu/government-affairs/FY12AppropChart.

American Association of Nurse Anesthetists. (2007, September 20). *AANA announces support of doctorate for entry into nurse anesthesia practice by 2025.* Retrieved November 12, 2011, from http://www.aana.com/news.aspx?id=9678.

American College of Nurse Midwives. (2009, July 1). *Mandatory degree requirements for entry into midwifery practice.* Retrieved November 12, 2011, from http://www.midwife.org/ACNM/files/ACNMLibraryData/UPLOADFILENAME/000000000076/Mandatory_Degree_Req_for_Entry_Midwifery_Practice_7_09.pdf.

American Midwifery Certification Board. (2009, May 1). *Letter from AMCB board president, Barbara Graves.* Retrieved November 11, 2011, from http://www.amcbmidwife.org/assets/documents/FINAL%20CMP%20LETTER3.pdf.

American Nurses Association. (2011). *Advanced nursing practice: A new age in health care.* Retrieved August 15, 2012 from http://nursingworld.org/FunctionalMenuCategories/MediaResources/MediaBackgrounders/APRN-A-New-Age-in-Health-Care.pdf.

Apold, S. (2008). The doctor of nursing practice: Looking back, moving forward. *Journal for Nurse Practitioners, 4,* 101–107.

Beckstead, J. (2010). DNP = PhD-light, or old wine in new bottles? *International Journal of Nursing Studies, 47,* 663–664.

Bellini, S., & Cusson, R. M. (2011). The role of the practitioner. In H. M. Dreher & M. E. Smith Glasgow, *Role development for doctoral advanced practice nursing* (pp. 123–140). New York: Springer.

Bennis, W. G., & O'Toole, J. (2005). How business schools lost their way. *Harvard Business Review, 83,* 96–104.

Bloch, J. (2007). *The DNP degree as entry into nurse practitioner practice: Is this nursing's answer to eliminate disparities in health care access to vulnerable populations?* Paper presented at The First National Conference on the Doctor of Nursing Practice: Meanings and Models, Drexel University, Annapolis, MD.

Boston University Sargent College of Health and Rehabilitation Science. (2004). *Programs: Audiology, doctor of science.* Retrieved June 8, 2005, from http://www.bu.edu/sargent/programs/graduate/audiology/research_track.html.

Broome, M. E. (2005). Constructive debate and dialogue in nursing. *Nursing Outlook, 53,* 167–168.

Center for Nursing Advocacy. (2008). *How many nurses are there? And other facts.* Retrieved June 13, 2008, from http://nursingadvocacy.org/faq/rn_facts.html.

Consensus Model for APRN Regulation: Licensure, Accreditation, Certification & Education. (2008, July 7). Retrieved November 1, 2011, from http://www.aacn.nche.edu/education-resources/APRNReport.pdf.

Council on Accreditation of Nurse Anesthesia Educational Programs. (2003). *Trial standards for accreditation of nurse anesthesia programs.* Park Ridge, IL: Author.

Council on Accreditation of Nurse Anesthesia Educational Programs. (2004). *Standards for accreditation of nurse anesthesia programs.* Park Ridge, IL: Author.

Cronenwett, L., Dracup, K., Grey, M., McCauley, L., Meleis, A., & Salmon, M. (2011). The doctor of nursing practice: A national workforce perspective. *Nursing Outlook, 59,* 9–17.

Dahnke, M. D., & Dreher, H. M. (2011). *Philosophy of science for nursing practice: Concepts and application.* New York: Springer.

Dracup, K., & Brown, C. (2005). Doctor of nursing practice: MRI or total body scan? *American Journal of Critical Care, 14,* 278–281.

Dracup, K., Cronenwett, L., Meleis, A. I., & Benner, P. E. (2005). Reflections on the doctor of nursing practice. *Nursing Outlook, 53,* 77–182.

Dreher, H. M. (2011a). Nursing as a practice discipline. In H. M. Dreher & M. D. Dahnke, *Philosophy of science for nursing practice: Concepts and application* (pp. 23–54). New York: Springer.

Dreher, H. M. (2011b). Next steps toward practice knowledge development: An emerging epistemology in nursing. In H. M. Dreher & M. D. Dahnke, *Philosophy of science for nursing practice: Concepts and application* (pp. 301–331). New York: Springer.

Dreher, H. M. (2011c). *Educating "clinicians" to be influencers in the new interprofessional healthcare environment.* 2011 Summer Institute on Evidence-Based Practice, Transforming Care: Friction, Heat, and Light, San Antonio, TX, June 29–July 2, 2011.

Dreher, H.M., Donnelly, G.F., & Naremore, R.C., (2005). Reflections on the DNP and an alternate practice doctorate model: The Drexel DrNP., *Online Journal of Issues in Nursing,* Retrieved June 10, 2012 from www.nursingworld.org/ojin/topic28/tpc28_7.htm.

Dreher, H. M., Fasolka, B. & Clark, M. (2008). Navigating the decision to pursue an advanced degree. *Journal of Men in Nursing, 3*(1), 51–55.

Dreher, H. M., & Montgomery, K. E. (2009). Let's call it "doctoral" advanced practice nursing. *Journal of Continuing Nursing Education, 40*(12), 530–531.

Dreher, H. M., & Smith Glasgow, M. E. (2011). Global perspectives on the professional doctorate. *International Journal of Nursing Studies, 48,* 403–408.

Fink, D. (2006). The professional doctorate: Its relativity to the PhD and relevance for the knowledge economy. *International Journal of Doctoral Studies 3,* 35–44.

Fitzpatrick, J. (2003). The case for the clinical doctorate in nursing. *Reflections on Nursing Leadership, 8,* 37.

Florczak, K. L. (2010). Research and the doctor of nursing practice: A cause for consternation. *Nursing Science Quarterly, 23*(1), 13–17.

Ford, L. (1975). An interview with Dr. Loretta Ford. *Nurse Practitioner, 1*(1), 9–12.

Harris, G. (2011, October 1). When the nurse wants to be called "doctor." *New York Times,* October 1, 2011. Retrieved November 11, 2011, from http://www.nytimes.com/2011/10/02/health/policy/02docs.html?_r=2&ref=todayspaper.

Horrocks, S., Anderson, E., & Salisbury, C. (2002). Systematic review of whether nurse practitioners working in primary care can provide equivalent care to doctors. *British Medical Journal, 324,* 819–823.

Institute of Medicine. (1999). *To err is human: Building a safer health system.* Washington, DC: National Academy Press.

Institute of Medicine. (2001). *Crossing the quality chasm.* Washington, DC: National Academy Press.

Institute of Medicine. (2003). *Health professions education: A bridge to quality.* Washington, DC: National Academy Press.

Institute of Medicine. (2010). *The future of nursing: Leading change, advancing health.* Committee on the Robert Wood Johnson Foundation Initiative on the Future of Nursing at the Institute of Medicine. Washington, DC: National Academies of Science.

Kinslow, K. (2005, September). *Practice doctorate in nursing: American Association of Nurse Anesthetist's perspective.* Paper presented at the Pennsylvania State Nurses Association Pre-conference Session on "The dilemma over the doctor of nursing practice (DNP): Different perspectives," Harrisburg, PA.

Landro, L. (2008). Making room for "Dr. Nurse." *Wall Street Journal Online,* April 2, 2008. Retrieved June 13, 2008, from http://www.physicianassistantforum.com/forums/showthread.php?t=15539.

Levine, S., & Marek, A. (2005). Nurses step to the front. *US News & World Report, 138,* 66–71.

McKenna, H. (2005). Doctoral education: Some treasonable thoughts. *International Journal of Nursing Studies, 42*(3), 245–246.

Meleis, A. I., & Dracup, K. (2005). The case against the DNP: History, timing, substance, and marginalization. *Online Journal of Issues in Nursing, 10,* 1–8.

Miller, J. E. (2011). Reflective response 2. In H. M. Dreher & M. E. Smith Glasgow, *Role development for doctoral advanced nursing practice* (pp. 388–392). New York: Springer.

Montgomery, O. C. (2011). Reflective response 1. In H. M. Dreher & M. E. Smith Glasgow, *Role development for doctoral advanced nursing practice* (pp. 384–387). New York: Springer.

Mundinger, M. O. (2005). Who's who in nursing: Bringing clarity to the doctor of nursing practice. *Nursing Outlook, 53,* 173–176.

Mundinger, M. O., & Kane, R. L. (2000). Health outcomes among patients treated by nurse practitioners or physicians. *Journal of the American Medical Association, 283,* 2521–2524.

Mundinger, M., Kane, R., Lenz, E., Totten, A., Tsai, W., Cleary, P., et al. (2000). Primary care outcomes in patients treated by nurse practitioners or physicians: A randomized trial. *Journal of the American Medical Association, 283,* 59–68.

Murray, B. (2000, January). The degree that almost wasn't: The PsyD comes of age. *Monitor on Psychology, 31,* 1–5. Retrieved April 4, 2005, from http://www.apa.org/monitor/jan00/ed1.html.

National Academy of Sciences. (2005). *Advancing the nation's health needs.* Committee for monitoring the nation's changing needs for biomedical, behavioral, and clinical personnel. Washington, DC: National Academies Press.

National Association of Clinical Nurse Specialists (NACNS). (2011, May 2). *Criteria for the evaluation of clinical nurse specialist master's, practice doctorate, and post-master's certificate educational programs* [draft]. Retrieved November 12, 2011, from http://www.nacns.org/docs/EvalCriteria.pdf.

National Institutes of Health. (2005). *Summary of the FY 2006 president's budget.* February 7, 2005. Washington, DC: Author.

National League for Nursing Accrediting Commission, Inc. (December 1, 2005). *NLNAC statement on clinical practice doctorates.* Retrieved July 1, 2008, from http://www.nlnac.org/statementClinPrac.htm.

Nyquist, J., & Wilff, D. H. (2000). *Recommendations from national studies on doctoral education. Re-envisioning the Ph.D. project.* Retrieved March 18, 2005, from http://www.grad.washington.edu/envision/project_resources/national_recommendhtml.

Oldfield, S. (2011). The doctor of nursing practice graduate and the use of the title "doctor." In H. M. Dreher & M. E. Smith Glasgow, *Role development for doctoral advanced nursing practice* (pp. 369–383), New York: Springer.

O'Sullivan, A. L. (2005). The practice doctorate in nursing. *Mentor, 16,* 2–3, 12.

O'Sullivan, A. L, Carter, M., Marion, L., Pohl, J., & Werner, K. (2005). Moving forward together: The practice doctorate in nursing. *Online Journal of Issues in Nursing, 10,* 1–14.

Peterson, D. R. (1976). Need for the doctor of psychology degree in professional psychology. *American Psychologist, 31,* 792–798.

Peterson, D. R. (1982). Origins and development of the doctor of psychology concept. In G. R. Caddy, D. C. Rimm, N. Watson, & J. H. Johnson (Eds.), *Educating professional psychologists* (pp. 19–38). New Brunswick, NJ: Transaction Books.

Pittman, E. (2005). *Luther Christman: A maverick nurse—A nursing legend.* Victoria, BC: Trafford Publishers.

Potempa, K. M., Redman, R. W., & Anderson, C. A. (2008). Capacity for the advancement of nursing science: Issues and challenges. *Journal of Professional Nursing, 24,* 329–336.

Robert Wood Johnson Foundation. (2007). *Charting nursing's future.* Retrieved November 13, 2011, from http://www.rwjf.org/files/publications/other/nursingfuture4.pdf.

Smith Glasgow, M.E., Dreher, H. M. (2010). The future of oncology nursing science: Who will generate the knowledge? *Oncology Nursing Forum*, 37, 393-396.

Trossman, S. (2008). BSN in ten. *American Nurse Today*. Retrieved November 15, 2011, from http://www.americannursetoday.com/Article.aspx?id=5272&fid=5244.

University of Alabama at Birmingham Department of Physical Therapy, School of Health Related Professions. (2005). *Doctor of science in physical therapy.* Retrieved June 8, 2005, from http://main.uab.edu/shrp/default.aspx?pid=80258.

University of Washington. (2008). *Doctor of audiology program.* Retrieved June 13, 2008, from http://depts.washington.edu/sphsc/aud2/index.html.

Upvall, M., & Ptachcinski, R. (2007). The journey to the DNP program and beyond: What can we learn from pharmacy? *Journal of Professional Nursing, 23,* 316–321.

Valiga, T. (2004). *The nursing faculty shortage: A national perspective.* Congressional briefing presented by the A.N.S.R. Alliance, Hart Senate Office Building, Washington, DC.

Wheaton College. (2004). *Clinical dissertation manual for the doctor of psychology degree (Psy.D).* Wheaton College Psychology Department. Wheaton, IL: Author.

Widener University. (2004). *Manual for the clinical dissertation for the doctor of psychology degree (PsyD).* Widener University Institute of Graduate Clinical Psychology. Chester, PA: Author.

Wittmann-Price, R., Waite, R., & Woda, D. L. (2011). The role of the educator. In H. M. Dreher & M. E. Smith Glasgow, *Role development for doctoral advanced practice nursing* (pp. 161–180). New York: Springer.

5

Global Perspectives on Advanced Nursing Practice

Madrean Schober

INTRODUCTION

There is growing international recognition that advanced nursing practice (ANP)* should be developed, acknowledged, and legitimized. Factors contributing to a greater willingness to explore ANP options are multifaceted. Physician shortages, increased demand for highly specialized nurses, a greater emphasis on primary health care (PHC) and home-based services, and the increased acuity and complexity of hospitalized patients are motivating decision makers to rethink health service provision (Bryant, 2005; New Zealand Ministry of Health, 2002; Schober, 2008; World Health Organization [WHO], 2002a, 2002b; WHO–Eastern Mediterranean Region [EMR], 2001). Professional factors are also influencing developments in this field. The acquisition of higher professional qualifications as nursing education moves into the higher education sector is matched by a demand for choice in clinical career ladders that acknowledges professional advancement and gives nurses a reason to remain in practice (International Council of Nurses [ICN], 2007; Zurn, Dolea, & Stilwell, 2005).

The estimated global deficit of 2.4 million doctors, nurses, and midwives has stimulated a renewed examination of skill mix, including options for introducing new types of health-care workers, task shifting, and expanding current roles of health professionals (WHO, 2006, 2007). Buchan and Calman (2005) identify several drivers in health systems in countries belonging to the Organization for Economic Co-operation and Development (OECD), contributing to a heightened interest in the advanced practice nursing role. In addition to staff shortages faced by these countries, these authors suggest that health-sector reform and new initiatives have stimulated serious consideration of the appropriateness of current role definitions for health-care workers and skill mixes. Aspects affecting these deliberations include cost containment measures, actions to improve service quality, the introduction of technological innovations and new therapeutic interventions, and alterations in the legislative/regulatory environment. See **Box 5-1** for a summary of factors contributing to ANP growth.

This chapter examines some of the issues influencing the development of ANP globally. The emergence of the role in different regions of the world, the International Council of Nurse's (ICN's) role in setting international standards, role development, and some of the controversial practice issues affecting the nature of ANP are explored. Country illustrations provide examples of growth and progress worldwide.

***Advanced nursing practice (ANP)* is used as a comprehensive "umbrella" term for the discipline or functions of APNs. The term *advanced practice nurse (APN)* is used in reference to APN roles, APN practice, APN curriculum, or APN positions or individuals who are APNs.

BOX 5-1
Factors Contributing to International Growth in Advanced Nursing Practice

Escalating disease burden worldwide
Increased inpatient acuity and complexity of treatment
Impact of technological innovations and new therapeutic approaches
Increased emphasis on primary health-care and community-based services
Increasing requests for and complexity of home care
General global shortage of health-care workers stimulating new consideration of skill mix and task-shifting options
Physician shortages
Increased demand for specialized nurses
Nursing's desire for a clinical career ladder and professional advancement
Better-informed health-care consumers
Intensified demand for options to address out-of-control health-care costs
Search to improve quality of services

THE ROLE OF THE INTERNATIONAL COUNCIL OF NURSES

Since ICN set up the International Nurse Practitioner/Advanced Practice Nursing Network (INP/APNN) in 2000. As shown in **Box 5-2,** it has consulted extensively to reach consensus on the definition, characteristics, scope of practice, standards, and core competencies for advanced practice nurses (APNs). The ICN (2002) position is that the APN is

> *a registered nurse who has acquired the expert knowledge base, complex decision-making skills and clinical competencies for expanded practice, the characteristics of which are shaped by the context and/or country in which s/he is credentialed to practice. A master's degree is recommended for entry level.*

BOX 5-2
Goal of the International Council of Nurses International Nurse Practitioner/ Advanced Practice Nursing Network

The key goal of the network is to become an international resource for nurses practicing in nurse practitioner (NP) or advanced nursing practice (ANP) roles and interested others (e.g., policy makers, educators, regulators, and health planners) by
Making relevant and timely information about practice, education, role development, research, policy, regulatory developments, and appropriate events widely available
Providing a forum for sharing and exchanging knowledge, expertise, and experience
Supporting nurses and countries that are in the process of introducing or developing NP or ANP roles and practice
Accessing international resources that are pertinent to this field

Retrieved June 13, 2011, from www.icn-apnetwork.org.

See **Table 5-1** for ICN-recommended role characteristics.

Although ICN does not specifically define the scope of practice, it draws on the definition and characteristics described in Table 5-1, in recommending countries to keep the following points in mind when developing scopes of practice for the APN:

- Requires cognitive, integrative, and technical abilities to put into practice ethical and culturally safe acts, procedures, protocols, and practice guidelines
- Has the capacity for delivery of evidence-based care in primary, secondary, and tertiary settings in urban and rural communities
- Practices a high level of autonomy in direct patient care and management of health problems, including case management competencies
- Accepts accountability for providing health promotion, patient and peer education, mentorship, leadership, and management of the practice environment
- Maintains nursing practice current and seeks improvement through the translation, use, and implementation of meaningful research
- Engages in partnerships with patients and health team members for determining resources needed for continuous care and partnering with stakeholders in influencing policies that direct the health-care environment (adapted from ICN, 2008a, p. 13)

Core competencies have been identified and published in the following ICN documents: *The Scope of Practice, Standards and Competencies of the Advanced Practice Nurse* (ICN, 2008b) and *Nursing Care Continuum—Framework and Competencies* (ICN, 2008a).

TABLE 5-1

International Council of Nurses Characteristics for the Advanced Practice Nurse

Educational Preparation	Nature of Practice	Regulatory Mechanisms (Country-Specific Regulations That Underpin Advanced Practice Nursing Practice)
Educational preparation at an advanced level	The ability to integrate research, education, and clinical management	Right to diagnose Authority to prescribe medications and treatments
Formal recognition of educational programs A formal system of licensure, registration, certification, or credentialing	High degree of autonomy and independent practice Case management Advanced assessment and decision-making skills Recognized advanced clinical competencies The ability to provide consultant services to other health professionals Recognized first point of entry for services	Authority to refer to other professionals Authority to admit to hospital Title protection Legislation specific to advanced practice

International Council of Nurses. (2002). Definition and characteristics of the role. Retrieved June 13, 2011, from http://www.icn-apnetwork.org.

ADVANCED NURSING PRACTICE: A GROWING GLOBAL PRESENCE

Since 2000, ICN has monitored the progress of ANP globally. In 1999, 33 countries reported nursing roles with advanced practice elements in response to an ICN survey sent to 125 members (Schober & Affara, 2006). In a follow-up, Roodbol (2004) reported 60 countries claiming to be implementing, or in the process of developing, advanced practice roles. Information on the state of ANP globally and associated developmental issues was obtained from a Strength/Weakness/Opportunities/Threats (SWOT) analysis carried out with participants attending the 2006 ICN APN network conference. This analysis highlighted important areas of concern affecting the evolution of ANP in many of the participating countries (Affara, 2006). Issues surfacing were similar to those uncovered by Schober and Affara (2006) from their survey of key informants and the literature, published and unpublished, on the status of ANP internationally. An ICN survey of 32 countries conducted in 2008 provides additional support for the expansion of the NP-APN roles internationally while highlighting some of the challenges encountered globally (Pulcini et al., 2010). At the 2011 ICN Congress in Malta, Roodbol (2011) reported that membership in the ICN International NP/APN Network represents 78 countries indicating an interest in advanced nursing practice.

CHALLENGES AND CONTROVERSY

This section identifies some of the key challenges in APN role development from the international perspective.

An Uncertain Identity Contributing to Poor Role Clarification

The uncertainty of identity and lack of role clarity appear to center largely on an inability to define the scope of practice for the APN. In the absence of a clearly defined scope of practice, it is difficult to delineate accountability and responsibility for the APN. In addition, as the participants in the SWOT analysis noted (Affara, 2006), the lack of a clear identity affects the ability of APNs to communicate clear messages about the nature of ANP to others, such as clients, policy makers, other health professionals, regulators, and educators. Findings from the Canadian Decision Support Synthesis on Clinical Nurse Specialists and Nurse Practitioners in Canada further indicate that regulators, educators, government officials, and administrators consistently raised concerns regarding the lack of clarity surrounding APN roles and the potential of losing the role during economic downturns or when other roles were introduced if the contributions of the APN role were not clear (DiCenso & Bryant-Lukosius, 2010).

Proliferation of Titles

Advanced nursing practice (ANP) is plagued by a proliferation of titles globally. In studying this role internationally, Schober and Affara (2006) found that functions and responsibility vary considerably from one setting to another even when the same title is used in the same country. Extensive confusion has resulted from the lack of consensus as to what title should be applied to ANP. Titles currently being used throughout the world include nurse practitioner (NP), family nurse practitioner (FNP), adult NP, advanced NP, primary care practitioner, nurse-midwife, clinical nurse specialist (CNS), nurse anesthetist (NA), community health NP (CHNP), and women's health nurse practitioner (WHNP). Pediatric NP, gerontological NP, emergency room NP, and acute care NP are also titles applied to APN roles. Some titles indicate the specialty of the APN; other titles have been developed to fit the context of the systems or the situations in which the APN role exists. The ICN survey of 32 countries discovered 14 different titles being used to designate ANP (Pulcini et al., 2010). The variety of titles being used reveals the explorative nature of advanced practice internationally with respect to the parameters of the role and where it sits in relation to other roles in the health-care system.

Lack of Recognition by Others in the Health-Care System

Medical dominance and the control of medicine over health care are cited as some of the main obstacles to implementing advanced nursing roles. In addition, scope of practice conflicts with other health professionals' scope, especially medicine, contributes to APNs feeling unwelcome within the health-care team. Interestingly, one of the particular problem areas brought up during the SWOT analysis conducted by Affara (2006) was a mistrust that may exist between APNs and other nurses. In many cases it seems that APNs may feel more at ease with medical rather than nursing values. Affara and Schober (2006) uncovered a similar sentiment in information obtained from key informants who reported obstacles to the APN role arising more frequently from nurse rather than physician colleagues. In the Netherlands, Roodbol (2005) found that even though physicians believed that the APN presence had a positive effect on the social identity of nurses in general, nurses as a whole did not share this view and were not prepared to accept them into their professional group.

Varied Levels of Autonomy

The degree of autonomy afforded to APNs varies from country to country and even within the country. This appears to be related to the degree of recognition and acceptance of the role and to the type of regulatory mechanisms in place (Schober & Affara, 2006).

Fragmented and Variable Standards and Quality of Education Programs

Historically and up to the present time, educational qualifications for the APN role have varied from the awarding of certificates for postbasic courses of various lengths to undertaking a formal university program and obtaining a master's degree. Information from an ICN INP/APNN survey indicates that of the 31 responding countries, 50% replied that the most prevalent credential was the master's degree (Pulcini et al., 2010). Because education beyond the preparation of the generalist nurse is a critical component in the development of the APN role, the ICN Board of Directors approved an organizational position that entry-level education should be set at the master's level (ICN, 2002). See **Box 5-3** for the ICN-recommended educational standards.

Issues of Regulation, Credentialing, and Standard Setting

Standards, regulations, and supportive legislation ultimately provide the underpinnings of successful ANP implementation, but they are also likely to contribute to conflict, discussion, and lengthy debate. The lag between actual APN practice and supportive legislation can be attributed to uneven starts in initiating new roles and the diversity of health issues challenging the communities and countries where these roles seek to grow. Also, restrictive regulations that unnecessarily limit the expertise and scope of practice for APN roles can considerably affect to what extent advanced practice will be embraced by a health-care system and permit APNs to contribute to their fullest capacity. Thus, a process of evaluation and revision of regulations may be the only option to follow when

BOX 5-3
International Council of Nurses Standards for Education of the Advanced Practice Nurse

Programs prepare the student, a registered/licensed nurse, for practice beyond that of the generalist nurse by including opportunities to access knowledge and skills, as well as demonstrate their integration in clinical practice as a safe, competent, and autonomous practitioner.

Programs prepare the authorized nurse to practice within the nation's health-care system to the full extent of the role as set out in the scope of practice.

Programs are staffed by faculty who are qualified and prepared at or beyond the level of the student undertaking the program of study.

Programs are accredited or approved by the authorized national or international credentialing body.

Programs facilitate lifelong learning and maintenance of competencies.

Programs provide student access to a sufficient range of clinical experience to apply and consolidate under supervision the theoretical course content.

International Council of Nurses. (2002). *Definition and characteristics of the role.* Retrieved June 13, 2011, from http://www.icn-apnetwork.org

they are found to hinder optimum professional practice. This, in turn, poses another set of problems as to who has the authority to initiate and the power to supply leverage in provision of solutions in the credentialing and regulatory arena.

National nursing associations and nursing leadership would seem to be the likely foundation for development and exploration of education requirements and standards, especially because the core of ANP is viewed to be grounded in nursing theory and nursing science. However, there appears to be a lack of consensus among nursing academics and leaders as to what ANP really means, and at times, overt support by nursing bodies is lacking as the roles develop.

Key decision makers and advisors have begun to provide regulatory and credentialing guidance. International organizations, such as the ICN, are taking official organizational positions regarding ANP and offer publications (ICN, 2008a, 2008b) to facilitate a better understanding of these new nursing roles. **Box 5-4** identifies the minimal regulatory standards recommended by ICN (2008b).

Flexible regulatory language has been encouraged to ensure quality health-care services that are protective of the populations receiving those services. However, at times restrictive regulatory legislation affecting APNs is promulgated or supportive protocols for APN practice are blocked to protect the practice of other health-care professionals. Clarity and consistency in defining the process and structure of credentialing for APNs and accreditation of educational programs worldwide is essential as the APN investigates intercountry choices for employment and educational opportunities. Professional mobility will potentially shape a move toward consensus for credentialing among countries as APNs relocate, immigrate, or accept temporary assignment. The capability of agencies and organizations in addressing legislative issues, standards, and regulations will increasingly come under scrutiny as the international nursing community looks for authorities to provide guidance.

In ANP development and implementation, regulation often needs to catch up with innovation, a necessary step if understanding and confidence in the role is to be established for the benefit of key decision makers and the public. However, the setting up of suitable regulatory mechanisms needs to

BOX 5-4
International Council of Nurses Minimal Standards for Regulating the Advanced Practice Nurse

Develop and maintain sound credentialing mechanisms that enable the authorized nurse to practice in the advanced role within the established scope of practice.

Establish relevant civil legislation or rules to acknowledge the authorized role, monitor the competence, and protect the public through issuance of guidance, assessment processes, and when necessary, fitness to practice procedures and processes.

Periodically revise regulatory language to maintain currency with nursing practice and scientific advancement.

Establish title protection through rule making or civil legislation.

Source: International Council of Nurses. (2008). *Nursing care continuum—framework and competencies.* Geneva: Author.

be approached in such a manner that new problems are not created, health-care systems made less efficient, or access is reduced to those who need APN services.

Authority to Prescribe Medicines and Therapeutics

Nurse prescribing of medicines or therapeutics describes various types of nursing practice currently undertaken in different countries or regions of the world. In general, discussion of this issue focuses on the suitability of prescriptive authority for nurses and the appropriateness of nurse prescribing as it relates to defined characteristics and expected competencies for APN roles. Discourse and comment reveal that nurses have been prescribing medicines, treatments, and other therapies in certain health-care settings, but the reality of carrying out these activities within a legal framework and in a supportive health-care environment such as, having enabling workplace policies in place, often lags behind the requisites of actual practice. However, as more countries implement APN roles in a variety of settings, the issue of nurse prescribing looks as if it is becoming less of a controversial issue.

It appears that advancement for APN and NP roles necessitates prescriptive authority, but it is worth noting that health-care services in some areas of the world have for some time included nurse prescribing of a range of essential drugs at the first level of practice in primary health-care systems (WHO-EMR, 2001). Thus, nurses may carry prescriptive authority in the absence of the other elements that characterize APN practice.

Buchan and Calman (2009) review nurse prescribing prototypes internationally and provide models by which nurses may potentially be involved in prescribing. Although nurse prescribing is not always associated with APN or NP roles, countries or regions with authority for nurses to prescribe, such as Sweden, Australia, United States, United Kingdom, Canada, and New Zealand, have well-established community nursing or general nursing roles supportive of this capability.

In their appraisal of the key global issues associated with nurses' prescribing, Buchan and Calman (2009) indicate that there is little uniformity as to what role nurses should have with regard to prescriptive authority. Educational programs to prepare nurses for prescribing range from master's degree preparation to a designated program of a few study days. Although these issues are varied, there are common approaches when considering nurses' prescriptive authority. These include the acceptability of nurse prescribing within the health-care setting, designation of which nurses will prescribe, strategies for implementation, and feasibility from an administrative and health policy perspective.

GLOBAL PERSPECTIVE—COUNTRY ILLUSTRATIONS

The development of APN and NP roles internationally has progressed to the point where a global review is best accomplished using examples drawn from experiences of specific countries introducing and developing advanced practice nursing roles. Country illustrations are arranged according to regions designated by the World Health Organization (WHO). Descriptions of country progress and expansion in this field are intended to provide representative examples and not meant to portray all activity in a region or a country.

Africa: WHO-AFRO

Botswana

In Botswana, a poorly developed health-care system and a severe shortage of physicians following independence in 1966 triggered the need for nurses with advanced skills and decision making to provide services usually associated with physician practice. Nurses accepted these increased responsibilities but demanded further education to enhance their ability to meet the health-care needs of the country.

The Ministry of Health, through the National Health Institute (NHI), responded by establishing the first FNP program in 1986 with the aim to educate nurses in advanced skills in diagnosis and management of PHC problems common in Botswana. The program evolved to 18 months of post-basic education in 1991, followed by a revision and update in curriculum in 2001 with increased emphasis on comprehensive family health services (NHI, 2002). In 2007, a four-semester format was introduced (Pilane, Neube, & Seitio, 2007). An MSN/FNP is now offered by the University of Botswana, which has begun to graduate students while simultaneously the diploma program at the Institute of Health Sciences (IHS) continues to offer a four-semester format (O. Seitio, personal communication, June 26, 2011).

Because the University of Botswana now offers a master's degree in nursing, a comparative analysis of the master's and FNP curricula is underway to identify how the two programs could articulate common course work and remove redundant or repetitious study, while still supporting educational advancement for the FNP. Possibilities for credit transfer and opportunities for challenge examinations or applying for exemption from retaking courses when seeking further study at the University of Botswana are being considered (Pilane et al., 2007).

Nurse practitioners provide care in outpatient departments, clinics, industry, schools, and private practice throughout the country. The environment in Botswana supports autonomy in provision of PHC services as evidenced in nurse-managed facilities and prescribing privileges. Challenges continue to be lack of specific regulations, the absence of clear qualifications, no designated career advancement for FNPs, and lack of availability of qualified faculty for the educational programs (O. Seitio, personal communication, June 26, 2011).

Republic of South Africa

The "key challenges for NPs in South Africa lie in lobbying for enabling legislation, obtaining access to education and training opportunities, and managing risks within the rapidly changing environment" (Geyer, Naude, & Sithole, 2002, p. 11). Even though this statement was made in 2002, the commentary remains true today (N. Geyer, personal communication, March 4, 2008).

The move since 1994 from a mainly hospital-based health-care service to increased emphasis on PHC and community-based services increased the visibility of the NP. The creation of a more unified health-care system, while dealing with rapid change in the health-care environment, posed challenges and opportunities for the primary clinical practitioner (PCP). PCP is the title that has been used for NPs in the RSA; however, with the development and introduction of new qualifications in 2008, the title will become family nurse practitioner (FNP) over time (N. Geyer, personal communication, March 4, 2008).

The 2005 Nursing Act and its regulations call for NPs to possess required competencies. Standards for the education and training of nurses and midwives have also been established. Postbasic preparation for FNPs follows either acquisition of a 4-year diploma or 4-year degree for general nursing, midwifery, psychiatry, or community health nursing. However, the rapid acceleration in use of nurses in PHC services has resulted in FNPs that have not received specialist education. Therefore, one of the challenges is providing sufficient access to education to ensure nurses in the NP role have the required competence to provide high-quality care.

The scope-of-practice regulations provided by the South African Nursing Council in 1984 provided practice principles that support nurses and midwives to "perform any acts for which they have been trained" (Geyer et al., 2002, p. 13). The FNP scope of practice is written in such a way that it emphasizes the provision of comprehensive clinical services such as the following:

- Comprehensive assessment
- Diagnosis of health and disease, especially diseases common in the RSA
- Treatment and management (pharmacological and nonpharmacological)
- Referral to other professionals
- Counseling
- Leadership and management
- Health promotion and disease prevention

However, the legal framework for the FNP has not evolved as rapidly as practice. A new scope of practice for nursing has been developed and was promulgated in 2008. See first numbered item in **Box 5-5**. This scope will make a clear distinction between the roles for professional nurses, staff nurses, and auxiliary nurses while also providing the basis for progression to specialist nurse and NP scopes of practice.

The FNP scope of practice overlaps with aspects of scopes of practice for other health practitioners, such as physicians and pharmacists in the case of medicines. Dispensing of drugs falls under the pharmacist's function, and the control of drugs as associated with prescribing is exclusive to the physician, unless the practitioner or professional, such as a nurse, has been authorized to prescribe by their respective councils or regulatory bodies. Nurses are listed as one of these professions (see numbered items 3 and 4 in Box 5-5). A nurse who wishes to dispense medicines must undergo a course accredited with the pharmacy council. Application for a license to dispense medication is made through the national department of health. The license is valid for 3 years, after which reapplication is required.

NPs in RSA are mainly employed in the public health sector at the provincial and local authority level. The majority of health services are provided by nurses and midwives, with nurses identified as the first point of contact for preventive health and minor ailments. With the growing need for home-based care, resulting mainly from the epidemic proportions of HIV and AIDS, nurses and NPs are increasingly holding leadership and supervisory responsibilities for other workers and volunteers in health-care systems.

BOX 5-5
New Developments for the Nurse Practitioners in the Republic of South Africa

1. The new scope has been structured for three categories of nurses within a framework of professional-ethical practice, clinical practice, and quality of practice. This lends itself to developing a structured scope that progresses to the next levels of specialist nurses and nurse practitioners.
2. New educational programs linked to this scope will prepare staff nurses who will be independent/autonomous practitioners able to plan and execute comprehensive care for stable and uncomplicated patients. Professional nurses can specialize in a variety of areas, including family nurse practice. A criterion has been built in that no nurse can specialize until he or she has a 2-year clinical experience (this includes 1 year of community service after completion of basic training plus 1 additional year of clinical practice).
3. Although there is a new Nursing Act, the profession has not managed to get rid of government control regarding the authorization of nurses to prescribe. Section 56 of the new Nursing Act of 2005 places more controls into the system; nurses will now be licensed to prescribe and reapply for licensing.
4. Work is currently in process on regulations for nurse prescribing. The thinking has been that there will be three levels of prescribing where nurses will have access to specified drugs to manage minor injuries and diseases—likely according to protocols. These levels are

   Staff nurse = level one
   Professional nurse = level two
   Specialist nurse = level three (only access for specialist area)

N. Geyer, personal communication, March 14, 2008.

Establishing collaborative practice in the RSA context is fraught with difficulty because language contained in separate practice acts and regulations governing practice of each category of health-care professionals poses a significant barrier. Health-care practitioners can employ each other, but stipulations within regulations prohibit group practice. Such limitations either discourage formation of multiprofessional groups or require developing involved legal contracts to bypass the rules. Conflict arises when existing scopes of practice are seen to overlap with other professions, thus contributing to lack of agreement supportive of the development of advanced nursing roles. This situation has interfered with legislative support for FNP practice and expanded nurse dispensing and prescribing (N. Geyer, personal communication, March 4, 2008).

Western Africa

Madubuko (2001) describes the scope of practice of an NP in West Africa (WA) as very similar to that of registered nurses (RNs) who also possess a postbasic nursing education and clinical training in midwifery (a registered midwife [RM]). Advanced education is not recognized in the nursing register, but hopefully with time, explanation, lobbying, and pressure, the nurses in WA will obtain recognition for advanced education and clinical practice.

All RNs have additional advanced education in at least one specialty area—for instance, in the psychiatric, perioperative, nurse education, orthopedic, gynecological, thoracic, or pediatric field. More than 1,000 RNs have a master's degree in a nursing specialty. The WA College of Nursing has accredited the University of Benin Teaching Hospital's School of Ophthalmic Nursing for an 18-month master's degree for ophthalmic NPs. Madubuko (2001) considers this to be consistent with the global NP movement.

Madubuko (2001) clarifies that an RN or RM is certified by national certification examination and provides direct PHC. The practice description includes obtaining a history, performing a physical examination, diagnosing and treating common illnesses, performing illness prevention screenings, and health promotion. Education and counseling are provided in collaboration with other health professionals. The reforms globally have supported the concern for more relevant health-care services in WA, providing an opportunity for NPs and other health professionals.

Americas: WHO-AMRO

Canada

The Canadian Nurses Association (CNA) has been instrumental in providing leadership for the development and implementation of ANP in Canada. In 1999, the CNA developed a framework for ANP that was revised in 2002 and 2008. The framework provides the following definition (CNA, 2008, p. 5):

> *Advanced nursing practice is an umbrella term describing an advanced level of clinical nursing practice that maximizes the use of graduate educational preparation, in-depth nursing knowledge and expertise in meeting the health needs of individuals, families, groups, and populations. It involves analyzing and synthesizing knowledge; understanding, interpreting and applying nursing theory and research; and developing and advancing nursing knowledge and the profession as a whole.*

According to this framework, it is the combination of graduate education and clinical experience that allows nurses to develop the competencies required in advanced nursing practice (CNA, 2008, p. 6). Core competencies are described as essential to ANP with a list of competencies in four categories outlined in the framework as clinical, research, leadership, and consultation/collaboration.

The implementation of the NP role gained momentum following an 18-month federally funded, CNA-led Canadian Nurse Practitioner Initiative (CNPI) conducted from 2004 to 2006. This initiative helped in the development of a framework for the integration and sustainability of the NP role in Canada's health-care system. Recommendations for practice, education, legislation, regulation, and health human resources planning were provided as a result of findings from the CNPI.

In 2009, the CNA consulted with stakeholders on the progress made in meeting the recommendations generated from the 2006 CNPI. The main purpose of the consultation was to compile information on the activities of governments, nongovernmental organizations, and other stakeholders at the federal/provincial levels in relation to the CNPI recommendations.

The consultation process revealed that while more than half of the actions concerning the CNPI recommendations had been fully or partially completed to date, several key actions remain ongoing. The findings of the consultation process are outlined in *Recommendations of the Canadian Nurse Practitioner Initiative Progress Report.* Among the remaining challenges to NP integration, continued advocacy is needed on federal legislative or policy barriers (e.g., prescribing of controlled drugs and substances, distribution of drug samples, completion of medical forms for disability claims, and workers' compensation) (CNA, 2009a).

Nurses in Canada are regulated at the provincial or territorial level. Specific titles used in reference to ANP may vary among provinces and territories. Currently, the only advanced practice nursing role with additional regulation and title protection, beyond RN, is the NP. NPs can autonomously make a diagnosis, order and interpret diagnostic tests, prescribe pharmaceuticals, and perform specific procedures within their legislated scope of practice (CNA, 2009a, p. 1). Nurse practitioner legislation currently exists in all provinces and territories in Canada and national core competencies for the nurse practitioner role were revised in 2010.

Clinical nurse specialists (CNSs) in Canada are "registered nurses who hold a master's or doctoral degree in nursing and have expertise in a clinical nursing specialty" (CNA, 2009b). They provide support for high-quality practice and health system strengthening across the health-care continuum. The CNS role was introduced to respond to increased patient need, a demand for nursing specialization, and to support nursing practice at the point of care. However, despite the fact that it has been part of the Canadian health-care system for the past four decades (DiCenso, 2008), CNSs continue to face challenges. The CNA in partnership with its members and the Canadian Association of Advanced Practice Nurses continue to promote understanding and use of the CNS role. Outcomes and the impact of both the CNS and NP roles have been highlighted in the new national ANP framework.

Several tools have been developed to assist with the implementation of Canadian ANP roles: the CNPI implementation and evaluation toolkit (CNA, 2006) and the Participatory, Evidence-Based, Patient-Centered Process for Advanced Practice Role Development, Implementation and Evaluation (PEPPA framework [Bryant-Lukosius & DiCenso, 2004]). These tools serve as a structured and practical guide in assessing the need and readiness for ANP roles based on the population health needs of Canadians. In 2010, research titled the *Clinical Nurse Specialists and Nurse Practitioners in Canada: A Decision Support Synthesis* was published (DiCenso & Bryant-Lukosius, 2010). The report provides an understanding of the roles of advanced practice nurses, the contexts in which APNs are being used, and the health system factors that influence the way in which advanced practice nursing is being integrated into the Canadian health-care system.

Although there continues to be a lack of understanding among health professionals and the public in relationship to ANP, the professional and policy environment in Canada is generally receptive and looking to integrate a variety of ANP roles into the health-care system. Policy makers, decision makers, and nursing are working together to face future challenges as they refine and coordinate what this means in terms of services for the country (C. Buckley, personal communication, July 4, 2011).

Jamaica

The NP program in Jamaica started in 1977 as a response to the shortage of physicians needed to provide cost-effective health care to the poor in rural and underserved areas. Since 1978, graduate NPs have been providing nursing and medical care to all age groups within the health-care delivery systems and in communities. Most NPs function from health centers in primary health-care settings. Presently there are three specialties: family, pediatric, and mental health/psychiatric nurse practitioner. The training of pediatric nurse practitioners has been discontinued. Since the inception of the program, Jamaica has trained NPs from at least 10 Caribbean countries.

In 2002, the education program was upgraded from certificate to the master's degree level and is now taught at the University of the West Indies (UWI) School of Nursing, Faculty of Medical Sciences. Nurse anesthetists (NAs) are technically classified as NPs; however, even though the NA program started many years before the NP program, it has yet to evolve to the master's level.

Despite these achievements, NPs and NAs are not registered or licensed as APNs and have no prescriptive privileges. All NPs and NAs are registered as nurses and/or midwives. They have no official authority in the expanded role. Prescriptions have to be countersigned by doctors. NPs, NAs, the Nursing Council of Jamaica, and other stakeholders on the island are working diligently to move forward an agenda to enact policies supportive of advanced nursing roles. This is to be entrenched in law (D. Less, personal communication, May 1, 2011).

Cayman Islands

The emergence of ANP services in the Cayman Islands provides an example of how NP-like roles evolve and develop in response to the needs of the people, as well as within geographical circumstances. The initiation of NP-like services started in 1930 with provision of care by a local midwife to meet community health needs. Physician services were scarce and conditions were primitive, with populations residing in remote locations. NP services progressed with the official employment of a nurse experienced in midwifery and community health to provide PHC. Comprehensive health-care services were provided in homes, schools, and clinic settings (Slocombe, 2000).

Expansion of clinical expertise progressed rapidly during subsequent years, with the nurse as the main health-care provider on the islands. The nurse diagnosed, treated, prescribed, and dispensed what was viewed to be necessary. Conditions receiving care were "whatever walked in through the door" (M. Slocombe, personal communication, 2002). Immunization, antenatal, well-baby, nutritional, diabetic, and hypertensive clinics were held, with backup consultation and collaboration provided by phone call to the nearest hospital or by appointment with periodic visiting physicians. The nurse took on the multifaceted role and duties of counselor, administrator, staff supervisor, health educator, accountant, and secretary. Absence of adequate support by other professionals, lack of resources, and limited educational opportunities created frustration and obstacles to professional development.

The location of the three Cayman Islands, situated in the Caribbean Sea between Jamaica and Cuba, contributes to the diversity, as well as the uniqueness, of presenting conditions. Cuban refugees and rafters trickle in for health screening and health care; periodic care for prison inmates is provided; and hurricane evacuation preparedness is essential for the health centers. The tourist industry, with visitors from more than 80 countries, requires the nurse to be knowledgeable about trauma and injuries related to deep sea diving (Slocombe, 2000).

Eastern Mediterranean: WHO-EMRO

In June 2001, the Regional Director for Nursing for the WHO—Eastern Mediterranean Region (EMR) convened the Fifth Meeting of the Regional Panel on Nursing to discuss ANP and nurse prescribing (WHO-EMR, 2001). Countries represented at the 3-day workshop in Islamabad, Pakistan, included Bahrain, Cyprus, Islamic Republic of Iran, Iraq, Jordan, Lebanon, Oman, Pakistan, Saudi Arabia, Sudan, Syrian Arab Republic, United Arab Emirates, and the Republic of Yemen. Twenty-two representatives from nursing, medicine, pharmacy, and ministries of health gathered to begin to develop a regional policy framework for ANP and mechanisms for nurse prescribing. The regional panel highlighted factors leading to development of the roles, as well as identifying strategies for the region (WHO-EMR, 2001). Obstacles and factors identified as supportive of development for ANP and nurse prescribing are provided in **Table 5-2**.

Strategies formulated for ANP development include the following:

- Assessment of need and cost-effectiveness for APN roles in the region
- Development of APN curriculum and standards of practice
- Definition of the role and identification of related revision of nurse practice acts to cover ANP

Significantly, there was consensus that authority for nurse prescribing within a range of essential drugs is an activity that could be allocated at some level to the competent general nurse and does not

TABLE 5-2

WHO-EMR Consensus on Factors Influencing Advanced Practice Nursing Development

Obstacles	Support
Lack of a regional definition and role ambiguity	Increased population and community needs for health-care services
Absence of country-level educational or regulatory systems to support such roles	Improving levels of nursing education
No feasibility studies for advanced nursing practice needs	Desire in the region to improve quality of care and access
No awareness of the role among the public and health professionals	Research studies from outside the region supportive of advance nursing practice
Absence of nursing leadership at the policy level	Commitment of WHO toward development and use of nursing roles

Adapted from World Health Organization—Eastern Mediterranean Region. (2001). *Fifth meeting of the regional advisory panel on nursing and consultation on advanced practice nursing and nurse prescribing: Implications for regulation, nursing education and practice in the Eastern Mediterranean.* WHO-EM/NUR/348/E/L. Cairo: Author.

necessarily depend on the development of ANP. On the other hand, authority to prescribe was acknowledged as one of the many areas of expertise associated with APN roles. In addition, it was agreed that these nursing roles require advanced education, regulatory changes, and expansion of traditional nursing.

Recommendations were made for WHO-EMR (2001) to provide guidelines to assist countries in the region who are in the process of developing and strengthening ANP at all levels of health care. Additional assistance was requested from WHO to initiate and coordinate pilot projects to evaluate the impact and cost-effectiveness of related change when introducing new nursing roles and nurse prescribing.

Bahrain

As a result of the WHO-EMR meeting in Pakistan in 2001, Bahrain received additional consultative support coordinated by WHO-EMRO to assess the country's readiness for ANP (Schober, 2007b). Consultation services found a stable organizational structure for health-care service provision within PHC. Two pediatric APNs educated in NP programs in the United States have recently started working in pediatric specialties in a hospital. Additional NPs, also educated in the United States, are faculty at the College of Health Sciences (CHS).

The CHS has had an RN-bachelor of science in nursing (BSN) degree for some years and established a 4-year BSN program in 2003. The BSN is now considered entry-level education for nursing practice in Bahrain. With proper planning, this places the CHS in an ideal position to develop an ANP master's degree program. Although the associate degree (AD) nursing programs have been discontinued, the majority of the current Bahraini nursing graduates come from these programs. Postbasic 1-year education, called *advanced practice programs,* is available in the country. Lacking a current option for a master's program within Bahrain, nurses interested in obtaining ANP education are sponsored by the Ministry of Health to study in the United States or elsewhere (A. Matooq, personal communication, March 14, 2008).

Bahrain faces certain challenges in developing an APN role suitable for its health services:

- Identifying services that could be provided by APNs
- Developing an educational plan that meets the needs of the current workforce while properly planning for the potential APN roles
- Constructing strategies to ensure faculty are adequately qualified to deliver ANP education
- Establishing standards and regulations supportive of APN roles

Iran

In Iran, the degree of master's in nursing sciences (MNS) was initiated in 1976, in the areas of nursing education and nursing administration. Graduate students focus on any of four subspecialties: (a) psychiatric, (b) pediatric, (c) community health, and (d) medical–surgical nursing. Fourteen schools of nursing offer graduate nursing degrees, and as of 1995 the 10 PhD programs in Iran had graduated nearly 40 individuals. The majority of these graduates were hired for clinical and educational positions in hospital, community, or academic settings.

The Farsi term *Karshenasae-e-Arshad* translates to "advanced specialist". In the urban areas physicians and advanced specialist nurses share role responsibilities and functions. In rural regions of Iran, these nurses work in an autonomous manner much like APNs in the United States.

Nurses in Iran obtain a practice permit from the Ministry of Health and can open a private practice clinic (center for nursing services). Medical supervision by physicians is not required because the state Ministry of Health monitors health-care practices. However, the scope of practice is set and supervised by physicians. Society needs determine curriculum content in the nursing programs. Recent changes include additional emphasis on geriatric, rehabilitation, women's health, neonatal health, military, and oncology nursing at the graduate level. Short-term continuing nursing education courses are available for school nursing, home health, intensive care, burn care, ostomy care, and HIV/AIDS, and geriatric courses are also being developed for graduate nurses (M. Fooladi and F. Sharif, personal communication, March 12, 2008).

Israel

Almost 100 years ago two U.S. nurses arrived in Israel to help improve the health of the Jewish nation in Palestine and established the Hadassah Medical Organization. The aim was to educate nurses to care for a population desperate for adequate health-care services. This tradition of innovation and professionalism continues to this day.

In 2002, the Hadassah-Hebrew University School of Nursing established a master's degree program in advanced practice nursing, the first of its kind in Israel. Its founders and supporters worked hard for many years to develop and set up a program that took the best of theoretical and clinical nursing knowledge from around the world and implemented it within the framework of the Israeli health-care delivery system.

Changes in Israel have created a demand for health-care practitioners who can provide optimal care within the context of the present health-care system. The graduate of the program, known as an APN, is a clinician who can integrate advanced clinical skills with systems knowledge, educational commitment, and leadership ability using clinical judgment and knowledge gained from graduate studies to promote evidence-based practice at the bedside and to persuade other nurses to integrate this practice. The view of the school of nursing is that master's education in general has been shown to develop and refine analytical skills, broad-based perspectives, articulation of viewpoints and positions, and the ability to more clearly connect theory to practice.

Economic and professional processes have led to the development of a new model of practice that combines characteristics of the roles of both the NP and the CNS. The new nurse practice role is called the APN. Nursing practice according to this model applies to the entire continuum of health-care delivery (from the hospital to the community) and requires learning and a knowledge base gleaned from both roles. The model attempts to create a balance between the responsibility and authority associated with direct patient care of individuals and groups with an advanced professional role at the level of change agent, teacher, and researcher. A list of clinical competencies for the entry-level graduate of a clinical master's program has been delineated. However, certain aspects of an APN role, such as diagnostic and prescriptive authority, are not possible in Israel at this time. The master's program is based on a combination of the NP and CNS roles, taking into account the realities of the Israeli health-care system.

At present there is no formal standing in Israel for any of the ANP models. Program graduates assume roles in a variety of settings, using their increased knowledge and leadership capacities to clinically improve health care (B. Reznick and M. Rom, personal communication, March 10, 2008).

Oman

Oman is exploring the possibility of community nursing (CN) and community nurse practitioner (CNP) roles. Consultations, discussions, and reports of a successful nurse home-visiting project preceded WHO-EMRO–supported consultation services. External consultation and related recommendations advise that progressing to CN and CNP roles would be a logical approach to strengthen community health-care services in the country (Schober, 2007a).

However, difficulties have arisen as (a) physicians are emphatically lobbying the Ministry of Health for highly specialized nurses to assist them in specialty areas such as diabetic clinics, (b) there is a lack of qualified people to educate for and supervise community service provision, and (c) there is limited understanding of the reality of what services a CN or CNP could provide. Nurses in more remote area health centers are already providing NP-like services but lack the necessary advanced skills and qualifications. This is a major cause of concern for the director of nursing services at the Ministry of Health.

These dilemmas pose challenges for the Ministry of Health and nursing leaders as they consider options for ANP, while at the same time needing to address issues such as bridging the educational gaps of the current nursing workforce and meeting community health-care needs and the demands of the multidisciplinary workforce (Schober, 2007a).

Europe: WHO-EURO

The European Union (EU) is comprised of 27 culturally and linguistically different member states. By 2010, the total EU population had reached 501 million and approximately 20.1 million (4%) of the population were immigrants from non-EU countries (European Migration Network [EMN], 2011). The partner countries represent different histories and health-care systems as well as variations in nursing education and roles. In Europe nursing roles, including the advanced practice nursing (APN) roles, are connected with the historical and societal characteristics of each country. Due to the dominance of the public health-care sector in most of the European countries, APNs are rarely licensed, independent practitioners who practice autonomously.

The European countries are at different stages in implementing the APN roles. The development started in 1991, as the first NP educational program was introduced in the Royal College of Nurses in the United Kingdom (UK) (Sheer & Wong, 2008), thus catalyzing the development in the UK. In

Ireland, the first "advanced nurse practitioner" was accredited in 1996, and a career pathway toward advanced nursing practice was established following a Commission on Nursing in the late 1990s (National Council for the Professional Development of Nursing and Midwifery, 2005).

Currently, many European universities have established APN degree programs at the master's level. For example, the University Medical Center, Groningen in the Netherlands, has had a program since 1997 (Donato, 2009) with specialties on managing chronic illness, critical and intensive care, acute care, illness prevention, and psychiatric care. The University of Basel in Switzerland (a non-EU country) has had a program since 2000, with emphasis on managing chronic illness (Sheer & Wong, 2008). Finland and other Nordic countries have extensive experience with advanced collaboration between doctors and nurses in primary care health centers (Delamaire & Lafortune, 2010) and master's-level APN programs have been established since 2009 in several applied science universities.

After the political crises in Eastern Europe in the 1990s followed by the persecution in the Balkans, several Eastern European countries still have obstacles and severe financial problems in organizing health-care services and education (Wright et al., 2005). However, they are rapidly adopting new economic and political reforms that affect many sectors, including health care and advanced practice nursing (L. Loskinen, personal communication, July 12, 2011).

Finland

A physician shortage in Finland stimulated enhanced clinical roles for nurses in many municipalities and organizations. A Ministry of Education study in 2004 supported the need for APNs who could provide care and follow-up of patients with chronic illness. The APN role within secondary prevention will be increasingly important with an increase in the aging population.

Based on the ICN definition of NP/APN, the educational program is a part-time master's level lasting 2.5 years and was developed with a first cohort of 19 students. Curriculum for the program focuses on acute care, advanced nursing assessment, and follow-up for chronic diseases. The APN, known as a clinic expert nurse, is expected to be responsible for comprehensive patient care and treatment, and is also the first point of contact for acute health-care problems. Salaries and legislation continue to be addressed as these nurses in new roles take their place within the Finnish health-care system (ICN-APNetwork, 2007).

France

France is facing an increase in health-care needs similar to many other Western countries. Current characteristics challenging the health-care system in the country include aging of the population, significant increase in chronic disease, scarcity of medical services, and emerging absence of medical services in some regions. National strategies are being developed to respond to these challenges, including the introduction of advanced practice nurses.

As early as 2003 the report "Cooperation of the Health Professions: The Transfer of Tasks and Competencies" (Berland, 2003) listed strategies aimed at addressing the medical scarcity and envisioned the feasibility of the transfer of tasks in the French context. Pilot projects then followed. A series of reports ensued, allowing the *Haute Autorité de Santé (HAS)*, the French authority for health, to formulate recommendations in 2008 (HAS, 2008). **Table 5-3** lists strategies for the adaptation of health-care services to compensate for challenges associated with implementing APN roles.

Two leading health organizations, *Haute Autorité De Santé* (HAS) and *Observatoire National De La Demographie Des Professions De Santé* (ONDPS), appointed by the Minister of Health in 2007, formed a working group to explore future education for NPs, or *infirmiere cliniciennes,* and to generate recommendations. They examined how roles of health-care professionals may be redefined through

TABLE 5-3

Steps in Development of Advanced Practice Nursing in France

Year	Steps
2003	Berland Report: consideration of task transfer between medical and nonmedical health professionals
2004	First trials aiming to transfer medical activities to nonmedical health professionals (5 pilot projects)
2006	Second trials (10 new pilot projects and 3 renewed projects)
2007	Reports from a group of experts as to the modification of the fields of health professional competencies (focus: economic, legal, formation) of the *Haute Autorité de Santé (HAS)*
2007 (May/December)	Public consultation of the *HAS*, aiming to determine the functions between health professionals (334 testimonies)
2008	Recommendations of the *HAS* in the matter of the new cooperation between health professionals Mission: reflection around the sharing of tasks and the competencies between health professionals (report not circulated)
2009	Adoption of the law for the patient health territories hospitals, introducing the new cooperation between health professionals (article 51 and application texts) Launching of the first master's of science in clinical nursing intended for the education of advanced practice nurses *(EHESP/Université de la Méditerranée)*
2010	Circulation of the *HAS* guide manual: "New Cooperation Between Health Professionals" and Ministry of Health guide (DGOS) intended for health professionals wishing to write a protocol of new cooperation Reflections on the evolution of three clinical nursing specialties toward advanced practice in a framework to reestablish diplomas certified by the Ministry of Health Registration and instruction for the first files of the new cooperation by health professionals.
2011	Report related to midlevel professionals.

Source: C. Debout, personal communication, July 12, 2011. With permission.

the transfer of tasks and competencies with a view of improving care and adapting interventions to actual health-care demands (*HAS*, 2007). Preceding the formation of this working group, 5 research projects in dissimilar areas of the country had been completed and 10 additional projects concerning role redefinition followed (ICN-APNetwork, 2007).

Historically, although French nurses did acquire increased autonomy in 1978, they are still not considered a point of entry into the health-care system. Private practice nurses *(infirmières liberales)* depend on a medical order to deliver professional nursing care. Recognizing that the current arrangement of the health-care workforce will be inadequate to respond to future health-care needs, the health authorities considered alternatives that included implementation of APN roles. Capitalizing on this situation, the French nurses association (ANFIIDE) conducted a public information campaign on ANP, targeting nurses, authorities, and the public (Schober & Affara, 2006).

New cooperation: a model of substitution between medicine and advanced practice nurses The law "*Hôpitaux-Patients-Santé-Territories,*" voted in 2009, authorizes in a local way and by name more flexibility in the competencies of the medical and nonmedical health professions while introducing the concept of "new cooperation" (Article 51, 2009). See **Figure 5-1.**

While the question of transfer of activities of the medical profession toward the paramedical professions feeds the public debate, it is important to note that France is undecided about several structuring models. New cooperation, intermediary professions, and advanced practice nurses are three concepts that coexist currently without succeeding to be stable in France. Although the validation of a protocol of cooperation imposes on the "delegated" nurse to combine required competencies to implement the designated activities, no qualifying education is required currently from a regulatory perspective.

The processes of revision of the diplomas of specialties certified by the Ministry of Health The Ministry of Health engaged a vast project aimed at revising the competencies and the education programs for three clinical specialty diplomas that it currently certifies: pediatric nurse, surgical nurse, and nurse anesthesiologist. This project is in line with the vast reformation of nursing education that seeks reconciliation with the university-based model coming from the Bologne agreements.

Initially, this project will develop a competence framework for every function from a descriptive and retrospective analysis of the activities of the professionals in these positions. The intent is to adopt a long-term approach that anticipates the evolution of the functions and activities of the professions wherein they address the health needs of the public. Leaders representing the professional specialty organizations requested that the specialties be viewed as advanced practice and that the recommendations developed by this network guide the revision of both education and practice

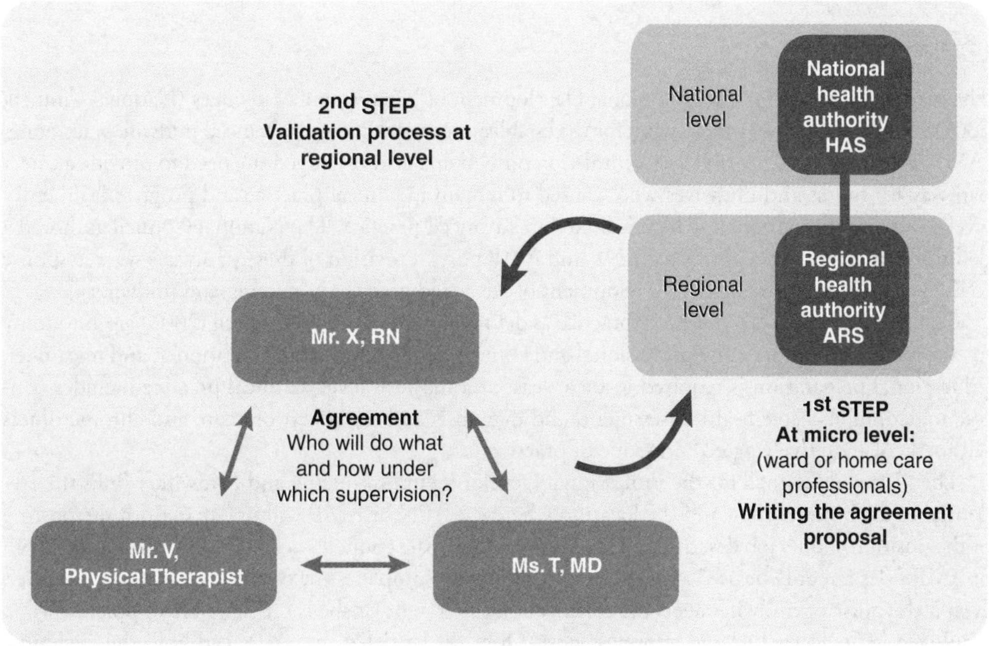

FIGURE 5-1 Visualizing the concept of "new cooperation" in the French law, "Hôpitaux-Patients-Santé-Territories."

(regulations, design of master's education, definition of autonomy). The negotiations related to the various points of view are in process, and decisions should be made in 2011 (C. Debout, personal communication, July 10, 2011).

Toward intermediary professions A report relating to the new intermediary-level health professions, published in 2011, defines the characteristics of the advanced practice nurse in France (Henard et al., 2011). As of July 2011, no political decision had been made to establish the recommendations proposed in this report.

A master of science in clinical nursing The first master in science for clinical nursing was launched in 2009 jointly by the department of nursing sciences and the paramedical section of *l'Ecole de Hautes Etudes en Santé Publique (EHESP)* and *l'Université de la Méditerranée* (faculty of medicine). This program, a forerunner in France in the domain of the education of advanced practice nurses, rests on a vision of advanced practice nursing in the international context but specific to France. Currently three specialties are proposed: oncology, gerontology, and coordinator of complex healthcare conditions.

Unresolved issues When examining the position of France, key words such as "protected title", "qualifying education", and "specific regulations", often associated with the APN roles are not observable. The methodology in the framework for the protocols of cooperation, while showing a response to local needs, makes development of national competencies difficult. Currently, no qualification is required to function as an APN other than a diploma verifying preparation to work as a nurse.

In addition, it is currently possible for any French university to develop programs for master's-level education. No national directive exists in relation to this. What is needed is a national position to stabilize the APN concept and a defined regulatory process, including both education and practice. Reports to date indicate that France is moving in that direction (C. Debout, personal communication, July 12, 2011).

Ireland

The National Council for the Professional Development of Nursing and Midwifery (National Council, 2001) in Ireland provides a framework for the establishment of APN and advanced midwife practitioner (AMP) roles and posts. In 1998, a Commission on Nursing acknowledged the need to provide a career pathway for nurses and midwives who wanted to remain in clinical practice and progress from entry level to clinical specialization, which is linked to advanced practice. The National Council authored a definition and core concepts for the ANP and AMP posts. Provision of these pathways was a response to the national and international development of advanced practice in nursing and midwifery.

Core concepts for ANP and AMP practice as defined by the National Council (2001) are autonomy in clinical practice, pioneering professional and clinical leadership, expert practitioner, and researcher. Educational preparation is required to be at least at a master's level. Clinical practice includes conducting comprehensive health assessment, and diagnosis and treatment of acute and chronic illness within a collaboratively agreed on scope of practice.

The National Council for the Professional Development of Nursing and Midwifery links the credential to a job description and the location where the APN or AMP will practice. Both the posting of the position and its job description require approval by the council's accreditation committee. ANP or AMP titles can only be used after the nurse or midwife completes the certification process; however, even if the nurse or midwife meets the certification criteria, he or she is only eligible to practice when employed in an accredited and approved post. Once credentialed, the APN can hold the credential so long as he or she continues to work at the approved post in the designated specialty (Schober & Affara, 2006).

Netherlands

As of May 2011, there were approximately 2,000 NPs working in the Netherlands in all fields, including general practice. Since 2002, there have been bachelor's and master's programs for nursing education. Currently, there are master's programs in nine cities with waiting lists for potential students to enter the NP programs.

The shortage of physicians that prompted the introduction of NP roles in the Netherlands has been resolved, but the numbers of NPs continue to increase in contrast to physician assistant (PA) numbers. At one point it was thought that the introduction of PAs would threaten NP development, but this has not been the case.

NPs have been accepted as professionals providing high-quality care and friendly advice. Each year the government financially supports the education of 250 new NP students, funding 20% of their salary and the cost of their preceptors. Legislation including title protection, prescriptive authority, and practice autonomy is almost realized, and as of May 2011 was in the Senate awaiting final approval.

In 2008, the national description of the NP was authorized, resulting in the opening of an official national register. NPs that are registered with the option for prescribing will be allowed to work independently from physicians. In this capacity the NP will be responsible for a clearly defined patient load. Nurse practitioners who graduated before 2006 will need to be reassessed and complete an additional pharmacology course. The financial structure in the country is not yet accustomed to NP services, but the insurance companies are becoming more powerful and supportive of the ANP model. It is envisioned that they will contract directly with NPs in the future (P. Roodbol, personal communication, May 23, 2011).

Sweden

Sweden is exploring the use of NPs as a strategy to improve access to PHC, including care of the elderly in the community. Educational programs have been established with these clinical foci in mind.

In Skaraborg, the PHC authorities worked with the University of Skovde to develop a model and educational program that met the requirements of the National Board of Health and Welfare. Community PHC, care of the elderly, and the NP as the vehicle to address these needs was the primary consideration (Schober & Affara, 2006).

The initial batch of students enrolled in 2003 faced challenges to introduce a new nursing role that fits the Swedish health-care system and is acceptable to all stakeholders. In the process, a definition for the ANP was negotiated (Schober & Affara, 2006, p. 6):

> *An Advanced Nurse Practitioner in Primary Health Care is a registered nurse with special education as a district nurse with the right to prescribe certain drugs, and with a post graduate education that enables [the advanced nurse practitioner] an increased and deepened competence to be independently responsible for medical decisions, prescribing of drugs and treatment of health problems within a certain area of health care.*

It is interesting to note that prescriptive authority for nurses in Sweden was in place approximately 10 years before the consideration and development of ANP.

Switzerland

The Institute of Nursing Science (INS) at the University of Basel, Switzerland, introduced course material including formal clinical assessment, physical examination skills, and clinical reasoning for bachelor nursing education in 2001. As of 2006, six universities of applied science either offer or plan to offer the BSN degree including similar content (ICN-APNetwork, 2007). Such changes are significant for APN development as moving from diploma-based education to the BSN will provide a stronger foundation for the generalist nurse and thus a sounder educational background for APN studies.

The INS at the University of Basel has also invested in ANP through a master's degree in nursing science, research, and clinical development activities. The momentum to create APN positions originated with insightful nurse leaders who could envision an advanced nursing role and physicians who showed interest in working with nurses with higher levels of clinical skills. Exploration of ANP coincides with a general call for nurses to expand their role functions in anticipation of a physician shortage. In the absence of a clear model for nursing evolution, this change could mimic the PA as opposed to the APN. Enlightened decision makers hope to strengthen nursing at this challenging time. However, it should be noted that the drive to ANP development is occurring in the absence of a framework that addresses regulatory, educational, practice, or reimbursement issues (Schober & Affara, 2006).

United Kingdom (England, Northern Ireland, Scotland, and Wales)

Within the United Kingdom, the countries of England, Northern Ireland, Scotland, and Wales are developing advanced nursing practice in different ways. White (2001) describes the emergence of the NP movement in the United Kingdom as a response to the changing demands within health-care systems and acknowledgment that the traditional medical model alone is not sufficient to provide comprehensive health care for community populations.

A reduction in doctors' hours and an overall shortage of general practitioners in some areas accelerated the move toward NPs in acute-and primary-care settings. In addition, government-initiated pilot programs to address the needs of special groups, such as refugees, the homeless, the mentally ill, traveling families, and the elderly, increased the use of NPs and provision of services in a range of settings. All of these changes must be seen in the context of the Labour and subsequent Conservative/Liberal Democrat coalition, a demand for government's modernization of health service, and the expectation of clinical effectiveness and high service quality.

The year 2002 represented a milestone in NP roles, celebrating the 10th anniversary of the first graduates from the Royal College of Nursing (RCN) NP program. The initial 15 graduates paved the way for NPs now practicing throughout the United Kingdom. The NP degree program, originally developed by the RCN in 1990, formed the basis for RCN accreditation of NP programs, using 15 standards and associated criteria as the basis for approval (RCN, 2008). Currently, seven universities have used this framework to explicitly demonstrate the quality of their programs. Different pathways of preparation exist, ranging from a generic approach to a more specific focus including primary, acute, emergency, pediatrics, neonatal, and cancer care. However, as demand for NPs and APNs increases, the number of universities providing such programs has escalated. For example, the Association of Advanced Nursing Practice Educators (AANPE) now has 43 higher education institutions in its membership from across the UK (AANPE, 2007). Though there may not be fully developed ANP programs in each of these institutions, this is a huge demonstration of interest.

NPs are present in all types of health-care settings, including general practice, walk-in centers, accident and emergency units, and many other hospital-based specialties. NP practice in the United Kingdom includes diagnosis with prescribing rights, which increasingly include prescription of medication. The move, originating in England, to enable nurses to undergo a specified nonmedical prescribing program has resulted in over 10,000 nurses who are now classed as *independent prescribers,* and as a consequence, can prescribe almost everything from the British National Formulary (Nursing and Midwifery Council [NMC], 2006).

This has resulted in NPs being able to deliver more autonomous care and greatly opens up the opportunities for NP innovation; however, it is worth noting that not all nurses classed as independent prescribers are NPs.

Despite all this activity, regulation of NP practice has not yet been introduced into the United Kingdom. In 2007, the Nursing and Midwifery Council (NMC) submitted proposals to the Department of Health for regulation of ANPs to provide greater public protection (NMC, 2007). Within their proposals, it is notable that the NMC has used the term *ANP* to make explicit the level of practice that should be expected from a nurse working in this role.

The term *advanced nurse practitioner* has been adopted by many NPs and is now the preferred term. The NMC proposal was scrutinized by the Department of Health and the Council for Healthcare Regulatory Excellence (CHRE, 2010). It was concluded that there was insufficient grounds for additional regulation for NPs who were already registered as nurses. Despite this, debate on the need for regulation of advanced nursing practice continues (K. Maclaine, personal communication, June 13, 2011).

Southeast Asia: WHO-SEARO

Thailand

The Nursing Council of Thailand adopted the ANP concept in 1998, and in 2003, the first group of 49 APNS was certified and awarded the title APN. There are five specialties for certification: medical/surgical, pediatrics, maternal/child, community, and psychiatric/mental health (ICN-APNetwork, 2007).

In response to an urgent need for community health-care services, the country identified short- and long-term goals to offer 4-month education programs for general NPs to work in the community as primary care providers. Even though one of the first postbasic NP programs was established in the 1970s, it was health-care reform and the drive for a universal health-care coverage system, implemented in the country in 2002, that accelerated the development of NP educational programs.

To develop strategic planning for enhancing capacity among NPs, a study was conducted by Hanucharurnkul, Suwisith, Piasue, and Terathongkum (2007) that explored characteristics and work settings of 1,928 NPs and provided a picture of those certified by the Thailand Nursing and Midwifery Council. Strategies derived from this study are as follows:

- Extend within 5 years the entry-level education to a master's level by acknowledging the 4-month programs that were originally initiated to respond to PHC needs of the country.
- Establish NP positions in the health-care system such that when APNs are master's graduates and certified, they would be eligible for the title of APN/MN (midwife nurse) and have an associated increase in salary.

Findings are consistent with those in other illustrations in this chapter that confirm the perceived usefulness of the NP role. However, at times NPs were functioning at levels beyond their defined scopes of practice; their position were not adequately distinguished from those of other nurses; and administrators did not support them sufficiently.

Western Pacific: WHO-WPRO

Australia

Australia first considered the development of nurse practitioner (NP) roles in 1990 (Offredy, 1999). Pilot projects were conducted first in New South Wales (NSW) and then in most other states and territories of Australia. The results from the initial projects support the findings that NPs are feasible, safe, and effective in their ability to provide high-quality health-care services in a range of settings (NSW Health Department, 1998; Gardner & Gardner, 2005).

In Australia, the NP title is protected and only nurses who have been authorized by the National Nursing and Midwifery Registration Board of the Australian Health Practitioner Regulation Agency may use the NP title. A study by Gardner and colleagues (2006b) recommended the master's degree as the required educational preparation for the role from two perspectives. Findings suggested that a master's education is needed to meet the demands of the role and to also provide the necessary credibility with the community and other health-care disciplines, regarding the professional standing of these clinicians. The new national registration board adopted this recommendation and mandates that a specific master's for the NP is the minimal level of education required to practice.

The Nursing and Midwifery Board of Australia (Board) has two pathways for nurses to fulfill their educational requirements at the master's level for endorsement as an NP:

1. Nurses who have successfully completed a Board-approved nurse practitioner program of study at the master's level
2. Nurses who have completed a program of study at the master's level that is clinically relevant to the nurses' context of advanced practice nursing for which they are seeking endorsement as a nurse practitioner and supplementary education that demonstrates equivalence and meets the national competency standards for a nurse practitioner

Having the two educational pathways provides flexibility for nurses to choose an educational program that best meets their individual learning needs (A. Green, personal communication, July 18, 2011).

The Mutual Recognition Act of 1992 and the Trans Tasman Mutual Recognition Act of 1999 recognize nurses educated in all states of Australia and those educated in New Zealand, regardless of differences within programs. In 2004, the Australian Nursing and Midwifery Council (ANMC) in conjunction with the Nursing Council of New Zealand commissioned a project to develop competency standards for the NP to further ensure delivery of safe and competent care (Gardner et al., 2006a). These competency standards are now used to assess NPs educated overseas and by the Australian Nursing and Midwifery Accreditation Council (ANMAC, 2010) for accrediting universities and nurse practitioner master's programs.

In 2011, there were more than 400 endorsed NPs in Australia. A recent study (Gardner et al, 2010) found that two-thirds of NPs in Australia reported their role was "extremely limited" because of a difference between state and federal governmental laws. These results were similar to those from an earlier survey undertaken in 2009 (Gardner et al). Until late 2010, NPs were able to write prescriptions and refer patients to other health-care professionals at a state level; however, at a federal level, NPs did not have access to the pharmaceutical benefits scheme (PBS) or the Medicare benefits schedule (MBS). This resulted in patients having to pay a premium when their prescription was filled at a pharmacy or when they had pathology tests undertaken, placing these patients at a disadvantage because they did not have equal access to government subsidies for health care. In November 2010, national legislation was enacted to enable nurse practitioners to obtain provider numbers, potentially reducing costs to patients. To date this legislation is primarily limited to nurse practitioners in private practice but the initiative is likely to improve access for all patients of nurse practitioners within the next few years (A. Gardner, personal communication, June 23, 2011).

In Australia, NPs are steadily being introduced throughout the country, while continuing to face country-specific challenges. The Australian College of Nurse Practitioners (http://www.acnp.org.au/) has been established to provide a representative voice for NP role development in Australia (A. Green, personal communication, July 18, 2011).

Brunei Darussalam

The Nursing Services Department, Ministry of Health, Brunei Darussalam is proceeding forward in exploring advanced nursing practice (ANP) for the nurses in Brunei and for the health-care services in the country. To motivate the nurses and provide a strategic action plan to the Minister of Health, a workshop and symposium were held in July 2011 to gain an understanding of ANP as the practice is positioned for the future of the public. A resolution and recommendations have been presented to the Minister for development of a nursing career pathway for clinical practice along with organization of a task force to promulgate criteria, standards, and regulations for ANP. Debate has been focused around alignment of nurse practitioner roles with nurse-midwives under the ANP umbrella, as well as clarification of where the specialist nurse fits in the future scheme for Brunei Darussalam (M. Schober, site visit, July 2, 2011).

Hong Kong, China

Hong Kong has been pursuing the concept of the APN/NP for many years, while facing complicated governmental, clinical, and academic challenges. Although there is evidence of strong nurse-led clinics at Queen Elizabeth Hospital, educational initiatives have found it difficult to coordinate appropriate didactic courses and clinical practicua for advanced roles. Hong Kong has still to find a champion for APN roles to catch a foothold within the health-care systems.

The Hospital Authority of Hong Kong, eager to motivate nurses to remain in clinical practice, introduced the nurse specialist position in 1994. The introduction of new nursing roles without regulatory oversight resulted in uneven clinical, education, and research development (Chang & Wong, 2001). Development for APNs continues to be linked to the enhancement of basic nursing education and efforts by the Hong Kong Hospital Authority to introduce a new grading structure and career ladder intended to improve the clinical focus for nursing (Schober & Affara, 2006).

Islands of the Western Pacific (Fiji and Samoa)

NPs and other midlevel practitioners have provided health-care services for the populations of the Pacific Island countries for more than 20 years. The rural and remote nature of this region and a shortage of physicians encouraged governments to explore the most appropriate models to provide comprehensive health-care services. Demographics help determine the best approach for the Pacific Islands in initiating education and practice guidelines for NPs. Reasons for educating nurses for NP roles in the Pacific Islands include the following (WHO—Western Pacific Region [WPR], 2001):

- Nurses are already present in the workforce of most countries and usually compose the largest category of health professionals.
- Nurses are currently living and working in underserved areas.
- Nurses are providing a wide range of preventive and curative services.
- Nurses are considered to be an adaptable, multitalented resource of the workforce.

Strategies recommended by WHO-WPR for developing and sustaining a midlevel practitioner workforce include the following (WHO-WPR, 2001):

- Legal protection
- Standard treatment guidelines
- Ongoing clinical supervision
- Continuing education
- Career structure or career ladder

Fiji

Fiji is made up of over 300 islands, with over 60% of the population living in rural or remote settings. Through an arrangement of health centers and nursing stations, authorities have attempted to address health-care challenges by providing preventive and PHC services supported by subdivisional and referral hospitals.

Staffing of facilities has been a major problem, especially in rural and remote areas. In 1988, an NP program was developed in response to this difficulty. The Fiji School of Nursing is the base for the NP program, admitting RNs and nurse-midwives. The first NPs graduated in 1999; in March 2007, the fourth class completed their academic program and progressed to a 6-month internship. The program has now become regional, including nurses from Tonga and the Marshall Islands. The immediacy of health-care needs prohibited education at the master's level initially, but efforts are being made to increase educational levels. Part of this strategy is enhancing the educational level of the program faculty through a cooperative program with James Cook University in Australia.

NPs in Fiji have an established scope of practice and work under published protocols, allowing them prescriptive privileges. Postings for positions are listed by the Public Service Commission, with most NPs employed by the Ministry of Health. These nurses have been widely accepted by communities and other health-care providers. There is strong support from the directors of health services to continue the educational program. Access to continuing education and career pathways are among the challenges facing NPs in Fiji (ICN-APNetwork, 2007).

Samoa

Education for nurse specialist practice in Samoa is a year of postgraduate study following a generalist nurse preparation. Clinical practice for a nurse specialist reflects in-depth knowledge and relevant skills that are focused on a specific area of nursing and directed toward a defined population or a defined area of activity. Specialist practice may occur at any point along a continuum, from beginning to advanced.

Nurse specialists are considered to be APNs, with practice focusing on health assessment and clinical decision making. Physicians are consulted or accept referrals for confirmation of findings and prescribing of medications. Currently nurses prescribe in life-threatening situations, but the nursing law is being reviewed with respect to wider prescribing rights. Mental health specialist nurses provide community-based family-focused services with minimal assistance from the volunteer part-time psychiatrist. This service is totally developed and steered by a nurse consultant and her small team of nurses (I. Enoka, personal communication, April 1, 2008).

New Zealand

ANP was initially recognized in 1988 at two levels in New Zealand. The New Zealand Nurses' Organization's (NZNO's) credentialing process certified nurses as nurse-clinicians or nurse consultants (clinical). Once the NP model was introduced in 2000, NZNO phased out and ceased its certification process in 2006, when regulation of NPs came under the jurisdiction of the Nursing Council of New Zealand (S. Trim, personal communication, March 11, 2008).

A task force established in 1997 studied barriers to nursing practice and recommended the development of an advanced role. The Nursing Council of New Zealand (NCNZ) then set up a working group to develop a regulatory framework. Following significant consultation, a framework was agreed on and published (NCNZ, 2001). The framework includes standards for the approval of specific master's programs and process for such approval, a title (NP), competencies, and a description of the role and a process for endorsement. The role was defined as follows (NCNZ, 2001, p. 9):

> *A Nurse Practitioner is a registered nurse practicing at an advanced practice level in a specific scope of practice, who has been recognized at Master's level of education and has been recognized and approved by the Nursing Council as a Nurse Practitioner.*

The New Zealand NP model is depicted in **Figure 5-2.**
The requirements for endorsement are as follows:

- Completion of an approved master's program (or approved equivalent)
- A minimum of 4 years of clinical experience in a specific specialty area
- Successful assessment against the NP competencies by an approved panel, which includes an NP (or clinical specialist if there are no NPs in the specialty area of practice) and an experienced medical clinician in the same specialty

The applicant formally applies to the council and must present a portfolio that includes a curriculum vitae, transcript of education preparation, research, publications, and evidence of clinical practice that includes descriptions, case studies, case notes from assessments, and endorsements of practice. The panel interview includes a presentation by the applicant describing relevant clinical practice and a response to panel questions that include clinical vitae and scenario testing (M. Clark, personal communication, March 4, 2008).

The first NP in New Zealand was endorsed in late 2001, and initially title protection was achieved through trademarking. Following the enactment of the Health Practitioners Competence Assurance Act of 2003, the Nursing Council of New Zealand established a part of its official register for NPs, and formally stated, as required under the legislation, the following description of the role (New Zealand Government, 2004, p. 2959):

> *Nurse Practitioners are expert nurses who work within a specific area of practice incorporating advanced knowledge and skills. They practice both independently and in collaboration with other*

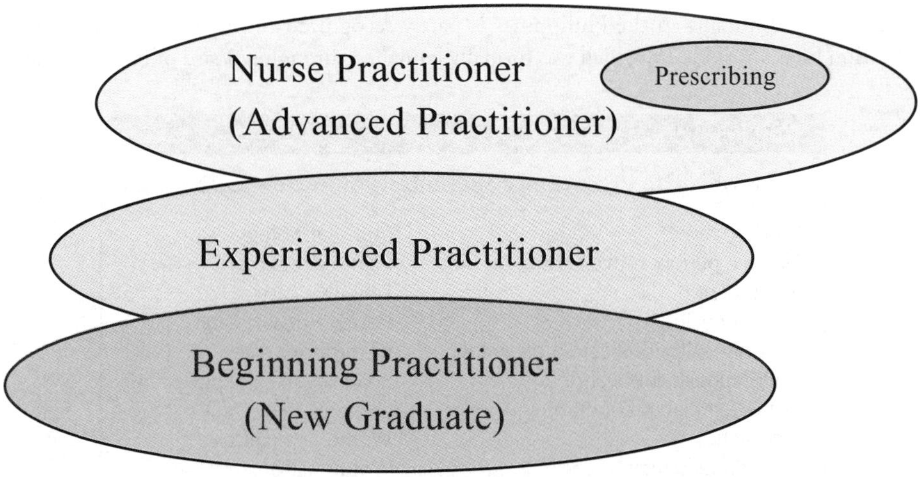

FIGURE 5-2 The New Zealand Framework is depicted in an illustration that portrays a view of the stages of practice that a nurse pursues to become an NP. *(Adapted from Nursing Council of New Zealand, with permission.)*

health care professionals to promote health, prevent disease and to diagnose, assess and manage people's health needs. They provide a wide range of assessment and treatment interventions, including differential diagnoses, ordering, conducting and interpreting diagnostic and laboratory tests and administering therapies for the management of potential or actual health needs. They work in partnership with individuals, families, whanau *(indigenous health workers) and communities across a range of settings. Nurse Practitioners may choose to prescribe medicines within their specific area of practice. Nurse Practitioners also demonstrate leadership as consultants, educators, managers and researchers and actively participate in professional activities, and in local and national policy development.*

NPs choose their area of practice (scope of practice), which is placed on the register as a condition. This is done to reflect the New Zealand legislation. **Table 5-4** provides details on specialized areas (scopes of practice) in New Zealand.

A report released by the Ministry of Health for district health boards outlined the future use of NPs (New Zealand Ministry of Health, 2002). A variety of activities to assess and provide visibility for advanced practice continue to be in progress. The Nurse Practitioner Advisory Committee of New Zealand, composed of four professional groups (NZNO, National Council of Maori Nurses, College of Nurses Aotearoa, and Australia New Zealand College of Mental Health Nurses), is driving the implementation of the role.

In 1999, an amendment to the Medicines Act of 1981 enabled the government to issue regulations allowing prescribing for "designated prescribers," and thus set a pathway for nurses to prescribe. This was followed in 2002 by regulations to allow NPs to prescribe in child health and aged care. These regulations were very restrictive and only one NP (a U.S. citizen qualified NP in child health) obtained the right to prescribe under them. Extensive lobbying by the profession resulted in much broader regulations in 2005, which allowed all NPs who are authorized by the Council to prescribe from an extensive formulary following established and published criteria (*New Zealand Gazette,* November 10, 2005).

The uptake of NPs has been slower than expected but seems to be gaining momentum. As of May 2011 there were 96 NPs in New Zealand (P. Maybee, ICN conference presentation, Malta, May 12, 2011).

Philippines

Advanced practice nursing in the Philippines is partly recognized through the Nursing Specialty Certification Program (NSCP), which was formally launched through a Board of Nursing resolution

TABLE 5-4

Areas of Nurse Practitioner Specialization in New Zealand

Cardiac care	Ophthalmology
Elective perioperative care	Pain management
Aging care	Palliative care
Mental health	Primary health care
Mental health/intellectual disability	Respiratory care
Child/adolescent health	Solid organ transplantation
Diabetes/related conditions	Urology
Emergency	Women's health
High dependency	Wound care
Neonatal care	

M. Clark, personal communication, March 4, 2008.

in 1999 (Board of Nursing Resolution, 2002). Nursing leaders introduced the Nursing Specialty Certification Council, which credentials nurses and accredits organizations and educational programs highlighting the practice of specialized nursing. This is further enforced through the Comprehensive Nursing Specialty Program stipulated under the Philippine Nursing Law of 2002. Qualified nurses may be given certification in three levels: Nurse Clinician I, Nurse Clinician II, and Clinical Nurse Specialist, and may work under four major groups of Nursing Specialties: Medical-Surgical, Community Health, Maternal and Child Health, and Mental Health/Psychiatry (Philippine Board of Nursing, 2008).

These policies provide for an informal category of nurses working in specialty areas across secondary, tertiary, and specialty hospitals. These nurses may or may not be credentialed under the NSCP. Most of these nurses are prepared through formal or informal education within their home institutions.

Currently, there is no policy that formalizes the position of an "advanced practice nurse" in the Philippines; neither are there explicit standards of practice for those who may be working as "advanced practice nurses." In most health institutions, the generalist and specialty area nurses have the same job descriptions, with a similar sense of patient and professional accountability. These developments provide the motivation to formulate an APN framework in the Philippines that would define systems, scopes, and standards of practice, and ultimately contribute to better health for the public (V. Manila, personal communication, July 26, 2010).

There are a large number of baccalaureate entry-level programs for nursing in the Philippines, with an emphasis on education for export of its graduates, not only to the United States, but even more to the Middle East. In the midst of this situation, we find many master's degree programs in nursing, and at least three well-established nursing doctoral programs in the Philippines.

Singapore

The National University of Singapore, under the auspices of the Yong Loo Lin School of Medicine, established an APN program in Singapore in 2003, offering an academic preparation in acute care, adult health, and mental health, while viewing the course of studies as generic in emphasis. The fifth group of APNs graduated in 2010. As of 2011 specialty offerings have now extended to critical care and oncology/palliative care. Following graduation from the 2-year master's program, students must complete a 1-year internship in their specialty before applying for certification and registration with the Singapore Nursing Board (SNB). Registration to practice as an APN is renewed on an annual basis with the SNB.

The APN Register established in 2005 by the Ministry for Health is expected to help with the systemic development of this category of clinical nurse, educated to a master's level in nursing, in becoming a key player in Singapore's drive to keep health care affordable while maintaining high-quality services. Consistent with this view and to support developing professionalism for nursing, the Ministry of Health established a clinical nursing career path for the APN, similar to the career paths that exist for management and education.

Key decision makers in education, policy, and administration are working to adapt models and frameworks from the United States, while at the same time attempting to introduce APN roles to the public that are suitable for hospital and community settings in the country. Visibility and support for this advancement in nursing is evidenced up to the Ministry of Health level, where a request has been made to have 200 APNs in place in various specialties in Singapore by 2014 (M. Schober, on site, 2011).

South Korea

It could be said that NP-like nursing roles have been in place in Korea since the time of the "medicine lady" in the 15th century. Care provided by the medicine ladies included deliveries, physical examinations, acupuncture, and prescribing of herbal medicines (J. Kang, personal communication, November 15, 2007).

Community health nurse practitioners (CHNPs) have been providing comprehensive primary health-care services in rural communities of South Korea since the health-care law for provision of health care for rural residents was legislated in 1980. CHNPs provide PHC to approximately 28% of the rural population in South Korea; however, this number is decreasing because it is more difficult to attract nurses to work in the rural areas (J. Tang, personal communication, November 15, 2007).

Haho Clinic, located 2 hours from Seoul between Yoju and Ichon, has provided clinic services for the community and the surrounding area since 1985. The scope of practice for the CHNPs includes diagnosis, prescriptive authority, and referral to other practitioners. In addition, home visits, health education, disease management, immunizations, school health services, and care for the elderly are part of the health-care service provision with additional support from nurses and community helpers. The nurse specialist system was formalized in Korea to fulfill changes in the medical environment. Anesthesia, public health, mental health, and home health-care nurses are approved for practice under the Medical Service Law. A special law for agriculture approves the CHNP for practice as a nurse specialist.

Discussions attempting to clarify issues related to APNs began in the 1990s. In 2003, the medical law revision identified qualifications for the APN and designated 13 areas of specialization. Qualifications include master's-level education, passage of the certification examination, and experience in a chosen specialty. The first certification examination was given in 2005 (J. Kang, personal communication, 2007). As in many countries, the Korean Nurses Association faces difficulty obtaining consensus from the nursing community on scope of practice, educational requirements, and titling (Schober & Affara, 2006).

Taiwan

Taiwan has a long history of nursing education and practice evolving from apprenticeship hospital-based programs to academic professional education in institutions of higher learning. Following the country's release from Japanese rule in 1945, nursing rapidly evolved in its development of university programs. The first master's of science (MS) program was started in 1979, with the first doctoral program in nursing offered in 1997.

In 1990 "nurse practitioners" were listed along with "professional nurse" as a legal position in nursing. In 1991 the Nurses Act was passed in an attempt to alleviate the nursing shortage and allow nurses to practice independently. Nurse practitioner programs were started in 2000 after an amendment to the Nurses Act made the "nurse practitioner" title official (Yu-Mei Chao [YU], 2008).

Nurse practitioners have been educated in hospital training programs since the 1990s in an attempt to alleviate the shortage of physicians and lessen their workload. However, the NPs were functioning at first without guidelines and standards. The Department of Health (DOH), in conjunction with the National Health Research Institute (NHRI) and the Taiwan Association of Nurse Practitioners (TANP), has established standards for approving programs, curriculum guidelines, and preceptor guidelines. NP preparation remains predominantly based in hospitals with the faculty made up of physicians and health providers from other disciplines, and the education focused on the medical and surgical domains.

The main work settings for NPs are in acute care hospitals with some positions in emergency room and ambulatory care settings. Continuing education is required for an NP to apply for a 6-year extension of the certification period. As of 2008 there were 857 certified NPs in Taiwan. Similar to other countries, certified NPs in Taiwan are seeking additional academic preparation to achieve professional status and credibility in their work settings and among professional colleagues. Several schools of nursing within universities are responding by offering master's-level NP programs. Additional universities are offering post-NP certificate transition programs toward a master's in nursing (R. Goodyear, personal communication, June 13, 2011).

In a country with a national health insurance system that enrolls 99% of its citizens, it is estimated that there will be a health problem associated with an increase in the aging population expected to escalate to 4.76 million by 2026 (Shiow-Luan Tsay & Su-Zhen Kuo, 2008). Health promotion, disease prevention, integrated health care, and chronic disease management are all areas of upcoming need that will be addressed by nurses with advanced knowledge and skills. Advanced practice nursing has a beginning with guidelines that have been established to ensure that nursing graduates will have sound preparation to provide quality care in Taiwan.

CONCLUSION

In reviewing country illustrations, it appears that research and description of APN development confirms the usefulness of ANP and supports the view that these nursing roles are feasible, sustainable, and able to provide high-quality, competent health care. Legislation and regulations often lag behind actual practice; disagreement exists among practice acts; and progression presents as more of an intricate maze or puzzle than a picture of coordinated forward motion. International momentum supportive of ANP services is increasing; however, NP and APN initiatives are fraught with frustrations, obstacles, and challenges as leaders attempt to activate schemes that will ultimately change the profile of the health-care workforce and delivery systems worldwide. Role ambiguity and confusion regarding titling, scope of practice, educational preparation, and credentialing continue to present obstacles that must be addressed. A consistent definition and related terminology will enhance possibilities for sound standards for credentialing and legislation, an essential component to legitimatizing the ANP concept globally.

For ANP to thrive in health systems, the author believes that a number of areas related to role development need to be confronted and managed successfully. This includes being able to embrace the diversity of health-care systems worldwide without losing ANP core characteristics and reaching international consensus on a scope of practice founded on the core values of nursing. A well-developed scope of practice engages APNs in a wide range of activities, including advocacy, health planning, and policy development, in addition to health promotion, disease prevention, and diagnosis and treatment of illness.

Challenges lie in the capacity of ANP advocates and implementers to achieve consistency across clinical and educational models. Continually evaluating and reviewing practice by adding new competencies that reflect dynamic changes in health care will be essential. Finally, APNs will be asked to provide evidence that they are a cost-effective, valued, and sustainable addition to health-care teams and provision of services. Evidence that demonstrates the ability to provide care in partnership with patients and their families, within communities, and in collaboration with other health-care professionals will provide a strong foundation for an innovative addition to comprehensive health-care services.

REFERENCES

Affara, F. A. (2006). *SWOT analysis in relation to advanced nursing practice becoming recognized as a valid part of nursing and health care provision globally.* Retrieved June 13, 2011, from http://www.icn-apnetwork.org.

Article 51. (July 21, 2009). *Portant réforme de l'hôpital et relative aux patients, à la santé et aux territories.* loi #2009-879.

Association of Advanced Nursing Practice Educators. (2007). *Membership census autumn 2007: Advanced nursing practice courses results.* Retrieved January 10, 2008, from www.aanpe.org/AANPHome/tabid/448/Default.aspx.

Australian Nursing and Midwifery Accreditation Council. (2010). Retrieved May 13, 2011, from http://www.nursingmidwiferyboard.gov.au/Accreditation.aspx.

Berland, Y. (2003). Mission: Cooperation des professions de santé: le transfert de taches et de competences. Rapport d'etape presente par le Professeur Yvon Berland.

Board of Nursing Resolution. (2002). *Nursing specialty certification program BON RES. NO. 14 s 1999* and *Guidelines for implementation BON RES. No. 118-s 2002.* Manila: PRC Printing Office.

Bryant, R. (2005). *Regulation, roles and competency development* (ICN global nursing review initiative Issue paper No. 1). Retrieved February 25, 2008, from www.icn.ch/global/Issue1Regulation.pdf.

Bryant-Lukosius, D., & DiCenso, A. (2004). A framework for the introduction and evaluation of advanced practice nursing roles. *Journal of Advanced Nursing, 48*(5), 530–540.

Buchan, J., & Calman, L. (2005). *Skill-mix and policy change in the health workforce: Nurses in advanced roles.* (Working paper). Retrieved February 25, 2008, from www.oecd.org/dataoecd/30/28/33857785.pdf.

Buchan, J., & Calman, L. (2009). *Implementing nurse prescribing* (Monograph No. 25). Geneva: ICN.

Canadian Nurses Association. (2006). *Canadian nurse practitioner initiative: Implementation and evaluation toolkit for nurse practitioners in Canada.* Ottawa, Ontario: Author.

Canadian Nurses Association. (2008). *Advanced nursing practice: A national framework.* Ottawa, Ontario: Author.

Canadian Nurses Association. (2009a). *Recommendations of the Canadian nurse practitioner initiative: Progress report.* Ottawa: Author.

Canadian Nurses Association. (2009b). *Clinical nurse specialist* [position statement]. Ottawa: Author.

Chang, K. P. K., & Wong, T. (2001). The nurse specialist role in Hong Kong: Perceptions of nurse specialists. *Journal of Advanced Nursing, 36*(1), 32–40.

Council for Healthcare Regulatory Excellence. (August, 2010). *Right-touch regulation.* London, United Kingdom: Author.

Delamaire, M., & Lafortune, G. (2010). *Nurses in advanced roles: A description and evaluation of experiences in 12 OECD countries.* OECD Health Working Paper No. 54. Retrieved July 12, 2011, from www.oecd.org/els/health/workingpapers.

DiCenso, A. (2008). Roles, research and resilience: The evolution of advanced practice nursing. *Canadian Nurse, 104*(9), 37–40.

DiCenso, A., & Bryant-Lukosius, D., et al (December, 2010). Clinical nurse specialists and nurse practitioners in Canada: A decision support synthesis. *Nursing Leadership,* 23(Special Issue), 15-34.

Donato, A. S. (2009). Nurse practitioners in Holland: Definition, preparation, and prescriptive authority. *Journal of the American Academy of Nurse Practitioners, 21*(11), 585–587.

European Migration Network. (2011). Retrieved July 3, 2011, from http://emn.intrasoftintl.com/Downloads/prepareShowFiles.do?entryTitle=2%2E%20Annual%20Reports%20on%20Asylum%20and%20Migration%20Statistics.

Gardner, G., Carryer, J., Gardner, A., & Dunn, S. (2006a). Nurse practitioner competency standards: Findings from collaborative Australian and New Zealand research. *International Journal of Nursing Studies, 43*(5), 601–610.

Gardner, G., Dunn, S., Carryer, J., & Gardner, A. (2006b). Competency and capability: Imperative for nurse practitioner education. *Australian Journal of Advanced Nursing, 24*(1), 8–14.

Gardner, A., & Gardner, G. (2005). A trial of nurse practitioner scope of practice. *Journal of Advanced Nursing, 49*(2), 135–145.

Gardner, A., Gardner, G., Middleton, S., & Della, P. R. (2009). The status of Australian nurse practitioners: The first national census. *Australian Health Review, 33*(4), 679–689.

Gardner, G., Gardner, A., Middleton, S., Della, P., Kain, V., Doubrovsky, A. (2010) The work of nurse practitioners. *Journal of Advanced Nursing, 66, 10, 2160-2169.*

Geyer, N., Naude, S., & Sithole, G. (2002). Legislative issues impacting on the practice of the South African nurse practitioner. *Journal of the American Academy of Nurse Practitioners, 14*(1), 11–15.

Hanucharurnkul, S., Suwisith, N., Piasue, N., & Terathongkum, S. (2007). *Characteristics and working situation of nurse practitioners in Thailand.* Retrieved March 14, 2008, from www.icn-apnetwork.org.

Haute Autorité de Santé [HAS]. (2007). *Délégation, transfert, nouveaux métiers...: Conditions des nouvelles formes de coopération entre professionnels de santé.* Paris: Author.

Haute Autorité de Santé [HAS]. (2008). Retrieved January 10, 2012 from http://www.has-sante.fr/portail/upload/docs/application/pdf/reco_cooperation_vvd_16_avril_2008_04_16_12_23_31_188.pdf.

Henard, L., Berland, Y. & Cadet, D. (January, 2011) Rapport relatif aux métiers de niveau intermediare, Professionnels d'aujourd'hui et nouveaux métiers: des pistes pour advancer. Retrieved January 30, 2011 from http://translate.google.com/translate?hl=en&sl=fr&u=http://www.net-iris.fr/veille-juridique/actualite/26447/proposition-elargissement-des-competences-medicales-de-certains-praticiens.php&prev=/search%3Fq%3Dhenard%2Bberland%2Bnursing%26hl%3Den%26qscrl%3D1%26rlz%3D1T4DKUS_enUS251US251%26biw%3D1024%26bih%3D507%26site%3Dwebhp%26prmd%3Dimvnso&sa=X&ei=YRQvUMisF4Xs0gGqtoDACQ&sqi=2&ved=0CE0Q7gEwAw{.

International Council of Nurses. (2002). *Definition and characteristics of the role.* Retrieved June 13, 2011, from http://www.icn-apnetwork.org.

International Council of Nurses. (2007). *Positive practice environments: Quality workplaces=quality patient care.* Retrieved June 13, 2011, from http://www.icn.ch/indkit2007.htm.

International Council of Nurses. (2008a). *Nursing care continuum—framework and competencies.* Geneva: Author.

International Council of Nurses. (2008b). *The scope of practice, standards and competencies of the advanced practice nurse.* Geneva: Author.

International Council of Nurses–APNetwork. (2007). Retrieved June 13, 2011, from http://www.apnetwork.org.

Madubuko, G. (2001). *NP/ANP development in West Africa.* Retrieved March 11, 2008, from www.icn-apnetwork.org.

National Council for the Professional Development of Nursing and Midwifery. (2001). *Framework for the establishment of advanced nurse practitioner and advanced midwife practitioner posts.* Dublin: National Council for the Professional Development of Nursing and Midwifery.

National Council for the Professional Development of Nursing and Midwifery. (2005). *A preliminary evaluation of the role of the advanced nurse practitioner.* Retrieved May 26, 2011, from http://www.ncnm.ie/items/1314/85/6200145527%5CANP%20Evaluation%2012_05.pdf.

National Health Institute. (2002). *Curriculum for the training of family nurse practitioners: Post-basic course.* Gaborone, Botswana: National Health Institute.

New South Wales Health Department. (1998). *Nurse practitioner services in NSW.* Sydney: Author.

New Zealand Gazette. November 10, 2005. No. 188, p. 4750. Notice No. 7428.

New Zealand Government. (2004). *New Zealand Gazette.* Issue No. 120. Wellington: Author.

New Zealand Ministry of Health. (2002). *Nurse practitioners in New Zealand.* Wellington: Author. Nursing and Midwifery Council. (2006). *Standards of proficiency for nurse and midwife prescribers.* Retrieved March 10, 2008, from www.nmc-uk.org/aFrameDisplay.aspx?DocumentID=1312&Keyword=.

Nursing and Midwifery Council. (2007). *Advanced nursing practice update—19 June 2007.* Retrieved March 10, 2008, from www.nmc-uk.org/aArticle.aspx?ArticleID=2528.

Nursing Council of New Zealand. (2001). *The nurse practitioner: Responding to health needs in New Zealand.* Wellington: Author.

Offredy, M. (1999). The nurse practitioner role in New South Wales: Development and policy. *Nursing Standard, 13*(43), 38–41.

Philippine Board of Nursing, Professional Regulations Commission. (2008, August 19). Updates on the Nurse Certification Program. *BON Newsletter, 3,* 7.

Pilane, C., Neube, P., & Seitio, O. (2007). *Ensuring quality in affiliated health training institutions: Advanced diploma programmes in Botswana.* Retrieved March 17, 2008, from www.icn-apnetwork.org/.

Pulcini, J., Jelic, M., Gul, R., & Loke, A. L. (2010). An international survey on advanced practice nursing education, practice and regulation. *Journal of Nursing Scholarship, 42*(1), 31–39.

Roodbol, P. (2004). *Survey carried out prior to the 3rd ICN-International Nurse Practitioner/Advanced Nursing Practice Network Conference.* Network Conference. Gronigen, The Netherlands.

Roodbol, P. (2005) *Willing o'-the-wisps, stumbling runs, toll roads and song lines: Study into the structural rearrangement of tasks between nurses and physicians.* Unpublished summary of doctoral thesis.

Roodbol, P. (2011). *Update report on the global status of advanced practice nurses and nurse practitioners for the APN Network Session.* ICN Congress, Malta.

Royal College of Nursing. (2008). *Advanced nurse practitioners—an RCN guide to the advanced nurse practitioner, role, competencies and programme accreditation.* London: Author.

Schober, M., & Affara, F. (2006). *Advanced nursing practice.* Oxford: Blackwell Publishing.

Schober, M. (2007a). Development of advanced community nursing/nurse practitioner roles and educational programmes in Oman, EM/NUR/392/E/R/07.07. Cairo: WHO-EMRO. Unpublished.

Schober, M. (2007b). Development of a framework for advanced practice nursing in Bahrain, assignment report EM/NUR/394/E/R07.7. Cairo: WHO-EMRO. Unpublished.

Schober, M. (2008). *Advanced nursing practice: The global experience, reflections on nursing leadership, first quarter.* Indianapolis: Sigma Theta Tau.

Sheer, B., & Wong, F. K. Y. (2008). The development of advanced nursing practice globally. *Journal of Nursing Scholarship, 40*(3), 204–211.

Shiow-Luan Tsay & Su-Zhen Kuo. (2008). *Nursing care in Taiwan.* Section VII: Advanced nursing practice (177–183). Taiwan: Department of Health.

Slocombe, M. (2000). *Development of community health services in the Cayman Islands.* International NP/APN Conference, San Diego, CA.

White, M. (2001). *Emergence of the nurse practitioner in the UK.* Geneva: Centre for Nursing Roles.World Health Organization. (2002a). *Human resources, national health systems: Shaping the agenda for action.* (Final report.) Geneva: Author.

World Health Organization. (2002b). *Nursing and midwifery services: Strategic directions 2002–2008.* Geneva: Author.

World Health Organization. (2006). *Working together for health: World health report 2006.* Geneva: Author.

World Health Organization. (2007). *The global recommendations and guidelines on task shifting.* Geneva: Author.

World Health Organization—Eastern Mediterranean Region. (2001). *Fifth meeting of the regional advisory panel on nursing and consultation on advanced practice nursing and nurse prescribing: Implications for regulation, nursing education and practice in the Eastern Mediterranean.* WHO-EM/NUR/348/E/L. Cairo: Author.

World Health Organization—Western Pacific Region. (2001). *Mid-level and nurse practitioners in the Pacific: Models and issues.* Manila: Author.

Wright, S., Cloonan, P., Leonhardy, K., & Wright, G. (2005). An international programme in nursing and midwifery: Building capacity for the new millennium. *International Nursing Review, 52*(1), 18–23.

Yu-Mei Chao [YU]. (2008). *Nursing care in Taiwan* (p. 30). Taiwan: Department of Health.

Zurn, P., Dolea, C., & Stilwell, B. (2005). *Nurse retention and recruitment: Developing a motivated workforce.* Retrieved July 15, 2011, from www.icn.ch/global/Issue4Retention.pdf.

UNIT 2

The Practice Environment

6

Payment for Advanced Practice Nurse Services

Karen R. Robinson

INTRODUCTION

History has shown that nurse practitioners (NPs), clinical nurse specialists (CNSs), certified nurse-midwives (CNMs), and certified registered nurse anesthetists (CRNAs), collectively referred to as advanced practice registered nurses (APRNs), have made significant contributions to the health-care delivery system in terms of providing high-quality, cost-effective, and safe care. With the passage of the Balanced Budget Act of 1997 (Public Law 105-33), APRNs achieved Medicare professional provider status and became part of the mainstream health-care payment system. Achieving this status assisted APRNs in being recognized as legitimate independent providers of primary and specialty care. With this status came responsibilities for APRNs to develop new skills to meet growing demands in the reimbursement arena. To a certain degree, they have been able to achieve additional reimbursement gains, but barriers remain that impede use of APRNs in mainstream health-care delivery and that stifle development of innovative care models (Sullivan-Marx & Keepnews, 2010). APRNs need to continue to be vigilant in addressing the reimbursement challenges that they encounter in their practices.

BACKGROUND

APRNs have been practicing for many years. In fact, nurse anesthesia, the oldest advanced nursing specialty, has been in existence since the mid-1800s when nurses became involved in administering anesthesia (Bigbee & Amidi-Nouri, 2000). In 1925, Mary Breckenridge established the Frontier Nursing Service in the Appalachian area of Kentucky, which became a futuristic model of nurse-midwifery advanced nursing practice. The psychiatric CNS is the oldest and perhaps the most highly developed of the CNS specialties. By 1970, graduate-prepared psychiatric CNSs assumed roles as individual, group, family, and milieu therapists, and obtained some direct third-party reimbursement for their services (Robinson, 2009).

In the early 1960s, physicians began to mentor nurses who had clinical experience. At the same time, increasing specialization in medicine led to a large number of physicians leaving primary care, creating a shortage of primary care physicians. This led to many areas, especially rural areas, being medically underserved. In addition, in 1965, the Medicare and Medicaid programs began to provide health-care coverage to low-income women, children, the elderly, and people with disabilities, thereby increasing the demand for more primary care services. Because physicians were unable to meet this demand, nurses answered the call to become NPs. Loretta Ford, a nurse, and Henry Silver, a physician, created the first training program for NPs (O'Brien, 2003).

However, even though these four advanced practice roles have been well established for decades, direct reimbursement for their services has been difficult to obtain (Robinson, 2009). Historically, nurses were not paid directly for their services, but rather this cost was included with the overhead that facilities and medical providers charged their patients. In 1948, the American Nurses Association (ANA) began a campaign for direct reimbursement of nursing services; however, it faced many barriers and did not achieve major success until approximately 40 years later when significant changes in federal laws governing health programs granted direct reimbursement to APRNs for their services. These changes assisted in breaking down some barriers for full use of APRNs as primary care providers, and they enabled them to have a more direct role in the delivery of health care (Mittelstadt, 1993).

In 1965, Congress amended the Social Security Act to establish Medicare and Medicaid (Frakes & Evans, 2006). Medicare reimbursed home care agencies for skilled nursing services. Physician orders were required to initiate the services, but the reimbursement was specifically for nursing care. In the 1970s, NPs established some success in being reimbursed for primary care and CRNAs began their attempt to secure third-party reimbursement (Bigbee & Amidi-Nouri, 2000). In 1973, the first legislation mandating private insurance reimbursements of nurse-midwifery services was passed in the state of Washington. Since 1979, CNMs have received direct reimbursement through both Medicare and Medicaid (Brucker & Reedy, 2000).

In the early 1980s, 25 states had enacted legislation enabling direct reimbursement for specific groups of nurses; however, little data existed regarding the implementation of these laws. A case study of legislation providing direct third-party reimbursement to NPs in Maryland was conducted in 1983 and in Oregon in 1986 (Griffith, 1986). The study investigated the degree to which NPs in these two states were receiving direct third-party reimbursement and how it affected health-care costs. Findings revealed that 4 years after enactment of legislation in Maryland, 1% of NPs in the study had been directly reimbursed by a third-party payer in contrast to 21% of NPs in Oregon, 7 years after enactment of the law.

In 1983, Congress adopted the prospective payment system (PPS) in an effort to control hospital costs to the Medicare program. All services by providers other than those reimbursed through Medicare Part B were assembled into a hospital diagnosis-related group (DRG) payment (Bruton-Maree & Rupp, 2001). This fixed rate was to cover all costs associated with a hospital admission, including services provided by nonphysician providers. Under this system, CRNAs were placed in jeopardy because, in an effort to cut costs, hospitals had no incentive to hire CRNAs because their cost would come directly from the hospital DRG payment (Faut-Callahan & Kremer, 2000). Congress had created reimbursement disincentives for the use of CRNAs while strengthening incentives for the use of anesthesiologists. Lobbying efforts by CRNAs caused the Health Care Financing Administration (HCFA) to revise portions of this legislation that allowed CRNAs to obtain direct Medicare reimbursement or to sign over their billing rights to their employer (Robinson, 2009).

A report to U.S. Congress by the Office of Technology Assessment in 1986 found that NPs and CNMs, as well as physician assistants, provided a high quality of care and patient satisfaction. The focus on health promotion and disease prevention by these providers made them a good potential provider for the managed care models in the 1980s (Sullivan-Marx, 2008). However, barriers to the use of APRNs were evident in physician resistance, legal restrictions, lack of reimbursement, and limited coverage for health promotion/preventive care (U.S. Congress Office of Technology Assessment, 1986).

The Physician Payment Review Commission (PPRC) was created in 1986 to advise Congress on reforms of the methods used to pay physicians under the Medicare Part B program, a program that includes the payment regulations for health-care professionals who are eligible to receive direct reimbursement through the Medicare program. Nursing groups such as the ANA and the American Association of Nurse Anesthetists (AANA) lobbied the PPRC to consider their contributions when they revised the payment system (Robinson, 2004, 2009).

In 1989, Congress, incorporating the PPRC recommendations, passed legislation that changed physician payment from a reasonable charge payment method to a Medicare Fee Schedule based on a resource-based relative value scale (RBRVS). In response to the lobbying done by nurses, the legislative package included a recommendation that the PPRC study the effect of the Medicare Fee Schedule on nonphysician providers (PPRC, 1991; Robinson, Griffith, & Sullivan-Marx, 2001).

In its annual report to Congress, the PPRC made a recommendation that *nonphysician providers,* including NPs, CRNAs, and CNMs, should be paid a percentage of physician payment levels reflecting differences in physicians' and nonphysicians' resource costs: work, practice expense, and malpractice expense (Griffith & Robinson, 1993). The ANA counterproposed that APRNs should be paid the same as physicians for the same services (Mittelstadt, 1991).

Anticipating that APRNs would be included in the emerging RBRVS payment system, Griffith and Robinson (1993) studied nine nurse specialty groups, including CNMs and family NPs, to demonstrate that APRNs were providing some of the current procedural terminology (CPT) coded services being considered by the PPRC and universally used for physician payment by government and private insurers. Findings of these exploratory studies provided documentation of the degree to which family NPs and CNMs performed, with little or no supervision, the same services and procedures for which physicians were being reimbursed.

Amendments to the Social Security Act passed by Congress and signed by President Clinton as part of the Balanced Budget Act of 1997 (Public Law 105-33) gave direct Medicare reimbursement to NPs and CNSs in all geographical areas and health-care settings at 85% of the physician rate. This enactment precipitated a study by Sullivan-Marx and Maislin (2000) to ensure that there were no significant differences in how NPs and physicians assessed work values for commonly used primary codes. The researchers compared relative work values between NPs and family physicians for commonly used office visit codes and found no significant difference between the two groups for establishing relative work values, thus providing an indication that services provided by NPs could be reliably valued in the Medicare Fee Schedule.

To establish relative values for the practice expense component of CPT codes, the Center for Medicare and Medicaid Services (CMS), formerly the Health Care Financing Administration (HCFA), developed and now relies on recommendations from the American Medical Association's (AMA's) Relative Value Practice Expense Advisory Committee (PEAC). Specialty societies that serve on PEAC survey their members to obtain accurate "direct input" data for the CPT codes, and then society representatives present the data to the PEAC. The PEAC members critique the data, making modifications as needed. Following PEAC approval, data are forwarded to the CMS to use to calculate the practice expense relative values (AMA, 2011). The ANA has a voting seat on this committee and the nurse representative became chair of the PEAC in 2006 (Sullivan-Marx, 2008).

On March 9, 2000, the HCFA announced that removal of the federal requirement in which CRNAs must be supervised by physicians when administering anesthesia to Medicare patients was forthcoming. Delays in the final rule continued until July 5, 2001, when CMS published a proposed rule that would maintain the existing supervision requirement, but allow a state's governor, in consultation with the state's boards of medicine and nursing, to request an exemption from the physician supervision requirement or to "opt out" (Bruton-Maree & Rupp, 2001; Edmunds, 2002). By 2005, fourteen states had exercised this option. An analysis of Medicare data for 1999–2005 found no evidence that opting out of the oversight requirement resulted in increased inpatient deaths or complications (Dulisse & Cromwell, 2010). Based on their findings, the study authors recommended that CMS allow CRNAs in every state to work without surgeon or anesthesiologist supervision.

The Patient Protection and Affordable Care Act, the health-care reform legislation signed into law by President Obama on March 23, 2010, will expand health insurance coverage to 31 million uninsured Americans in 2014. This was good news for millions of Americans, but the country could face logistical difficulties in providing high-quality care services to the newly insured citizens at a time when the nation's supply of primary care physicians is decreasing (Hansen-Turton, Bailey, Nagle, Torres, & Ritter, 2010; Robinson & Griffith, 2012). The underserved areas of the country could be affected the most.

Attention is now focused on the ability of NPs and CNMs to assist in solving the nation's shortage of primary care providers (Summers, 2011). ANA is currently engaged with "The Negotiated Rulemaking Committee on the Designation of Medically Underserved Populations" to determine, among other things, if and how NPs and CNMs will be counted as primary care providers in the federal government designation of health professional shortage areas. Even though these two groups of APRNs have a long history of providing care to vulnerable populations, they have not been included in the "provider-to-population ratio," a critical aspect of the health professions shortage and medically underserved area formula. A variety of federal and state programs use these designations to target resources such as eligibility for the National Health Service Corps scholarship and loan repayment program for which NPs and CNMs are eligible. Medicare also makes bonus payments to primary care physicians working in these designated areas, but not to NPs or CNMs.

In May 2010, a nurse was appointed to the prestigious federal policy commission, the Medicare Payment Advisory Commission (MedPAC). Congress established MedPAC in 1997 to analyze access to care, cost and quality of care, and other key issues affecting Medicare. MedPAC advises Congress on payments to health plans participating in the Medicare Advantage program and providers in Medicare's traditional fee-for-service programs (U.S. Government Accountability Office, 2011). It is anticipated that the appointee's unique perspective as an innovative nurse leader will enhance the Commission's work.

APRNs have been part of the health-care system for decades and are now, with other providers, entering a time of change aimed at revolutionizing care delivery and reimbursement (Kennerly, 2007). This section provides some of the history behind the various APRN roles as well as their gains and challenges over time in terms of reimbursement autonomy.

PAYMENT MECHANISMS AND IMPACT ON ADVANCED PRACTICE REGISTERED NURSES

Most third-party payers, whether a managed care organization (MCO), Medicare, or Medicaid, to name a few, will recognize APRNs, in varying degrees, as qualified providers of health care. However, the reimbursement and coverage policies may differ considerably. Finerfrock and Havens (1997) stressed that differences exist between how individual health plans "treat" APRNs as well as how they are permitted to practice under state law and the criteria the plan may impose as a precondition for payment. These differences in billing for services still exist today; therefore, this section will detail some of the current billing options and discuss the challenges for APRNs within each of those options, including the following:

1. **Medicare,** created as part of the Social Security Act of 1965, is a federally funded health-care program that consists of four parts. Part A (Hospital Insurance) covers inpatient hospital services, skilled nursing facility services, home health agency services, and hospice care. Medicare Part B (Supplemental Medical Insurance) covers services to physicians (i.e., medical doctors,

optometrists, dentists, and podiatrists) and nonphysician providers, including NPs, CNSs, CRNAs, and CNMs. Part B also covers laboratory and diagnostic services, renal dialysis, outpatient hospital procedures, chemotherapy, medical equipment, and supplies. Medicare Part C is known as Medicare Advantage and is a program through which Medicare beneficiaries can choose to receive their Parts A, B, and D services through a private health plan, most often a managed care plan. Medicare Part D covers prescription drugs (Frakes & Evans, 2006; Robinson, 2009; Sullivan-Marx & Keepnews, 2010).

For institutional care such as hospital and nursing home care, Medicare uses prospective payment systems. A prospective payment system is one in which the health-care institution receives a set amount of money for each episode of care provided to a patient, regardless of the actual amount of care used. The actual allotment of funds is based on a list of diagnosis-related groups (DRGs).

The Primary Care Health Practitioner Incentive Act, which was included in the Balanced Budget Act of 1997, removed Medicare Part B restrictions on the settings and practices in which APRNs could provide professional services. This allowed direct Medicare reimbursement to the APRN, but at 85% of the physician fee rate (Frakes & Evans, 2006).

Under the current reimbursement system, which allows CRNAs or their employers to receive direct reimbursement from Medicare Part B, a process titled *pass-through* occurs (Broadston, 2001; Robinson, 2009). The pass-through process allows a facility to be reimbursed for its CRNA expense from the Medicare program over and above the DRG payment of the prospective payment system. It was created by Congress in an attempt to restore the equal playing field between anesthesiologists and CRNAs. The pass-through process is available only to small health-care facilities that meet specific criteria. A rural hospital can qualify and be paid on a reasonable cost basis for one full-time employed CRNA providing 500 or fewer inpatient and outpatient anesthesia procedures without anesthesiologist services provided at the hospital. The hospital and/or CRNA receiving pass-through funding is prohibited from billing a Medicare Part B carrier for any anesthesia services furnished to patients of that hospital (AANA, 2011).

Payment to clinical providers under Medicare fee-for-service or managed care is categorized in the CPT coding system, developed by the AMA in 1966. Approximately 8,000 procedures are listed in the CPT publication, which mainly describes physician procedures and is intended to provide a uniform language that accurately describes medical, surgical, and diagnostic services (AMA, 2011). The CPT is used extensively by payers for fee-for-service reimbursement and tracking services in managed care. It is revised annually to reflect changes in medical practice and technology. Reimbursement for a service represented by an individual CPT code is based on the RBRVS, which was originally implemented to establish a Medicare fee schedule for Part B physician payment. This system now extends to payment for services provided by APRNs, physician assistants, and other Part B providers (Robinson et al., 2001). In this system, a total relative value that incorporates work, practice expense, and malpractice insurance is established for each CPT code. The total relative value for a code is multiplied by a standard dollar amount and adjusted geographically to determine the allowable Medicare charge for that code (AMA, 2011).

The CPT system has been criticized for confining codes to physicians' services, thereby limiting its usefulness to the current health-care system, which uses multiple providers, many of whom are directly reimbursed by Medicare such as APRNs (Robinson, 2009; Robinson et al., 2001).

Section 3114 of the Patient Protection and Affordable Care Act (ACA) of 2010 increased the amount of payment that the Medicare program will make to CNMs for their personal professional services and for services furnished incident to their professional services. Since 1992, payment has been made at 80% of the lesser of the actual charge or 65% of the physician fee schedule amount that would be paid for the same service furnished by a physician. Effective January 1, 2011, payment is being made at 80% of the lesser of the actual charge or 100% of the physician fee schedule amount that would be paid for the same service furnished by a physician. When a CNM is providing care to a Medicare beneficiary and the collaborating physician provides some of the services, the fee paid to the CNM is based on the portion of the global fee that would have been paid to the physician for the service provided by the CNM (CMS, 2011).

2. **Medicaid** provides health insurance coverage for certain groups of individuals and families with low incomes and resources. It is a means-tested program that is jointly funded by the state and federal governments, but is managed by the states. Even within the groups, certain requirements must be met to include age; whether the person is pregnant, disabled, blind, or aged; income and resources; and U.S. citizenship or a lawfully admitted immigrant. The rules for counting income and resources vary from state to state and from group to group. This program is a state-administered program, and each state sets its own guidelines regarding eligibility and services (CMS, 2011). Medicaid does not pay money directly to the patient; instead, the payments are sent directly to the patient's health-care provider. In some states, Medicaid beneficiaries are required to pay a small copayment for medical services. The Patient Protection and Affordable Care Act of 2010 will expand Medicaid eligibility starting in 2014; people with income up to 133% of the poverty line qualify for coverage, including adults without dependent children.

   Before 1989, reimbursement of APRNs varied according to individual state policy and legislation. To increase access to primary care services for low-income families and children, the U.S. Congress included a provision in the Omnibus Budget Reconciliation Act of 1989 requiring Medicaid payment for certified pediatric and family NPs, regardless of whether they are supervised by or associated with physicians. Since 1989, some states have opted to reimburse more broadly than required by federal law, allowing Medicaid payment for all NPs and some CNSs. Payment varies from 70% to 100% of the prevailing physician fee (Chapman, Wides, & Spetz, 2010; Sullivan-Marx & Keepnews, 2010).

   APRN reimbursement is mainly provided under a fee-for-service approach in which the state pays the lesser of the provider's charge or a defined maximum amount for a specific service (Frakes & Evans, 2006). Some states provide APRN reimbursement at a percentage of the physician's fee-for-service reimbursement rate, and some restrict the reimbursement to a specific patient population (statutorily defined as needy compared with individuals demonstrating medical necessity) or APRN specialty (i.e., family, adult, geriatric, or pediatric). At least 38 state Medicaid programs, responding to a 2008 survey, indicated that they reimburse CRNAs directly for their services. The remaining 12 states either did not respond to the survey, responded that they reimburse facilities (but not CRNAs directly) for CRNA services, or responded that they reimburse for medically directed CRNA services (AANA, 2011).

3. **MCOs** are insurers that provide both health-care services and payment for services. There is a continuum of organizations that provide managed care, each operating with slightly different business models. Some organizations are made of physicians, whereas others are combinations of physicians, hospitals, and other providers. There are several types of network-based managed care programs. These range from more restrictive to less restrictive, and include health maintenance

organizations (HMOs), independent practice associations (IPAs), preferred provider organizations (PPOs), and point-of-service (POS) plans. See **Table 6-1** for specific details of these network-based managed care programs.

Hansen-Turton and Torgan (2008) surveyed MCOs in 2005 and again in 2007 to determine the insurers' credentialing and reimbursement policies regarding primary care NPs. Compared to the 2005 survey, credentialing policies generally improved. For example, in 2005, only 33% of all companies surveyed had credentialed NPs as primary care providers, whereas in 2007, 53%

TABLE 6-1

Managed Care Organizations

Categories	Chararacteristics
Health maintenance organizations (HMOs)	One of the oldest forms of managed care. Members are provided comprehensive health care. The primary care provider of the HMO member, acting as a "gatekeeper," coordinates all of the medical care for that individual. If specialist care is needed, the primary care provider refers the member to a specialist generally within the HMO. Nonemergency hospital admissions also require preauthorization by the primary care provider.
Independent practice associations (IPAs)	Legal entity contracts with a group of physicians to provide service to the HMO's members. The physicians are generally paid on a basis of capitation, which means a set amount for each enrolled person assigned to that physician or group of physicians, whether or not that person seeks care. The contract is not usually exclusive, allowing individual doctors or the group to sign contracts with multiple HMOs. Physicians who participate in IPAs generally also serve fee-for-service patients not associated with managed care.
Preferred provider organizations (PPOs)	Composed of physicians, hospitals, or other providers who have contracted with an insurer or a third-party administrator to provide health care at reduced rates to the insurer's or administrator's clients. A PPO is a subscription-based medical care arrangement. PPOs earn money by charging an access fee to the insurance company for the use of their network (unlike the usual insurance with premiums and corresponding payments paid either in full or partially by the insurance provider to the medical doctor). PPOs can offer more flexibility to patients, but they tend to have slightly higher premiums. They have utilization review and precertification requirement features.
Point of service (POS)	Uses features of each of the other plans. Members of a POS plan do not make a choice about which system to use until the point at which the service is being used. The plan has levels of progressively higher patient financial participation as the patient moves away from the more managed features of the plan. For example, if the patient stays in a network of providers and seeks a referral to use a specialist, the patient may have a copayment only. However, if the patient uses an out-of-network provider, but does not seek a referral, the patient will pay more. POS plans offer more flexibility and freedom of choice than standard HMOs.

had instituted pro-NP credentialing policies. Although progress had been made in the 2 years, nearly half of all MCOs surveyed in 2007 refused to credential NPs as primary care providers. The researchers did find that MCOs in states that grant prescription authority to NPs without a requirement for physician involvement were more likely to credential NPs as primary care providers than MCOs in states that require physician oversight for prescription authority.

If APRNs become a member of the provider panel of an MCO, they have a contract for providing care, credentialing, directory listing, and reimbursement (Buppert, 1998). The APRN has full responsibility for the patient's primary care, which includes (a) complying with the organization's quality, use, and patient satisfaction standards; (b) coordinating care with specialists or hospitals; (c) approving or disapproving specialty care referrals; (d) providing a system for 24-hour access to care; and (e) keeping costs as low as possible while maintaining quality. MCOs reimburse providers on a fee-for-service basis, a capitated basis, or a combination of both. Each organization negotiates a payment arrangement with each group or provider on its panel. Most private health plans, including fee-for-service (FFS) plans, PPOs, HMOs, and health benefits administrators that are not health insurance programs per se, reimburse directly for CRNA services (AANA, 2011).

4. **Incident-to billing** enables APRNs to provide services that are "incident to" those of a physician and applies only to the office setting. Services that qualify as an "incident to" must be part of the patient's normal course of treatment during which a physician personally performed an initial service and remains actively involved in the course of treatment. The physician does not need to be present in the examination room, but he or she must be present in the office suite and ready to assist if needed (CMS, 2011). The claim can be submitted under the physician's provider number as if the physician performed the service and is paid at 100% of the physician fee schedule (Kleinpell, French, & Diamond, 2007). Documentation must include that the physician supervised the visit.
5. **Indemnity insurance companies** pay providers on a per visit, per procedure basis. They have fee schedules based on "usual and customary" charges; however, some insurers may pay more than others for the same procedure. If a provider charges more than what an insurer considers to be usual and customary, the insurer will pay only according to its fee schedule; the patient then becomes responsible for the difference between what the provider charges and what the insurance company pays (Barone & Paniagua-Ramirez, 2006). It becomes dependent on the provider to collect the difference from the patient. Some providers agree to accept the usual and customary payment, whereas others will not (Buppert, 1998; Robinson, 2009).
6. The **shared visits** provision by Medicare allows groups employing APRNs to combine services and can occur in an office or inpatient setting. A stipulation for shared visits is that the APRN and physician must have an employment or other type of contractual business relationship (Kleinpell et al., 2007; Magdic, 2006). The shared service concept does not apply to critical care services. An example of a shared visit would be if the NP or CNS sees a hospital inpatient in the morning and the physician follows with a later face-to-face visit with the patient on the same day, in which case the physician or the NP or CNS may report the service (CMS, 2011).

To allow direct billing of NPs and CNSs in hospital and inpatient settings, CMS issued a policy change in 2007 stating that "direct billing and payment for the professional services of NPs and CNSs furnished to hospital patients (inpatients and outpatients) must be made to the NP or the CNS. However, if NPs or CNSs reassign payment to the hospital for their professional services to hospital patients, payments must be made to the hospital for these services at 85% of the physician fee schedule" (U.S. Department of Health and Human Services, 2007).

Medicare issued critical care billing clarifications in 2008 that would mainly be pertinent to acute care NPs. When NPs adhere to scope of practice and licensure requirements as well as meet the specifications for providing time-based critical care services, they can bill for their services and receive payment directly. Time spent in delivering critical care services must be at the bedside or in the immediate vicinity (Sullivan-Marx & Keepnews, 2010; U.S. Department of Health and Human Services, 2008).

7. **TRICARE**, operated by the Department of Defense, is the government's "managed care" program for active duty military personnel, their families, and retired members of the military. It includes the following: (a) TRICARE Prime is similar to an HMO that provides the lowest out-of-pocket cost, in return for the requirement that enrollees use only providers and hospitals that are part of the TRICARE network. Enrollees are assigned a primary care provider who supervises all medical care and authorizes referrals for specialty care. Active duty service members and their families pay no enrollment fees and no out-of-pocket costs for any type of care as long as care is received from the primary care provider or with a referral. All other beneficiaries pay enrollment fees and the cost for care is based on where the care is received. Care received without a referral is subject to point-of-service fees. (b) TRICARE Standard and Extra is a fee-for-service plan available to all non–active duty beneficiaries. Enrollees may visit any TRICARE authorized provider, network or nonnetwork. Care at military treatment facilities is on a space-available basis only. Enrollees do not need a referral for any type of care, but some services may require prior authorization. The type of provider seen determines which option the enrollee is using and how much will be paid out-of-pocket. If the enrollee visits a nonnetwork provider, the Standard option is used. If the enrollee visits a network provider, he or she is using the Extra option. When using the Extra option, the enrollee will pay less out-of-pocket and the provider will file the claims for the enrollee (TRICARE, 2011).

   NPs, psychiatric CNSs, CNMs, and CRNAs are authorized to provide TRICARE services and are directly reimbursed (Mittelstadt, 1993; Robinson, 2009). The TRICARE plans directly reimburse CRNAs and anesthesiologists at the same rates, using similar payment modalities as the Medicare Part B program (AANA, 2011).

8. **Indian Health Service (IHS)** is an Operating Division within the U.S. Department of Health and Human Services. IHS is responsible for providing medical and public health services to members of federally recognized Tribes and Alaska Natives. APNs provide primary and specialty care in IHS facilities. They operate under the IHS National Scope of Practice for APRNs, which preempts state licensure guidelines. However, state licensure laws do apply to IHS-APRNs related to the prescribing of controlled substances. In the IHS, APRNs work as licensed, independent practitioners (Sahota & Rose, 2009).

   Specialty APRNs such as CNMs, CRNAs, and psychiatric NPs are employed in IHS facilities. IHS and tribal health programs are not able to bill Medicare and Medicaid for all services provided by APRNs. In some cases, less compensation is provided (e.g., 85%) than if the same services were delivered by a physician (Sahota & Rose, 2009).

STRATEGIES BY ADVANCED PRACTICE REGISTERED NURSES THAT HAVE BEEN SUCCESSFUL IN PURSUING REIMBURSEMENT PAYMENT

Over the last 35 years or so, APRNs have forged ahead to achieve reimbursement for their services and have achieved some degree of success by using various strategies such as the following **Box 6-1:**

BOX 6-1
Advanced Practice Registered Nurse Reimbursement Successes

Rural Health Clinic Act of 1977 mandated that 50% of services in rural health clinics be provided by NPs and CNMs.

Office of Technology Assessment issued a report to the U.S. Congress in 1986 that revealed that NPs and CNMs provided high-quality care and patient satisfaction.

Omnibus Reconciliation Act of 1989 mandated a study of nonphysician providers and Medicare reimbursement.

Balanced Budget Act of 1997 granted direct Medicare reimbursement to NPs and CNSs in all geographical areas at 85% of the physician rate.

Numerous outcomes-based research studies were conducted by APRNs and their colleagues that demonstrated improved patient outcomes and patient satisfaction.

Nurse-managed health centers (NMHCs) have been established.

VA home-based primary care program meeting the comprehensive needs of the veteran population.

APRNs established key political contacts and lobbying campaigns.

Increased sophistication in grassroots efforts and activities.

Documented reduction in the direct and indirect costs of professional liability/malpractice.

1. APRNs working in underserved rural areas took advantage of the reimbursement available under the Rural Health Clinic Act of 1977 (O'Brien, 2003). This Act mandated that 50% of services in funded rural health clinics be provided by NPs and CNMs.
2. The Omnibus Reconciliation Act of 1989 provided limited reimbursement for NPs collaborating with physicians in rural areas and established Medicaid payments for pediatric or family NPs. In addition, it mandated a study of nonphysician providers and Medicare reimbursement. These changes were influenced by an NP appointee to the 14-member Physician Payment Review Committee, as well as by nursing organizations (O'Brien, 2003).
3. APRNs and nurse researchers conducted numerous outcomes-based research studies that demonstrated improved patient outcomes and patient satisfaction, as well as improved access and demonstrated cost-effectiveness benefits of APRN care. For example, a study conducted in Tennessee revealed that university community health NPs delivered health care at 23% below the average cost of other primary care providers with a 21% reduction in hospital inpatient rates, 42% decrease in prescription drug use, and 24% lower laboratory use rates compared to physicians. Additionally, 82% of patients reported that they were well satisfied with their quality of care (Spitzer, 1997).

   Another example of NP effectiveness was demonstrated by Mundinger and colleagues (2000). They studied 1,316 primary care patients who were randomly assigned to either NPs or physicians. Their findings revealed that patients' outcomes were comparable in the two groups. In yet another example, following an extensive literature review, three Department of Veterans Affairs researchers concluded that NPs compare equally to or better than physicians with patients who have various health-care needs. Many studies in their review documented less costly care, while at the same time maintaining high-quality and effectiveness (Feldman, Ventura, & Crosby, 1987).

Johantgen and colleagues (2011) conducted a systematic review of articles from 1990 to 2008 in which processes or outcomes of care were quantitatively compared between CNMs and physicians. For measures that related to the processes of care (e.g., epidural, labor induction, episiotomy), lower use was found for CNMs. For many of the infant outcomes (e.g., low Apgar, low birth weight, neonatal intensive care unit admission), there were no differences between physicians and CNMs. The group concluded that care by CNMs is safe and effective.

Chenowith, Martin, Pankowski, and Raymond (2005) analyzed the health-care costs associated with an on-site NP practice for 4,284 employees and their dependents. Annualized cost of the NP program was about $83,000. Savings in health-care costs were $1,313,756 per year, yielding a benefit-to-cost ratio of 15 to 1. Paez and Allen (2006) compared NP and physician management of hypercholesterolemia following revascularization. Patients in the NP-managed group were more likely to achieve their goals and comply with a prescribed regimen, with decreased medication costs. A collaborative NP/physician group was associated with decreased length of stay and costs, and higher hospital profit, without altering readmissions or mortality (Cowan et al., 2006).

4. Approximately 250 nurse-managed health centers (NMHCs), staffed by APRNs, have been primarily established in places that are medically underserved such as low-income urban neighborhoods and rural areas. They have 2.5 million patient encounters on an annual basis (Hansen-Turton, Bailey, Nagle, Torres, & Ritter, 2010; King & Hansen-Turton, 2010; Ritter & Hansen-Turton, 2008). Specific services of NMHCs generally include primary care, prenatal care, laboratory and diagnostic tests, access to free or low-cost pharmaceuticals, family planning, midwifery, behavioral health, and dental care. Referrals to specialists, hospital services, and radiologic services are accomplished via contracts.

   A study of 11 NMHCs in Pennsylvania, conducted by the National Nursing Centers Consortium (NNCC), reported that these centers are of critical importance as "safety net providers" for the medically underserved (Rothman & Hansen-Turton, 2006). They have a reputation for providing high-quality, cost-effective care and achieving high patient satisfaction rates. In fact, the NNCC study revealed their patients had higher rates of generic medication fills and lower rates of hospitalization than other "safety net providers."

5. APRNs in the U.S. Department of Veterans Affairs (VA) have met the challenges and taken advantage of meeting the comprehensive needs of the veteran population (Robinson, 2010). For example, the Eastern Colorado Health Care System Home-Based Primary Care Program, based at the Denver VA Medical Center, targets frail, chronically ill, older veterans who often have prolonged hospital and rehabilitation stays and inadequate home support (North, Kehm, Bent, & Hartman, 2008). The interdisciplinary team, including an NP as the patient's primary care provider, makes home visits for evaluation and management purposes. In a longitudinal study to assess the effects of the program, the group reported that the number of hospitalizations, emergency department visits, and "no show" appointments were all significantly lower compared with use by the same group for 1 year before enrollment in the program. Most impressive was the 84% reduction that occurred in the number of hospitalizations. Total cost savings was over $1 million, with hospitalization reductions accounting for 98% of the cost savings.
6. Nursing professional organizations are becoming more sophisticated in their grassroots activities. They are able to do this through their association journals, seminars, and Web sites. An example of these efforts involved the passage of Public Law 105-33, which included expansion of Medicare reimbursement for NPs and CNSs to all geographical areas. The ANA and APRNs

came out in force by assembling and packaging outcome data to show how APRNs make a difference in cost and quality, establishing political action partnerships, coordinating state and regional legislative volunteers, and lobbying "the Hill" (Robinson, 2009).

7. It has been documented that NPs reduce the direct and indirect costs of professional liability/malpractice (Bauer, 2010). Analysis of data from 1991 through 2009 in the United States National Practitioner Data Bank revealed that NPs do not increase liability claims or costs. NPs have lower rates of malpractice claims and lower costs per claim.

FUTURE REIMBURSEMENT OPPORTUNITIES AND CHALLENGES FOR ADVANCED PRACTICE REGISTERED NURSES

Despite many years of providing safe, high-quality cost-effective health care and achieving some remarkable reimbursement accomplishments (as detailed in the previous section), APRNs are continuing to fight some of the same battles that they were fighting many years ago and they will be facing some new opportunities and challenges. See **Box 6-2**.

Some of these long-standing battles and new opportunities/challenges include the following:

1. The Patient Protection and Affordable Care Act, the health-care reform legislation that was signed into law by President Obama in 2010, will expand health insurance coverage to 31 million uninsured Americans in 2014. With the passage of this legislation, the country could face difficulties in providing high-quality primary care services to newly insured citizens at a time when the nation's supply of primary care physicians is decreasing (Hansen-Turton et al., 2010). Attention has turned to NPs and CNMs to help solve this shortage problem (Summers, 2011).

BOX 6-2
Future Advanced Practice Registered Nurse Reimbursement Opportunities and Challenges

The Patient Protection and Affordable Care Act will expand health insurance coverage to 31 million uninsured Americans in 2014. At a time when supply of primary care physicians is decreasing, APRNs can solve this shortage problem.

Nursing groups must continue to unite and lobby any new bills, as well as those that have been reintroduced.

The Physician Quality Reporting System (PQRS), a quality improvement program implemented by CMS, deserves APRN attention.

Lack of reimbursement knowledge and skills limits the abilities of APRNs to be key players in practice and business ventures.

Implement a regulatory model that will establish clear expectations for licensure, accreditation, certification, and education for all APRNs.

Data on the reimbursement issue must be updated by conducting additional studies directly related to the topic.

Continue to focus on informing legislators and consumers about APRN education, requirements for licensure, and regulatory procedures in place.

As a result of Section 5602 of the Act, the Health Resources and Services Administration (HRSA) was directed to establish a committee to review and update the criteria used to define *health professions shortage area* (HPSA) and *medically underserved area* (MUA). The committee was subsequently titled "The Negotiated Rulemaking Committee on the Designation of Medically Underserved Populations." ANA has closely monitored the work of this rulemaking committee because it is this group who will determine if and how NPs and CNMs will be counted as primary care providers in the federal government designation of HPSAs. ANA, through formal testimony and responding to committee members' inquiries, has been strongly advocating that accurate assessment of primary care shortage areas requires the inclusion of NPs and CNMs *on par* with physicians.

Hansen-Turton and colleagues (2010) emphasize that nurse-managed centers have the potential to play a significant role in meeting this nation's growing population of patients seeking primary care services, particularly for the low-income and medically underserved groups. To do this, it is crucial that the centers get the needed funding.

In April 2010, CMS requested that the American Academy of Nursing (AAN) provide them with a nursing perspective on the Affordable Care Act. In response, AAN submitted a document, "Implementing Health Care Reform: Issues for Nursing," to CMS officials, other federal health agencies, and the White House. Ways to remove barriers to innovative models of nursing care, particularly those that relied on APRNs, were highlighted. Mason and Keepnews (2011) reported that there was substantial agreement on most of the recommendations in the document; however, more dialogue was needed in the following two areas: (a) federal options for reducing state barriers to full utilization of APRNs; and (b) whether and when to press for 100% reimbursement of NPs and CNSs under Medicare.

2. Even though some key bills have not passed, APRN organizations and other nursing groups must continue to unite and lobby any new bills, as well as those that have been reintroduced. For example, the Home Health Care Planning Improvement Act of 2007, which would have changed the Medicare law to grant NPs, CNSs, and CNMs the ability to order and certify home health services and to sign home health plans, did not pass. However, in 2011, Congress reintroduced the Act (S. 227/H.R. 2267) as previously stated in 2007 and added a section that clarifies the new requirement for a face-to-face encounter between a patient and a provider before certification for home health services. Current law allows APRNs to substitute for a physician for the purpose of the face-to-face requirement, but it does not allow them to sign the final plan of care at the end of the process. S. 227 would give APRNs this authority (Conant, 2011). A study commissioned by ANA and the National Association for Home Care and Hospice (NAHC) determined that S. 227, if passed, would yield a 1-year cost savings estimate of $6.3 million and a 10-year estimate of $273.1 million for Medicare. The most recent major action on this bill in the Senate was on January 31, 2011, when it was referred to the Senate Committee on Finance where it remains as of October 2011. The House referred the bill to the House Subcommittee on Health on June 3, 2011 (Library of Congress, 2011).

   Another key bill that did not pass was S. 59 (H.R. 2066), the Medicaid Advanced Practice Nurses and Physician Assistants Access Act of 2007. It would have amended title XIX (Medicaid) of the Social Security Act to eliminate the state option to include NPs, CNMs, and physician assistants as primary care case managers. However, in 2011, the Act was reintroduced as S. 56 (H.R. 2134). If passed, it will revise the coverage of certain NP services under the Medicaid fee-for-service program to remove the specification of certified pediatric NP and certified family NP to extend such coverage to services furnished by an NP or CNS.

The Act includes NPs, CNSs, CNMs, CRNAs, and physician assistants in the mix of service providers that Medicaid managed care organizations are required to maintain. The most recent action on the bill was June 3, 2011, when the House referred it to the House Subcommittee on Health. The Senate referred it to the Senate Committee on Finance on January 25, 2011 (Library of Congress, 2011).

3. The Physician Quality Reporting System (PQRS), a quality improvement program implemented by CMS, deserves attention by APRNs. The 2006 Tax Relief and Health Care Act mandated the establishment of a reporting system featuring incentive payment for eligible professionals who satisfactorily report data on quality measures for covered services provided to Medicare beneficiaries. In 2011, the program name was changed to PQRS. Each measure has specific criteria for documentation, evidence, and frequency of reporting. For 2011, CMS has established 194 PQRS measures. To participate, an eligible person can report information on an individual PQRS quality measure or measure groups. Those who meet the submission criteria of PQRS quality measures will earn an incentive payment equal to 1% of their total estimated Medicare B Physician Fee Schedule (PFS) allowed charges. A group practice may also qualify to earn incentive payment equal to 1% of the group practice's total estimated Medicare B–PFS allowed charges (Lavoie-Vaughan, 2011).

   It is important for APRNs to get involved in this program as it is a method of improving patient care while receiving a financial incentive. In addition, it provides the tools and guidelines to evaluate best practices and appropriate documentation. CMS is planning pay-for-performance programs in the future, and the PQRS is a model for these programs. Therefore, by participating in PQRS now, APRNs will be better prepared for the future CMS programs.

4. APRNs are well prepared for patient care, but they still are not prepared for the financial aspects of practice. APRNs have had difficulty in acquiring the business skills and knowledge of reimbursement relevant to their practices (Kennerly, 2006; Zuzelo et al., 2004). Rapid changes are occurring in reimbursement because of enhanced federal monitoring of provider billing and coding error rates, provider pay-for-performance reimbursement measures, and increased public attention to the quality of outcomes. Since financial responsibility is now linked with provision of quality of care, if APRNs are going to be viable providers of care, they must take an active part in policy and business (Sullivan-Marx & Keepnews, 2010).

5. The changing landscape of health care and population demographics provides APRNs the opportunity to assume a more prominent role in care delivery and demonstrate the impact of APRN practice on patient outcomes. Currently, however, there is no uniformity across states in defining what an APRN is, what advanced practice nursing and education encompasses, and licensing and credentialing requirements. These realities lead to potential confusion among the public, weaken the APRN position in the public policy arena and health-care community, and limit access to APRNs across states and settings (Stanley, 2009).

   Since 2005, consensus bodies of regulatory and professional organizations have been meeting to reestablish the regulatory environment for APRNs (Graham, 2011; Johnson, Dawson, & Brassard, 2010; Stanley, 2009). The proposed model distinguishes licensure, regulation, credentialing, and education regulation from professional specialization certification, so that consistency across legal entities can occur.

   A common definition for advanced practice and for regulatory requirements across all states has the potential to have a significant impact on APRN utilization and practice. It will make the collection of workforce data possible. Without common licensing and credentialing requirements, it is difficult to obtain accurate APRN information about their practice settings.

Standardization is key because health professions workforce data are used by policy makers to develop national health-care policy and make federal and state funding allocations (Stanley, 2009). To date, the model has been endorsed by 48 organizations (Graham, 2011).

If the proposed model is to be implemented by 2015, considerable work needs to be done. An organizational structure will need to be developed to bring all aspects of regulation together in an effort to increase communication and resolve issues of concern (Johnson et al., 2010). Each individual state board of nursing, school of nursing, certification entity, and accrediting body will need to examine what changes are needed and what actions they specifically need to that in an effort to make this model a reality (Stanley, 2009).

6. As one can see from the historical review of the research on the reimbursement system, the landmark studies by Griffith, Robinson, and others are dated. Just as Carol Lockhart, PhD, RN, FAAN, in 1989, issued a call for data showing how much of a particular service, billed by a physician, is done by a nurse, we, today, strongly believe that data on this reimbursement issue must be updated by conducting additional studies directly related to the topic. If the profession is going to continue its lobbying efforts for reimbursement, it must provide up-to-date, meaningful data to policy makers and payers (Robinson & Griffith, 2012).
7. Continue to focus on informing legislators and consumers about APRN education, requirements for licensure, and regulatory procedures in place (Phillips, 2008). If APRNs are to influence changes in health care and protect reimbursement, they must have personal contact with policy makers at the state and federal levels. This goes beyond knowing the names of legislators and what districts or states they represent. APRNs must get to know the legislators, as well as their staff who manage the local offices or campaign headquarters (Milstead, 1997; Pearson, 2002; Pruitt, Wetsel, Smith, & Spitler, 2002). The majority of local staff members have limited knowledge on the many issues that surface, so they often turn to individuals with whom they have developed relationships to obtain reliable, factual information. APRNs can provide this vital information by using fact sheets, statistics, case examples, outcomes-based research findings, and other key resource material.

CONCLUSION

The growing demand for health-care services, the increasing number of newly insured citizens, and growing shortages of health professionals, particularly primary care physicians, all demand an increased number of APRNs. This group of health-care providers must be expertly prepared, allowed to practice to the full extent of their knowledge and skills, readily accessible to patients in all settings, and reimbursed to the maximum extent.

Even though the number of APRNs has been increasing and APRNs are producing studies that reveal they are able to provide care at a high quality, reimbursement for their valuable work continues to be a struggle. Restrictive policies of programs such as Medicaid and private insurers, as well as numerous state laws and regulations that limit direct reimbursement and supervision required by another health-care provider, result in significant barriers for APRN reimbursement. The proposed Regulatory Model, due for implementation in 2015, is intended to define regulatory requirements across all states. It shows significant promise in having a major impact on APRN utilization and practice in the future.

REFERENCES

American Association of Nurse Anesthetists. (2011). Retrieved October 1, 2011, from www.aana.com.
American Medical Association. (2011). Retrieved September 7, 2011, from www.ama-assn.org.

Barone, C. P., & Paniagua-Ramirez, C. T. (2006). Coding and reimbursement. *AACN Advanced Critical Care, 17*(2), 116–118.

Bauer, J. C. (2010). Nurse practitioners as an underutilized resource for health reform: Evidence-based demonstrations of cost-effectiveness. *Journal of the American Academy of Nurse Practitioners, 22*, 228–231.

Bigbee, J. L., & Amidi-Nouri, A. (2000). History and evolution of advanced nursing practice. In A. B. Hamric, J. A. Spross, & C. M. Hanson (Eds.), *Advanced nursing practice: An integrative approach* (2nd ed.) (pp. 3–32). Philadelphia: WB Saunders.

Broadston, L. S. (2001). Reimbursement for anesthesia services. In S. D. Foster & M. Faut-Callahan (Eds.), *A professional study and resource guide for the CRNA* (pp. 287–312). Park Ridge, IL: American Association of Nurse Anesthetists.

Brucker, M. C., & Reedy, N. J. (2000). Nurse-midwifery: Yesterday, today, and tomorrow. *American Journal of Maternal Child Nursing, 25*(6), 322–326.

Bruton-Maree, N., & Rupp, R. M. (2001). Federal healthcare policy: How AANA advocates for the profession. In S. D. Foster & M. Faut-Callahan (Eds.), *A professional study and resource guide for the CRNA* (pp. 357–379). Park Ridge, IL: American Association of Nurse Anesthetists.

Buppert, C. (1998). Reimbursement for nurse practitioner services. *Nurse Practitioner, 23*(1), 67–81.

Centers for Medicare and Medicaid Services. (2011). Retrieved August 24, 2011, from www.cms.hhs.gov.

Chapman, S. A., Wides, C. D., & Spetz, J. (2010). Payment regulations for advanced practice nurses: Implications for primary care. *Policy, Politics, and Nursing Practice, 11*(2), 89–98.

Chenowith, D., Martin, N., Pankowski, J., & Raymond, L. W. (2005). A benefit-cost analysis of a worksite nurse practitioner program: First impressions. *Journal of Occupational and Environmental Medicine, 47*(11), 1110–1116.

Conant, R. (2011). Home Health Care Planning Improvement Act of 2011. *American Nurse Today, 6*(5), 20.

Cowan, M. J., Shapiro, M., Hays, R. D., Afifi, A., Vazirani, S., Ward, C. R., et al. (2006). The effect of a multidisciplinary hospitalist physician and advanced practice nurse collaboration on hospital costs. *Journal of Nursing Administration, 36*(2), 79–85.

Dulisse, B., & Cromwell, J. (2010). No harm found when nurse anesthetists work without supervision by physicians. *Health Affairs, 29*(8), 1469–1475.

Edmunds, M. (2002). Keeping nurses in their place. *Nurse Practitioner, 27*(2), 11.

Faut-Callahan, M., & Kremer, M. J. (2000). The certified registered nurse anesthetist. In A. B. Hamric, J. A. Spross, & C. M. Hanson (Eds.), *Advanced nursing practice: An integrative approach* (2nd ed.) (pp. 521–548). Philadelphia: WB Saunders.

Feldman, M. J., Ventura, M. R., & Crosby, F. (1987). Studies of nurse practitioner effectiveness. *Nursing Research, 36*(5), 303–308.

Finerfrock, W., & Havens, D. H. (1997). Coverage and reimbursement issues for nurse practitioners. *Journal of Pediatric Health Care, 11*(3), 139–143.

Frakes, M. A., & Evans, T. (2006). An overview of Medicare reimbursement regulations for advanced practice nurses. *Nursing Economic$, 24*(2), 59–65.

Graham, M. C. (2011). Building a national consensus for APRN regulation. *Nurse Practitioner, 36*(5), 8.

Griffith, H. (1986). Implementation of direct third party reimbursement legislation for nursing services. *Nursing Economic$, 4*(6), 299–304.

Griffith, H., & Robinson, K. R. (1993). Current procedural terminology (CPT) coded services provided by nurse specialists. *Image: Journal of Nursing Scholarship, 25*(3), 178–186.

Hansen-Turton, T., Bailey, D., Nagle, D., Torres, N., & Ritter, A. (2010). Nurse-managed health centers. *American Journal of Nursing, 110*(9), 23–26.

Hansen-Turton, T., & Torgan, R. (2008). Insurers' contracting policies on nurse practitioners as primary care providers. *Policy, Politics, and Nursing Practice, 9*(4), 241–248.

Johantgen, M., Fountain, L., Zangaro, G., Newhouse, R., Stanik-Hutt, J., & White, K. (August, 2011). Comparison of labor and delivery care provided by certified nurse-midwives and physicians: A systematic review, 1990 to 2008. *Women's Health Issues.* Retrieved September 28, 2011 from http://womenshealth.about.com. .

Johnson, J., Dawson, E., & Brassard, A. (2010). Consensus model for advanced practice nurse regulation: A new approach. In E. Sullivan-Marx, D. McGivern, J. Fairman, & S. Greenberg (Eds.), *The evolution and future of advanced practice* (5th ed.) (pp. 125–142). New York: Springer.

Kennerly, S. (2006). Positioning advanced practice nurses for financial success in clinical practice. *Nurse Educator, 31*(5), 218–222.

Kennerly, S. (2007). The impending reimbursement revolution: How to prepare for future APN reimbursement. *Nursing Economic$, 25*(2), 81–84.

King, E. S., & Hansen-Turton, T. (2010). Nurse-managed health centers. In E. Sullivan-Marx, D. McGivern, J. Fairman, & S. Greenberg (Eds.), *The evolution and future of advanced practice* (5th ed.) (pp. 183–198). New York: Springer.

Kleinpell, R. M., French, K. D., & Diamond, E. J. (2007). Billing for NP provider services: Updates on coding regulations. *Nurse Practitioner, 32*(6), 16–17.

Lavoie-Vaughan, N. (2011). CMS incentives for quality care: Get started now. *Advance for NPs and PAs, 2*(4), 18.

Library of Congress. (2011). Retrieved October 4, 2011, from www.congress.gov.

Magdic, K. S. (2006). Acute care billing: Shared visits. *Nurse Practitioner, 31*(11), 9–10.

Mason, D. J., & Keepnews, D. (2011). Implementing health care reform: A nursing perspective. *Nursing Outlook, 59*(1), 57–58.

Milstead, J. A. (1997). Using advanced practice to shape public policy: Agenda setting. *Nursing Administration Quarterly, 21*(4), 12–18.

Mittelstadt, P. (1991, March 1). PPRC recommends payment levels for non-physician providers. *Capitol Update* (pp. 7–8). Washington, DC: American Nurses Association.

Mittelstadt, P. (1993). Federal reimbursement of advanced practice nurses' services empowers the profession. *Nurse Practitioner, 18*(1), 43–49.

Mundinger, M. O., Kane, R. L., Lenz, E. R., Totten, A. M., Tsai, W., Cleary, P. D., et al. (2000). Primary care outcomes in patients treated by nurse practitioners or physicians. *Journal of the American Medical Association, 283*(1), 59–68.

North, L., Kehm, L., Bent, K., & Hartman, T. (2008). Can home-based primary care cut costs? *Nurse Practitioner, 33*(7), 39–44.

O'Brien, J. M. (2003). How nurse practitioners obtained provider status: Lessons for pharmacists. *American Journal Health-System Pharmacists, 60*(22), 2301–2307.

Paez, K. A., & Allen, J. K. (2006). Cost-effectiveness of nurse practitioner management of hypercholesterolemia following coronary revascularization. *Journal of the American Academy of Nurse Practitioners, 18*(9), 436–444.

Pearson, L. J. (2002). Fourteenth annual legislative update: How each state stands on legislative issues affecting advanced nursing practice. *Nurse Practitioner, 27*(1), 10–22.

Phillips, S. J. (2008). After 20 years, APNs are still standing together. *Nurse Practitioner, 33*(1), 10–34.

Physician Payment Review Commission. (1991). *Annual report to Congress.* Washington, DC: U.S. Government Printing Office.

Pruitt, R. H., Wetsel, M. A., Smith, K. J., & Spitler, H. (2002). How do we pass NP autonomy legislation? *Nurse Practitioner, 27*(3), 56–65.

Public Law 105-33. *Balanced Budget Act of 1997.* Washington, DC: U.S. Congress.

Ritter, A., & Hansen-Turton, T. (2008). The primary care paradigm shift: An overview of the state-level legal framework governing nurse practitioner practice. *Health Lawyer, 20*(4), 20–28.

Robinson, K. R. (2004). Payment for advanced practice nursing services: Past, present, and future. In L. Joel (Ed.), *Advanced practice nursing* (1st ed.) (pp. 99–121). Philadelphia: F. A. Davis.

Robinson, K. R. (2009). Payment for advanced practice nursing services: Past, present, and future. In L. Joel (Ed.), *Advanced practice nursing: Essentials for role development* (2nd ed.) (pp. 102–118). Philadelphia: F. A. Davis.

Robinson, K. R. (2010). Roles of nurse practitioners in the U.S. Department of Veterans Affairs. In E. Sullivan-Marx, D. McGivern, J. Fairman, & S. Greenberg (Eds.), *The evolution and future of advanced practice* (5th ed.) (pp. 223–238). New York: Springer.

Robinson, K. R., & Griffith, H.M. (2012) . Current procedural terminology-coded services. In J. J. Fitzpatrick (Editor-in-Chief) & M. Wallace (Associate Editor), *Encyclopedia of nursing research* (3rd ed.). New York: Springer.

Robinson, K. R., Griffith, H. M., & Sullivan-Marx, E. M. (2001). Nursing practice reimbursement issues in the 21st century. In N. L. Chaska (Ed.), *The nursing profession: Tomorrow and beyond* (pp. 501–513). Thousand Oaks, CA: Sage.

Rothman, N. L., & Hansen-Turton, T. (2006). Nursing center model of health care for the underserved. Retrieved October 4, 2011, from http://apha.confex.com.

Sahota, P., & Rose, A. (2009). Non-physician practitioners in Indian Health Service. Retrieved September 7, 2011, from www.ncaiprc.org.

Spitzer, R. (1997). The Vanderbilt University experience. *Nursing Management, 28*(3), 38–40.

Stanley, J. (2009). Reaching consensus on a regulatory model: What does this mean for APRNs? *Journal for Nurse Practitioners, 5,* 99–104.

Sullivan-Marx, E. M. (2008). Lessons learned from advanced practice nursing payment. *Policy, Politics, and Nursing Practice, 9*(2), 121–126.

Sullivan-Marx, E. M., & Keepnews, D. (2010). Systems of payment for advanced-practice nurses. In E. M. Sullivan-Marx, D. McGivern, J. Fairman, & S. Greenberg (Eds.), *The evolution and future of advanced practice* (5th ed.) (pp. 271–294). New York: Springer.

Sullivan-Marx, E. M., & Maislin, G. (2000). Comparison of nurse practitioner and family physician relative work values. *Image: Journal of Nursing Scholarship, 32*(1), 71–76.

Summers, L. (2011). ANA works to get APRNs counted as primary care providers. *American Nurse,* July-August, 8.

TRICARE. (2011). Retrieved October 2, 2011, from www.tricare.mil.

U.S. Congress Office of Technology Assessment. (1986). *Nurse practitioners, physician assistants, and certified nurse-mid-wives: A policy analysis.* (Health technology Case Study 37, OTA-HCS-37). Washington, DC: U.S. Government Printing Office.

U.S. Department of Health and Human Services, Center for Medicare and Medicaid Services. (2007) *Medicare carriers manual* (Transmittal No. 1168. Sec. 120.1).

U.S. Department of Health and Human Services, Center for Medicare and Medicaid Services. (2008). *Medicare carriers manual* (Transmittal No. 1548. Sec. 30.6.12).

U.S. Government Accountability Office. (2011). Retrieved October 4, 2011, from www.gao.gov.

Zuzelo, P. R., Fallon, R., Lang, A., Lang, C., McGovern, K., Mount, L., et al. (2004). Clinical nurse specialists' knowledge specific to Medicare structures and processes. *Clinical Nurse Specialist, 18*(4), 207–217.

7

Advanced Practice Nurses and Prescriptive Authority

Jan Towers

DEVELOPMENT OF AUTHORITY TO PRACTICE

As professional nurses expanded their role to cross into traditional medical domains, the ability to prescribe medications became increasingly important. Although certified registered nurse anesthetists (CRNAs), certified nurse-midwives (CNMs), and clinical nurse specialists (CNSs) had practiced in advanced roles for some time before the birth of nurse practitioners (NPs), the advent of NP practice in primary care influenced the authorization of all advanced practice registered nurses (APRNs) to prescribe medications. Before that time, CRNAs selected and administered anesthesia, but not other medications. Likewise, CNMs traditionally focused on childbirth and did not require extensive prescriptive authority. CNSs functioned in advanced practice nursing roles with diagnosed patients who were under the care of a physician. Although professionals in each of these roles made judgments regarding medications used by patients under their care, they relied mainly on physicians to provide prescriptions for medications when they were needed.

Nurse Practitioners and Prescriptive Authority

As NPs began to provide primary care services, they used these same traditional processes to provide medications for the patients that they served. Although there is an emphasis on health promotion and disease prevention in primary care practice, most patients coming for primary care services do so with a health problem for which they are seeking assistance. As time went on, it became evident that depending on physicians to prescribe medications created problems in the areas of patient access to care, continuity of care, and patient flow. When providing primary care, NPs assessed and diagnosed patients who needed prescription medications and treatments for their care.

The inability to sign one's own prescription, even if a physician was on site, was inconvenient for NP, physician, and patient alike. It caused interruptions in the physician's interactions with patients, unnecessary delays each time NPs had to wait to get signed prescriptions from physicians, and often interfered with the credibility of NPs by rendering them dependent on physician signatures for medications that were being ordered based on their own diagnostic decision making. These problems were exacerbated when a physician was not on site. Then patients had to wait for prescriptions to be signed before they could be filled. If a physician was not available for a day or more, the implications for patient safety and health care were serious.

Methods were found to get around this stumbling block, such as calling prescriptions in to pharmacies or using other more questionable methods for obtaining a physician signature on the prescription so that the patient could pursue treatment in a timely manner. The need for the authority of NPs to prescribe under their own names became evident and pressing.

In the early days, NPs did not have title recognition other than that of registered nurse (RN) in their state regulatory systems. They were not alone; with the exception of CNMs and CRNAs in a number of states, no APRNs had title recognition in statutory or regulatory language in the state nurse practice acts or administrative rules. Likewise, there was no authority to prescribe medications. In fact, many nurse practice acts clearly prohibited the prescribing of medication by nurses regardless of specialty or status. And so began the long journey of convincing legislators and regulators to change state statutes and regulations to give title recognition and prescriptive authority to APRNs.

Because licensure for all professions occurs at the state rather than the federal level, the movement to achieve these goals moved unevenly, as states with the most need moved forward to make changes. The movement was enhanced in the early days by an acute shortage of primary care physicians, and some states with higher primary care needs moved forward more rapidly than others. At that time, rural states were more likely to initiate statutory and regulatory adjustments than were states with large urban populations.

Convincing decision makers in the states was not without its problems. Then, as now, NPs had to demonstrate that they had the knowledge base to safely diagnose illnesses and prescribe medications. This meant that educational programs had to demonstrate that their curriculums prepared NPs for an independent prescribing role. Advanced pathophysiology and pharmacology and the development of differential diagnosis and clinical decision-making skills needed to be visible in the programs. With the advent of federal grants to prepare NPs, the content and quality of the preparatory programs was increasingly standardized.

In addition, to be credible in health-care systems, it was necessary for members of the medical community to advocate for the recognition of these professionals and their ability to prescribe medications independently. Many did, and through this window of opportunity, NPs began to gain prescriptive authority state by state over subsequent years.

Initially, the authority to practice and prescribe was limited. In many of the early states where some form of prescriptive authority was conferred, boards of medicine and boards of nursing were authorized to jointly promulgate rules and regulations governing NP actions, including prescriptive authority. States such as North Carolina and Idaho were among those first states with jointly promulgated rules. Even today a few states still fall under the regulation of both boards of nursing and boards of medicine. Some of those states (where the highest degree of controversy over scope of practice has traditionally existed) are limited to joint regulation of prescriptive authority. Recent attempts to change that regulatory pattern have been harder to achieve. Pennsylvania is the most recent state to move away from joint promulgation of rules to regulation solely by the board of nursing.

Initially, NPs were authorized to prescribe a limited number of medications under physician supervision. North Carolina was one of the first states to develop a limited drug formulary. Subsequently, states developed combinations of formularies and physician oversight under jointly promulgated rules or under rules developed by boards of nursing. The form of those rules depended largely on the persuasiveness of NPs and the attitudes of the legislators and governors of those states.

Currently, NPs prescribe legend drugs under their own signature in 50 states and the District of Columbia. In addition, they prescribe controlled drugs in 48 states and the District of Columbia. Variation exists among states in the area of the authorization to prescribe controlled drugs and the relationship, if any, that must be maintained with a physician. Currently, there exists plenary prescriptive authority (no requirement for any physician involvement) in 16 states and the District of Columbia (American Academy of Nurse Practitioners [AANP], 2012). See **Figure 7-1.**

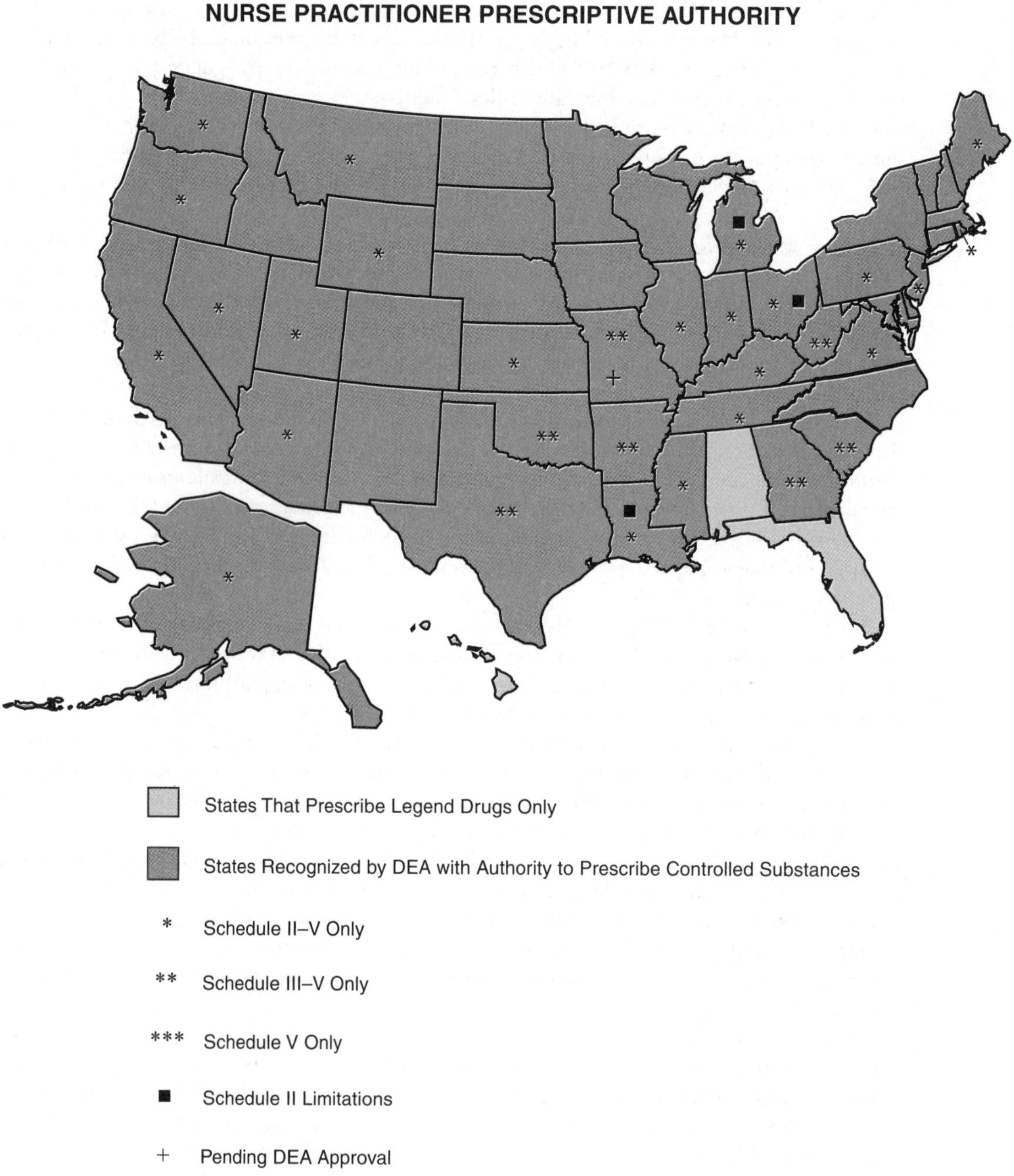

FIGURE 7-1 Nurse practitioners' authority to prescribe medications. *(Source: Drug Enforcement Administration, Washington, DC, 2012; © American Academy of Nurse Practitioners, 2012.)*

Nurse-Midwives and Prescriptive Authority

CNMs have had to undergo the same process as other APRNs to attain prescriptive authority. Because their educational preparation and role developed to include not only obstetrical and newborn care, but also the general health management of their patients, the need to prescribe a broader range of medications also increased, making the previously described arrangement for prescribing under the physician's signature unreasonable.

Federal funding of CNM educational programs helped to implement the standards established by this discipline and facilitate the passage of statutes and rules that allow them to prescribe in 50 states and the District of Columbia with variable limitations in the area of controlled drugs (American College of Nurse-Midwives [ACNM], 2008). See **Figure 7-2.**

Other factors that have assisted in this endeavor include an enthusiastic consumer population, especially pregnant women, who spread the word about the skills of CNMs. They have often packed hearing rooms and legislative chambers, bringing their babies and children, providing testimony regarding the worth and skill of the services provided to them by CNMs. CNMs have the same

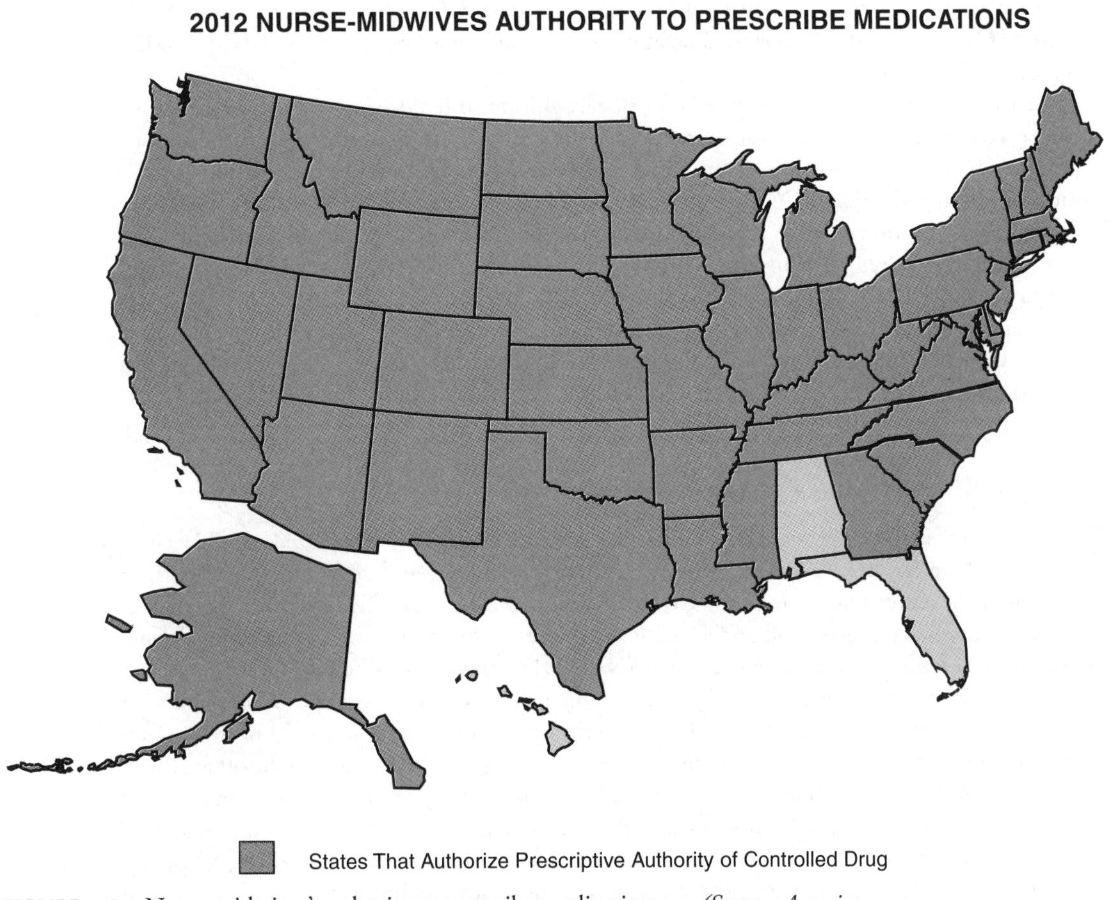

FIGURE 7-2 Nurse-midwives' authority to prescribe medications. *(Source: American College of Nurse Midwives, 2008; © American Academy of Nurse Practitioners, 2012.)*

state-to-state variability regarding authorization to prescribe controlled drugs and required relationships, if any, with physicians.

Clinical Nurse Specialists and Prescriptive Authority

CNSs have more recently felt the need to prescribe medications for the patients they serve. Those particularly desirous of the authorization are the psychiatric and mental health CNSs who often have their own practices or function autonomously in mental health clinics and other specialty practices. The prescriptive authority need for practitioners in this field is particularly acute in agencies serving vulnerable populations.

The remainder of the CNS community has mixed responses to the need for authorization to prescribe medications. At the core of this ambivalence is the role played by the CNS in the employment setting, the scope of prescriptive authority needed when working in a particular specialty with patients who have already been diagnosed, the educational preparation required to allow for this authorization, and the risk of being unnecessarily placed under the supervision of physicians in states where such supervision is required. Some states do not provide title recognition for CNSs. There has been controversy regarding whether an additional title recognition is actually needed for CNSs. As a result, the issue of prescriptive authority for CNSs has been more cloudy than that of NPs or CNMs (National Association of Clinical Nurse Specialists [NACNS], (2002); NACNS, 2005).

Nevertheless, CNSs have begun to obtain title recognition (often driven by the need for recognition to receive reimbursement for services) and the authority to prescribe within their scope of practice. Currently, two-thirds of the states authorize CNSs to prescribe medications in one fashion or another (National Council of State Boards of Nursing [NCSBN], 2012).Variability in recognizing who may qualify, scope of prescriptive authority, ability to prescribe controlled substances, and required relationships with physicians occur from state-to-state. In some states the statutes and regulations are similar to those of NPs and in others they are not. A few states have extended prescriptive authority to psychiatric and mental health CNSs only. A few have grouped all APRNs under one set of regulations, whereas most have kept the four clinical groups separated under an APRN umbrella that allows for regulatory variability among APRNs in their states.

Nurse Anesthetists and Prescriptive Authority

The authority of CRNAs to select and administer anesthesia has long been recognized. Until recently, CRNAs have been less involved in the struggle to obtain prescriptive authority than the other three disciplines. Some representatives from the CRNA community have maintained that ordering and administering anesthesia does not fall under the rubric of prescriptive authority in its traditional sense (American Association of Nurse Anesthetists [AANA], 2011). Increasingly, however, CRNAs are becoming involved in pain management of patients in the practices they serve and thus have the need to prescribe. Currently, nurse anesthetists have prescriptive authority in 30 states; 23 of those states still require collaboration with or supervision by a physician (AANA, 2011). As with the other APRN groups, CRNAs have found that they have to work to convince legislators and governors of their knowledge and skills. Their availability in rural areas has enhanced their ability to obtain these privileges even in the presence of opposition from the medical community. As with NPs, CNMs, and CNSs, they have had to demonstrate the strength of their educational programs and the safety of their practice to obtain privileges in this area.

THE ROAD TO STATUTORY AND REGULATORY CHANGE TO AUTHORIZE PRESCRIPTIVE AUTHORITY

To alter state statutes and regulations, APRNs had to educate state legislatures, executive offices, and regulators regarding the role of the APRNs they represented. In addition, they had to demonstrate a need for APRNs to prescribe and prove that prescribing by APRNs was safe and contributed to the well-being of the population.

There are a variety of ways to authorize prescriptive authority within a state. Changes (amendments) may be made to nurse practice acts (statutes); new statutes may be developed separate from nurse practice acts; or changes may be made in states' administrative codes through the development of regulations promulgated by the appropriate regulating board (in most cases the board of nursing).

In the case of new statutes or statutory changes, legislation must be introduced that amends or adds to current law to give title recognition and prescriptive authority to APRNs (NPs, CNMs, CNSs, or CRNAs). Once legislation is introduced, it is referred to a committee of jurisdiction (usually a professional licensure committee) for consideration. Once the legislation is in committee, the chair of that committee generally calls for a hearing to allow proponents and opponents of the legislation to give testimony regarding the introduced legislation. After hearings are conducted, at the chair's discretion, the committee votes on the legislation and passes it out of committee. In some states, proposed legislation must also go through the appropriations committee of at least one of the voting chambers to determine cost and evaluate fiscal impact on the state. After passing through all appropriate committees, the legislation, at the discretion of the majority party leadership, is taken to the floor of the voting chamber for a vote. Sometimes this is done simultaneously in both chambers of the state legislature; in others, the legislation passes through one chamber at a time. Once the legislation has been agreed on (passed) by both chambers of the legislature, it is sent to the governor to be signed or, in the case of some states, to be vetoed.

It is during this process that language changes in proposed legislation are often made or negotiated to satisfy other interested parties. For this reason, the language of authorizing statutes varies to a certain extent from state to state. This is particularly true in the sections (a) defining procedures to be followed and requirements that must be met to be recognized as an APRN; (b) defining the relationship, if any, that must be held with a physician to prescribe; and (c) determining the scope of prescriptive authority of the APRN, particularly the authorization to prescribe controlled drugs (schedules I through V). As statutes are passed, much time and energy goes into attempting to negotiate language that is acceptable to the advanced practice community, involved legislators, governors, regulatory bodies, and other interested parties. Once statutes have been passed and signed by the governor of a state, rules and regulations are developed and approved by the authorized regulatory body or bodies.

Several states have not introduced or altered statutes to authorize APRN prescriptive authority, but rather have developed and instituted regulatory changes in the administrative code by which the advanced practice disciplines must abide. Although regulation cannot override statute, statutes are often worded broadly enough for regulations regarding title recognition and authorization to prescribe drugs to be developed by the regulatory body or bodies without disturbing statutes.

When regulations are developed, they are first written as proposed rules and are placed in a public register for comment. The comment period covers a limited time, after which the promulgating boards consider the comments and make appropriate changes in the proposed rule at their discretion before publishing a final rule. In most states, such regulations must then be approved by some arm of the legislature, often committees of jurisdiction, sometimes by one or the other legislative chamber, before approval by the governor. For this reason, APRNs and regulatory bodies are often embroiled in negotiations similar to those encountered in the legislative process that result in alterations that make for variance in regulations from state to state. These variations are in the same general areas where there is variability in statute.

Because the purpose of state regulatory bodies, such as boards of nursing, is to protect the public (in this case, the public health), boards of nursing vary in their advocacy of advanced practice roles in the regulatory process. In most states governors appoint the members of the professional licensure boards. Having APRNs, who understand the roles of NPs, CNMs, CNSs, and CRNAs, appointed to these positions can help the regulatory process when issues such as prescriptive authority are considered.

Patterns of Statutory and Regulatory Authority

Four basic patterns of regulation regarding prescriptive authority have evolved over time:

- The use of an established formulary or lists of drugs that the APRN can prescribe
- A negative or exclusionary formulary that allows the APRN to prescribe all drugs with a short list of forbidden drugs
- An individualized collaborative formulary established by the APRN with a collaborating physician
- Unlimited authority with no formulary or collaborative requirements

Regulator Established Formulary

An established formulary was used in the early days of NP prescribing activity to determine an agreed-on list of drugs that NPs could prescribe. As new drugs came onto the market, these formularies had to be updated to allow NPs to prescribe according to current practice standards. Although this quickly became a cumbersome process, it is still in use today in a few states.

Negative or Exclusionary Formulary

Exclusionary formularies were found to be a more practical approach to regulation of prescriptive authority of NPs. By creating a short list of forbidden drugs (e.g., cancer drugs and gold treatments), the NP had more flexibility in choosing appropriate treatments for patients. This has been particularly important in the primary care setting.

Collaborative Formulary

More flexible than the established formulary, and to a certain extent more flexible than a negative formulary, a collaborative formulary allows the APRN to create a formulary most useful to his or her practice in collaboration with an identified physician who serves as a collaborator. Although this has worked well in some states, in others, where the formulary must be shared with the regulatory board, it has sometimes become a nightmare. Requirements regarding information to be included in formularies and updating formularies can be, to say the least, cumbersome and obstructive.

Open Formulary

The most flexible framework for prescriptive authority is the open formulary, in which APRNs have no limitations regarding what they can prescribe. In these cases, APRNs prescribe according to their own specialty scope of practice, just as physicians prescribe within their own scope of specialty practice. The majority of states that have implemented this framework in their regulations have done so without difficulty or negative repercussion. Over all, the trend toward the removal of barriers to prescribing has resulted in the removal of limitations of drugs to be prescribed and the requirement for physician collaboration to do so. Although barriers still exist in the authorization to prescribe controlled substances in a few states, the limitations of authorization to prescribe legend drugs have disappeared.

Advanced Practice Nurse–Physician Relationships in Statute and Regulation

Often, the requirement of some sort of collaborative arrangement with physicians to prescribe is coupled with the prescriptive authority patterns discussed previously. Whereas many states do not require formal collaborative arrangements with physicians, the remainder have some requirement for collaborative or supervisory agreements with physicians to practice or prescribe medication. For NPs, approximately one-third of the state statutes and regulations have no requirements, less than one-fourth require supervision or have delegated authority, and the remainder require some kind of collaborative or consulting arrangement with a physician. These arrangements range from identifying a consulting physician to submission of a written agreement to the regulatory board(s) for filing or approval (AANP, 2012). CNMs have a similar pattern: approximately one-fourth have no requirements; approximately one-fourth require a supervising physician; and the remainder require some kind of collaborative/consulting relationship in statute or administrative rule (ACNM, 2001). CRNAs have supervising or cooperating physicians in most states (AANA, 2011), whereas CNSs, in the states in which they have prescriptive authority, tend to have the same requirements as NPs (NCSBN, 2012).

Some of these requirements stem from a desire on the part of legislators or interested and influential parties for physician oversight to prescribe; others have been driven by reimbursement laws and policy that calls for physician oversight of APRNs. Sometimes rules are made for APRNs that reflect the supervisory relationship required of physician assistants, without considering the fact that APRNs are accountable under their own license, carry their own liability insurance, and in the majority of states are not required to be supervised by physicians, as are physician assistants.

BARRIERS TO PRESCRIPTIVE PRACTICE

The roads traveled by APRNs to obtain prescriptive authority have not been without struggle. There is no denying that the majority of barriers to practice have roots in organized lobbying by certain parts of the medical community to limit the autonomy of APRNs. This move has often been couched in the language of "protecting public safety." As a result, some legislators and governors have seen fit to set limitations in statute and administrative rules governing APRNs. The literature is replete with studies that report on the clinical safety of APRNs. In the studies that have been conducted, APRNs have been found to be as safe as physicians and often have been found to be safer than physicians (Brown & Grimes, 1995; Laurent et al., 2006; Office of Technology Assessment [OTA], 1986). The ratings on quality of care have been consistently high in the studies that have been conducted over the years. APRNs, particularly NPs, have been studied and scrutinized in multiple studies with consistently positive reports (AANP, 2010).

The biggest barriers to practice for all groups have been the limitations set in state statute and regulation. Of those, the requirements for formalized agreements with physicians to prescribe or practice have created the most frustrating barrier for APRNs. This has been particularly true for NPs and

CNMs who, to practice and receive reimbursement, must find physicians who will agree to serve as collaborators. CRNAs, particularly in rural areas, suffer from similar problems.

Once a physician has agreed to serve as a consultant, both the APRN and physician often find the reporting rules to be frustratingly cumbersome. Although it now occurs infrequently, requirements to list types of patients that may be seen, consultation patterns to be maintained, types of drugs to be prescribed, and identification of physicians to serve as backup in the absence of the identified collaborating physician still plague APRNs. Although, generally speaking, pharmacists have been cooperative and NPs report a good working relationship with pharmacists, issues such as continued use of the collaborating physician name as the prescriber on a medicine bottle label and requests for the name of the "supervising physician" before dispensing a prescription have frustrated APRNs, physicians, and patients through the years. The requirement of a Drug Enforcement Administration (DEA) number by insurance companies to pay for prescriptions is still problematic, particularly in the two states where APRNs are not yet authorized to prescribe controlled drugs. This problem lands on the pharmacists' doorstep when they cannot obtain reimbursement for dispensed drugs from insurance companies without an accompanying DEA number. Although this practice is a misuse of the DEA number, which is to be used for the prescription of controlled drugs only, it has become common practice for insurance companies and pharmacies to use this number as an identifier because of its uniformity for physician identification throughout the country. Mail-order pharmacies sometimes create barriers for APRNs. Occasionally, patients cannot obtain prescriptions from these entities without the name or signature of a physician. Although this is no longer a problem with most mail-order pharmacies, those with warehouses located in states where laws for this form of dispensing require the order of a physician still occasionally pose difficulties for patients with prescriptions written by APRNs.

Confusion about the role and scope of practice of an APRN through the grouping of NPs, CNMs, and physician assistants as "midlevel practitioners" has created problems for APRNs. It is often assumed that the required supervisory arrangements for physician assistants is the same for NPs and CNMs, so that policies related to practice, including prescriptive authority and ordering of medications for patients, are often based on the statutes and rules governing physician assistants rather than the APRNs. Because most regulation of physician assistants stems from a state's medical practice act, insurance companies, institutions, accreditation entities, and pharmaceutical companies sometimes assume that the physician assistant administrative rules apply to APRNs and do not seek information regarding APRNs from a state's nurse practice act and supporting regulations. Because APRNs are authorized to practice more autonomously in most instances, this assumption, and the actions taken based on it, create barriers for the APRN, particularly in relation to prescribing controlled drugs.

PRESCRIBING PATTERNS

The AANP has conducted several national surveys that examined the prescribing patterns of NPs throughout the United States (Goolsby, 2005, 2009; Towers, 1989, 1999a, 1999b). In those studies it was found that an NP's prescription patterns reflected the specialty and the practice setting of the NP. In these studies the mean number of prescriptions per day for all NPs was approximately 19, with family, adult, and emergency NPs among the highest daily prescribers.

Drugs most frequently prescribed by all specialties in these studies were antimicrobials, anti-inflammatories, and analgesics. Antihypertensives, bronchodilators, and cardiovascular drugs were prescribed most frequently by adult, family, and gerontological NPs. Contraceptives were most often prescribed by women's health NPs. The vast majority of NPs practicing in emergency department settings prescribe analgesics, anti-inflammatories, and antimicrobials most often, and in the Department of Veteran's Affairs (VA) hospital setting, the vast majority of NPs prescribe antihypertensives and cardiovascular drugs most frequently, followed by diabetic medications, gastrointestinal medications, and analgesics. Among NPs authorized to prescribe controlled drugs, the majority of adult, family, gerontological, and psychiatric and mental health NPs prescribe them at least once a week, the highest percentages being in the hospital and VA hospital setting.

CNM prescriptive activities center on medications needed for prenatal care, such as vitamins, and intrapartum and postpartum care, such as analgesics. In addition, their prescribing practices are similar to those of women's health NPs. They include contraceptives and other hormone therapies, vaginal preparations, and antimicrobials, as well as anti-inflammatories, analgesics, and vitamin therapies (Towers, 1999a). The CNSs who most often prescribe medications at this time are the psychiatric and mental health specialists. In a study conducted by Talley and Richens (2001), psychiatric and mental health CNSs authorized to prescribe controlled drugs were reported to most frequently prescribe antidepressants (selective serotonin uptake inhibitors and tricyclic antidepressants). The next most frequently prescribed medications were antiparkinsonian drugs and antihistamines for neuroleptic side effects and sleep, followed by mood stabilizers such as lithium and carbamazepine.

Among CNSs of other specialties, prescribing activities appear to function around already diagnosed conditions and altering, adjusting, or refilling physician-prescribed medications in stable patients. The lack of authorization and the desire to maintain autonomy in nursing practice led many CNSs to choose not to obtain authorization in settings in which such authorization is attainable. The position of the National Association of Clinical Nurse Specialists (NACNS) is that CNS prescriptive authority should be optional and that when prescribing is to be undertaken, the CNS should meet the requirements of any other APRN (Lyon & Minarik, 2001; NACNS, 2005).

THE FUTURE FOR APRN PRESCRIBING

While authorizing APRNs to prescribe medications is no longer a controversial issue, obsolete statutes and regulations still need to be changed in some states to guarantee the unencumbered ability for APRNs to prescribe needed medications for all patients. Toward this end, two important documents have been developed that reinforce the authorization of APRNs to function at their full educational scope, which includes unrestricted prescriptive authority for APRNs. The APRN Consensus Model (2008), endorsed by 46 states, provides recommendations for the education and certification of APRNs. Likewise, the Institute of Medicine (IOM) *Future of Nursing* report (2010) reinforces the need for APRNs to be authorized to practice to the full extent of their education and training. Both documents reflect the culmination of the APRN's evolution to full prescriptive authority that generally exists today.

CONCLUSION

Prescriptive authority is now generally recognized as an integral part of advanced practice nursing. Although totally unfettered authority by all APRNs has not yet been achieved, the experience of prescribing medications for patients under the care of these providers has been found to be safe and beneficial. The arguments put forth to limit their prescribing activities grow weaker with each advance that APRNs make. The practicality, the enhancement of quality of care, and the cost-effectiveness of the practice of these groups has enhanced the logic and desirability of giving prescriptive authority to APRNs nationwide.

REFERENCES

American Academy of Nurse Practitioners. (2012). *Statutory and regulatory authority for nurse practitioners.* Washington, DC: Author.

American Academy of Nurse Practitioners. (2010). *Cost effectiveness of nurse practitioners.* Washington, DC: Author.

American Association of Nurse Anesthetists. (2011). *Prescriptive authority by state.* Vol. 79, no 3. Retrieved February 14, 2012 from www.aana.com/aana/journalonline.aspx. American College of Nurse-Midwives. (2001). *State laws governing the relationship between CNMs and physicians.* Washington, DC: Author.

American College of Nurse-Midwives. (2008). *Midwives and prescriptive authority.* Washington, DC: Author.

APRN Consensus Workgroup. (2008). *Consensus model for APRN regulation: Licensure, accreditation, certification and education.* Washington, DC: Author.

Brown, S. A., & Grimes, D. E. (1995). A meta-analysis of nurse practitioners and nurse midwives in primary care. *Nursing Research, 44*(6), 332–339.

Drug Enforcement Administration. (2012). Retrieved August 15, 2012 from http://www.deadiversion.usdoj.gov/pubs/manuals/pract/pract_manual012508.pdf.

Goolsby, M. (2005). 2004 AANP national nurse practitioner sample survey, part II: Nurse practitioner prescribing. *Journal of the American Academy of Nurse Practitioners, 17*(12), 506–511.

Goolsby, M. (2009). *National nurse practitioner survey.* Austin, TX: American Academy of Nurse Practitioners.

Institute of Medicine. (2010). *The future of nursing.* Washington, DC: Author.

Laurent, M., et al. (2006). Substitution of doctors by nurses in primary care. *Cochrane Database Reviews,* Issue 1.

Lyon, B., & Minarik, P. (2001). Statutory and regulatory issues for clinical nurse practitioner practice. *Clinical Nurse Specialist, 15*(3), 30–39.

National Association of Clinical Nurse Specialists. (2002). *Assuring the public's access to CNS services: Model statutory/regulatory language to regulate CNS practice.* Mission Aliso, CA: Author. National Association of Clinical Nurse Specialists. (2005). *NACNS position statement on advanced pharmacology: Practice, curricular and regulatory recommendations.* Harrisburg, PA: Author.

National Council of State Boards of Nursing. (2012). Retrieved November 30, 2012 from https://www.NCSBN.org/2567.htm.

Office of Technology Assessment. (1986). *Nurse practitioners, physician assistants and certified nurse-midwives: A policy analysis.* (Policy No. OTA-HCS-37). Washington, DC: U.S. Government Printing Office.

Talley, S., & Richens, S. (2001). Prescribing practices of advanced practice psychiatric nurses: Part I—Demographic, educational and practice characteristics. *Archives of Psychiatric Nursing, 15*(5), 205–213.

Towers, J. (1989). American Academy of Nurse Practitioners National Survey. Part II. *Journal of the American Academy of Nurse Practitioners, 1*(4), 137–145.

Towers, J. (1999a). *American Academy of Nurse Practitioners National Survey: Prescribing practices.* Washington, DC: American Academy of Nurse Practitioners.

Towers, J. (1999b). *American Academy of Nurse Practitioners National Survey: Prescribing practices in hospital settings.* Washington, DC: American Academy of Nurse Practitioners.

8

Credentialing and Clinical Privileges for the Advanced Practice Registered Nurse

Ann H. Cary
Mary C. Smolenski

INTRODUCTION

Credentialing and privileging of health-care providers, and advanced practice registered nurses (APRNs) in particular, is the initial and ongoing mechanism employed by regulatory and voluntary oversight bodies and delivery systems to ensure protection of the public and high-quality patient care during the delivery of health-care services. The independence and autonomy of APRN services necessitate the same degree of attention to the processes of credentialing and privileging as accorded to physicians and other providers. The process is a critical dimension of any risk management plan and is reflected in the level of responsibility assumed by the governing board, medical staff organization, or top administrator of the institution. APRNs are increasingly being granted privileges in acute care and hospice settings, and participate in provider networks as primary care practitioners. For example, in Maryland alone, over 3,500 APRNs are eligible to bill as primary care providers (HCPro, 2011a, p. 3). Based on data from 2010 and 2011, it is estimated that at least 43% of nurse practitioners (NPs) and 67% of certified nurse-midwives (CNMs) have hospital privileges (Goolsby, 2011; Schuiling, Sipe, & Fullerton, 2010). Membership data from the American Association of Nurse Anesthetists (AANA) reveal that 37% of certified registered nurse anesthetists (CRNAs) are employed by hospitals and another 34% are employed by an anesthesia group (with the assumption that this would necessitate credentialing by the facility of practice).

The Institute of Medicine (IOM) report *The Future of Nursing: Leading Change, Advancing Health* has challenged nursing and society "to allow nurses to practice to the full extent of their education and training" (IOM, 2011, p. 4). Recommendation 1 asserts that to master this challenge, we must remove barriers to the scope of practice through actions in Congress, state legislatures, the Centers for Medicare and Medicaid Services (CMS), the Federal Trade Commission, and the Department of Justice. In addition, organizational barriers created by the APRN employer may be equally oppressive. APRNs who experience these barriers often realize them during the process of credentialing and as an outcome of the privileging process. Credentialing and privileging outcomes have a dramatic and common impact on the ability of the APRN to execute the full scope of practice and thus have resulted in the American Association of Retired Persons (AARP) issuing a warning: "barriers (to APRNs) . . . are short-changing consumers" (IOM, 2011, p. 106).

There appear to be relief and progress to removing barriers to APRN practice with the issuance of the *Consensus Model for APRN Regulation* (National Council of State Boards of Nursing [NCSBN], 2008) and the newly issued credentialing and privileging processes for providers by CMS (Manos, 2010) and The Joint Commission (TJC, 2011). The *Consensus Model for APRN Regulation: Licensure, Accreditation, Certification and Education* (NCSBN, 2008), or LACE (**L**icensure, **A**ccreditation, **C**ertification, **E**ducation of APRNs), proposes uniformity of national standards and regulation to promote mobility of APRNs and access to APRN care. Since credentialing verification includes the APRN education, certification, licensure, and accreditation of the educational institution from which the APRN graduated, this model, which is under consideration by the states for uniform APRN preparation and credentialing, can reduce APRN barriers to practice in the near future. Each state board with jurisdiction over APRN education and practice will need to adopt the LACE approach to foster a standard approach to APRN education and practice regulation. The reader can access the model and explanation at www.ncsbn.org.

CMS and TJC support rule/regulatory changes related to the issuance of uniform processes for the credentialing and privileging of medical and allied health professionals (including APRNs and physician assistants) to ensure consistency of standards and processes for providers, as well as to reduce duplication of effort in the case of interstate telemedicine site provider credentialing and privileging. Since CMS no longer recognizes an equivalent process for credentialing and privileging of certain providers who provide "medical level of care," certain APRNs providing this level of care must now be processed through the medical staff standards process at the institution or system (Cheung, 2011). This process will include recommendations of the medical staff, approval of the governing body, and the institution of peer review performance processes such as focused professional practice evaluation (FPPE) and ongoing professional practice evaluation (OPPE). If the APRN does not provide "medical level of care," the APRN can be processed through an "equivalent" process (Cheung, 2011).

This chapter discusses credentialing and privileging as separate mechanisms, with the understanding that analysis of the data about the APRN's application (credentialing) is a precursor to the decision about the nature of activities (specific procedures or treatment of specific conditions) for which privileging will be awarded (Pelletier, 2011). Issues related to credentialing and privileging for APRNs within the health-care arena are also presented. The reader is advised to maintain access to new developments in these areas since barriers to executing full scope of practice for APRNs appear to be rapidly changing in federal and state regulations, voluntary standards, and provider groups.

CREDENTIALING

Credentialing involves the collection, verification, and assessment of information that determines the eligibility and qualifications of the APRN provider to execute health-care services. It includes three categories: current licensure/certification; education and training; and experience, ability, and current competence to perform the work (TJC, 2008). Whereas privileging decisions are based on evaluation of the applicant's credentials and performance competencies, the credentialing process itself guarantees the integrity of the data issued for the APRN and is the basis of decisions regarding authorization for scope of practice and appointment of the APRN in a facility or system.

The types of data gathered during the credentialing process are directed by federal and state regulations; professional standards; facility requirements, policies, and procedures; and voluntary oversight bodies. Medicare Conditions of Participation (CoP) guide the federal and many state-regulated processes; standards of practice guide the professional standards; institutional bylaws, policies, and procedures mandate the specific application of the credentialing and privileging processes for the employed, independent contractor or a licensed independent provider (LIP) (an APRN can be an LIP); and voluntary or semiregulatory accreditation standards mandate the institutional processes. At a minimum, TJC standards require credentialing and privileging of all LIPs and APRNs who deliver a "medical level of care" permitted by law for the organization to provide patient care without supervision or direction (Pelletier, 2011). Regardless of the array of data that must be provided to support the APRN application, there are common data elements that the APRN can expect to complete for the application.

Credentialing Application and Procurement of Data

General categories of data are required to support the application for APRN appointment or reappointment to a clinical position. Typically, a written application is required to be submitted to the authorizing department or person in an institution. The application may be lengthy, and completeness and accuracy of information are critical to ensure timeliness of processing. Review of the application examines both the submission of information by the APRN and verifies sources as well as consistency of information among all sources. Any gaps in information or inconsistencies are further investigated by the institution before a decision is made for appointment. The APRN has the responsibility to add information as needed and to answer queries for incomplete or inconsistent data. In circumstances where changes in status for the APRN occur (e.g., licensure renewal, registration, additional education and certifications, recertification, voluntary or involuntary termination of staff membership, reduction or loss of privileges), the provider is obligated to submit the respective information to the credentialing body immediately for review of appointment status. Falsification of information or intentional omission of information on the application may be grounds for termination of the process, disciplinary action, or dismissal. If credentialing is denied, this is typically reported to the National Practitioner Data Bank (NPDB) (Pelletier, 2011). Credentialing of APRNs in managed care organizations with most health plans is largely conducted by the Council for Affordable Quality Healthcare (CAQH) (Buppert, 2012).

Verification of Advanced Practice Nurse Application Data

Two types of verification of data sources, primary and secondary, are conducted on an application in accordance with the rules and regulations of the accountable body for credentialing within the institution and as directed by the institutional accreditation process. Primary source verification attests to the accuracy and authenticity of the APRN's credentials based on evidence obtained from any source issuing the credential or the attestation of clinical performance. Examples include verification of licensure by state agency and certifications by certifying bodies, letters by authorized personnel at the professional school, letters from individuals personally acquainted with the APRN's skills, and database queries. Secondary source verification relies on verification actions of the APRN credentials based on data obtained by means other than direct contact with the issuing source of the credential (Utilization Review Accreditation Commission [URAC], 2011a, 2011b). Examples include unofficial copies of documents or reports on patient satisfaction statistics by the applicant. Verification processes may also include obtaining peer references or quality information from past employer organizations.

Some credentialing processes allow for Internet or telephone verification if documented. State nursing licensure boards are evolving technologically and many have online license verification processes. In addition, some health-care institutions contract with credentialing verification organizations (CVOs) to collect the primary and secondary data on which the decision for appointment will be made. For example, CAQH has over 800,000 physicians and other healthcare professionals engaged in the online Universal Provider Datasource (UPD). UPD allows providers to electronically submit and update standard training, experience, and practice information required by health plans and hospital medical staffs. Providers complete one form and update it three times annually to ensure the data are current in the searchable database (CAQH, 2010). The institution contracting with the CVO has adjunctive accountabilities to monitor the quality of service provided by the CVO and may require the CVO to be accredited by one of the national accrediting bodies such as URAC. The institution is not relieved of liability resulting from decisions based on contracted CVO data and processes for credentialing of APRNs. In addition, the institution remains accountable for the accreditation standards issued by its accreditation bodies such as TJC.

Analysis of Credentialing Application

On completion of the APRN application review and verification processes, the institutional decision on appointment constitutes the final step. This is guided by institutional policies and procedures related to the structure of the decision-making body; roles of the members; risk management and legal reviews; due process mechanisms; documentation requirements for decisions; and reporting mechanisms to the institutional board of directors, clinical directors, and the applicant. In some institutions, the human resource department processes the data for credentialing, while in other institutions certain providers are credentialed by the medical staff. In examining an organizational model at the University of Rochester, the Margaret D. Sovie Center functions as a centralized coordination point for core APRN functions related to regulation, institutional requirements, and credentialing with a direct line to the medical staff office. The center also functions as a repository for credentialing information, state licensure, prescriptive authority, and Drug Enforcement Administration (DEA) numbers (Ackerman, Mick, & Witzel, 2010). In most institutions, the credentialing committee is composed of physicians. As more APRNs become credentialed, their representation on medical staff committees should be embraced and the bylaws adjusted to expand governance for APRNs on provider panels and teams. The credentialing process is time consuming due to the importance of adhering to principles of good data integrity and decision making. It can often take 90 to 120 days for processing (Monarch, 2002). It behooves the APRN to obtain a copy of the policy and procedures for the credentialing process, committee member list, schedule of meetings, anticipated action on the application, and due process mechanisms. Rapid response to queries facilitates the completion of data collection and decision making.

When a credentialing process results in an appointment to the staff, the length of appointment and reappointment procedures are guided by institutional policy. It is wise to obtain copies of the reappointment process and criteria so that the APRN can continuously compile the necessary evidence and documents to meet the criteria for reappointment.

Decisions for emergency credentialing of volunteer LIPs have been revisited since 2002. For example, in 2002, TJC created a standard that allows the institutional chief executive officer, medical staff president, or his or her designee to grant emergency privileges when an emergency management plan has been activated. Implications for credentialing focus on data integrity: acceptable sources of identification including a current license to practice, current hospital identification with the license number, or verification of identity by a current hospital or medical staff member (American Hospital Association [AHA], 2002; TJC, 2008). Time limitations are typically imposed for credentialing.

Sources of Organizational Standards for Credentialing of Advanced Practice Nurses in Institutions

APRN practices can be found in almost all venues of health-care delivery. Appointment and privileging mandates from credentialing organizations have broadened the standards to include LIPs in hospitals, ambulatory care organizations, subacute long-term care, mental health, and managed care organizations (MCOs), regardless of practice structures. Credentialing for other delivery systems is on the horizon. Because the standards of sponsoring organizations can change annually, the reader is advised to consult the list of Web sites related to this chapter on DavisPlus to obtain the most current information on standards for accreditation as they relate to credentialing and privileging of the APRN's practice.

Once the application for credentialing is approved, a subsequent decision is made by the institution to authorize the specific practice activities (privileges) of the APRN. In some instances a separate privileging application is required. Consult institutional policies for their procedures.

PRIVILEGING

Privileging, once a process that hospitals used to "award" physicians the right to admit and perform clinical activities within their facility, is now a process that many APRNs are facing as they apply for positions within health-care facilities, and even doctors' offices (if the APRN will be following private patients in the acute-care setting). Privileging is used by a facility or employing organization to monitor the clinical activities a provider is authorized to perform in that facility and is the process of authorizing a health-care professional to perform (order) specific diagnostic or therapeutic services within well-defined limits. The granting of privileges is based on the following factors: state practice acts, agency regulations, license, education, training, experience, competence, health status, and judgment. It should be noted that just because the state practice act authorizes a particular activity (e.g., prescribing narcotics), the particular institution may not allow this privilege, or may require a secondary signature by a physician. Institutional policies may be more rigorous, but not less rigorous than the law.

Rationale and Background

Privileging is a component of the credentialing process of health-care facilities. As mentioned previously, national accrediting bodies such as URAC, the National Committee for Quality Assurance, TJC, and the Accreditation Association for Ambulatory Care establish both the credentialing and privileging standards and processes by which organizations are accredited. In the early 1980s TJC (then called the Joint Commission on the Accreditation of Healthcare Organizations [JCAHO]) revised its definition of medical staff and broadened scope of practice rules with permissive language to allow hospitals to include other licensed individuals, permitted by law and by the hospital, to provide patient care services independently. These privileges usually include clinical and admitting practices. TJC also established a mechanism to monitor these privileges and charged the hospital to establish criteria and processes for clinical privileging to ensure that competent individuals are providing patient care. Some facilities may have a list of "core privileges" that are appropriate for a particular type of provider or specialty practice. For example, HCPro provides sample core privilege forms that facilities can use for APRNs in dermatology and emergency departments, acute-care nurse practitioners, clinical nurse specialists in psychiatric mental health, and CNMs (HCPro, 2011b). HCPro is a leading provider of integrated information, education, training, and consulting products and services in the vital areas of health-care regulation and compliance (www.hcpro.com).

TJC is not prescriptive as to what process should be used for privileging, nor does it endorse or devalue the use of "laundry lists" or core privileges. However, TJC requires evidence that the facility does indeed evaluate whether individual providers are qualified and competent to perform the privileges they are granted by the process (http://www.jointcommission.org/standards_information/jcfaqdetails.aspx?StandardsFAQId=42&StandardsFAQChapterId=74).

- Standards of TJC (2011) speak to the issue of hospital privileging in sections MS 4.0 through MS 4.13. TJC 2011 standards in the Section B3, BoosterPak™ addition to MS.08.01.01 and MS.08.01.03, additionally eliminates the use of an "equivalent process" of credentialing for most APRNs except for those who do not provide "medical level of care" services. The standards speak to the process itself and to the mechanisms that must be in place and outlined in the hospital bylaws. These processes must include the time frames, the appeals processes, criteria for appointment and determination of specific privileges, persons responsible for the credentialing and privileging process, the reappointment process, temporary privileging, telemedicine privileges, disaster privileges, and the quality improvement process. Section B3 of the Joint Commission BoosterPak™ states, in part:

Those who provide "medical level of care" must use the medical staff process for credentialing and privileging, making all [medical staff] standards applicable (including recommendation by the organized medical staff and approval by the governing body, OPPE, and FPPE). APRNs and PAs who provide "medical level of care" must be credentialed and privileged through the medical staff standards process.

- APRNs and PAs who do not provide "medical level of care" use the human resources "equivalent" process detailed in HR.01.02.05, EPs 10-15.

Another standard speaks to those individuals providing patient care via telemedicine and introduces the concept of credentialing and privileging by proxy. The proxy approach recognizes the burden of credentialing for the originating site (where the patient is located) when privileges are bestowed to providers at the distant site (where providers of care are located) and for which there is more relevant information to base a decision. The proxy acknowledges that the originating site may have little experience with how to privilege certain specialty providers (TJC, 2008). This proxy approach had been a concern for TJC and the CMS, especially regarding the more stringent telemedicine credentialing requirements for Medicare participation. However, as of May 3, 2011, CMS CoP were changed to allow medical staff of the originating hospital to use the credentialing verification process of the telemedicine physician's home-base hospital as a basis for decisions on privileging. Thereby CMS decreased the duplication and burden placed on the many small rural hospitals in need of telemedicine services and in essence approved TJC's "proxy" process (Lowes, 2011). The reader is referred to CMS CoP for more detail and specific requirements (CMS, 2011). APRNs, as well as other practitioners, providing telemedicine diagnostic and treatment services may be subject to the credentialing process of the organization receiving the telemedicine services, but the process is becoming more streamlined.

In the case of disaster privileges, an APRN may be granted disaster privileges through a modified process. This process is typically granted for two conditions: when a disaster management plan has been activated and when the organization is unable to meet immediate patient care needs. At a minimum, verification of license and oversight of care treatment and services must be provided (TJC, 2011). Continuing education is also mandated in TJC standards, as are four core criteria: current licensure, relevant training or experience, current competence, and ability to perform the privileges requested.

Six areas of competence inform the evaluation of a practitioner in TJC standards for the credentialing and privileging process:

1. Patient care
2. Medical and clinical knowledge
3. Practice-based learning and improvement
4. Interpersonal and communication skills
5. Professionalism
6. System-based practice

In addition to incorporating the aforementioned concepts into the overall evaluation of an individual's credentialing and privileging file, there are also two other processes that allow for closer evaluation. The first is a focused professional practice evaluation (FPPE). The FPPE might be used when an individual has the credentials on paper, but there is a need to evaluate the individual more closely to determine competence. The second is an ongoing professional practice evaluation (OPPE) that allows for a more evidence-based approach to credentialing rather than just the formal process every 2 years. If any issues are apparent during the ongoing evaluation, a more focused evaluation can be done.

When the evaluation processes are executed correctly, they can provide protection for the facility, the patient, and the practitioner. The process of credentialing and privileging attempts to decrease chances of liability for the facility and the practitioner by ensuring that the practitioners providing care to patients are currently licensed, have been educated for the role in which they are working, and are safe and competent in the scope of care they are authorized to provide. The process in an accredited organization also provides some security for the practitioner since federal law regarding participation in Medicare requires that staff membership and professional privileges in a hospital are not dependent solely on certification, fellowship, or membership in a specialty body or society (42 C.F.R. 482.12 (a)7) (Buppert, 2012). TJC also spells out that an appeals process must be in place if privileges are denied. The appeal process provides for time frames and feedback to the practitioner, as well as mechanisms for temporary or emergency privileging. Finally, privileging provides data for determining the economic effect of provider practice on the health-care system.

As stated in the definition, several factors affect the outcome of privileging: state practice acts, agency regulations, license, education, training, experience, competence, health status, judgment, the culture of the medical staff, and its bylaws. The factor that affects APRNs most is the scope of practice outlined in the state practice act for the state of licensure and authorization. Each state regulates the practice of APRNs differently at this time (although it may dramatically change with full implementation of the Consensus Model by 2015). Some practice acts define what APRNs can do and what specific drugs they may or may not be able to prescribe, if they have prescriptive authority. As mentioned in the introduction, the NCSBN worked for several years with stakeholders to support the Consensus Model for APRN Regulation (NCSBN, 2008), an advanced practice uniform model that all states are encouraged to adopt for recognition of APRN practice by 2015 as a way to standardize credentialing. Agency regulations are usually defined by the medical staff and hospital board, and may restrict APRNs from performing certain procedures. The license is tied to scope of practice issues outlined in the state practice act. Education provides the theoretical and experiential components to develop specific outcome competencies (as determined by the professional organization and the profession in scope and standards of practice). For example, the outcome competencies for a pediatric nurse practitioner (NP) would not be the same as those for a geriatric NP, although there may be some overlapping competencies.

It is important to document training and experience as practitioners progress in their careers because not everything essential for practice can be learned in the formal education process. However, just because a practitioner learned a particular procedure does not mean he or she is legally allowed to perform it since it may be outside the scope of practice and license.

Health requirements (both physical and mental) for the practitioner are evaluated and certain restrictions may apply. Untreated substance abuse problems and physical impairments may interfere with the performance of a particular role.

Competence and judgment become a little more subjective when evaluating and reviewing a privileging file. Many of the components of the file are taken into consideration when making an overall determination of competence and judgment, and the credentialing panel may want to establish a period of observation and performance evaluation.

Process

Therapeutic and diagnostic patient care services that fall under the privileging framework are usually defined by the particular medical or surgical specialty area within the health-care facility, and criteria are established to outline safe practice. Delineation of the specific types of privileges may be presented in a variety of ways, and each facility may have its own guide of core privileges. Among the basic types of approaches are the following: category, "laundry list," severity or complexity of care, and hybrid form. The first, category, usually defines privileges along specialty lines and can vary significantly across types of specialty programs because of curriculum. The listing of privileges and skills, or the laundry list approach, is used mainly for procedures and is less appropriate when specific diseases are referenced because of the variability of presentation. Severity or complexity of care is the third form. The fourth is a variation or hybrid form of those previously mentioned.

The credentialing panel or peer review panel reviewing credentialing files may or may not also determine the applicant's privileges, or there may be a separate panel composed of members, including peers, from the particular service or area. The ideal panel includes an interdisciplinary group including APRNs. This group determines if a candidate applying for particular privileges meets the criteria based on the information submitted in his or her credentialing package and application. The panel may allow the practitioner independent privileges or supervised privileges, depending on the evaluation. Other strategies that provide support for the credentialing and privileging of APRNs besides representation on the credentialing panel include representation in the development of any policies and procedures relevant to the process, and communication networks for periodic updates on changes or alterations in APRN credentialing and privileging practices (Kleinpell, 2008).

Clinical privileges are reviewed, revised, or updated for a variety of reasons other than at the time of reappointment. Evaluations of provider performance may warrant privileges being expanded or reduced. Nonuse of privileges may indicate that specific privileges are not needed and competency cannot be maintained. Finally, as technology and innovation emerge across hospital procedures and in the treatment of various diseases, the scope of privileges also change. Privileging is an ongoing process. New privileges may be added and some may be removed based on performance. Accreditation requires that the privilege and credential files be reviewed every 2 to 3 years to ensure currency and competence.

As an example, some of the specific tasks or procedures identified by Kleinpell (2008) in a sample privilege request form for which an acute-care NP might want to obtain hospital privileges include ventilator adjustments, managing resuscitation, digital block, chest tube insertion, and insertion of arterial or central venous catheters. Another exemplar of clinical privileges is identified in the Guidelines for Clinical Privileges developed by the American Association of Nurse Anesthetists (AANA,

2005). CRNAs, one of the four types of APRNs, have been completing credentialing and privileging processes for years, and other APRNs can learn from their experience.

Temporary privileging may need to occur from time to time when a particular provider becomes ill or disabled, necessitating that another provider be recognized to take over certain duties of care. Recently recruited providers whose skills are specialized and needed in the facility may be awarded temporary privileges while the formal process of credentialing continues. These privileges are time limited, and primary source verification of licensure and competence is allowed through phone calls until the full credentialing process occurs.

The National Practitioner Data Bank (NPDB) serves an important role in the credentialing process. In a survey of NPDB users, Waters, Warnecke, Parsons, Almagor, and Budetti (2006) found that most institutions use this inquiry process to make decisions about credentialing and subsequently privileging in a timely manner. Less than 10% of institutions indicated they had reached a credentialing decision before receiving the NPDB report, whereas up to 30% of respondents receiving an NPDB report did not grant privileging applications as requested. However, the issue of incidents not being reported to the NPDB still remains a barrier to the NPDB process. Clearly, multiple methods of data access and analysis are needed to achieve the goals of any credentialing and privileging system.

THE PROFESSIONAL CAREER PORTFOLIO

Portfolios continue to play a role in the world of competence assessment. Portfolios are used in a variety of ways by facilities, regulators, nursing organizations, certifying bodies, and educational institutions. Hospitals use them for evaluation and career ladder programs. Regulatory agencies use them for ensuring the public of competent practitioners (e.g., in Ontario, Canada). Dietitians use them for their recertification processes. Certifying bodies use them for recertification or reactivation of credentials. Educational institutions use them for advanced placement of RNs into bachelor of science and graduate programs, and for compiling clinical practice evidence for doctoral projects. Professional career portfolios serve as the foundation of the credentialing and privileging application process used in today's health-care system.

Evidence-based practice provides a scientific, justifiable rationale for patient care therapeutics, while "practice-based evidence" provides a rationale for authorizing a practitioner to perform specific patient care therapeutics. Documentation of this practice-based evidence provides the information needed to make decisions regarding the privileging component of the credentialing process as currently outlined.

Tracking professional events accurately becomes more and more complex, even with the available technology. Establishing a professional credentialing portfolio as the APRN begins his or her advanced practice education and career can make the credentialing and privileging process easier and save time and money. It may even help the APRN to be more adequately compensated by allowing him or her to achieve a higher status within a health-care facility because of practice-based evidence. The credentialing and privileging portfolio described here can build on this process. For students or early professionals building a portfolio, Beauchesne (2007) suggests including some of the following items (pp. 34–35):

- Résumé
- Personal statements on practice and scholarship
- Case studies and research activities
- Health-care project descriptions

- Brief papers and assignments
- Publications and presentations
- Evidence-based examples; meaningful use performance measures
- Clinical practice logs or reflections
- Video clips
- Certificates of participation
- Letters of support and recommendation
- Continuing education activities
- Evaluations and competency reviews
- Course syllabi and transcripts

An online portfolio is an excellent way to build a professional career history that can serve multiple purposes, including the credentialing and privileging process. Licenses, certificates, transcripts, and documents can be scanned and/or uploaded to the online portfolio, eliminating the need for paper copies. Although some of the materials collected during the student educational process (course syllabi, clinical logs, reflections) may not seem pertinent for the professional career portfolio, it is easy to archive these data with an online portfolio for availability only if necessary at a later time. It is better to collect more information and not use it than to need it and not have it. The individual can have access to his or her file anytime, anywhere Internet access is available. Fear of misplacing documents or having them destroyed by unforeseen natural disasters (i.e., floods, hurricanes, or fires) can be eliminated. Stronger security of online materials has resulted in files that can be password protected. In addition, compilation of particular documents can be sent to credentialing committees via e-mail or through Internet access to them. Updates can be added to the portfolio as new knowledge and skills are acquired, making the portfolio a living document.

The purpose for which a portfolio is used determines the elements it should contain. Although many of the components are similar across portfolio types, some things are unique to the credentialing and privileging portfolio. Keeping the idea of credentialing and privileging in mind, the following format is suggested for developing this type of professional career portfolio. The professional career portfolio is composed of 4 major components: (a) the practitioner contact information page; (b) the practice-based evidence component, used to assist in determining specific privileges; (c) the credentials component section; and (d) the attestation page.

Practitioner Contact Information

An introductory page with name, address, contact information, practitioner's identity, and photo (if desired) is included.

Practice-Based Evidence Component

This area provides evidence to support the six areas of general competencies being evaluated during the hospital credentialing process and includes aspects of patient care, medical and clinical knowledge, practice-based learning and improvement, interpersonal and communication skills, professionalism, and system-based practice.

The practice-based evidence component should include the following:

1. Copy of the state practice act governing scope of practice in the state of licensure
2. Core competencies for the APRN specialty
3. A sampling of references on the cost-effectiveness and quality of care provided by APRNs

4. Copies of job descriptions held in the past, especially those where clinical privileges were held
5. Specialty procedures or processes learned and verified:
   a. In the educational process
   b. On the job
   c. Through continuing education
   (See sample of verification form, **Figure 8-1,** which could be used to validate these procedures.)
6. Letters of support and verification of practice competence in the areas outlined; include both peers and supervisors or employers; meaningful use compliance
7. Employment history, identifying significant responsibilities
8. Any performance outcome data that may have been collected at places of employment (e.g., number of patients seen per day, revenue generated)
9. Copy of the Consensus Document

Credentials Component

The credentials component should include the following:

1. Education (transcripts and diplomas)
2. Military history (if any)
3. Licenses (numbers and expiration dates or copies)
4. Certification(s) (national specialty)
5. Certification(s) (e.g., advanced cardiac life support, basic cardiac life support, pediatric advanced life support, trauma nurse coordinator)
6. Drug Enforcement Administration (DEA) and Medicare/Medicaid numbers
7. Insurance coverage, any liability history, disclosures of physical, mental, substance, or criminal problems
8. Immunizations and dates
9. Languages spoken, written, and understood (identify beginning, average, or advanced levels)
10. Research in progress or completed
11. Publications
12. Continuing education (no more than 5 years worth or length of certification)
13. Professional organization membership and offices held in those organizations
14. References (professional and personal)
15. Certified Background Report results
16. Any previous denials of hospital credentialing/privileging

Attestation Page

The final page, or the fourth component, should include a statement that is signed and dated by the provider attesting to the information contained in the portfolio. This should be updated every 2 years or more often as any changes occur. The entire portfolio should reflect real-time data.

Sample:

I, ______________________, attest to the authenticity of the information contained in this portfolio and verify that I am in good health and able to perform the clinical privileges I am requesting. I permit the employer or gaining party of this portfolio to verify any of the information provided if necessary.

Signed______________________________ Date______________________

Provider Name:

Specialty:

License Number and Certification:

____

Date(s) of performance ____________________

Procedure(s) or activity:

Description/elaboration:

Verification:

I, the undersigned, have observed ________ *(name)* ________ and can verify that he/she can safely perform the above outlined procedure(s) independently/with supervision *(circle one)*.

Provider/verifier: ______________________________

Title: ______________________________

License: ______________________________

Facility: ______________________________

Address: ______________________________

____

____

Phone: ____________________ **Date:** ____________________

FIGURE 8-1 Sample verification of practice form.

ISSUES

Although APRNs are joining the staff of various facilities in greater numbers, several areas continue to challenge the APRN's full scope of practice and the process to achieve it in clinical settings. The six issues presented here are not exclusive, but provide a springboard for fuller discussion and solution generation in a manner in which APRN scope of practice can benefit consumers.

Maintaining Data About Performance

APRNs are held to standards of performance that include clinical practice and administrative standards. Both have economic implications for decisions to appoint or reappoint APRNs to an institutional staff. The institution may find that clinical performance falls outside established benchmarks if patients under the APRN's care have excessive lengths of stay, repeated and lengthy delays in appointments, quality-of-care issues, and additional exposure to liability resulting from variation in performance. CMS incentives for "meaningful use" of electronic data is quickly becoming a metric of incentivized performance. Patient satisfaction may be easily tied to performance. Institutions will need to more closely track coding practices of APRNs to capture their actual practice and subsequent outcomes. Without this data and analysis, performance cannot be understood or managed in ways comparable to that of other providers.

APRNs are wise to document and monitor their performance against the targets of the organization and colleagues, and use the feedback to initiate personal or systems-wide performance improvement strategies. Maintaining documentation of accomplishments, patient acknowledgments, and cost savings are important assets for the APRN's portfolio. CMS "meaningful use" metrics are useful to include. It is also important that APRNs are aware of the information and reference data about activities that are required to be verified as part of the credentialing process. Losing track of certification and licensure renewals has immediate repercussions for the credentialing process. Determining the accuracy of any inputs into the NPDB or other databases is important to verify before an institutional query occurs.

Decreasing Barriers to Continuity of Care

Although the numbers of APRNs holding hospital privileges continues to slowly grow, two reasons stand out as rationale to seek/obtain privileges and consequently help decrease barriers to continuity and seamless patient care. One issue relates to the fact that some insurance companies and MCOs require their primary care providers (PCPs) (in this case APRNs) to hold hospital privileges as a prerequisite to credentialing and/or billing/payment. The other is that a PCP who does not have privileges within a hospital cannot review the chart or care provided for his or her patient once that patient is admitted to the hospital. PCPs may make a friendly visit and ask questions of the patient themselves, but they cannot validate or follow the treatment, tests, and outcomes in the patient record because of the Health Insurance Portability and Accountability Act (HIPAA). Being the provider of record and in many cases the one who will eventually continue to follow that patient after discharge, it would make the transition back to the community a much more seamless process and improve continuity of care (Brassard & Smolenski, 2011).

Managed Care Panels

Health-care providers work in a competitive environment where more than one type of provider is able to provide the same scope of practice or provide partial activities within another scope of practice.

The ability to be credentialed and apply for legal scope of practice privileges rests in the hands of the credentialing structure. Professional medical societies are flush with complaints from physicians who perceive they have been excluded from MCO provider panels, and these exclusions present a glass ceiling for APRNs as well.

Sometimes the exclusion of APRNs is due to lack of knowledge concerning the full scope of APRN practice parameters. At other times there is a perception of anticompetitive or restraint of trade action (IOM, 2011). APRNs are well advised to provide documentation about APRN performance outcomes compared with other providers through the use of evidence-based reports and articles, and quality reports especially published in the provider's representative journals. Seeking advocates and allies at the institution to which the APRN is applying can assist in the politics of selection for worthy candidates. Where warranted, legal consultation may prove helpful to understand the issues and the APRN's rights. Six legal cases related to the multiple dimensions of this concern are discussed by Monarch (2002), and more have emerged since then. Patient advocacy groups can be particularly helpful to informing and creating demand for APRN services. As more insurance plans regulated by the states embrace the use of APRNs as primary care providers and providers of "medical levels of care," it will become more difficult to exclude APRNs on provider panels.

Credentialing of the APRN Among Multiple Organizations

When working in a health-care system or between two or more entities, the APRN may be confronted with replication of the credentialing application process for each entity. This can be extremely time consuming and expensive in opportunity costs. It is important to gather perceptions from other providers and administrators about expectations and ramifications for productivity given duplication in processing of multiple credentialing applications. Create a solution team to construct alternative approaches that promote efficiencies and be prepared to gather support from colleagues on alternative proposals to present to the governing board. Maintaining an online professional portfolio will also help. Registering with a database such as UPD can assist in maintaining accurate and current information. Other regulations are on the horizon to limit redundancy in credentialing and privileging, such as those occurring in telemedicine with distant and originating site credentialing (Manos, 2010). The aim of these regulations is to prevent redundancy and administrative waste. Consulting the CMS rules and regulations intermittently can facilitate your ability to meet the changes in processes in a timely manner.

Uniform Adoption of the Consensus Model for APRN Regulation

Should all states accept the Consensus Model for APRN regulations by 2015, this movement may address barriers to mobility for the APRN workforce. Currently, credentialing requirements for APRNs vary among states as to the mechanism for title protection and scope of practice differences. The NCSBN proposed that it is appropriate for APRNs to be legally regulated through a second license for their role and population focus because their activities are complex and involve role and population competencies, independence, and autonomy (NCSBN, 2008). Adoption of the Consensus Model (NCSBN, 2008) would allow the APRN role and population focus to be regulated at the state level and the specialization focus to be credentialed by specialty organizations rather than by state licensures. One issue of contention is that of states' right, and may well be handled in the same manner as the nurse licensure compact, which allows mutual recognition of the RN license between states.

Most state models now require an application, RN licensure, completion of a graduate degree with a major in nursing or a graduate degree with a concentration in the advanced nursing practice category, and professional certification from a board-approved national certifying body. The requirement for graduate education also includes the addition of the doctor of nursing practice (DNP) degree.

There is a newer certification credential for DNPs proposed by the Council for the Advancement of Comprehensive Care (CACC) and promoted by Columbia University for DNP graduates. The Comprehensive Care Certification (CCC) administered by the American Board of Comprehensive Care (ABCC) for the first time on November 10, 2008, is currently not an NCSBN-approved certification nor is it recognized by the Consensus Document or Joint Dialogue Group as an appropriate certification for uniform regulation of APRNs. The CCC examination is purely voluntary. Forty-five NPs took the initial examination, and 50% earned a passing score. The examination test items are drawn from a pool of clinical test items created by the National Board of Medical Examiners for Step 3 of the medical education examination. Those who opposed this form of examination have claimed that it did not reflect the nurse practitioner role. APRNs will want to keep current on the evolution of this credentialing option.

APRN Representation on the Medical Staff and Bylaws Adjustment

As APRN privileging becomes more common, the APRN should seek governance representation on the medical staff and ensure that the medical staff bylaws embrace full representation of APRNs. There are exemplars for this movement, notably in Ellenville Regional Hospital in New York, where an APRN, Bob Donaldson, was invited to review and revise the medical staff bylaws; Donaldson was ultimately elected president of the medical staff in 2009–2010 (Hendren, 2011). Clearly this model can work to further the outcome of collaborative practice.

All 50 states currently address advanced practice in public policy in some manner. In most part, state boards of nursing hold authority over advanced practice. For example, additional education in advanced pharmacology may be required where the prescription of medications is a sanctioned activity. By this arrangement, many state boards of nursing have deferred to the profession's right to recognize APRNs and their specialties through certification and to develop and promulgate the standards of practice on which certification is based.

As you think about eventual changes in credentialing and privileging, be aware that no change is insignificant. Each readjustment holds both personal ramifications and implications for the profession as a whole. It is always wise to follow the dialogue and planning around national regulatory initiatives that will direct your scope of practice.

REFERENCES

Ackerman, M., Mick, D., and Witzel, P. (2010). Creating an organizational model to support advanced practice. *Journal of Nursing Administration, 40*(2), 63–68.

American Association of Nurse Anesthetists. (2005). *Guidelines for core clinical privileges: CRNA practice.* Park Ridge, IL: Author. Retrieved May 1, 2008, from www.aana.com/practice/clinical_priv.asp.

American Hospital Association. (2002). Retrieved August 15, 2012 from www.ahanews.com.

Beauchesne, M. A. (Ed.). (2007). *NP competency based education evaluation: Using a portfolio approach.* Washington, DC: National Organization of Nurse Practitioner Faculties.

Brassard, A., & Smolenski, M. (2011). Reducing barriers to advanced practice registered nurse care: Hospital privileges. *Insight on issues 55.* Washington, DC: AARP Public Policy Institute.

Buppert, C. (2012). *Business practice and legal guide* (4th ed.). Sudbury, MA: Jones & Bartlett.

CAQH. (2010). *More than 800,000 physicians and allied health professional now using the Universal Provider Datasource to save $92 million per year in administrative costs.* Retrieved April 15, 2011, from http://www.caqh.org/PR201004.php.

Cheung, K. (2011). *TJC changes MS.08.01.01 and MS.08.01.03: "Medical" APRN and PA to be privileged through med staff process.* Retrieved April 15, 2011, from http://blogs.hcpro.com/credentialing/2011/02tjc-changes-ms-08-01-01 and ms-08-01-03/.

Centers for Medicare and Medicaid Services. (CMS). Retrieved April 20, 2011 from http://www.cms.gov/Telehealth. Goolsby, M.J. (2011). 2009–2010 AANP national nurse practitioner sample survey: An overview. *Journal of the American Academy of Nurse Practitioners, 23*(5), 266–268.

HCPro. (2011a). *APRN privilege trends: Barriers fall as more nurses move to independent practice.* Briefings on credentialing. Retrieved April 13, 2011, from www.credentailingresourcecenter.com.

HCPro. (2011b). Sample forms available for NP Derm and ER, CNS PMH, ACNP and CNM. Retrieved May 2, 2011, from http://www.online-crc.com/core-privileges.cfm.

Hendren, R. (February 8, 2011). Nurse practitioner elected medical staff president. *HealthLeaders Media.* Retrieved August 15, 2012 from http://www.healthleadersmedia.com/page-3/NRS-262335/Nurse-Practitioner-Elected-Medical-Staff-President Institute of Medicine. (2011). *The future of nursing: Leading change, advancing health.* Washington, DC: National Academies Press.

Kleinpell, R. M., Hravnak, M., Hinch, B., & Llewellyn, J. (2008). Developing an advanced practice nursing credentialing model for acute care facilities. *Nursing Administration Quarterly, 32*(4), 270–287.

Lowes, R. (2011). CMS removes credentialing barrier to telemedicine. *Medscape Medical News.* Retrieved May 3, 2011 from http://www.medscape.com/viewarticle/742028.

Manos, D. (2010). CMS proposes easing telemedicine credentialing rules. *Healthcare IT News.* Retrieved April 15, 2011, from www.govhealthit.com/news/cms-process-easing-telemedicine-credentialing-rules.

Monarch, K. (2002). *Nursing and the law: Trends and issues.* Washington, DC: American Nurses Association.

National Council of State Boards of Nursing. (2008). *Consensus Model for APRN Regulation: Licensure, Accreditation, Certification and Education* Retrieved April 30, 2011, from www.ncsbn.org.

Pelletier, S. J. (2011). *Core privileges for AHPs* (2nd ed.). Danvers, MA: HCPro, Inc.

Schuiling, K. D., Sipe, T. A., and Fullerton, J. (2010). Findings from the analysis of the American College of Nurse-Midwives' membership surveys: 2006–2008. *Journal of Midwifery and Women's Health, 55*(4), 299–307.

The Joint Commission. (2008). *Comprehensive accreditation manuals.* Chicago: Author.

The Joint Commission. (2011). *2011 hospital accreditation standards.* Retrieved May 11, 2011 from http://www.jcrinc.com/Joint-Commission-Requirements/Hospitals/ and http://www.jcrinc.com/Accreditation-Manuals/HS11/1245/ (MANUAL).

Utilization Review Accreditation Commission. (2011a). *Credentials verification organization standards.3.1.* Washington, DC: Author. Retrieved May 4, 2011, from www.urac.org/docs/programs.

Utilization Review Accreditation Commission. (2011b). *Provider performance measurement and public reporting standards, version 1.0.* Washington, DC: Author. Retrieved May 4, 2011, from www.urac.org/docs/programs.

Waters, T. M., Warnecke, R. B., Parsons, J., Almagor, O., & Budetti, P. P. (2006). The role of the national practitioner data bank in the credentialing process. *American Journal of Medical Quality, 21*(1), 30–39.

9 The Kaleidoscope of Collaborative Practice

Alice F. Kuehn

The future of nursing and health care depends on partnership. One of the four key messages of the Institute of Medicine (IOM) report on the future of nursing states that "nurses should be full partners with physicians and other health professionals in redesigning health care in the United States" (2011, p. 7). In the 2011 annual legislative updates of the status of advanced practice registered nurse (APRN) practice, several states identified positive change in regulatory status for advanced practice nurses. The adoption of the APRN Consensus Model (APRN Joint Dialogue Group, 2008) is identified as a key factor in much of this ongoing regulatory reform, noting that the resulting consistency in regulation of advanced practice nursing across states is facilitating steady progress in legislative reform (Pearson, 2011; Phillips, 2011). Current trends in health care reflect an increasing call for collaborative practice, and the terms *interprofessional* and *consensus building* are becoming more commonplace (American Nurses Association [ANA], 2010a; Hughes, 2011; Rice et al., 2010). In the American Nurses Association's (ANA's) Social Policy statement, collaboration is described as a partnership in which all partners are valued for their expertise, power, and distinct areas of practice. The statement also acknowledges their shared areas of practice and mutual goals and emphasizes that the "nursing profession is particularly focused on establishing effective working relationships and collaborative efforts essential to accomplishing its health-oriented mission" (ANA, 2010a, p. 7). The role of the APRN has evolved along a continuum of collaborative interactive models of increasing complexity (Kuehn, 1998). Just as a kaleidoscope creates a constantly changing set of colors and patterns, collaboration is a constantly changing aspect of health-care practice, moving from little interest to a great demand, from frustration to success, and sometimes back again. The interactions among members of a health-care team present a new picture each time the group, situation, time, or environment changes. This chapter reviews the history and examines myriad aspects of collaborative practice. It compares and contrasts multidisciplinary, interdisciplinary, intradisciplinary, and transdisciplinary practices, using examples to clarify the distinctions and similarities. The values, barriers, and strategies by which collaborative practice is being successfully developed are presented, and the continuing and expanding evolutions of collaborative practice models are examined.

A HISTORY OF CHANGING RELATIONSHIPS

Our world continues to rapidly change to such an extent that change itself has become the constant. This sense of change in every aspect of life was described by Alvin Toffler in his classic 1970 publication, *Future Shock,* a term he created to describe the "shattering stress and disorientation" resulting from too much change too quickly. Our response to change has historically been slower than the change itself. However, in today's world of a rapidly increasing pace of change, the lag between the change and our response is growing, and this is what Senge (1994) calls *future shock.* Much of our human behavior flows from our ability to embrace or to fight the pace of life. Ours is a world of transience: a series of short-term relationships with people, things, places, workplaces, and information itself. In a situation in which the duration of relationships has been shortened, our sense of reality and of commitment and our ability to cope are seriously challenged. The flow of change is not linear, and we are being forced to adjust to novel situations for which we have not been prepared. Because we are living in a health-care world demanding collaboration, cost-effectiveness, and high-quality care, the relationships among professionals are rapidly changing, demanding flexibility and collegiality. A key recommendation of the IOM report *Keeping Patients Safe: Transforming the Work Environment of Nurses* (2004) was for health-care institutions to move away from a hierarchal approach to shared decision making and increased support of interdisciplinary collaboration. "Ultimately, the success of each discipline will be judged by how effectively it participates in a continuum of care that meets the needs of patients and of the health care system overall" (Cooper, 2001, p. 58).

Physician–Nurse Relationships Over Time

In 1859, Florence Nightingale described the role of nursing as a specific set of relationships to medicine and hospital administration set within the social structure of the times. Placing the nurse as a care provider subservient to the physician established and formalized a role structure that, after nearly 150 years, continues to define society's general sense of the nurse role as within the role of the physician (Partin, 2009; Workman, 1986). A statement issued at the 2009 American Medical Association (AMA) House of Delegates meeting supporting this hierarchical role structure called for physician supervision of nurses, noting that, although the nurse role is important, it must be supervised. The nursing response drafted by the ANA and some APRN organizations stressed that the concept of physician supervision of APRNs is out of date, is inappropriate, and creates a major barrier to the access of care (Partin, 2009; Sorrel, 2009). The challenges physicians face in understanding, supporting, and embracing the reality of the advanced practice role is a result of "cognitive dissonance," a rejection or denial of information that challenges their preconceptions of the nurse role. In examining the historical roots of collaborative experiences between physician and nurse, the years between 1873 and the 20th century saw the relationship of nurse to physician become more a scenario within a hospital setting. The triad of physician–nurse–hospital superintendent never truly evolved in equilibrium as the Nightingale model envisioned because the scenario of a nursing superintendent reporting separately to the hospital trustees challenged the deference given physicians and administrators in practice and would have undermined both their authority and the use of student nurses as workers. The ongoing development of hierarchical relationships within the hospital between physicians, nurses, and administrators resulted also from changes occurring in nursing itself. Nursing sought to gain more professional status through a rigid hierarchical management style of its own within a continuing hospital attitude of paternalism (Markowitz & Rosner, 1979; Reverby, 1979, 1987). Collaborative relationships with physicians, hospitals, and foundations serving the health-care system began to develop during and following the Great Depression as evidenced by the following: medical society participation in the Committee on Nursing of the Association of American Medical Colleges as they endorsed the Committee on the Grading of Nursing Schools; a manual on hospital nursing service administration, sponsored by the American Hospital Association (AHA) and the National League for Nursing Education (NLNE), published in 1935; and a survey of nursing schools in psychiatric hospitals under the auspices of a joint committee approach by the American Psychiatric Association (APA) and the NLNE. It should be noted, however, that these examples are not of individual collaborative relationships, but of organizations, and were tenuous at best; the medical society withdrew from the Committee on Nursing shortly after their endorsement (Roberts, 1959).

The ANA code of 1950 spelled out a relationship of nurse to physician as a complex mix of dependent and independent responsibilities. Roberts (1959) stated, "The nurse is obligated to carry out the physician's orders intelligently, to avoid misunderstandings or inaccuracies by verifying orders, and to refuse to participate in unethical procedures" (p. 563). However, if every nursing decision made must come from within the orders flowing from another profession, the relationship cannot be collaboration but instead becomes supervised delegation. Kinlein (1977) identified the dilemma in nursing as a blockage of the ability of nurses to initiate nursing diagnoses, design nursing care, or establish a distinctive practice when the power of the medical judgment is the prime source of all decision making regarding patient care. Nursing judgments thus become delegated medical judgments because they are aimed at a medical goal and have to agree with that goal. Kinlein describes an example of a physician snatching a chart from her hands while she was teaching a student regarding a treatment regimen. The doctor stated, "What are you doing, talking about that? That's none of your concern. Just teach those students to give bedpans and then to remove them" (1977, p. 30), leaving both nurse faculty and student to conclude that either the nurse has to learn more and become a doctor or learn less so that he or she is prepared merely to carry out orders. In this situation, Kinlein notes, the nurse was expecting the physician to be knowledgeable, the patient expected both physician and nurse to be knowledgeable, and the physician expected the nurse to have no knowledge. This is an unacceptable situation, as well as a clear example of noncollaborative, unidisciplinary practice, with no communication between the two sets of providers except through a hierarchical, supervisory relationship.

The current system of care delivery is described as supporting professional individualism, prerogatives, and separatism of roles, resulting in defensiveness, lack of continuity, competition, redundancy, excessive costs, fragmentation, little cooperation or teamwork, grossly inadequate and outdated systems of communication, and underutilization of APRNs (Fischman, 2002; Goodman, 2007; IOM, 2011; Norsen, Opladen, & Quinn, 1995; O'Neil & Pew Health Professions Commission, 1998). However, calls for collaborative practice have continued to grow and intensify, requiring physicians, nurses, and all health professionals to begin working through the relationship-building process required to establish a collaborative team approach. Pearson (2002) noted that "the irony of our continuing struggle with organized medicine is that, even while we fight against medicine's inappropriate domination over our practice, we must maintain and enhance our working relationship with individual physicians, for patients are best served when providers work together" (p. 22). This requires a team effort within an environment of mutual respect and valuing of each professional role. The 2011 Phillips report on the legal status of the APRN demonstrated continuing movement toward full autonomy across the country, noting that in 24 states, the board of nursing now has sole authority to define the scope of practice and there are no statutory requirements for physician collaboration, regulation, direction, or supervision (p. 32). This movement toward full autonomy of practice does not necessarily equate to solo practice. "The credible evidence showing that collaboration improves health care outcomes for patients entreats the two professions to put cooperation before professional roles" (Phillips, Green, Fryer, & Dovey, 2001, p. 1,325). An increasing number of health-care studies continue to affirm the need for and value of collaboration, emphasizing that efficient delivery and high-quality of care may depend on the level of collaboration among professional care providers (Donald et al., 2009; Hojat et al., 2003; Hughes, 2011; Rice et al., 2010; Zwarenstein & Bryant, 2000).

Status of Collaborative Practice in Advanced Practice Roles

The growth and acceptance of the APRN role has hinged on the willingness of the profession to acknowledge and support the role; provide advanced education and experience; and promote a clarity of role that facilitates development of a sense of identity and clear understanding by other disciplines, policy makers and legislators, and the public. As each of the four APRN practices—certified registered nurse anesthetists (CRNAs), certified nurse-midwives (CNMs), clinical nurse specialists (CNSs), and nurse practitioners (NPs)—has moved toward autonomy in practice, establishing positive relationships with the medical community has been key. Stanley (2005, p. 34) notes that "consumer satisfaction and physician advocacy have proved to be powerful stimuli" for operationalizing the APRN role. Applying Benner's (1984) competencies and domains of nursing practice from novice to expert levels to advanced practice, Fenton and Brykczynski (1993) identified additional domains and competencies and verified the high level of expertise of APRNs. However, the scope of practice flowing from this model of expertise needs to be clearly identified. It is critical for the practice of all APRNs, while maintaining clinical practice distinctions, to be conceptually united, stressing commonalities while acknowledging differences in practice patterns but promoting an interdisciplinary focus in their practice (Stanley, 2005). Once the role is clarified, scopes of practice delineated, common practice elements of APRNs made known, and support from professional colleagues and consumers ongoing, the challenges faced in establishing collaborative practice will be greatly minimized. This is the hope of the APRN Consensus Model (APRN Joint Dialogue Group, 2008). Without these foundational components, the challenges of creating truly functional teams will continue to be significant. The following section provides a brief overview of role development challenges, achievements, and approaches to collaboration for each of the four APRN practices.

The Certified Registered Nurse Anesthetist

Clarity of role and a reach for autonomous practice were forged early in the development of nurse anesthetists. Alice Magaw, a pioneer in the field who worked at the Mayo clinic in the early 1900s, supported the separation of nurse anesthesia from nursing service administration, emphasizing its need for recognition and requirements for specialized education. During World War II, the role was identified as a clinical nursing specialty within the military field, and in 1945 a formal national certification process was established.

The scope of practice of the CRNA has been described as a practice in collaboration with legally required professional health-care providers (American Association of Nurse Anesthetists [AANA], 2006. This description noting a "legally required collaborator" has led some to regard the legal status of nurse anesthesia as a "dependent function" under physician control and continues to result in considerable challenges in development of a high-level collaborative practice model (Bigbee, 1996; Faut-Callahan & Kremer, 1996; Taylor, 2009). Some states use the term *collaboration* to define a relationship in which each party is responsible for his or her field of expertise while maintaining open communication on anesthetic techniques. Other states require the consent or order of a physician or other qualified licensed provider to administer the anesthetic. The Centers for Medicare and Medicaid Services (CMS) required physician supervision for nurse anesthetist services to Medicare patients. However, in late 2001, a rule published in the *Federal Register* allows a state to be exempt from this physician supervision requirement for nurse anesthetists after appropriate approval by the governor. By 2007, 14 states had opted out of this federal requirement (Blumenreich, 2007, p. 93). Recent literature focuses on the term *anesthesia care team (ACT)* to indicate a practice by a CRNA with an anesthesiologist in a medically directed environment. Jones and Fitzpatrick (2009) identified four possible types of current inpatient anesthesia team arrangements in the United States: an all-anesthesiologist staff, an all–nurse anesthetist staff, a mixed staff of the above, and a team of anesthesiologist and anesthesiologist assistants (p. 431). In their study of collaboration among members of these teams, they found satisfaction with collaboration expressed by both nurse-anesthetists and physicians. However, they noted that there are still issues with role conflict; unclear expectations and/or limits on scope of practice with mixed teams; and a component of exclusion from hospital, departmental, and anesthesia group responsibilities when only physicians can participate in hospital committees or represent the group. The challenge for CRNAs is to work with physician colleagues to achieve fullness of practice for each member of the anesthesia team.

The Certified Nurse-Midwife

In the colonial and pioneer history of the United States, midwives were respected members of both settler and Native American communities. However, since the early 1900s the role has had a stormy history caused in no small part by the low status of women, sparse education, religious intolerance, and increased domination of physician obstetricians with the movement toward birthing in hospitals. In 1921, the Maternity Center Association of New York and the Henry Street Visiting Nurse Association proposed establishing a school of nurse-midwifery. However, strong opposition from medicine, nursing, and the public arose, mainly because of a generally held negative view of the role of midwife as an exemplar of inadequacy, little education, and social incompetence. In 1925, the role moved to a new level of recognition and respect with the inauguration of the Appalachian clinics of Kentucky (Frontier Nursing Service) by Mary Breckenridge (Dorroh & Norton, 1996).

The number of CNMs has increased from just 275 in 1963 to over 4,000 by 1995 and 7,000 in 2011 (American College of Nurse-Midwives [ACNM], 2011). CNMs consider interdisciplinary practice as a *sine qua non* of their practice, and this position has been affirmed in their standards of care and formal definitions of practice (ACNM, 2008). In 1971, the American College of Nurse-Midwives (ACNM), the American College of Obstetricians and Gynecologists (ACOG), and the Nurses Association of the ACOG issued a joint statement supporting the concept of obstetrical team practice. However, the teams were to be "directed by a physician," formalizing a hierarchical practice pattern that continues to pose challenges to development of a collaborative approach to practice (Bigbee, 1996). The ACNM statement on collaborative management defines *collaboration* as "the process whereby a CNM or certified midwife (CM) and physician jointly manage the care of a woman or newborn that has become medically, gynecologically or obstetrically complicated" (ACNM, 1997). The need for collaboration is indicated by the health status of the client rather than by statute or edict. However, the number of viable practices currently differs considerably state-by-state because of legal and legislative requirements for collaboration and the parameters of required collaborative practice protocols, which vary from state to state.

Because of lack of support from physicians and hospitals, CNMs are often unable to practice or their practice is severely limited due to economic competition and differing views on the meaning and value of collaboration. A study from New Zealand offers a model of midwifery care in which midwifery-led maternity care is the dominant model and 75% of the New Zealand women choose a midwife as their "lead maternity caregiver" (LMC). When midwives did refer to an obstetrician, 74% indicated they continued providing care in collaboration with the obstetrician, and the relationships between professionals were satisfying (Skinner & Foureur, 2010). This model starkly contrasts with the description by Goodman (2007) of the "marginalization of certified nurse-midwives in the United States" where in 2007 midwives attended only 7% of births.

The issue of economic competition is another hindrance to CNM practice. In a conversation between a nurse-midwife and an obstetrician with whom she had a good working relationship, the physician commented, "I don't have any problems with you personally, but the fact is that my practice is not full, and until it is there is not going to be a nurse-midwife that will get privileges at this hospital" (Goodman, 2007, p. 616). Another economic factor threatening the future of the collaborative relationship is malpractice insurance cost. For example, in a discussion with one CNM/physician practice group, the CNMs noted that the cost of malpractice insurance increased from $18,000 to $40,000 during 1 year, and their practice group could not afford to cover the additional costs. Individual CNMs did not get paid for all the calls they took, nor were they able to perform enough births to cover the cost of their own insurance. This inequity of practice compensation coupled with the lack of 100% support of a practice by their physician group resulted in the midwives no longer practicing midwifery but being limited to providing other women's health services.

In October 2002, the joint statement between the ACNM and the ACOG was revised for the fifth time in 30 years. An ongoing concern of many CNMs and physicians had been the language and the inferences of previous documents, readily open to multiple interpretations. The leadership of ACNM and ACOG decided to develop a statement more reflective of the current status of each profession, as well as contemporary realities within the women's health-care system. The 2002 ACNM/ACOG joint statement was endorsed by both parties as a document "that promotes respect and collaboration between CNMs/CMs and [medical doctors] and encourages individual practices to work collegially together to meet the needs of individual patients" (Shah, 2002, p. 2). The simplicity of the statement was perhaps its greatest asset. By not dictating specific protocols or responsibilities, professional accountability is placed where it rightfully belongs: "on each respective profession and the individual women's health care professional" (p. 3). The most recent joint statement of the ACNM/ACOG alliance in 2011 reaffirms their shared goals regarding women's health and continues its simplicity of language and approach, emphasizing the need for a health-care system that facilitates communication among providers and across settings (ACNM/ACOG, 2011). The positive take on this statement, in addition to the review of APRN outcomes by Newhouse and colleagues (2011) confirming the high-quality care delivered by certified nurse-midwives in the United States, might begin to facilitate a more collaborative approach in the practice setting.

The Clinical Nurse Specialist

The CNS role, which originated in the late 1930s, was formalized as a nurse-clinician to be prepared in graduate nursing programs. Its emergence represented a major shift of focus in graduate education from the choice of a functional role of primarily teacher or administrator to the selection of a clinical specialization in practice. Of the multiple specialties represented by the CNS role, psychiatry was the first to move to graduate education and is among the most highly respected. Some have attested that collaborative activities with physicians seemed to come more naturally for this group because of their graduate-level education, which allowed CNSs and physicians to more readily relate to each other as peers (Bigbee, 1996). A review of literature published between 1990 and 2008 on care provided by clinical nurse specialists gave supporting evidence of their value in acute care settings in reducing length of stay, cost, and rates of complications (Newhouse et al., 2011).

Key elements of CNS practice identified by the American Association of Critical-Care Nurses (AACN, 2007) include "collaborating with other disciplines to provide interdisciplinary best practices" (p. 7). Collaboration is one of the eight CNS competencies considered essential for nurses providing care in the acute-care setting. These competencies are part of the AACN synergy model for patient care, recommended as a guide for clinical practice in acute care. The model is predicated on the fact that patient outcomes are optimal when patient characteristics and nurse competencies are in synch (Kaplow, 2007). One CNS described her collaborative practice level as a real partnership with a great deal of mutual caring and respect between providers. Each partner grounded interactions in self-confidence and personal mastery, and they planned together "always." Yet another CNS noted that her collaborating physicians needed some education on what the CNS could and could not do, but they learned as they jointly practiced, and a real comfort level occurred after about 6 months. A hematology-oncology APRN group, which formed a successful collaborative practice over a period of 7 years, identified effective leadership, shared development of goals, and communication as critical for establishment of a viable structure (Schaal et al., 2008). Another collaborative partnership of the CNS and the nurse manager of an oncology unit described the key element of success as development of mutually acceptable goals (Gaguski & Begyn, 2009). The key to the future of a positive and productive collaborative practice for the CNS with other health professionals is a relationship that becomes more mutually valued and partner driven.

The Nurse Practitioner

The role of the NP has been described as an innovative role in primary care, grown from the role of the public health nurse, and possessing a high degree of autonomy in practice (Bigbee, 1996). Since its inception in the 1960s, a considerable expansion of the concept of the NP role has occurred, as NPs have moved into a multitude of settings that are not necessarily primary care, such as long-term and acute care. Because of the unique and varied ways in which the role has developed, coming from certificate programs, many within medical schools, and gradually moving into graduate nurse programs, the history of collaboration is a patchwork quilt. Support of and opposition to the role has come from both medicine and nursing. Martha Rogers (1972) opposed the role as demeaning to nursing in deference to medical practice, and this view, supported by many nurse educators at the time, created serious divisions within the nursing profession as NP educators worked to enhance the role and move it into graduate-level education. Medical opposition, which existed from the beginning, is often couched in terms of *patient safety,* despite the fact that it often is more related to issues of control and competition in practice. Because of these powerful sources of opposition, the focus on collaboration has been both a boon and a boondoggle to NP practice. The importance of the interdisciplinary team and the responsibility of the NP to assist in collaborative team development have been consistently emphasized (Buerhaus, 2010; Hanna, 1996). However, as the term *collaboration* found in some state nursing practice acts often conveys a concept of "supervision," there are many who would strike the word from any statutory documents. The evolving acute-care NP (ACNP) role requires a very explicit differentiation of medical and nursing domains within a collaborative practice. Strong support from nursing service, and better yet, having the ACNP housed within the nursing department, allows for easier differentiation of role by each partner. This promotes a team in which each partner comes from a solid professional sense of self and can then join with others to fuse into an autonomous, interdependent team of providers. In contrast, when the ACNP is "supervised" by a resident or is employed by a medical specialty department, it becomes more difficult for the practitioner to participate equally in decision making and to be considered a full partner in the practice (Lott, Polak, Kenyon, & Kenner, 1996).

The role of the NP within managed care systems has evolved into a process of collaboration, coordination, and negotiation, requiring the creation of new relationships among a wide range of personnel. Role negotiation is a key component of this type of practice, in which the required interaction between professionals for the specific purpose of changing the other's expectation of one's role can result in increased job satisfaction, reduced role conflict, and a more positive team relationship (Miller & Apker, 2002). A professional partnership promoting collaboration replaces competition with shared responsibilities, in which each partner brings a unique and necessary set of knowledge and skills to the practice. The fear of loss of professional uniqueness is met head on by a practice in which the expertise and unique abilities of each team member, when combined into a synchronous whole, deliver a high level of care not possible through the efforts of a single provider (Norsen, Oplanden, & Quinn, 1995).

A review of two rural Ontario primary care practices between NPs and family physicians (FPs) found comparable involvement of both in health-promotion activities and considerably greater focus of NPs on disease prevention and supportive care. However, the review also found NPs underutilized in relation to curative and rehabilitative services, with referral patterns being largely unidirectional, from NP to FP. The authors noted that such a one-sided referral process does not reflect collaboration, which demands shared, reciprocal practice patterns (Way, Jones, Baskerville, & Busing, 2001). In addition, the regulated drug list required for Ontario NPs does not permit NPs to renew medications for stable chronic illnesses, limiting their scope of practice and hampering the ability of the NP to assist patients in the management of their chronic illnesses (Way et al., 2001). Rationale offered for drawbacks to a full collaborative practice included unclear medico-legal issues affecting the ability to "share responsibility," an absence of interdisciplinary education at both undergraduate and graduate levels, and lack of knowledge and practice experience regarding the scope of NP practice. Despite challenges to NP practice, their value is continuing to be acknowledged. The Missouri Nurses Association (2011) reported that the health-care access and needs of rural Missourians are currently strained and any discussion of solutions must include considering the role of nurse practitioners and physician assistants. They stressed that the "future economic stability and health status of rural Missourians depends on . . . [considering] options that allow for increased use of the expertise of advanced practice registered nurses" (Becker & Porth, 2011, p. 9). Panelist Charlene Hanson, in a recent interview of "NP Thought Leaders," summarized the current state of nurse practitioner practice when she noted that "physicians and NPs at the grassroots have worked out a comfortable, collaborative, professional relationship that benefits both. But the relationship at the policy and organizational state and national levels is much more divisive" (Buerhaus, 2010).

A FRAMEWORK FOR COLLABORATION

The Concept

Collaboration is a "dynamic, transforming process of creating a power-sharing partnership" (Sullivan, 1998, p. 6). As a dynamic process, it includes the flexible distribution of both status and authority, and requires both relationship building and shared decision making. A distinctive interpersonal process, it requires that the partners recognize and acknowledge their shared values and commit to interact constructively to solve problems and accomplish identified goals, purposes, or outcomes. Using the consensus process, where participants are not coerced as in compromise or "majority vote" but helped to reach an agreement they can approve, even if they do not agree with all points, facilitates high levels of agreement and team satisfaction. Shared power, a key component within a collaborative practice, requires the active contribution of each participant, respect for and openness to each other's contributions, and use of consensus in forming new approaches to practice that use the strengths of each participant (ANA, 2010b; APRN Joint Dialogue Group, 2008; IOM, 2011; O'Brien, Martin, Heyworth, & Meyer, 2009; Rice et al., 2010).

The Components

A viable and high-level collaborative practice may be readily identified by the existence of four essential components: separate and unique practice spheres, common goals, shared power control, and mutual concerns. **Table 9-1** presents the components essential for a positive practice, the key attributes of a highly collaborative practice, and practitioner competencies contributing to success. A phenomenological study of how APRN and physicians perceive and describe their sense of collaboration identified

TABLE 9-1

Components of Collaborative Practice

Essential Components	Key Attributes	Competencies
Separate and unique practice spheres Common goals Shared power control Mutual concerns	Autonomous, trusting relationship Confidence in a partner's skill Bidirectional referrals and consultation Consensus-driven decision making Equitable reporting lines and evaluators Mutually defined goals of the practice Open, informal communication Parity between providers (physical space, caseload, and support staff) Positive support by colleagues, support staff, and consumers	Assertiveness Communication skills Conflict management Cooperation Coordination Clinical skills Mutual respect Decision-making skills Positive attitude Trust Willingness to dialogue

four key behaviors identified as essential for collaboration: approachability, interpersonal skills, listening, and verbal message skills, each of which reflects either the attributes and/or competencies identified by O'Brien, Martin, Heyworth, and Meyer (2009).

1. *Separate and unique practice spheres.* Both physician and nurse must identify components of their practice that are separate and unique, and components that they share. A high-level collaborative practice requires an autonomous, trusting relationship within which bilateral consultation and referrals are the norm. Autonomy exists within each practitioner's skill and competence, and allows for confident decision making. It is the trust of the team that empowers that person to practice independently within his or her defined scope of practice. As one APRN noted, "You must be willing to expand your boundaries but know your limitations and where you feel comfortable in your practice" (Bailey & Armer, 1998, p. 243). The existence of bidirectional referral and consultation reflects a high level of trust between practice partners. In one instance, the physician response to a consultation request was, "Now this is not what you have to do; this is what I'd recommend. But the final decision is yours because it's your patient" (Bailey & Armer, 1998, p. 243).
2. *Common goals.* When both partners agree to responsibilities for practice goals, the partners are well on their way to a synchronous relationship. As one provider in a highly collaborative practice noted, "Care by all providers is based on mutually defined goals of the practice" (Bailey & Armer, 1998, p. 245). All of the participants cited by Bailey and Armer (1998) stressed that responsibility for patient outcomes was the key driving force in their collaborative actions. One APRN noted, "If there's a patient [I treated] who calls in and . . . says 'I'm just not better,' she'll [the physician] say things like 'If I had treated you, I would have given you the same thing.' It just sets the patient at ease because they realize that we're working together" (p. 245).
3. *Shared power control.* Each physician and nurse partner assumes individual accountability along with a shared responsibility for actively participating in the decision-making process as well as supporting the consensus-driven decisions and sharing in their implementation. In one

situation, a nurse, commenting on a physician perceived as very collaborative, stated, "We started when the MD and PA called me to discuss his patient's care and asked for suggestions. . . . We examined the patient together, the MD described what we were seeing in the wound . . . and I identified potential strategies for wound healing. . . . The MD/PA team acknowledged my expertise and came to me for assistance to assist the patient" (McGrail, Morse, Glessner, & Gardner, 2008, p. 201). Ongoing and consistent communication is key to building a shared-power practice. Providers must be comfortable sharing information both about patient care, issues of collaboration, and team functioning. Collaboration is a powerful tool to build a team, but without shared decision making, collaboration cannot exist (Gaguski & Bagyn, 2009; Maylone et al., 2011; O'Grady & Ford, 2009; Sullivan et al., 1998).

4. *Mutual concerns.* To ensure mutual concerns are met, providers need to have skills of assertiveness, cooperation, and coordination. Assertiveness can be described as the ability to express a viewpoint with confidence and with attention to being factually accurate and focused on the patient need. The key aspect of team success is the knowledge and utilization of each member's expertise by the others. For example, in a surgical care situation, the physician is in charge of the operation; the physician and NP or CNS jointly care for the patient postoperatively; the NP or CNS is in charge of discharge planning; and, in some settings, the CRNA might also be on the surgical team, assuming full responsibility for anesthesia delivery, each one confident in his or her skills and able to speak up regarding patient needs and care direction as he or she sees it. Acknowledgment and respect of other opinions and viewpoints while maintaining the willingness to examine and change personal beliefs and perspectives stresses the interdependence of the practitioners on the team and underlies true cooperation. Collegial relationships replace hierarchical authority with equality and shared decision making. Decisions made by consensus are based on the expertise of each member; there are different levels of input, but it is always in the best interest of the patient. One APN noted, "There are many times the physician will say to me 'This is a nurse practitioner patient,' and it's somebody that has all kinds of sociological problems. Problems that I could coordinate, and that's good; that's a compliment to nursing. He actually has learned what we do" (Bailey & Armer, 1998, p. 243). Trust is the bond that unites all the components of collaboration. "Without the element of trust, cooperation cannot exist, assertiveness becomes threatening, responsibility is avoided, communication is hampered, autonomy is suppressed, and coordination is haphazard" (Norsen et al., 1995, p. 45).

The Intensity Continuum

The level of collaboration within a practice can be found by identifying the intensity of professional relationships (high to low) and the type of collaborative structure found along a complexity continuum of unidisciplinary, multidisciplinary, interdisciplinary, or transdisciplinary practice. See **Figure 9-1.** The interactive complexity of the practice will increase as the structure becomes more complex, offering greater challenges to the team but resulting in even more positive and productive outcomes of practice.

Professional staff in any health setting (e.g., licensed practical nurse [LPN], RN, social worker, APRN, physician, radiology technician, and so on) are coming from a *unidisciplinary* base. As students, they were prepared for the interactive world of practice within the security of working with students, faculty, and practitioners of their discipline and program. They begin to develop personal mastery of professional knowledge and skill, an essential requirement for functioning effectively at the more complex levels of interactive relationships found in collaborative practice. Educational experiences with students of other professions are generally very limited, usually to clinical encounters. As the

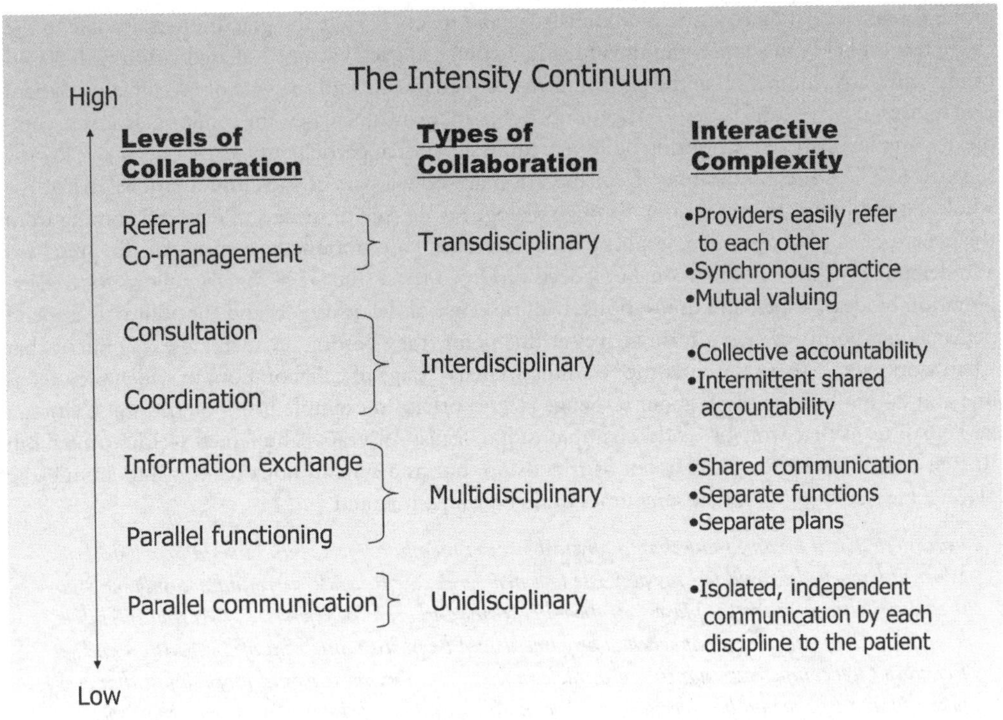

FIGURE 9-1 Intensity continuum. *(Data from Blais et al., 2002; Kuehn, 1998.)*

professionals begin to share responsibilities for the same patient or patient populations, they begin to interact with each other and a *multidisciplinary* practice model emerges. This is a level of information exchange, with no presumption of shared planning. Each fulfills a discipline-specific role but communicates with others on an as-needed basis. This level exemplifies the "chimneys of excellence" approach in which work is accomplished not by team effort but by a collection of professionals working for the most part in "isolated splendor" (Kuehn, 1998, p. 27). However, within this multidisciplinary framework, an *interdisciplinary* relationship can begin to develop as two or more members begin to coalesce their roles toward a common vision or goal. There begins to be a sense of shared investment and a desire to plan together for a better outcome. As each professional shares discipline-specific expertise, cross-fertilization of ideas starts to occur and group ownership of the practice begins to emerge. The dynamics that revolve around the emerging practitioner-to-practitioner relationships concern issues of leadership, power control, norms, values, group behavior, and conflicts, and demand skills in communication, collaboration, and conflict resolution. Major growth in the complexity of interactive practices can be seen by the increased use of the terms *interdisciplinary* and *interprofessional* to describe this third level of team dynamics as a key requisite for high-quality care (American Medical Directors Association [AMDA], 2011; Donald et al., 2009; Rice et al., 2010). The second basic tenet of nursing practice (ANA, 2010b) notes that "nurses coordinate care by establishing partnerships . . . collaborative interprofessional team planning is based on recognition of each discipline's value and contributions, mutual trust, respect, open discussion and shared decision-making" (p. 4). The intensity of relationships is at a peak when a practice moves into a *transdisciplinary* level. It becomes a practice without professional boundaries, a synthesis of knowledge and practice. Here the practitioners are able to rise above fears of being subsumed and the individual visions of each become a shared vision with "laser-beam" intensity. All, including the patient, own the plan of care and the goal of high-quality patient care transcends any "turf" issues. As the number of participants increases, the resulting diversity, complexity, and intensity of relationship building requires that each participant feel that he or she "owns" the vision. The critical indicators of collaboration are now a part of each and a visible part of the whole. At this level, communication through dialogue is the key to success. *Discussion,* coming from the same root word as *percussion,* implies a hard exchange of ideas bouncing back and forth, presented and defended with the need to come to a decision. In contrast, the art of *dialogue* allows for free exploration of ideas, issues, and innovations, with no sense of defensiveness and the ability to suspend personal viewpoints. When a team arrives at this point, they become in such close alignment that when working together they enter the "transdisciplinary" stage of collaboration, in which they act as one and do not have to think about it. Senge (1994) offers an example using the Boston Celtics, a basketball team that won 11 world championships in just 13 years. The famed Celtics center Bill Russell described their team play not as friendship, but as a synchronous relationship among the players. He stated (p. 234) that sometimes during a game, it would

> *heat up so that it became more than a physical or even mental game . . . and would be magical. . . . When it happened I could feel my play rise to a new level. . . . It would surround not only me and the other Celtics but also the players on the other team, and even the referees. . . . At that special level, all sorts of odd things happened. The game would be in the white heat of competition and yet I wouldn't feel competitive, which is a miracle in itself. . . . The game would move so fast that every fake, cut and pass would be surprising, and yet nothing could surprise me . . . during those spells I could almost sense how the next play would develop and where the next shot would be taken.*

To develop positive relationships with other health-care practitioners, comprehensive care requires the collective contributions of many varied professionals with highly developed skills, including self-knowledge and traditions of knowledge in the health professions; team and community building; and work dynamics of groups, teams, and organizations. Practitioners must be familiar with the healing approaches of other professions and cultures, be aware of historic power inequities across professions, identify similarities and differences among traditions of community members, know the value of the work of others, and learn from having had experiences of working with people from other disciplines and healing traditions. The key to team building is the affirmation by all of a shared mission, tasks, goals, and values (ANA, 2010b; IOM, 2004, 2011; Jehn, Northcraft, & Neale, 1999; Senge, 1994).

The "Iceberg" Effect

Where the team of APRN and physician falls on the collaboration continuum, as well as the intensity of the relationships, is determined by a number of critical factors. These factors can be visualized as an iceberg, with many visible and openly known, and others that remain invisible or unacknowledged although still extremely significant in their affect on the success or failure of the collaborative effort (Pearson & Jones, 1994; Plant, 1987). See **Figure 9-2.**

The formal "visible" systems include many common components of practice such as organizational policies, clinic objectives, systems of communications, and role or job descriptions. These are accessible and changeable, and are readily addressed in open, rational discussion. In contrast, the "invisible," informal systems, including power networks, values, and norms, are not as accessible but subtly present, difficult to change, and often give a sense of being untouchable. Many of the barriers to collaboration are hidden here. Only through working together can a team become aware of the impact of this

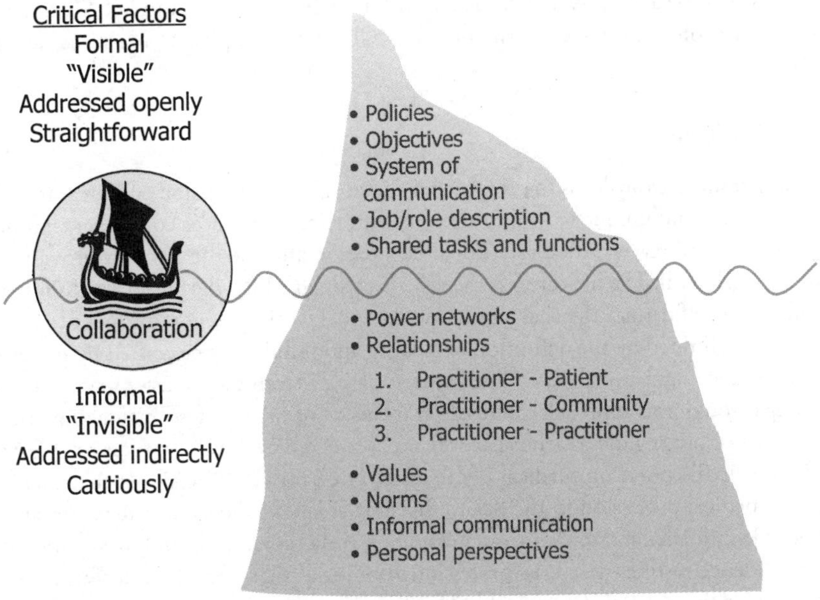

FIGURE 9-2 Iceberg factor. *(Data from Kuehn, 1998; Pearson & Jones, 1994; Plant, 1987.)*

invisible system and work to eliminate the barriers. The barriers must first be identified and acknowledged, and then strategies applied to remove or neutralize them as the partners in practice work to become a viable team (Donald et al., 2009; IOM, 2011; Paradise, Dark, & Bitler, 2011).

BARRIERS TO COLLABORATION

Barriers to collaboration hinder positive change and growth in our health-care system, frustrate the professionals trying to work as a team, and can negatively affect the future of health care (IOM, 2011; Kubota, 2011; Rice et al., 2010). Key barriers that continue to challenge collaborative efforts include educational isolation, professional elitism, organizational hierarchy, unrecognized diversity, role and language confusion, inadequate communication patterns, and professional dissonance.

Educational Isolation

Despite an increasing call for an interdisciplinary approach to education in the health professions, many educators continue to use a traditional linear approach with built-in assumptions of bureaucratic organizational structures, standardized sets of relationships and roles, and systematized methods of record keeping, billing, and payment for services. Past studies exploring the status of interdisciplinary education have noted many inherent problems associated with developing interdisciplinary educational programs, citing workload stress, intense workload demands, lack of academic and institutional support, and often seemingly insurmountable complications with clinical arrangements (Kuehn, 1998). In the past, some nurse educators have expressed concerns that the traditional concept of a nursing workforce is challenged by calls for health care to be delivered by interdisciplinary teams, fearing that this focus has the potential of obscuring the unique contribution of nursing to health-care delivery (National League for Nursing [NLN], 1997). However, shared educational experiences can actually help clarify roles because as faculty and students work together, they begin to better understand the contribution each profession makes to the practice (Glasgow, Dunphy, & Mainous, 2010; Hojat et al., 2003).

Professional Elitism

Educational isolationism easily leads to professional elitism as each profession educates "its own" with a sense of importance and unique worth. Professionalism consists of three components: professional ideals of knowledge and service, the professional occupation and the life career it provides, and the character of the work itself. The life career is the vehicle through which the ideals are put into practice, and the profession itself defines the character of professional work. The commitment to healing and to service is thereby limited by the definition of healing and public service crafted by the profession. Although "importance" and "worth" are valued aspects of self-identify, a pervasive sense of professional elitism running through this approach can result in the work of each professional taking priority over helping each other or putting the patient's needs first (O'Neil & Pew Health Professions Commission, 1998). In his classic discourse on medical dominance, Friedson (1970) claimed that the dominant position of the medical profession in the health division of labor "allows it to reinforce and protect itself from outside influence and to claim and maintain jurisdiction and control over many more areas than logic or evidence justifies. . . . It is 'professionalism' itself that seems to transform the ideal responsibility to serve the good of the general public into a limited concrete responsibility to serve the good of one's personal public" (p. 152). As Friedman (1970) cautioned, "A professional who is so qualified as to perform this extraordinary work of medicine . . . must himself be a rather extraordinary, gifted, person . . . as are his colleagues and his profession. . . . This professional pride leads the worker to consider himself to be quite different from, indeed superior to, those of other occupations. . . The thrust of professional activity becomes a mission to build barriers that keep the profession and its clientele safe from those beyond the pale while seeking jurisdiction over all that cannot be excluded" (pp. 154–155). In a recent intervention study to improve interprofessional collaboration, physicians reported that they expected orders would be carried out without discussion. Nurses and other health professionals in the study agreed that this was the medical expectation and it limited the possibility of much collaboration (Rice et al., 2010).

Nursing should acknowledge that it, too, has been guilty of elitism and of exhibiting professional dominance and defensiveness, both in relating to other nurses with different levels of education and expertise and in working with other health-care professionals. Lack of understanding, failure to acknowledge roles and responsibilities of other professionals, and the very isolated nature of health professional education is the basis for much of the elitism still prevalent today (Glasgow, Dunphy, & Mainous, 2010; Rice et al., 2010).

Organizational Hierarchy

The key to the inadequacy of health services is described as "professional dominance," a situation in which health services revolve around professional authority, with a foundational structure of dominance by a single profession over a variety of other "subordinate professions" (Friedson, 1970). The two lines of authority in medicine and health care have historically been the administrative authority of the "office" and the medical authority of professional skills and expertise. The medical profession as an occupation with institutionalized privileges and authority granted by others on a basis of faith and trust holds a special form of legal "power" based on "expert status" because their knowledge and work are considered very complex and nonroutine, and subsequently has a position of dominance among other occupations providing health care. This results in professional control of information and suspicion of the value of what lies "outside" their domain. Friedson (1970, pp. 231, 234) suggests that this autonomy and dominance need to be and can be controlled by an administrative structure that stresses accountability for effective and humane services, and is responsive to the patient:

> *For a profession to be true to the ideal of a profession, members must let go of the total authority and control over the terms and content of their work and cease total dominance in favor of a division of labor. The physicians must temper autonomy and dominance with administrative accountability, accountability to the patient, self-regulated peer review and encouragement of other providers to assume responsibilities of health care . . . [However] no service using other providers is possible . . . without the active cooperation of the dominant profession. If the profession does not trust them, or if it resents and fears them, it will not refer patients to them, nor will it graciously receive patients referred from them . . . Mere administrative fiat is not enough.*

Supervision is defined as critically watching and directing activities or a course of action and is a mainstay of any hierarchical structure. Rationales given for supervision of health care include documented inadequacy; lack of knowledge, experience, or skills in relation to the person supervised; legal requirements; a lack of trust or confidence despite no legal limits requiring supervision; perceived safety needs of patient or provider; and history, tradition, or local institutional policy. In exploring the difference between "under the supervision of" and "ownership of practice decisions," it may be most helpful to view them not as polar opposites but as different levels of collaboration along a continuum of autonomous practice. Kinlein (1977) stressed that if a physician, a member of one another profession, determines by his or her orders what actions a nurse, a member of a separate profession, will take, the practice is no longer the "essence of nursing" but becomes "medically directed care" delivered by nurses (p. 30). Supervised or medically directed care seems to fall within the framework of multidisciplinary interactions representing a very limited level of intensity of relationships and collaboration. Supervision may not preclude some level of collaboration, but it seems to severely limit its scope. The extent of collaboration possible within such a "delegated" mindset is questionable.

Unrecognized Diversity

Diversity in a health-care team can have a powerful impact on its success or failure as a cohesive workgroup. It can bring a wealth of helpful differences but can also be the cause of great conflict within the group. Cultural diversity may be easily recognized and acknowledged, but there are many complex aspects of diversity that may not be recognized and that can undermine team efforts. Three major categories of diversity are informational, social category, and value (Jehn et al., 1999). Informational diversity reflects the differences in knowledge and perspectives of team members, flowing from their education, experiences, and levels of expertise. Social category diversity relates to age, race, gender, and ethnicity and is the aspect we are most familiar with as cultural diversity. Value diversity reflects the differences in members' perspectives of the mission, goals, and values relating to the work at hand. A study of the impact of diversity on work-group performance found that different forms of diversity could result in different levels of performance within the team. Having high information diversity (differences in education and experience) can make a team quite effective because of the many professional perspectives that can be available to the team. However, if it is accompanied by high value diversity, the team may malfunction as a unit. Over time, age, gender, and race differences in a group become less important, but value diversity—differences in understanding of the mission, goals, and values—becomes the more important component as a predictor of conflict or success. The complexity of relationships within a team is heightened by the level and type of diversity. Often unrecognized or unacknowledged, value diversity may be the most critical factor in the success or failure of teamwork and collaboration (Jehn et al., 1999).

Role and Language Confusion

The increasingly expanded scopes of nursing practice being experienced across the United States continues to be hampered by inconsistencies of legal language and titling variations among states. In examining the role of "primary care provider," Starfield (1992b) identified three types of functions performed by nonphysician personnel: (a) supplementary, extending the efficiency of the physician by assuming the technical tasks, usually under the direction of the physician; (b) substitutive, providing services usually provided by physicians; and (c) complementary, extending the effectiveness of physicians by doing things physicians do not do at all, do poorly, or do reluctantly. Noting that the nonphysician role has not been clarified to the extent that the three functions can be differentiated, Starfield concluded that primary care is largely a physician-dominated effort. Although primary care cannot function without some teamwork involving other practitioner providers, she believed that there was little evidence supporting the concept of team practice and little research indicating when and under what conditions a team approach may be more effective than a singular practice approach. In conclusion, Starfield asserted that primary care should be provided by physicians and the concept of *teamwork* in primary care needed to be researched regarding (a) standards for different roles and relationships; (b) identification of which type of delegated function—substitutive, supplementary, or complementary—is most appropriately assumed by what level or type provider; and (c) how well the attributes of primary care are achieved by nonphysicians in comparison with care by physicians. Concerns raised by Starfield's discussion of primary care center on the language used, as well as her consistent adherence to the traditional medical viewpoint of the physician as the "captain of the ship." The use of the term *team* is quite perfunctory and seems to imply only a multidisciplinary collection of individuals gathered by the physician to facilitate his or her practice. The three functional types—supplementary, substitutive, and complementary—are each defined in relation to their ability to enhance physician effectiveness rather than as shared components of a joint practice. In addition, Starfield (1992a) frames the role of the nonphysician provider by tasks and functions, severely limiting the scope of advanced practice and the role of collaboration.

Collaboration, often used in statute, is frequently interpreted in rules and regulations as "supervision," implying a hierarchical relationship and a contradiction to the critical indicators of collaboration. For collaboration to consistently mean an egalitarian, collegial relationship, the legislative language must be more clearly defined. The question becomes whether power sharing can coexist with a supervision requirement in a practice. When collaboration is mandated, or termed *supervision,* the process of shared practice becomes one of forced negotiation in which the dominant profession, medicine, has the choice of collaboration, with no legal need for a collaborative partner, whereas the subjected profession, nursing, must obtain a collaborative partner to legally function within the full scope of its practice (Sullivan, Morgan, Heimerichs, & Scott, 1998). Physician involvement can be termed *collaboration, supervision, direction, delegation, or authorization,* and the meaning of each term can be ambiguous, particularly in statute.

Statutory requirements for collaboration for advanced practice nursing couched as "delegated" or "supervised" practice are not acceptable for a number of time-tested reasons. If patterns of practice are legislated, legislative judgment becomes limited by the parameters of the legal definitions, rules, and regulations of the state in which the practice is located. The flexibility needed for individual clinical situations may be seriously compromised by these legally defined parameters. The result is that, because of restrictive legislation, rules, regulations, and reimbursement policies, advanced nursing practice too often depends on the willingness of a physician collaborator, whereas the same limitations are not placed on the physician. "One can only imagine what the reaction of organized medicine would be if a state legislature attempted to delineate when and how internist physicians should refer patients to a specialist" (ANA, 1998, p. 4). Legislatively mandated collaboration often results in a conflict (Sullivan, 1998). In states where APRN practice is controlled by joint board decisions, the negotiation process of joint rule making can become very hostile because of an unequal balance of power among the parties. Further, when membership of the board of nursing includes representatives of each level of nursing, those members not in advanced practice may lack the knowledge base required for debating advanced practice issues such as prescriptive authority. The subsequent rules passed may be far more restrictive than had been imagined from the broader language of the statute. Reasons offered by Sullivan and colleagues (1998) for the failure of these disparate groups to accomplish an externally imposed power-sharing partnership are not difficult to understand. They state (p. 350),

> *Because the participants did not share a common purpose or vision, and were forced to meet, it is not surprising that they did not work well together or achieve a satisfactory result—by any standards. Because the representatives were forced to come together and their Boards had their budgets held hostage to the process, it was not unexpected that despite the need to reach some level of agreement there was little commitment to a win-win situation. . . . Instead, representatives of each discipline worked to protect their distinctly different professional agendas. It became not a collaborative process but a legalistic and formalized process of enforced negotiation.*

Collaboration has also been described as an interdependent, interdisciplinary practice in which the APRN role is "substitutive" in a primary care setting in contrast to the "complementary" role more applicable to acute-care settings (King, Parrinello, & Baggs, 1996). However, there are difficulties with the use of the term *substitutive* because it implies a temporary stopgap until the "regular" practitioner can be provided. More contemporary views of collaboration and interdisciplinary practice steer clear of the substitutive and complementary language and stress partnership and the unique areas of expertise of each member of the team (Donald et al., 2009; IOM, 2011). In the 23rd Annual Legislative Update, Phillips (2011) notes that 24 states now have no statutory or regulatory requirements for physician collaboration, direction, or supervision, reflecting a movement toward the autonomous nursing role and facilitating a teamwork approach to practice.

Another language issue relates to the use of protocols and clinical guidelines. *Protocols* are defined as the "detailed plan of a scientific or medical experiment, treatment, or procedure" (*Merriam-Webster's*, 1994). In research, they need to be followed "to the letter" to have accurate, consistent, and comparable sets of data. The concern with protocols comes with their use in statutes, rules, and regulations as a definitive set of boundaries restricting practice to sets of predetermined criteria. When the perception of nursing is a dependent practice under physician supervision, the mechanisms created for allowing advanced practice often include a system of protocols designed with the approval of the "collaborating" physician. However, this "solution" compromises the concept of nursing autonomy, suggests that the nurse is incapable of making accurate choices among treatment options, and becomes implicit "standing orders" reinforcing nursing dependency (Baer, 1993). In some states, neither protocols nor a collaborative practice agreement with a physician is required for full practice privileges. In others, if prescriptive authority is possible, a collaborative practice agreement with a physician may be required, but perhaps no protocols. Historically, clinical guidelines represented collective wisdom gathered over time and were considered no threat to autonomy. In contrast, guidelines today may not be as willingly accepted because of the fear that they might influence or "manage" provider behavior.

If guidelines or protocols allow room for the exercise of provider judgment, they will support provider autonomy as well. The Agency for Healthcare Research and Quality (AHRQ) uses the term *clinical practice guidelines* to describe systematically developed statements to assist practitioner and patient decisions about appropriate health care for specific clinical conditions. They may be broad or very detailed based on literature review as well as expert opinion. These are written by independent multidisciplinary panels of private-sector clinicians and other experts, supported by AHRQ. Practitioners must have clinical guidelines in place for reimbursement from Medicare (Newman, 1996), and they are viewed sometimes as an excellent tool for communicating the role to funding agencies (Way & Jones, 1994).

One additional aspect of language confusion is that of "titling" of APRNs. Many titles found in the different state statutes include advanced nurse practitioner (ANP), advanced practice nurse (APN), advanced practice professional nurse (APPN), advanced practice registered nurse (APRN), advanced registered nurse practitioner (ARNP), certified nurse practitioner (CNP), and registered nurse practitioner (RNP). The APRN Consensus Model for APRN Regulation, Licensure, Accreditation, Certification, and Education (LACE) defines advanced practice and each specialty, describes the regulatory model, and identifies titles to be used. This document was created by regulators, nurse educators, APRN certifiers, and representatives of a large number of APRN professional organizations with the goal of creating national consistency regarding laws and rules regulating APRN practice. With some physician groups still insisting on supervision, the challenge remains to get past the language barriers and clarify roles to foster a collaborative approach to care. *The Pearson Report* (2011) encourages NPs to share the updated legislative information with their legislators to help them understand that NPs are competent and high-quality clinicians, and to remove barriers to advanced practice nursing.

The launching of doctorate of nurse practice programs has also created some language difficulties. The fairly recent nursing doctorate (ND) has been phased out and the doctor of nursing practice (DNP) is now identified as the expectation for all APRNs by 2015. One expected benefit of the DNP is the greater opportunity to fully participate on the interdisciplinary team. However, there are challenges to the concept, suggesting that the educational and clinical residency requirements of the DNP do not prepare one for becoming faculty, assuming leadership roles, or conducting clinical research (Brar, Boschma, & McCuaig, 2010; Webber, 2008). In addition, the term *Dr. Nurse* is causing many physician groups to challenge not only the terminology but also the concept itself (Landro, 2008). In some states, legislation has directly challenged nurse ability to be called "Doctor" despite having doctoral credentials, simply because they are not "physicians." A report of a developing collaborative practice in the emergency department (ED) stated, "By performing the dual role of physician and nurse, the NP eliminates the fragmentation of care often seen in the ED," where patients see many different physicians, nurses, and staff members, and there is no consistent provider (Covington, Erwin, & Sellers, 1992, p. 124). Instances in which the APRN is described as assuming the "dual role of physician and nurse" can lead to a misconception of the nurse role. No nurse can assume the role of a physician, nor can a physician assume the role of a nurse. What is possible is that certain responsibilities, functions, and skills are learned and assumed by both providers. When the nurse assumes some of the responsibilities, functions, and skills traditionally assumed by the physician, if they fall within the scope of nursing practice, they are nursing. If they fall outside, they are considered medically directed acts, and the nurse in that instance is serving as assistant to the physician. It follows, then, that if a physician assumes some of the responsibilities, functions, and skills traditionally assumed by the nurse, they would be considered nurse-directed acts and the physician is serving as assistant to the nurse.

Inadequate and Inappropriate Communication Patterns

When physicians and nurses do not share information or concerns, when communication is a one-way street, or there is an inadequate system of written and verbal communication, quality of patient care suffers. Poor communication patterns also affect working relationships and seriously hinder any attempts at collaboration, often resulting in separate professional decision making that can create confusion and safety issues (Clarin, 2007; Zwarenstein & Bryant, 2000). Inappropriate communication patterns may reflect a pattern of "physician abuse." In a survey of nurse–physician relationships (Rosenstein, 2002), the level of respect for nurse input and collaboration was rated significantly higher by physicians than by nurses. However, physicians rated the findings on how important the physician's disruptive behavior was in contributing to nurse dissatisfaction and low morale much lower than nurses did. These findings reflect a dissonance in perception that is often a result of poor communication and lack of trust, creating a defensive, noncollaborative practice environment in which the number of errors rises and patient safety and positive patient outcomes are threatened. Magnet hospitals, emphasizing collaboration between physicians and nurses, have been documented as having better patient outcomes and fewer problems relating to shortages, turnovers, or abuse (Fischman, 2002).

Another aspect to consider is the line of reporting accountability. An NP-staffed "fast track" in the emergency department (ED) of Vanderbilt University Medical Center was designed using written protocols created collaboratively by the NPs and the medical director of the ED. Although the NPs reported to the ED nursing director and the physicians to the ED medical director, the collaborating practice was well established within a few months, with a growing sense of confidence and trust between these distinct professional providers. However, the report made no mention of the effect of a parallel reporting system (Covington, Erwin, & Sellers, 1992). If reporting is different for each practitioner, does that negatively affect the practice?

Professional Dissonance

When diversity is not recognized and acknowledged, the result is professional dissonance with a serious negative impact on the capacity for teamwork. Confusion of language, differing communication patterns and ways of interacting, and difficulty respecting each other's skills and roles are inevitable. In a study of attitudes regarding teamwork by critical care nurses and physicians, a seven-item "teamwork climate scale" was developed. It found that nurses and physicians had distinctly different attitudes toward teamwork. The source of the differences was found to be status/authority, responsibilities, gender, training, and professional culture (Thomas, Sexton, & Helmreich, 2003). In a study of nurses and physicians in a medical intensive care unit (ICU), Baggs and Schmitt (1997) found that collaboration would occur only if the time and place were appropriate, the physician believed the nurse had the knowledge needed, and trust, respect, and sincere interest in teamwork were present. For example, the physicians believed the general medical unit nurses did not have the same level of knowledge about medical illness as the medical ICU nurses. This perceived knowledge level was a precondition to the physician's willingness to collaborate more effectively with the nurses in the ICU.

A study by Jones (1994) explored the nature of nurse–physician collaboration, examining the differences and similarities in their perceptions related to the four indicators of nurse–physician collaboration identified in the ANA social policy statement of 1980: mutual power control, mutual safeguarding of provider concerns, responsibility for practice, and practice goals. The findings offer an interesting portrait of the collaborative perspective of the partners. Although nurses and physicians were in agreement on power control, most affirmed that the physician initiated more communications than the nurse, indicating a lack of mutual power control. In another study examining provider concerns, nurses and physicians were rated on the degree to which they achieved both assertiveness and cooperativeness, with high levels of both dimensions indicating collaboration. Nearly half of the responses reflected competition, compromise, or accommodation as the preferred method of safeguarding concerns. They did not agree on where responsibility for practice should rest—nurse, physician, or both—and they agreed on only 4 of 24 practice goals (e.g., maintain elimination patterns, promote cardiovascular healing). The conclusion reached was that nurses and physicians who cannot agree on provider responsibility regarding areas of practice and patient goals reflect a lower level of collaboration and will not be able to deliver the same high level of coordinated patient care as those nurse–physician teams who agree on the areas of responsibility (Norsen et al., 1995).

The Bottom Line

Barriers to collaboration hinder positive change and growth in our health-care system but do not need to be perpetuated. Organizational climate and culture are a living, growing aspects of institutional work life that bind the organization together. Professions and professionals are not static. They can and must work to eliminate barriers to collaboration and create a new culture of team practice in health care.

STRATEGIES FOR SUCCESS

Collaboration is a developmental process that emerges slowly through a series of sensitive and delicate interactions. Members of a newly forged partnership join forces in the belief that the common need they recognize can best be met through their combined efforts. Levels of collaboration achieved depend on context, ability, and the desire of the prospective partners to skillfully develop the practice. Based on the conceptual framework of collaboration described in this chapter, some key strategies are offered for developing a successful collaborative team.

Create a Collegial Team

Teamwork is a critical need for today and the reality of tomorrow's practice. Peters and Waterman (1982), focusing on people as the means to achieve productivity, noted that coworkers should be treated as partners. The reality of this shift of power from an authoritarian command structure to one of collegial teamwork can result in innovation, rapid response, and greater access by the customer. However, it requires a considerable mind shift by participants. The redesign of a health-care delivery model that supports a collegial, interdisciplinary team approach requires a radical way of thinking to acknowledge that this new model is not something "out there," but belongs to each of the participants as they confront their learned beliefs and perspectives. In addition, the participants must realize that they must undergo a significant cultural shift in accepting that they must become a community of learners, a "learning organization" that never "arrives" but continues to translate a shared vision into an ever-evolving practice (O'Brien, Martin, Heyworth, & Meyer, 2009; Rice et al., 2010; Senge, 1994). The key feature of this type of learning organization is a realization that the role of the "grand strategist" at the top is no longer possible because of the complexity and dynamic status of work. Instead, each individual participant's commitment and capacity to learn is tapped. Unlike a linear approach, the learning organization forges ahead based on shared understandings of interrelationships and patterns of change creating a common bond of commitment to the practice. The following five qualities are needed for participants in the learning organization:

1. *Personal mastery.* The practitioner is true to a personal vision while staying committed to the truth of the current reality.
2. *Use of mental models.* Learning is accelerated as we mentally consider alternative scenarios for care delivery. Participants do not become so attached to one scenario because it could freeze them into rigid adherence to outdated approaches to care.
3. *Shared vision.* Shared vision is described by Senge (1994) as the "first step in allowing people who mistrusted each other to begin to work together as it creates a common identity and sense of purpose" (p. 208).
4. *Team learning.* Nurses, physicians, and others on the team learn to think together about complex issues, acknowledging that the whole is truly greater than any of the individuals. They develop what is termed *operational trust* and master the practice of both dialogue and discussion. The apex of "team" is at the transdisciplinary level.
5. *Systems thinking.* Foundational in teamwork, systems thinking forces a focus on the whole pattern of the collaborative practice, rather than any isolated role. The structure or key interrelationships of the practice pattern influence behavior and decision making and are examined collectively.

Accept Growth and Development as a Joint Responsibility

For the concept of collaborative practice to grow and flourish, interdisciplinary education must be supported, affirming the values and roles of both physician and nurse. Educational institutions must reaffirm the value of education for interdisciplinary practice and research studies of the effect of collaboration on clinical outcomes. In practice, bidirectional referrals must be promoted and must include the expanded APRN scope of practice and "skill set" found in the APRN role description. Professionals and the public must be educated regarding the roles by both physician and nurse partners. Strategies recommended for physicians to address physician abuse and improve collaboration include physician education, zero tolerance policies, role playing, and changing the culture of the environment from defensive and hierarchical to supportive and collegial. Nurse responsibility for the problem—in tolerating the behavior, perpetuating the inequalities in the nurse–physician relationship, and sometimes countering with abusiveness—should be addressed with education, role playing, assumption of accountability, and an assertive capability to share the nursing perspective (Buerhaus, 2010; Fischman, 2002; Glasgow, Dunphy, & Mainous, 2010).

Use Protocols and Guidelines Wisely

In clinical practice, *protocol* is often used synonymously with *clinical guidelines* and is representative of a statement of agreement between an APRN and his or her collaborating physician. When the providers agree on a standard of care acceptable to both, the guidelines or protocols stand as their codification of acceptable criteria for diagnosing and managing an illness or condition. Texts such as *Patient Care Guidelines for Nurse Practitioners* (Hoole, Pickard, Ouimette, Lohr, & Powell, 1999) and *Gerontological Protocols for Nurse Practitioners* (Brown, Bedford, & White, 1999) offer excellent resources for practitioners, as well as sometimes serving as the basis for legal documentation to allow for treatment and prescriptive privileges through incorporation into the collaborative agreement as the agreed-to standard of care.

Clinical practice guideline development needs three aspects to accomplish its goal. Identification of key decisions and their consequences must first be outlined. In the case of the APRN, there are decisions to be made about when to call the physician with questions and when referral to an outside specialist is in order. The process of reviewing charts and prescriptions is another aspect. Finally, reimbursement from insurance providers must be defined because of strict insurance policies and legislative mandates. Although state and federal statutes may allow for certain billing practices, the viability of the practice may be hampered when nurse professionals are limited to lesser reimbursement amounts or are refused reimbursement. Legislative language in many states must continue to be reworked to clarify the meaning of the terminology, role and scope allowed, and the effect on practice viability of protocols and clinical guidelines. Progress is ongoing regarding legislative and statutory language changes needed for clarification and full scope of practice. *The Pearson Report of 2011* named 31 states reporting an expanded scope of practice for APRNs through legislative or regulatory changes in 2009, compared to 22 in 2008 and 19 in 2007. However, many states still need to remove barriers to autonomous scope of practice for APRNs. The annual legislative reports of Phillips (2011) and Pearson (2011) provide a benchmark and an incentive for regulatory reform and language clarity (Pearson, 2011; Phillips, 2011).

Watch Your Language

Language is one of the most significant facets of relationships. In an editorial from *American Family Physician* (Phillips et al., 2001), a physician professor took aim at the use of the term *health-care provider,* noting that "calling me a 'provider' lumps my physician colleagues and me with individuals who are frankly less qualified and yet aspire to do the same work we do . . . the use of terms . . . although 'politically correct' diminish us as professionals" (p. 1,342). That same year an article in the *Annual Review of Medicine* (Cooper, 2001) was titled "Health Care Workforce for the Twenty-First Century: The Impact of Nonphysician Clinicians." No APRN I have ever known has positively embraced the concept of his or her practice as being that of a "nonphysician clinician." In a forecast study of Missouri nursing (Kuehn & Porter, 1993), the first round of the Delphi brought together both nurse and nonnurse participants. One physician commented that it was the first time he had ever been called a *nonnurse* and found it rather demeaning. When he was reminded of the nurse correlative, being termed a *nonphysician,* a shared understanding of the awkwardness of either term in supporting a sense of collegiality emerged. In stark contrast to Starfield's (1992) language of dependency flowing from "delegated medical functions," nursing language stresses the need to avoid definition by function or tasks when describing role. Orem (1995) stresses that a task orientation for nursing disallows the focus on the person. To define oneself as a nurse, the following questions must be answered:

What do I do (scope of practice)?
How do I do it (methods of practice, tasks)?
Whom do I care for?
Why do they need or want my care?

The ANA social policy statement of 2010 reaffirmed collaboration as a standard of practice. Although advanced practice nursing texts have consistently addressed the concept of collaborative practice, undergraduate nursing texts on professional practice have not historically addressed collaboration. Often the word is not even found in the index, and if it is, it has nearly always referred to collaboration between nursing practice and education or between types of nurses within the same setting. However, this too is changing. A chapter in the 2002 text *Professional Nursing Practice,* "The Nurse as Colleague and Collaborator," noted, "changing models of health care have created a need for modification of traditional roles. Nurses and physicians have been especially affected by these changes and work more collaboratively" (Blais et al., 2002, p. 199).

In a spring 2001 report, *The Health Care Workforce in Ten States: Education, Practice and Policy* (American Federation of Teachers [AFT] Healthcare, 2001), 10 pilot states were studied regarding the status of their health-care workforce. Aspects compared were data collection status and process, practice issues, influences, and policies. In describing licensure and regulation of practice, the extent of physician supervision varied considerably among states and among types of providers. In one state, APRN practice called for both "independent judgment" and "collaborative interaction with other health-care professionals." However, neither collaborative interaction nor other health-care professionals was defined in their practice act (AFT Healthcare, 2001, p. 50). Although the effect of the enforced collaboration and supervision on APRN practice (noted in 9 of 10 states studied) was not addressed, researchers (AFT Healthcare, 2001, p. 2) affirmed that

> *the greatest opportunities for influencing the various environments affecting the health workforce lie within state governments. States are the key actors in shaping these environments as they finance and govern health profession education; license and regulate health profession practice and health insurance; purchase service; pay designated providers under Medicaid programs; and often assume responsibility for design and/or subsidy of programs providing incentives for health professionals to choose specialties and practice location.*

The 2011 legislative updates report a number of state boards of nursing working to amend regulations, and many state nurses organizations are reporting new legislative changes to address regulatory or statutory issues. For example, the North Carolina APRN Advisory Committee, appointed by the board of nursing, met for the first time in August 2010 with the charge to assist and support the board in practice and regulation issues relating to APRN practice (APRN Advisory Committee, 2010). Over 200 Missouri nurses met in June 2011 to attend the Missouri Teamwork Summit, sponsored by the Missouri Nurses Association, Missouri Health Advocacy Alliance, and Missouri League of Nursing. The summit was in response to the IOM report (2011) and focused on plans for the future of nursing in their state, with an emphasis on advanced practice (Missouri Nurses Association, 2011).

Socialize Students to Communication Skills Needed for Collaborative Interactions

When education includes the process of establishing an interdisciplinary team, this practice helps create a system for promoting collaborative practice and facilitates the use of essential communication skills. Group dynamics, role theory, organization theory, change theory, negotiation strategies, team interactions, networking, and focus on the need for organizational leadership for supporting interdisciplinary programs are key factors in preparing students for a collaborative world.

One point highly stressed is the insistence that interdisciplinary teams should be already delivering care and have a solidly positive practice in place before integrating students into the teams (Hanson & Spross, 1996; Hughes, 2011; Norsen et al., 1995). Alberto and Herth (2009) explored in depth the history, benefits, and challenges of interprofessional collaboration in education and practice, offering an excellent review of their experiences with collaboration in health-care education. An interdisciplinary professional education initiative has medical, APRN, pharmacy, and social work students learning together at Vanderbilt beginning March 2010 (Buerhaus, 2010). A study to determine the level of physician–nurse collaboration in pediatrics using simulation training reported positive value in assisting pediatric residents and staff nurses to improve collaborative skills (Messmer, 2008). A transdisciplinary medical, nursing, and health professional simulation center has been proposed for students to learn teamwork within simulated clinical settings (Glasgow, Dunphy, & Mainous, 2010).

COLLABORATIVE MODELS

Primary Nursing Model

A national project conducted by the National Joint Practice Commission (NJPC, 1981) required hospitals to demonstrate 100% registered nurse staffing within a primary nursing model of practice, individual clinical decision making by the nurse, a joint practice committee with equal representation of providers, an integrated patient record, and joint evaluation of patient care. The structural elements of integrated records, joint practice committees, and joint care review reflect the common goals, mutual concerns, and shared control identified as critical indicators of a high-level collaborative practice (see Table 9-1). Primary nursing, "the performance of clinical nursing functions by registered nurses with minimal or no delegation of nursing tasks to others" (NJPC, 1981, p. 11), is considered essential for enabling the nurse to better enter into a collegial relationship with the physician. The emphasis on the primary nurse role, coupled with the element of increased nurse responsibility for decision making, relates accountability directly with collegiality and individual clinical decision making by nurses, and is considered to be a prerequisite for shared decision making—you cannot share what you do not have (Devereux, 1981; Sullivan, 1998). The results from the four participating hospitals were positive in relation to improved doctor–nurse communications, increased mutual respect and trust between physicians and nurses, increased job satisfaction for physicians and nurses, and highly satisfied patients.

Differentiated Practice Model

In recent years, the cost-effectiveness of the primary nurse model has been challenged, with the reality of achieving it amidst a nursing shortage. However, newly developing models of differentiated practice have converted the "primary nurse" concept into that of a patient care coordinator (PCC) who assumes 24-hour accountability for specific patients. The PCC, however, does not deliver all the care personally. Instead, a team of other nurses and ancillary help assume major responsibility for care delivery, each with specific roles and levels of accountability. Each nurse is paired with certain physicians and his or her patients, and trust and collaboration are more readily developed as nurse and physician work together. This collaborative system model of patient care delivery has reported higher levels of coordination, cost-effectiveness, and patient and provider satisfaction than previously seen in less collaborative models (Devaney, Kuehn, & Jones, 2002; Koerner & Karpiuk, 1994).

Collaborative Practice Model in a Clinic

A collaborative practice model established in the early part of 2000 in an inner-city clinic in Beirut, Lebanon, reported a positive impact on quality of care of patients with diabetes mellitus type 2 that was nothing less than amazing (Arevian, 2005). The researchers first identified four key elements essential for the model—"collaborative defining of the problems; joint goal setting and planning; providing a continuum of self-management and support services; and maintaining active and sustained follow-up" (p. 446). In developing the model, they determined that thorough preparation of the professional team members would be an essential factor for success. In addition, they developed provider support systems, including standardized guidelines for care management; provided for patient education in illness management skills; and provided consistent access to a single team member. The development process was proven to be very effective because teams reported a high level of enthusiasm, cooperation, willingness to share expertise, and acknowledgment of skills of other colleagues. As one physician said, "We were treating each other like colleagues, with mutually respectful relationships," and another noted that he gained insights into "how much and how well the other team members contributed to patient care" (p. 449). Outcomes reported included improved documentation, increased patient recruitment, and improved glycemic control, as well as decreased cost of care. The most amazing aspect of the clinic was the positive response of team members to each other's skills and expertise in a Middle Eastern culture in which nurses are still considered as "handmaidens" to physicians. In addition, the positive patient response to active participation in their care was surprising in a Lebanese culture that encourages "passive submission" to the physician authority figure (Arevian, 2005, p. 450). The development process of this collaborative practice model can serve as an excellent template for clinics and provides additional proof of the value of interprofessional collaboration.

Collaboration in Long-Term Care

For over 30 years, collaborative practice models have been developing in long-term care (LTC). The positive impact of nurse practitioner–physician partnerships in LTC has been reported in studies of the Nursing Home Demonstration Project and the Teaching Nursing Home Project, among others. In the 1980s, two nurse practitioners developed the LTC model of care teams that focused on coordinated care of frail and elderly nursing home residents (Kappas-Larson, 2008). They founded the Evercare Company, which now is nationwide, and the model is used in both nursing homes and the community, where nurse–physician teams care for seniors who are still living independently at home. Seven specific practice roles of Evercare NPs include collaborator, clinician, care manager/coordinator, coach/educator, counselor, communicator, and cheerleader.

The NPs serve as the center of the interprofessional care team in which both physician and nurse are valued partners, and it is required by Evercare that each NP establish a positive relationship with his or her collaborating physician. As physicians become more aware of and comfortable with the NP's skill and expertise, they grow more supportive of the role. Active participation by physicians in LTC patient care is reported higher in Evercare programs; perhaps their increasing comfort in LTC care participation is due to their confidence in their NP partner. Physicians have said that "one of the most important components of their experience with Evercare is the personalized and coordinated care patients receive, thanks in part to the quality of Evercare's NPs and care managers" (Kappas-Larson, 2008, p. 135).

Shared Governance

Shared governance is an organizational model in which management and staff acknowledge their interdependence and power is balanced equally on issues relating to nursing practice (Porter-O'Grady, 1992). A recent model of shared governance on an oncology unit is focused on collaboration and mutually agreed on goals between the clinical nurse specialist and the nurse manager. It is described as an approach focusing on professional development, shared decision making, autonomy, use of evidence-based practice, and creating a "culture of excellence for nursing staff through role modeling, smart allocation of resources and the development of standards of excellence " (Gaguski & Bagyn, 2009, p. 385).

Additional Models

Examples of *collaborative models in long-term care* described by the AMDA (formerly the American Medical Directors Association) Ad Hoc Work Group (2011) include different employment scenarios, such as the APRN employed by the physician, self-employed, or employed by the nursing home; a specialty APRN collaborating with a specialty physician; and the care manager APRN model.

Innovative Care Models (www.innovativecaremodels.com), a program initiated in 2008, identified 24 successful collaborative care models for acute care and comprehensive aftercare developed as part of a research project funded by the Robert Wood Johnson Foundation. One example is "Collaborative Patient Care Management," a multidisciplinary case management model in which certified RN patient care coordinators and physicians co-chair practice groups targeting high-risk, high-cost patient populations.

CREATE THE FUTURE

The call for collaboration continues to accelerate, driven by consumer and insurer demands for high-quality care at low cost; the existence of fragmented, disorganized, impersonal, and inaccessible care; numerous reports and commissions recommending collaboration; and the demands of some accrediting agencies for collaboration (Bodenheimer, 2008; IOM, 2011; Zwarenstein et al., 1998). The Institute of Medicine Committee, in its call for the design of a new health-care system for the 21st century that better meets patient needs, recommended that health-care processes be redesigned in accordance with 10 new "rules" (IOM, 2001). The rules speak to a system of care delivery focused on continuous healing relationships, shared knowledge and decision making with patients, and cooperation among professional providers as reflected by active collaboration and communication, emphasizing cooperation in patient care as more important than professional prerogatives and roles. This emphasis on teamwork is repeatedly stressed in the IOM report, *The Future of Nursing* (2011). Collaboration is considered intrinsic to nursing, the norm for professional practice, and "a health care imperative" (Sullivan, 1998, p. 62). With health care increasingly provided in complex systems, the interactions of various providers are not only inevitable but also essential for high-quality holistic care. However, agreement on basic definitions of medical and nursing practice is the *sine qua non* of collaboration between the sets of providers.

During the tumultuous years of the mid-1990s, amidst national debates regarding comprehensive federal health-care reform, the leaders of the American Medical Association (AMA) and the ANA drafted the following joint definition of collaboration (ANA, 1998, p. 2):

> *Collaboration is the process whereby physicians and nurses plan and practice together as colleagues, working interdependently within the boundaries of their scopes of practice with shared values and mutual acknowledgment and respect for each other's contribution to care for individuals, their families and their communities.*

Although the ANA board of directors adopted this definition in 1994, it has yet to be adopted by the AMA. In considering strategies for successful collaboration, perhaps revisiting this mutually developed definition with medical and nursing organizations and practice boards on a state-by-state basis will provide the groundswell for a truly meaningful sense of shared practice relationships. The ongoing work of adopting the APRN Consensus Model state by state is a positive step in that direction (O'Grady & Ford, 2009).

REFERENCES

ACNM/ACOG. (2011). *Joint statement of practice relations between obstetrician gynecologists and certified nurse-midwives/ certified midwives.* American College of Nurse-Midwives. Retrieved August 22, 2011, from http://www.midwife.org.

Alberto, J., & Herth, K. (2009). Interprofessional collaboration within faculty roles: Teaching, service and research. *Online Journal of Issues in Nursing, 14*(2). Retrieved August 31, 2011, from http://www.nursingworld.org. DOI: 10.3912/ OHN.Vol14No2ppt02.

American Association of Critical-Care Nurses. (2007). *Acute and critical care clinical nurse specialists: Synergy for best practice.* Philadelphia: WB Saunders.

American Association of Nurse Anesthetists. (2006). *Scope and standards for nurse anesthesia practice.* Park Ridge, IL: Author. Retrieved August 30, 2011, from www.aana.com.

American College of Nurse-Midwives. (1997). *Collaborative management in midwifery: Practice for medical, gynecological and obstetrical conditions.* (Position Statement.) Washington, DC: Author.

American College of Nurse-Midwives (2011). *A brief history of nurse midwives in the U.S.* Retrieved August 30, 2011, from www.mymidwife.org.

American Federation of Teachers Healthcare. (2001). *The health care workforce in ten states: Education, practice and policy. A report of the state of the healthcare workforce 2001.* Washington, DC: American Federation of Teachers/American Federation of Labor—Congress of Industrial Organizations.

American Medical Directors Association (AMDA) Ad Hoc Work Group on the Role of the Attending Physician and Advanced Practice Nurse. (2011). Collaborative and supervisory relationships between attending physicians and advanced practice nurses in long-term care facilities. *Geriatric Nursing, 32*(1), 7–17.

American Nurses Association. (1998). Collaboration and independent practice: Ongoing issues for nursing. *Nursing Trends and Issues, 3*(5), 1–12.

American Nurses Association. (2010a). *Nursing's policy statement: The essence of the profession* (3rd. ed.). Silver Springs, MD: Nursebooks.org.

American Nurses Association. (2010b). *Nursing: Scope and standards of practice* (2nd ed.). Silver Springs, MD: Nursebooks.org.

1. APRN Advisory Committee (2010). *Meeting report,* North Carolina Board of Nursing Committee. Retrieved August 15, 2012, from www.ncbon.com/WorkArea/showcontent.aspx?id=2822.

APRN Joint Dialogue Group. (2008). *APRN Consensus Model.* Report. National Council of State Boards of Nursing. Retrieved August 15, 2011, from https://www.ncsbn.org/Consensus_Model_for_APRN_Regulation_July_2008.pdf.

Arevian, M. (2005). The significance of a collaborative practice model in delivering care to chronically ill patients: A case study of managing diabetes mellitus in a primary health care center. *Journal of Interprofessional Care, 19*(5), 444–451.

Baer, E. (1993). Philosophical and historical bases of primary care nursing. In M. Mezey & D. McGivern (Eds.), *Nurses, nurse practitioners: Evolution to advanced practice* (pp. 102–110). New York: Springer.

Baggs, J., & Schmitt, M. (1997). Nurses' and resident physicians' perceptions of the process of collaboration in an MICU. *Research in Nursing and Health, 20*(1), 71–80.

Bailey, J., & Armer, J. (1998). Registered nurse–physician collaborative practice: Success stories. In T. J. Sullivan (Ed.), *Collaboration: A health care imperative* (pp. 225–249). New York: McGraw-Hill.

Becker, M., & Porth, L. (2011). *Primary care physicians: The status in rural Missouri. Missouri Hospital Association.* Retrieved August 15, 2011, from http://www.mhanet.com.

Benner, P. (1984). *From novice to expert.* Menlo Park, CA: Addison-Wesley.

Bigbee, J. L. (1996). History and evolution of advanced nursing practice. In A. B. Hamric, J. A. Spross, & C. M. Hanson (Eds.), *Advanced nursing practice: An integrative approach* (pp. 3–24). Philadelphia: WB Saunders.

Blais, K. K., Hayes, J. S., Kozier, B., & Erb, G. (2002). *Professional nursing practice: Concepts and perspectives.* Upper Saddle River, NJ: Prentice Hall.

Blumenreich, G. (2007). Another article on the surgeon's liability for anesthesia negligence. Legal Briefs. *AANA Journal, 75*(2), 89–93.

Bodenheimer, T. (2008). Coordinating care—A perilous journey through the health care system. Health policy report. *New England Journal of Medicine, 358*(10), 1064–1071.

Brar, K., Boschma, G., & McCuaig, F. (2010). The development of nurse practitioner preparation beyond the master's level: What is the debate about? *International Journal of Nursing Education Scholarship, 7*(1). Retrieved August 22, 2011, from http://www.bepress.com/ijes/vol7/iss1/art9. DOI: 10.2202/1548-932X.1928.

Brown, J., Bedford, N., & White, S. (1999). *Gerontological protocols for nurse practitioners.* Philadelphia: Lippincott Williams & Wilkins.

Buerhaus, P. (2010). Have nurse practitioners reached a tipping point? Interview of a panel of NP thought leaders. *Nursing Economics, 28*(5), 346–349.

Clarin, O. (2007). Strategies to overcome barriers to effective nurse practitioner and physician collaboration. *Journal for Nurse Practitioners, 3*(8), 536–548.

Cooper, R. A. (2001). Health care workforce for the twenty-first century: The impact of nonphysician clinicians. *Annual Review of Medicine, 52,* 51–61.

Covington, C., Erwin, T., & Sellers, F. (1992). Implementation of a nurse practitioner–staffed fast track. *Journal of Emergency Nursing, 18*(2), 124–131.

Devaney, S., Kuehn, A., & Jones, R. (2002). The Fitzgibbon hospital experience. *Missouri Nurse, 14,* 29.

Devereux, P. M. (1981). Essential elements of nurse–physician elements. *Journal of Nursing Administration, 11*(5), 19–23.

Donald, F., Mohide, E. A., DiCenso, A., Brazil, K., Stephenson, M., & Akhtar-Danesh, N. (2009). Nurse practitioner and physician collaboration in long term care homes: Survey results. *Canadian Journal on Aging, 28*(10), 77-87.

Dorroh, M., & Norton, S. F. (1996). The certified nurse-midwife. In A. B. Hamric, J. A. Spross, & C. M. Hanson (Eds.), *Advanced nursing practice: An integrative approach* (pp. 395–419). Philadelphia: WB Saunders.

Faut-Callahan, M., & Kremer, M. (1996). The certified registered nurse anesthetist. In A. B. Hamric, J. A. Spross, & C. M. Hanson (Eds.), *Advanced nursing practice: An integrative approach* (pp. 421–444). Philadelphia: WB Saunders.

Fenton, M., & Brykczynski, I. (1993). Qualitative distinctions and similarities in the practice of clinical nurse specialists and nurse practitioners. *Journal of Professional Nursing, 9*(6), 313–326.

Fischman, J. (2002). Nursing wounds. *U.S. News and World Report, 132*(21), 54–55.

Friedson, E. (1970). *Professional dominance: the social structure of medical care.* New York: Atherton Press, Inc.

Gaguski, M., & Begyn, P. (2009, July). A unique model of shared governance. *Oncology Nursing Forum, 36*(4), 385–388.

Glasgow, M. E., Dunphy, L., & Mainous, R. (2010, November/December). Innovative nursing educational curriculum for the 21st century. *Nursing Education Perspectives, 31*(6), 355–357.

Goodman, S. (2007). Piercing the veil: The marginalization of midwives in the United States. *Social Science and Medicine, 65*(3), 610–621.

Hanna, D. (1996). Primary care nurse practitioner. In A. B, Hamric, J. A. Spross, & C. M. Hanson (Eds.), *Advanced nursing practice: An integrative approach* (pp. 337–355). Philadelphia: WB Saunders.

Hanson, C., & Spross, J. (1996). Collaboration. In A. B. Hamric, J. A. Spross, & C. M. Hanson (Eds.), *Advanced nursing practice: An integrative approach* (pp. 229–248). Philadelphia: WB Saunders.

Hojat, M., Gonnella, J. S., Nasca, T. J., Fields, S. K, Cicchetti, A., et al. (2003). Comparisons of American, Israeli, Italian and Mexican physicians and nurses on the total and factor scores of the Jefferson scale of attitudes toward physician-nurse collaborative relationships. *International Journal of Nursing Studies, 40*(4), 427–435.

Hoole, A., Pickard, C., Ouimette, R., Lohr, J., & Powell, W. (1999). *Patient care guidelines for nurse practitioners* (5th ed.). Philadelphia: Lippincott Williams & Wilkins.

Hughes, J. (2011, May 11). *New health care model emphasizes team work.* Retrieved August 22, 2011, from http://www.clinicaladvisor.com.

Institute of Medicine. (2001). *Crossing the quality chasm: A new health system for the 21st century.* Washington, DC: National Academies Press.

Institute of Medicine. (2004). *Keeping patients safe: Transforming the work environment of nurses.* Washington, DC: National Academies Press.

Institute of Medicine. (2011). *The future of nursing: Leading change, advancing health.* Washington, DC: The National Academies Press.

Jehn, K., Northcraft, G., & Neale, M. (1999). Why differences make a difference: A field study of diversity, conflict and performance in workgroups. *Administrative Science Quarterly, 44*(4), 741–763.

Jones, R. A. P. (1994). Nurse–physician collaboration: A descriptive study. *Holistic Nursing Practice, 8*(3), 38–53.

Jones, T., & Fitzpatrick, J. (2009). CRNA–physician collaboration in anesthesia. *AANA Journal, 77*(6), 431–436.

Kaplow, R. (2007). Synergy model: Guiding the practice of the CNS in acute and critical care. In American Association of Critical-Care Nurses, *Acute and critical care-clinical nurse specialists: Synergy for best practice.* Philadelphia: WB Saunders.

Kappas-Larson, P. (2008). The Evercare story: Reshaping the health care model, revolutionizing long-term care. *Journal for Nurse Practitioners, 4*(2), 132–136.

King, K. B., Parrinello, K. M., & Baggs, J. G. (1996). Collaboration and advanced practice nursing. In L. Hickey, R. Oimette, & S. Venegoni (Eds.), *Advanced practice nursing: Changing roles and clinical applications* (pp. 146–162). Philadelphia: Lippincott Williams & Wilkins.

Kinlein, L. (1977). *Independent nursing practice with clients.* Philadelphia: JB Lippincott.

Koerner, J., & Karpiuk, K. (1994). *Implementing differentiated nursing practice: Transformation by design.* Gaithersburg, MD: Aspen.

Kubota, S. (2011). *Missouri nurses attend summit for improved healthcare.* Posted June 28, 2011. Retrieved August 16, 2011, from http://www.komu.com/news/missouri-nurses-attend.

Kuehn, A. F. (1998). Collaborative health professional education: An interdisciplinary mandate for the third millennium. In T. J. Sullivan (Ed.), *Collaboration: A health care imperative* (pp. 419–465). New York: McGraw-Hill.

Kuehn, A. F., & Porter, R. (1993). Study design. In T. J. Sullivan (Ed.), *Missouri nursing 2000: Creating a positive future. A report of the Missouri Nursing 2000 Study Group* (pp. 42–54). Jefferson City, MO: Missouri Nurses Association.

Landro, L. (2008, April 2). Making room for "Dr. Nurse." In *The Informed Patient.* Retrieved April 8, 2008, from www.online.wsj.com/article.

Lott, J. W., Polak, J. D., Kenyon, T. B., & Kenner, C. A. (1996). Acute care nurse practitioner. In A. B. Hamric, J. A. Spross, & C. M. Hanson (Eds.), *Advanced nursing practice: An integrative approach* (pp. 351–373). Philadelphia: WB Saunders.

Markowitz, G., & Rosner, D. (1979). Doctors in crisis: Medical education and medical reform during the progressive era, 1895–1915. In S. Reverby & D. Rosner (Eds.), *Health care in America* (pp. 185–205). Philadelphia: Temple University.

Maylone, M., Ranieri, L., Griffin, M., McNulty, R., & Fitzpatrick, J. (2011, January). Collaboration and autonomy: Perceptions among nurse practitioners. *Journal of the American Academy of Nurse Practitioners, 23*(1), 51–57.

McGrail, K., Morse, D., Glessner, T., & Gardner, K. (2008). "What is found there": Qualitative analysis of physician-nurse collaboration stories. *Journal of General Internal Medicine, 24*(2), 198–204.

Merriam-Webster's Collegiate Dictionary (10th ed.). (1994). Springfield, MA: Merriam-Webster.

Messmer, P. (2008, July). Enhancing nurse–physician collaboration using pediatric simulation. *Journal of Continuing Education in Nursing, 39*(7), 319–327.

Miller, K. I., & Apker, J. (2002). On the front lines of managed care: Professional changes and communicative dilemmas of hospitals nurses. *Nursing Outlook, 50*(4), 154–159.

Missouri Nurses Association. (2011, June 28). *Missouri Teamwork Summit 2011: Summary of outcomes.* Retrieved August 29, 2011, from http://www.missourinurses.org.

National Joint Practice Commission. (1981). *Guidelines for establishing joint or collaborative practice in hospitals.* Chicago: Neely.

National League for Nursing. (1997). *Commission on a workforce for a restructured health care system.* Part 2. New York: NLN.

Newhouse, R., Stanik-Hutt, J., White, K., Johantgen, M., Bass, E., Zangara, G., et al. (2011). Advanced practice nurse outcomes 1990–2008: A systematic review. *Nursing Economics* (epub ahead of print). Retrieved August 17, 2011, from http://www.nursingeconomics.net/ce/2013/article3001021.pdf.

Newman, D. (1996). Program practice management for the advanced practice nurse. In A. B. Hamric, J. A. Spross, & C. M. Hanson (Eds.), *Advanced nursing practice: An integrative approach* (pp. 545–568). Philadelphia: WB Saunders.

Norsen, L., Opladen, J., & Quinn, J. (1995). Practice model: Collaborative practice. *Critical Care Nursing Clinics of North America, 7*(1), 43–52.

O'Brien, J., Martin, D., Heyworth, J., & Meyer, N. (2009). A phenomenological perspective on advanced practice nurse–physician collaboration within an interdisciplinary healthcare team. *Journal of the American Academy of Nurse Practitioners, 21*, 444–453.

O'Grady, E., & Ford, L. (2009, September). *The 5 NP political issues and the one solution.* Retrieved August 8, 2011, from http://www.webnponline.com.

O'Neil, E. H., & Pew Health Professions Commission. (1998). *Recreating health professional practice for a new century. Fourth report.* San Francisco: Pew Health Professions Commission.

Orem, D. (1995). *Nursing: Concepts of practice.* St. Louis: Mosby.

Paradise, J., Dark, C., & Bitler, N. (2011, March). *Improving access to adult primary care in Medicaid: Exploring the potential role of nurse practitioners and physician assistants.* Issue paper, Kaiser Commission on Medicaid and the Uninsured. Retrieved August 2011, from http://www.kff.org.

Partin, B. (2009). APRN/physician collaboration: A call to action. *Nurse Practitioner, 34*(11), 6.

Pearson, L. (2002). 14th annual legislative update. *Nurse Practitioner, 27*(1), 10–52.

Pearson, L. (2011). A national overview of nurse practitioner legislation and healthcare issues. In *The Pearson Report.* Retrieved August 22, 2011, from www.webNPonline.com.

Pearson, P., & Jones, K. (1994). The primary health care non-team? *British Medical Journal, 309*(6966), 1387–1388.

Peters, T., & Waterman, R. (1982). *In search of excellence.* New York: Warner Books.

Phillips, R. L., Green, L. A., Fryer, G. E., & Dovey, S. M. (2001). Trumping professional roles: Collaboration of nurse practitioners and physicians for a better U.S. health care system. *American Family Physician, 64*(8), 1325.

Phillips, S. J. (2011). 23rd Annual legislative update. *Nurse Practitioner, 36*(1), 30–52.

Plant, R. (1987). *Managing change and making it stick.* London: Fontana.

Porter-O'Grady, T. (1992). *Implementing shared governance.* St. Louis: Mosby.

Reverby, S. (1979). The search for the hospital yardstick. In S. Reverby & D. Rosner (Eds.), *Health care in America.* Philadelphia: Temple University.

Reverby, S. (1987). *Ordered to care: The dilemma of American nursing, 1850–1945.* New York: Cambridge University.

Rice, K., Zwarenstein, M., Conn, L., Kenaszchuk, C., Russell, A., & Reeves, S. (2010). An intervention to improve interprofessional collaboration and communications: A comparative qualitative study. *Journal of Interprofessional Care, 24*(4), 350–361.

Roberts, M. M. (1959). *American nursing.* New York: Macmillan.

Rogers, M. (1972). Nursing: To be or not to be. *Nursing Outlook 20*(1), 42–46.

Rosenstein, A. H. (2002). Nurse–physician relationships: Impact on nurse satisfaction and retention. *American Journal of Nursing, 102*(6), 26–34.

Schaal, A., Skalia, K., Mulrooney, T., Stearns, D., & Smith, E. (2008). Building a collaboration of hematology-oncology advanced practice nurses. Part II: Outcomes. *Oncology Nursing Forum, 35*(6), 875–878.

Senge, P. (1994). *The fifth discipline.* New York: Currency & Doubleday.

Shah, M. A. (2002). *Make way for a new ACNM/ACOG joint statement. The president's pen.* Retrieved July 1, 2002, from www.midwife.org/prof/display.cm/?id=274.

Skinner, J., & Foureur, M. (2010). Consultation, referral and collaboration between midwives and obstetricians: Lessons from New Zealand. *Journal of Midwifery and Women's Health, 55*(1), 28–37.

Sorrel, A. (2009, June 29). *AMA meeting: Physician supervision of nurses sought in all practice agreements.* Retrieved August 15, 2011, from http://amednews.com.

Stanley, J. (2005). *Advanced practice nursing* (2nd ed.). Philadelphia: F.A. Davis.

Starfield, B. (1992a). *Primary care: Concept, evaluation and policy.* New York: Oxford University Press.

Starfield, B. (1992b). The future of primary care in a managed care era. *International Journal of Health Science, 27*(4), 687–696.

Sullivan, T. J. (1998). Concept analysis of collaboration: Part 1. In T. J. Sullivan (Ed.), *Collaboration: A health care imperative* (pp. 3–42). New York: McGraw-Hill.

Sullivan, T. J., Morgan, S., Heimerich, S., & Scott, J. (1998). When collaboration is legislatively mandated. In T. J. Sullivan (Ed.), *Collaboration: A health care imperative* (pp. 325–357). New York: McGraw-Hill.

Taylor, C. (2009). Attitudes toward physician–nurse collaboration in anesthesia. *AANA Journal, 77*(5). Retrieved August 15, 2011, from http://www.aana.com/aanajournal.aspx.

Thomas, E., Sexton, J. B., & Helmreich, R. (2003). Discrepant attitudes about teamwork among critical care nurses and physicians. *Critical Care Medicine, 31*(3), 956–959.

Toffler, A. (1970). *Future shock.* New York: Random House.

Way, D., & Jones, L. (1994). The family physician–nurse practitioner dyad: Indications and guidelines. *Canadian Medical Association Journal, 151*(1), 29–34.

Way, D., Jones, L., Baskerville, B., & Busing, N. (2001). Primary health care services provided by nurse practitioners and family physicians in shared practice. *Canadian Medical Association Journal, 165*(9), 1210–1214.

Webber, P. (2008). The doctor of nursing practice degree and research: Are we making an epistemological mistake? *Journal of Nursing Education, 47*(10), 466–472.

Workman, L. (1986). No free lunches. *Missouri Nurse, 55*(5), 16.

Zwarenstein, M., & Bryant, W. (2000). Interventions to promote collaboration between nurses and doctors. *Cochrane Database of Systemic Reviews (2),* CD000072.

Zwarenstein, M., Bryant, W., Baillie, R., & Sibthorpe, B. (2000). Promoting collaboration between nurses and doctors [Cochrane Review]. *Cochrane Library: Issue 4.* Oxford.

10

Participation of the Advanced Practice Nurse in Health Plans and Quality Initiatives

Rita Munley Gallagher

Historically, advanced practice nurses (APNs) have been significant by their absence from health plan provider panels. In addition, their efforts are not fully recognized in activities within the national quality enterprise. Is this because of their predominantly employee status? Are they reticent to take on the full responsibility of a primary care provider, fearful of accepting accountability, hesitant to mobilize consumer support on their own behalf? On the other hand, is it a more fundamental issue—an issue of respect?

INTRODUCTION

Today's evolving health-care environment has transformed the way many health-care services are provided and compensated. The approach to health-care service delivery has undergone a significant alteration in both its contracting and reimbursement mechanisms. Fee-for-service is no longer the primary source of pricing; prospective payment, global pricing, capitation, and value-based purchasing are also prominent. Along with these changes comes a significant increase in financial risk to the provider. By taking on liability not only for service delivery costs, but also for level of use, providers have been "forced" into assuming roles historically reserved for insurance carriers. In addition, demonstration of practitioner accountability for quality has moved into the forefront of health-care delivery. More than 250,000 APNs (U.S. Department of Health and Human Services, 2010)—and their numbers are growing—are carving out a larger role in delivering safe, effective, patient-centered, timely, efficient, equitable health care. This chapter focuses on the involvement of APNs within health plans and within the national quality enterprise, and offers suggestions for increasing their visibility within both.

ADVANCED PRACTICE NURSES

APNs possess the education and expert clinical knowledge to enable them to practice in multiple settings. The expertise of APNs enables them to complement other practitioners within the health-care arena. "NPs are proven to be excellent healthcare providers. More than 40 years of research has established that NPs provide high-quality, cost-effective and personalized care. The body of evidence regarding the quality of NP practice supports the notion that NP care is at least equivalent to that of physician care. When NP care is compared with that of other providers such as physicians, NP patients are more satisfied with their care and say that, in addition to providing excellent healthcare, their NP excels in giving health advice. They are expert at assessing and diagnosing problems. The treatments they prescribe result in positive outcomes" (American Academy of Nurse Practitioners, 2010). Still they are often underused by health insurance plans.

HEALTH PLANS

Health plans (HPs) are rapidly becoming the overseers and administrators of health-care services for most Americans. HPs are nearly ubiquitous, having assumed the management and control of the overwhelming majority of health-care services provided throughout the entire United States. Nearly 85% of the U.S. population is currently covered under HPs, the majority (52.4%) in commercial plans with approximately 30% covered by Medicare or Medicaid (Managed Care Fact Sheets, 2010).

Almost all HPs have some sort of managed care program to help control health-care costs. Managed care includes programs "intended to reduce unnecessary health care costs through a variety of mechanisms, including: economic incentives for physicians and patients to select less costly forms of care; programs for reviewing the medical necessity of specific services; increased beneficiary cost sharing; controls on inpatient admissions and lengths of stay; the establishment of cost-sharing incentives for outpatient surgery; selective contracting with health care providers; and the intensive management of high-cost health care cases" (National Library of Medicine, 2011). At least in theory, managed care is designed to foster the effective, appropriate, and efficient monitoring of a specific population's health. Managed care calls for providers to assume responsibility and accountability for the health-care needs of a specifically defined population, while at the same time agreeing to accept the financial risk inherent in taking on that responsibility. In managed care, the insurer determines, under written standards, the medical necessity of medical services and directs care to the most appropriate setting so as to provide high-quality care in the most cost-efficient manner. To control benefits, HPs require preauthorization of certain services, careful review of payment of claims, and maintenance of a provider network. Each of these administrative functions contributes to lowering the cost of care by managing benefits closely (Richards, 2010). According to Katherine Baicker, a health economics professor at Harvard University, "From an economics perspective, there's no way around rationing. Some care is being rationed now. Everyone isn't getting everything" (PolitiFact, 2009).

In managed care, the burden of risk is shared. Unlike traditional indemnity plans in which the insurance company bears the financial risk and burden of enrollees requiring more complex and costly care, various incentive plans and capitation place the risk (and burden) on the managed care provider—whether that be a plan, APN, physician, mental health provider, or other practitioner (Himali, 1995). In addition to point-of-service (POS) plans, the most common types of HPs include health maintenance organizations (HMOs) and preferred provider organizations (PPOs), a component of which are exclusive provider organizations. All are grounded in provision of care to a specified cohort of enrollees at an established per member/per month rate. See **Box 10-1.**

The historical goal of managed care is to deliver value to the consumer by providing access to high-quality, cost-effective health care (Stahl, 1995). This mission is not always readily apparent in practice or necessarily shared by all HPs. However, as systems of managed care continue to develop, the goals are expanding to include, among others, a focus on outcomes analysis, development of practice guidelines, the creation of provider panels with a host of practitioners, and the coordination of service provision

BOX 10-1
Types of Managed Care Plans

Health maintenance organizations (HMOs) usually only pay for care within the network. The enrollee chooses a primary care provider who coordinates most of the enrollee's care.

Preferred provider organizations (PPOs) generally pay more if the enrollee receives care within the network, but a PPO still pays a portion if the enrollee goes outside the network.

Point-of-service (POS) plans let the enrollee choose between an HMO and a PPO each time care is needed.

among providers (May, Schraeder, & Britt, 1996). State governments have been moving to increase their regulation of HPs. Many states have passed laws expanding patient rights, guaranteeing access to care, requiring point-of-service options, including whistleblower clauses, and establishing provider due process protections. However, a number of self-insured HPs have successfully challenged state health insurance regulations under the Employee Retirement Income Security Act (ERISA), based on their contention that they are self-insured employee health benefit plans. As a result, these types of plans are exempt from many state regulations, such as any willing provider and nondiscrimination provisions (Chaikind, 2003). With a background in patient education and certification in a specialty at the master's level, the APN is well equipped to provide high-quality care in a cost-effective environment (American Academy of Nurse Practitioners, 2010). Yet APNs remain largely absent from HP panels, thereby limiting enrollee access to their services. This gives rise to suspicions of lack of respect for nursing overall. Managed care has become a way of life for all health-care practitioners and must include APNs.

Competencies Necessary in the Managed Care Environment

Despite naysayers' comments to the contrary (Stires, 2002), managed care is here to stay. However, although the fit between its stated care promotion and disease prevention goals is in line with those of the APN, HPs also place renewed emphasis on the "bottom line" in an often very competitive market. To prosper in such an arena, a number of skills are needed; these include marketing, advertising, and finance, which are generally considered as being beyond the components of the basic nursing curriculum.

Of great relevance to the APN is a process of self-assessment designed to assist in attaining an optimal level of success in the managed care arena (Leider & Bard, 1993). It has been said that to form an optimal system of "managed" care, a new paradigm of professional practice is needed. In this "new" system, the practitioner needs to be capable of integrating the traditional curing focus with an ability to manage the health of individual enrollees and the covered cohort, overall. In addition to appropriate credentials, to be successful in managed care, APNs must possess the following skills:

- Clinical accountability
- Communication skills
- Leadership skills
- Team-building abilities
- Negotiation and conflict resolution skills
- Ability to engage in quality management activities
- Financial acumen

APNs who see themselves as possessing these competencies can improve chances of successfully negotiating a contract with an HP by doing the following:

- Highlighting communication; enhancing documentation; becoming familiar with the "ins and outs" of the contract
- Being ready to follow through with commitments
- Educating HPs on the value—both quality value and efficiency value—of their services
- Improving fiscal and management system capacities
- Being creative, flexible, and willing to work with the HP to meet mutual goals

To operate successfully in the health plan environment, it is crucial that APNs work collaboratively with case managers, identify gaps in service that they are capable of filling, and hone the skills necessary to succeed in contracting with the HP as well as in securing needed benefits on behalf of their enrollees (Lachman, 1996).

HPs are interested in a provider's ability to furnish financial and cost data cross-referenced by client characteristics, including clinical complexity, resource utilization, therapy and pharmaceutical use, length of stay, and outcome criteria. In addition, the APN must be able to detail the processes established to ensure quality improvement and outcomes of activities. Administrative expertise, including quality and financial reporting mechanisms, must be in place. Operating standards focused on efficacy and outcome measurement criteria along with practitioner performance evaluations are also closely scrutinized by the HP (Walker, 1996). At a minimum, it is assumed that all parties preparing to enter into a contract do so voluntarily and knowingly having read, and understand fully, the document. Failing to read the contract critically, as well as failure to have it reviewed by an attorney, can result in significant problems at a later date.

Contracting with Health Plans

A number of challenges are inherent in providing health-care services, which makes the decision to enter into a contractual agreement with a health plan particularly attractive and also potentially difficult. For instance, working to move from the employee role by attempting to force HPs to bill directly for their services is seen by some NPs as counterproductive (Hill, Cohen, & Mason, 1999; Mason et al., 1999). They hold the perspective that, if the HP is unable to continue billing under the physician's name, the HP will experience a decrease in overall payment dollars that may result in further APN exclusion from provider panels. Such challenges may also result in a significant number of APNs continuing in the traditional role of employee, albeit with an HP as employer instead of the traditional hospital or nursing home. Approximately 1% of respondents to Goolsby's 2008 American Academy of Nurse Practitioners (AANP) compensation survey "reported having an independent practice, 2.4% reported being either self-employed or the practice owner, and 0.6% reported that they were a partner in their practice. Approximately 83% of respondents were salaried."

When an APN *does* consider entering into a contract with a health plan, numerous questions arise that require answers (Butler, 1995): Are there regulatory or legislative constraints or safeguards? Do they apply equally to APNs as well as to other practitioners? Will the HP require capital outlays to upgrade practitioner skills? How are client care protocols or treatment guidelines selected for adoption? How will the quality of client care be ensured? What are the processes for patient transfer? These and other relevant issues must be clarified by the APN before contractual integration into any HP system. Clearly, prospective planning is a critical choice in the decision-making process preparatory to contracting with an HP **Box 10-2.**

BOX 10-2
Tips for Contracting with Health Plans

Following are six tips for successful contracting with a health plan (HP):

1. Do your homework! Know as much about the HP plan as you can before you start to negotiate a contract. If you can, talk with other practitioners already on the provider panel.
2. Be a tough but fair negotiator up front and then a team player once you have signed on. If you want to make changes in the contract, do it before signing, not afterward.
3. Evaluate the "attitude" of the plan and cultivate a relationship with its officials. Do not expect plans to improve after you have signed on.
4. Work diligently at clarifying ambiguous language. Much of a contract's improvement comes from refining issues prospectively rather than negotiating substantive changes. Start with the less important issues when negotiating. It is important to know what you want and to know your limits. Before you go plunging into the most important or serious issues, start with the smaller ones (Caesar, 1995).
5. Particular attention should be paid to any specific processes required by the HP in relationship to the transfer of a patient (Buppert, 2008).
6. Finally, seek competent legal advice to avoid contracting pitfalls. The health plan does.

APNs must know whether the HP with which they are negotiating does the following:

- Confronts the realities of providing adequate care to clients
- Supports strong research and development programs
- Promotes health education and disease prevention
- Strongly integrates the perspectives of relevant enrollee groups
- Promotes collaborative care
- Collects and disseminates accurate data
- Advocates for financing reforms that better fund primary care
- Does a thorough job of attending to psychosocial factors
- Promotes palliative care, when appropriate
- Educates the public on the benefits of a healthy lifestyle
- Incentivizes APNs commensurate with the risks they accept

Reimbursement

When Medicare and Medicaid were first enacted in 1965 by amendment of the Social Security Act, few nurses were practicing independently; thus, no provisions were made for direct payment to them. Enactment of the Omnibus Budget Reconciliation Act (OBRA) of 1989 allowed for Medicaid coverage of services by family nurse practitioners (NPs) and pediatric NPs, and extended Medicare Part B coverage to NPs in skilled nursing facilities only (with no provision for coverage of services provided by clinical nurse specialists [CNSs]) and with the payment going to the facility, not directly to the NP. Medicare Part B coverage was extended to services provided by both NPs and CNSs in nonmetropolitan statistical areas (i.e., rural areas) by OBRA '90, establishing NPs and CNSs as Medicare providers. The 1990s saw a number of attempts by the American Nurses Association (ANA) and others to expand coverage for APN services (Abood & Keepnews, 2000), culminating with the signing of the Balanced Budget Act (BBA) of 1997 by President William Jefferson Clinton. The BBA extended reimbursement opportunities for APNs by removing geographical and practice site restrictions. However, significant barriers to full and autonomous practice for APNs remain firmly entrenched in the health-care delivery system. Federal (and many state) laws do not provide adequate support for the removal of barriers to practice for APNs that are created by policy makers, health-care institutions, insurance payers, or HPs. These barriers include denial of claims from third-party payers; failure to include APNs on preferred provider panels; institutional and provider policies that inhibit the objective and accurate assessment of the quality of care and benefits provided by use of APNs; and institutional and provider limitations on APN scope of practice, including contracting with HPs. Although the BBA did allow for direct Medicare reimbursement for services provided by NPs and CNSs regardless of geographical location or practice setting, it was at only 85% (80% for CNSs) of the amount Medicare reimbursed physicians. This inequity resulted in continued billing for APN services as "incident to" the physician (i.e., allowing a service provided by an APN to be billed at 100% of the fee schedule when the physician is on site and available for consultation, if necessary) adding to the "invisibility" of APNs.

Also of relevance is Medicare's payment system, which has historically rewarded quantity rather than quality of care, providing neither incentive nor support to improve health-care quality. Conversely, value-based purchasing (VBP) links payment more directly to the quality of care provided. This strategy will transform the payment system by rewarding providers for delivering high-quality, efficient clinical care. CMS launched its VBP initiative through a number of public reporting programs, demonstration projects, pilot programs, and voluntary efforts, in hospitals, physician offices, nursing homes, home health services, and dialysis facilities.

There is administrative as well as evidentiary support for VBP. Higher spending does not equate with higher quality, and VBP has the potential to improve quality and avoid unnecessary costs. In 2006, Congress passed Public Law 109-171, the Deficit Reduction Act of 2005 (DRA), which under Section 5001(b) authorized CMS to develop a plan for VBP for Medicare hospital services commencing with fiscal year 2009 when CMS added additional conditions to the hospital-acquired conditions provision (DRA Section 5001[c]). As a result, CMS (and a number of other third-party payers) no longer make higher payments for selected conditions that were not present at the time of hospital admission (CMS, 2012).

Although many VBP strategies are focused solely on hospitals, there are aspects directed to practitioners, including those related to resource use that should be particularly relevant to APNs. On December 20, 2006, Public Law (PL) 109-432, the Tax Relief and Health Care Act of 2006 (TRHCA), was signed. Division B, Title I, Section 101 of the law authorized the establishment of a physician quality reporting program by CMS. The Physician Quality Reporting Initiative (PQRI) is a voluntary reporting plan that provides an incentive payment to physicians and other eligible professionals who satisfactorily report data on quality measures for covered professional services. Included among the professionals eligible to participate in PQRI are physicians and physician assistants, NPs, CNSs, certified registered nurse anesthetists (CRNAs), anesthesiologist assistants, certified nurse-midwives (CNMs), therapists, and others. PQRI was first implemented in 2007. In 2011, the program name was changed to Physician Quality Reporting System (PQRS). CMS believes that changes to PQRI authorized under the Patient Protection and Affordable Care Act (PL 111-148) (ACA) lend permanency to the reporting program.

The Hospital Inpatient Value-Based Purchasing program payments will be made to hospitals that meet performance standards with respect to the fiscal year involved. The program will apply to discharges occurring on or after October 1, 2012, in accordance with ACA. Scoring in the hospital Inpatient VBP program will be based on whether a hospital meets or exceeds the performance standards established with respect to the measures. By adopting this program, CMS will reward hospitals based on actual quality performance measures, rather than simply reporting data for those measures (Department of Health and Human Services, 2011, May 6).

ACA links payment to the quality of patient outcomes and calls for transforming the health-care delivery system, in part through value-based purchasing, to foster improvement in the quality and efficiency of health care. "Demonstrations to test payment incentive and service delivery models that utilize physician- and nurse practitioner-directed home-based primary care teams designed to reduce expenditures and improve health outcomes are but one example of programs being instituted. P.L. 111-148 also allows nurse practitioners and clinical nurse specialists to order post-hospital extended care services. Access to care provided by certified nurse midwives is improved through increased reimbursement for their services. Nurse practitioners will have the ability to write orders so that patients can continue to receive hospice services" (Gallagher, 2010).

To participate in PQRS 2011, individual eligible professionals could choose to report information on individual quality measures or group measures: (1) to CMS on their Medicare Part B claims, (2) to a qualified registry, or (3) to CMS via a qualified electronic health record (EHR) product (this option is limited to 20 measures focusing on primary care and preventive services).

Individual eligible professionals who meet the criteria for satisfactory submission of quality measures data for services furnished during a 2011 reporting period will qualify to earn an incentive payment equal to 1.0% of their total estimated Medicare Part B Physician Fee Schedule (PFS) allowed charges for covered services furnished during that same reporting period. Incentive payments have been authorized for PQRS through 2014; however, the incentive is authorized on a declining scale (2011, approximately 1.0%; 2012 to 2014, approximately 0.5%). After 2014, a payment adjustment or penalty (2015, approximately 98.5%; 2016 and beyond, approximately 98%) will be made for professionals who do not successfully report on the quality measures (American College of Radiology, 2011).

Advanced Practice Nurse Participation in Health Plans

Great strides have been made in recent years to establish APNs as independent practitioners providing health-care services. APNs' practices are more widely accepted by health-care consumers than previously. During the past three decades, research has continued to demonstrate that APNs have established and built on a record of delivering high-quality health care. Despite this fact, there are continuing indications that APNs face significant barriers in the health-care marketplace, including the absence of full access to HP provider panels. APNs also experience significant barriers in the credentialing process with HPs, to inclusion on HP provider panels, and to being listed in HP provider directories. The result of these barriers is that consumers' choice of providers is limited. Furthermore, the APN's role is relegated to employee in many cases, as opposed to that of independent contractor, as is the case of most other classes of practitioners. In addition to barriers to inclusion on HP panels, insurers and employers have also added arbitrary restrictions to APNs' practices such as adding physician supervision or needless patient record cosignatory requirements. These requirements are not necessarily in adherence with state practice laws and increase the cost of APNs' services, thereby creating disincentives to employers and consumers to use APNs.

A secondary issue is that there is little, if any, data collection regarding the role of APNs in HPs. Most HMOs do not have formal methods for estimating and reporting nonphysician provider care, thus making it difficult to track APN use, efficiency, quality, and credentialing. With disparities in prescription labeling, it is equally hard to track APN prescribing patterns. These impediments make

APNs the "invisible providers," caring for many patients and generating revenue without recognition of their efforts (O'Grady, 2008).

The practice environment in the states in which they are chartered influences the policies of HPs. The legal definition of APN scope of practice, the type of physician collaboration required (or not required), prescription-writing authority, and state insurance laws may all affect the reimbursement and use of APNs. As health-care delivery systems evolve into increasing numbers of multistate HPs, the procedures and policies affecting APNs are not always clear. In some cases, the multistate corporations may elect to establish their own sets of rules instead of following state law. Multistate policies tend to diminish use of the separate states' APN scopes of practice, sometimes substituting stricter physician collaboration policies, or limiting nurses' prescriptive writing authority to HP formularies. "Managed care plans operating in more than one state must comply with the regulations of each jurisdiction . . . States may also require that out-of-state HMOs register to do business . . . Multi state operations can become expensive if plans are subject to numerous financial examinations and other regulatory requirements . . . Historically, group insurance policies have generally been subject to the laws of the state of issuance . . . This general rule has been eroded by extraterritorial application of state insurance law" (Kongstvedt, 2000, p. 1330). Inconsistent application and interpretation of state insurance law can adversely affect reimbursement and HP plan inclusion of APNs. To lend conformity and simplify regulatory compliance, HPs have generally resorted to application of the most rigorous (and hence, most restrictive) rules promulgated among the states in which they provide services.

Unfortunately, only a small (but growing) number of states require HPs to include NPs in provider panels and list them in directories provided to enrollees (Abood & Keepnews, 2002). APNs must now direct their efforts toward ensuring that additional states enact such legislation and that HPs allow them the recognition they so richly deserve. Whether the APN intends to work as an employee of an HP or to seek inclusion on an HP's provider panel by contracting with one, there is a need to develop a base of consumer support.

The issue is not one of APNs' competence or of the quality of the care they provide. Decades of reports have documented the high-quality of NP practice (American Academy of Nurse Practitioners, 2010). The Office of Technology Assessment (OTA) reported NPs as being especially valuable in improving access to primary care and supplementary care in rural areas, and in health programs for the poor, minorities, and people without health insurance (OTA, 1986). OTA found the quality of NP care to be as good as or better than care provided by physicians and found NPs superior at counseling, communications, and interviewing (OTA, 1986). Having an NP manage uncomplicated patients hospitalized for decompensated heart failure was associated with a significant decrease in total hospital costs, a trend toward decreased length of stay, and no significant change in the 30-day readmission rate (Dahle, Smith, & Wilson, 1998). The Gallup Organization has also noted the public's willingness to accept APNs as everyday health-care providers (Gallup Organization, 1993). Yet, it has been said that nurses—not just APNs, but all nurses—are invisible in health care (Hazzard, 2002). However, that perspective is changing. A 2002 poll commissioned by Johnson and Johnson found only 25% of those polled had ever heard of a nurse practitioner (Poll, 2002, p. 14). Conversely, most respondents (90%) to a later survey knew about NPs, and the majority had seen an NP for their care. Eighty-two percent of NP users were satisfied or very satisfied with the care they had received compared to a 70% satisfaction rate for other providers (Brown, 2007). Nevertheless, the skills of many APNs remain underused.

As ANA and the state nurses associations continue to advocate for the right of APNs to fully practice within their scope without arbitrary barriers, physicians have stepped up efforts to confine the practice of APNs. For over a decade, organized medicine has fostered comprehensive grassroots and media campaigns to promote supervised, collaborative practice between physicians and APNs, and has increased its public opposition to the expanded scope and independent practice of APNs (Japsen, 2006).

Yet another strategy that has been put forth by organized medicine is advocating for the relaxation of antitrust laws as they apply to health-care professionals. Legislation has also been introduced on both the federal and state levels to provide collective bargaining rights for health-care professionals. Only those employees deemed nonsupervisory under the National Labor Relations Act are accorded the rights to collectively bargain; however, these legislative proposals would provide physicians the right to enter into joint negotiations with insurance companies to work out payment arrangements, clinical practice conditions, and more. Such activity is currently forbidden under state and federal antitrust laws and is considered anticompetitive collaboration among competitors. In some instances, the courts have held that such collaboration on prices and market access are illegal boycotts. Changes in law being advocated by physician organizations would not only allow negotiation, but also would weaken the ability of the APN to prove antitrust violations by physician competitors, thereby ignoring their ability to take part equally in the competitive managed care arena, regardless of the quality of the care they provide.

In response to efforts by the American Medical Association (AMA) and other physician groups to limit the ability of licensed health-care professionals to provide care to millions of patients, the Coalition for Patients' Rights (CPR) was formed to ensure that the growing needs of the U.S. health system can be met and that patients have access to high-quality health-care providers of their choice. CPR urges all health-care professionals to work together to counter the AMA's actions. The coalition represents more than 3 million licensed professionals who provide a diverse array of safe, effective, and affordable health-care services. CPR has expressed concern about the negative impact on patients if their ability to seek care from APNs, psychologists, CNMs, chiropractors, and many other licensed, qualified health-care providers is limited. "The Coalition believes that limiting the ability of healthcare professionals to practice and provide appropriate care places an enormous and unnecessary burden on the American healthcare system. There is a tremendous need to combat the growing demands on the American healthcare system—including an aging population, health-care provider shortages, spiraling costs and more than 45 million uninsured Americans. The Coalition believes that it is inappropriate for organizations representing doctors of medicine and osteopathy (MDs and DOs) to advise legislators—as well as consumers, regulators, policy makers or payers—regarding the scope of practice of other licensed health-care professionals whose practices are authorized by law" (CPR, 2006). Among successful state initiatives are those in Colorado, which improve access to care, minimize the barriers to completing the paperwork associated with health status, and increase the number of available providers for Colorado Medicaid recipients. In Oklahoma, a bill placing the regulatory authority of APNs within the purview of the board of medicine was defeated. Not so in Georgia and Alabama, where limits imposed via the regulatory process call for APNs to include a written practice agreement and fee with the application to practice. As a result, only a fraction of eligible APNs have registered. Similar regulatory barriers are being faced by APNs in Pennsylvania. Examples of barriers include limitations on prescriptive authority, such as the ability to prescribe only a 30-day supply of Schedule II drugs, and opposition to removal of the APN-to-physician ratio. "This high degree of variation across the states for APN regulation has spotlighted the need to ensure that regulation serves the public, promotes public safety, and does not present unnecessary barriers to patients' access to care" (O'Grady, 2008, p. 8).

Alignment of all aspects of regulation is the goal of the Consensus Model for APRN/APN Regulation developed by the APRN Consensus Workgroup and the National Council of State Boards of Nursing APRN Advisory Committee (2008). The APN model of the future defines APNs as being NPs, CNSs, CRNAs, or CNMs, all of whom will be educationally prepared to provide care to patients across the health wellness-illness continuum. Population foci will include psychiatric/mental health; gender-specific; adult-gerontology; pediatrics, neonatal; and individual/family across the life span. The model calls for specialty practice, though optional, to build on the APN role and population-focused competencies with a target date for implementation of this regulatory model and all recommendations of 2015.

NATIONAL QUALITY EFFORTS

The public concern for error and patient safety together with the continuing "quest for quality" has created renewed responsibility and accountability for the outcomes of patient care. The National Quality Forum (NQF), a private, nonprofit, voluntary, consensus standard setting organization composed of approximately 400 organizations from federal and state governments and private sector entities, including a number of nursing organizations, the first of which was the ANA, is prominent in the national quality arena.

The mission of the NQF is to improve the quality of American health care by building consensus on national priorities and goals for performance improvement and working in partnership to achieve them, endorsing national consensus standards for measuring and publicly reporting on performance, and promoting the attainment of national goals through education and outreach programs (NQF, 2011). Nursing is active in all aspects of NQF efforts on steering committees and their technical advisory panels; the National Priorities Partnership, the Consensus Standards Advisory Committee (CSAC), and the NQF board of directors. The central activity of NQF is the endorsement of performance measures as "voluntary" consensus standards and the identification of gaps in health-care quality research.

Voluntary consensus standards, although relatively new in the health-care arena, are not new to other industries. Moreover, since passage of the National Technology Transfer and Advancement Act of 1995 (Public Law 104-113) voluntary consensus standards have legal standing. The voluntary consensus process, even in the face of strict requirements as to periods and transparency, is timelier than is the federal rule-making process. One key component of the act is the obligation of the federal government to use voluntary existing consensus standards, thus encouraging the federal government to take part in the NQF process. Federal agency involvement in the NQF serves to encourage both public and private purchasers, accrediting bodies, practitioners and providers, and the pubic to also take part. NQF is governed by a board of directors representing health-care consumers, purchasers, providers, health plans, and experts in health services research. The NQF board also includes representatives from two federal agencies, the CMS and the Agency for Healthcare Research and Quality (AHRQ).

The NQF recognizes the value of nursing to health-care quality. The NQF nursing care performance measures project established consensus on a set of evidence-based measures for evaluating the performance of nursing in acute-care hospitals (NQF, 2009). It also addressed the implementation of those measures within health-care organizations to improve nursing care and patient outcomes, and designated a subset of measures that are appropriate for public reporting (such as on the Web site, Hospital Compare, which was developed by the Hospital Quality Alliance [HQA] of which the ANA is a principal).

HQA developed and launched Hospital Compare to provide information to the public on hospital quality. Since its inception, HQA has worked to increase hospitals' voluntary participation in public reporting and expand the set of quality measures being reported. The information on Hospital Compare helps patients compare how often individual hospitals provide the specific care that most patients should receive for certain conditions, such as giving heart attack patients an aspirin on arrival at a hospital. Although nursing measures are not, as yet, included in Hospital Compare, the sheer number of nurses and their primacy in caregiving are compelling reasons for measuring their contribution to patients' experiences and the outcomes that are attained (NQF, 2007). See **Box 10-3.**

The Joint Commission engaged in a "comprehensive test of the NQF nursing-focused performance measures to determine whether they could be used nationally to identify opportunities to improve the quality of patient care provided by nurses. The project was funded by a grant from the Robert

BOX 10-3

The Value of Measuring Nursing Care

To increase the value of information provided to consumers regarding the quality of nursing care by nursing-sensitive measures, interested parties should focus on the following points:

1. Nurses represent the largest single group of health-care professionals.
   - Of the total licensed registered nurse (RN) population, in 2010 an estimated 2.74 million were employed in nursing (Bureau of Labor Statistics [BLS], 2012).
   - In initially endorsing voluntary consensus standards for nursing-sensitive care, the National Quality Forum (NQF) noted nurses, as the principal frontline caregivers in the U.S. healthcare system, have tremendous influence over a patient's healthcare experience (NQF, 2004).
2. A growing body of evidence demonstrates nursing's impact on the provision of care that is safe, effective, patient centered, timely, efficient, and equitable:
   - The adequacy of nursing staffing and proportion of RNs is inversely related to the death rate of acute medical patients within 30 days of hospital admission (Tourangeau et al., 2005).
   - Increasing RN staffing could reduce costs and improve patient care by reducing unnecessary deaths and reducing days in the hospital (Stone et al., 2007).
   - Patients hospitalized for heart attacks, congestive heart failure, and pneumonia are more likely to receive high-quality care in hospitals with higher RN staffing ratios (Landon et al., 2006).
   - Higher fall rates are associated with fewer nursing hours per patient day and a lower percentage of RNs (Dunton, Gajewski, Taunton, & Moore, 2004).
   - Nurses can accurately differentiate pressure ulcers from other ulcerous wounds in Web-based photographs, reliably stage pressure ulcers, and reliably identify community versus nosocomial pressure ulcers (Hart, Bergquist, Gajewski, & Dunton, 2006).
   - A 10% increase in the number of patients assigned to a nurse leads to a 28% increase in adverse events such as infections, medication errors, and other injuries (Weisman, 2007).
   - Understaffing of RNs in hospital intensive care units increases the risk for serious infections for patients, specifically pneumonia (Hugonnet, Uçkay, & Pittet, 2007).
   - According to The Joint Commission (2005), "quantifying the effect that nurses and nursing interventions have on the quality of care processes, and on patient outcomes, has become increasingly important to support evidence-based staffing plans, understand the impact of nursing shortages and optimize care outcomes."

Continued

BOX 10-3
The Value of Measuring Nursing Care—cont'd

3. Measures have been fully developed, are in use, and have been previously vetted. The endorsement of the nursing-sensitive measures by NQF was an initial (albeit significant) step toward standardized measurement of nursing care, detailing its relationship to the quality (and efficiency) of health care.
   - Scientific acceptability is a component of the NQF endorsement process; hence, NQF-endorsed nursing-sensitive measures are valid and reliable (NQF, 2002).
   - This initial measure set complements and extends existing hospital care measures of relevance to nursing care in the NQF *National Voluntary Consensus Standards for Hospital Care: An Initial Performance Measure Set* (NQF, 2003). For this reason, their implementation can be viewed as a natural, next step.
   - Collectively, the measures "provide consumers a way to assess the quality of nurses' contribution to inpatient hospital care, and they enable providers to identify critical outcomes and processes of care for continuous improvement that are directly influenced by nursing personnel" (NQF, 2004).
4. There has been a public call for information about nursing care quality.
   - Enhancing the initial nursing-sensitive measure set through the inclusion of additional measures will increase the overall value of the set.
   - Consumers will benefit from information regarding the impact of nursing care as they make decisions regarding care.
5. Evidence exists that public reporting stimulates quality improvement and choice.
   - Making performance data public results in improvements in the clinical area reported on (Hibbard, Stockard, & Tusler, 2005).
   - Making performance information public appears to stimulate quality improvement activities in areas where performance is reported to be low. This indicates that there is added value to making this information public (Hibbard, Stockard, & Tusler, 2003).
6. There is agreement among diverse health-care stakeholders that the NQF-endorsed nursing-sensitive measures should be incorporated into national and state hospital performance measurement and reporting activities.
   - Interviews were conducted with nearly three dozen national health-care, hospital, and nursing leaders, principles of nursing performance measurement efforts, and hospital representatives to determine their interest in and use of the NQF's nursing-sensitive measures. Recommendations derived from the data gathered from these interviews and published by NQF (2007) point to several complementary and incremental actions that can be collectively undertaken by health-care stakeholders to advance hospital performance measurement and accelerate our collective understanding of nursing's key role in quality. Among these recommendations is a "call" to health-care leaders to fully integrate the nursing-sensitive measures into national and state hospital performance measurement and reporting initiatives, including, but not limited to Hospital Compare (USDHHS, 2012) (NQF, 2007).

Wood Johnson Foundation. Testing of the integrated set of measures led to refined technical specifications. The resultant measures then underwent NQF investigation and most were re-endorsed. They are now available for use by hospitals nationwide and included in quality initiatives used by the Hospital Quality Alliance, the Centers for Medicare and Medicaid Services (CMS) and/or The Joint Commission" (Hill, 2007). The information available to assist consumer decision making (such as is provided on Hospital Compare) would be greatly enhanced by the inclusion of NQF-endorsed nursing-sensitive measures. See **Box 10-4.**

Advanced Practice Nurse Participation in Quality Initiatives

In addition to the NQF-endorsed nursing-sensitive measures, other clinician-level quality measures are of relevance to APNs, including those developed by the Physician Consortium for Performance

BOX 10-4
National Quality Forum–Endorsed® National Voluntary Consensus Standards for Nursing-Sensitive Care

Patient-centered outcome measures:

1. Death among surgical inpatients with treatable serious complications (failure to rescue): the percentage of major surgical inpatients that experience a hospital-acquired complication and die
2. Pressure ulcer prevalence (hospital acquired): the total number of patients who have hospital-acquired (nosocomial) stage II or greater pressure ulcers on the day of the prevalence measurement episode.
3. Patient fall rate: all documented falls, with or without injury, experienced by patients on eligible unit types in a calendar quarter.
4. Falls with injury: all documented patient falls with an injury level of minor or greater on eligible unit types in a calendar quarter. (Reported as injury falls per 1000 patient days.)
5. Restraint prevalence (vests and limb only): total number of patients who have vest and/or limb restraint (upper or lower body or both) on the day of the prevalence measurement episode.
6. Urinary tract infections: Standardized Infection Ratio (SIR) of healthcare-associated, catheter-associated urinary tract infections (CAUTI) will be calculated among patients in the following patient care locations: Intensive Care Units (ICUs) (excluding patients in neonatal ICUs [NICUs: Level II/III and Level III nurseries]), Specialty Care Areas (SCAs) adult and pediatric: long-term acute care, bone marrow transplant, acute dialysis, hematology/oncology, and solid organ transplant locations, other inpatient locations (excluding Level I and Level II nurseries). The standardized ratio is established by the National Healthcare Safety Network (NHSN, 2012).
7. Central line catheter–associated bloodstream infections (CLABSI): Standardized Infection Ratio (SIR) of healthcare-associated CLABSI will be calculated among patients in the following patient care locations: Intensive Care Units (ICUs), Specialty Care Areas (SCAs) adult and pediatric: long-term acute care, bone marrow transplant, acute dialysis, hematology/oncology, and solid organ transplant locations and other inpatient locations. Data from these locations are reported from acute care general hospitals (including specialty hospitals), freestanding long-term acute care hospitals, rehabilitation hospitals, and behavioral health hospitals. This scope of coverage includes but is not limited to all Inpatient Rehabilitation Facilities (IRFs), both freestanding and located as a separate unit within an acute care general hospital. Only locations where patients reside overnight are included, i.e., inpatient locations. The standardized ratio is established by the National Healthcare Safety Network (NHSN, 2012).
8. Ventilator-associated pneumonia for ICU and HRN patients: percentage of ICU and HRN patients who, over a certain number of days, have ventilator-associated pneumonia.

Continued

BOX 10-4
National Quality Forum–Endorsed® National Voluntary Consensus Standards for Nursing-Sensitive Care—cont'd

Nursing-centered intervention measures—system-centered measures:

9. Skill mix (registered nurse [RN], Licensed Vocational/Practical Nurse [LVN/LPN], Unlicensed Assistive Personnel [UAP], and contract): percentage of productive nursing hours worked by RN, LPN/LVN, UAP, and contract staff (RN, LPN/LVN, and UAP) with direct patient care responsibilities by type of unit.
10. Nursing care hours per patient day (RN, LPN, and UAP): the number of productive hours worked by nursing staff (RN, LPN/LVN, and UAP) with direct patient care responsibilities per patient day for each inpatient unit in a calendar month.
11. Practice Environment Scale–Nursing Work Index (composite and five subscales): Practice Environment Scale–Nursing Work Index (PES-NWI) is a survey measure of the nursing practice environment; completed by staff registered nurses; includes mean scores on index subscales and a composite mean of all subscale scores.
12. Voluntary turnover: total number of full-time and part-time RN, APN, LPN/LVN, and UAP voluntary uncontrolled separations occurring during the calendar month.

Endorsed by the National Quality Forum Board of Directors, based on recommendations of the Consensus Standards Approval Committee as updated or while undergoing endorsement maintenance and/or annual update, 2012.

Improvement (PCPI), convened by the AMA, whose goal is to improve patient health and safety by

- Identifying and developing evidence-based clinical performance measures.
- Promoting the implementation of clinical performance improvement activities.
- Advancing the science of clinical performance measurement and improvement.

Consortium activities are carried out through cross-specialty work groups established to develop performance measures from evidence-based clinical guidelines for select conditions. Membership is open to any organization or individual who is committed to health-care quality improvement or patient safety and who participates in the development, review, dissemination, or implementation of performance measures and measurement resources. More than 250 performance measures are available for implementation (AMA, 2011). See **Box 10-5.**

The Consortium's approach to measure development includes the following steps:

1. Identifying opportunities for improvement
2. Involving representatives from all medical specialties and other relevant health-care disciplines in the process
3. Linking measures to an evidence base
4. Supporting clinical judgment and patient preferences
5. Testing measures
6. Promoting a single set of measures for widespread use and multiple purposes

Practitioners of all relevant disciplines of medicine—as well as other health-care professionals for whom the care topic is within their scope of practice—are involved in each measure work group, APNs included (Kmetik, 2007).

BOX 10-5
Physician Consortium for Performance Improvement: Quality Measures Relevant to APNs

Physician Consortium for Performance Improvement (PCPI) measurement descriptions and specifications are available for the following 43 clinical topics and conditions:

1. Acute otitis externa (AOE)/otitis media with effusion (OME)
2. Anesthesiology and critical care
3. Asthma
4. Atrial fibrillation and atrial flutter
5. Care transitions
6. Chronic kidney disease
7. Chronic obstructive pulmonary disease
8. Chronic stable coronary artery disease
9. Chronic wound care
10. Community-acquired bacterial pneumonia
11. Diabetes—adult
12. Emergency medicine
13. End-stage renal disease—adult
14. End-stage renal disease—pediatric
15. Endoscopy and polyp surveillance
16. Eye care
17. Eye care II
18. Gastroesophageal reflux disease
19. Geriatrics
20. Heart failure
21. Hematology
22. Hepatitis C
23. HIV/AIDS
24. Hypertension
25. Major depressive disorder—child and adolescent
26. Melanoma
27. Nuclear medicine
28. Obstructive sleep apnea
29. Oncology
30. Osteoarthritis
31. Osteoporosis
32. Outpatient parenteral antimicrobial therapy
33. Palliative care
34. Pathology
35. Pediatric acute gastroenteritis
36. Perioperative care
37. Prenatal testing

Continued

BOX 10-5
Physician Consortium for Performance Improvement: Quality Measures Relevant to APNs—cont'd

38. Preventive care and screening
39. Prostate cancer
40. Radiology
41. Rheumatoid arthritis
42. Stroke and stroke rehabilitation
43. Substance use disorders

Nurses are the primary caregivers in all health-care settings. As such, they are critical to the provision of high-quality care. "Gaining a more in-depth understanding of the role that nurses play in quality improvement and the challenges nurses face can provide important insights about how hospitals can optimize resources to improve patient care quality" (Draper, Felland, Liebhaber, & Melichar, 2008). All nurses must have thorough evidence-based knowledge of the impact of the care they provide on the outcomes that patients experience. Measurement must be integrated into professional nursing practice at all levels, including the practice of APNs, and not simply considered to be a separate activity.

RECOGNITION AND CONSUMER SUPPORT

APNs are health-care professionals who do the following (AANP, 2011):

- Provide high-quality health-care services
- Diagnose and treat a wide range of health problems
- Stress both care and cure, using a unique approach
- Focus on health promotion, disease prevention, health education, and counseling
- Assist patients to make wise health and lifestyle choices

Simply put, APNs engage in many of the practices that patients are seeking. Why, then, are HPs not clamoring to engage their services? How can APNs increase HPs' demand for their services? In short, how can APNs market themselves (and their advanced practice roles) to both the HP and its enrollees? APNs focus primarily on health promotion and disease prevention—factors frequently overlooked by traditional primary care providers. They have significant experience in both the acute and ambulatory care arenas. These abilities coupled with APNs' possession of case management skills make them ideal for involvement in HPs not merely as employees but as fully credentialed members of the HP's provider panel. Although continuing emphasis is placed on quality, managed care's focus on reduction of costs has often resulted in a type of "managed competition" in which enrollees' benefits are restricted through limitation of their access to a variety of providers. It is within this trap that APNs frequently find themselves. To flourish in the managed care environment, APNs must market themselves to the HP and to enrollees.

Marketing begins with a survey of the desires, needs, and expectations of the "customer," which in managed care is the enrollee. Armed with that information, APNs should then structure a plan to meet those needs. Because most APNs practice in a specialty area, the marketing plan should focus on the provision of related services, known as a *market segment.* An APN can choose to focus on a population with a single condition (e.g., individuals with insulin-dependent diabetes), a specific enrollee need (e.g., rehabilitation following amputation), or a particular population (e.g., older adults). A primary decision centers on whether to engage in provision of services to a single population, a variety of populations, or to all plan enrollees.

Marketing principles are sometimes referred to as the "four Ps": product, price, promotion, and place (NetMBA, 2008). The first "P," product, encompasses the specialty practice services APNs provide, amplified by health promotion and disease prevention skills. The APN's product is self-evident. Thorough understanding of the second "P," price, is essential to the success of the APN, be it within an HP or in independent practice. Although the marketplace, itself, has a significant impact on demand for an APN's services as well as on how much it is willing to pay, the APN is the final arbiter as to price. It is critical that the APN has full knowledge of the costs of *all* of the components of the services delivered, not just personal compensation. The most difficult "P" for many nurses, not just APNs, to engage in is promotion. Nurses do not usually excel at "tooting their own horns." Self-promotion, or marketing, is unfamiliar to most nurses. Nurses generally operate from a mindset that views all health-care providers as doing their utmost to provide high-quality care. To increase recognition as well as consumer, or enrollee, support, APNs must be willing to call attention to the positive aspects of the safe, effective, patient-centered, timely, efficient, equitable care they provide. Finally, APNs must make an informed decision as to the last "P," place; that is, whether or not to engage in providing care as an employee, as an independent practitioner, or as a contractual partner in an HP.

CONCLUSION

Today's health-care delivery system, with increased merger activity between insurance companies and health-care systems, and the biased policies of providers and HPs, has created an environment in which APNs experience significant barriers to their ability to practice. Strategies are needed to unite the collaborative efforts of ANA, constituent member associations, other national APN organizations, and individual APNs. They need to identify trends related to exclusionary behavior and to develop an effective multipronged approach to address anticompetitive policies and practices, such as that proposed by CPR.

Nurses have looked to antitrust protections for relief from practices that block their full participation in the health-care market. CNMs and CRNAs used federal antitrust laws to limit boycotts and expand their market share. The Federal Trade Commission (FTC) has rendered opinions that provide the foundation for anticompetitive action by registered nurses. The Department of Justice and the FTC have issued joint guidelines for antitrust enforcement in the health-care industry that offer general direction about those practices that are (and that are not) likely to trigger action by these enforcement agencies.

Restrictive policies at the state level must be addressed by a comprehensive state-based strategy to better define and combat state-based anticompetitive behavior. Such strategies should include the state insurance commissions, state boards of nursing, and consumer and regulatory entities to enforce the law and to challenge anticompetitive activities.

It is crucial that nurses in general, and APNs in particular, work to gain recognition for the high-quality, cost-effective care they provide. ANA remains committed to monitoring state and federal activities of organized medicine to counteract their effectiveness. To the extent that organized medical societies focus their efforts on opposing or supporting legislation, even through the use of exaggerated arguments and legislative strategies, the major option available to nursing is to oppose those efforts and to respond to them by ensuring that legislators and the public hear the facts about APN practice.

APNs continue to be notably absent from HP provider panels and from the national quality enterprise. This is likely due, in part, to their predominantly employee status. In moving to contract independently with HPs, APNs can take on full responsibility as managed care providers. In addition, APNs can engage in the collection and reporting of data, using measures related to the quality of care they provide. Those data, in addition to informing nursing practice, can help purchasers and consumers decide where to look for high-quality, effective, efficient care. Using data, APNs can mobilize consumer support for their services, thereby increasing respect for themselves and on behalf of nursing overall. It is up to individual APNs, to professional nursing, to NQF, and to all who have interest in the provision (or receipt) of high-quality health care to advance quality in a collaborative, coordinated way. For after all, health-care quality really is an art—"more like ballet, than hockey" (Crosby, 1979).

REFERENCES

Abood, S., & Keepnews, D. (2000). *Understanding payment for advanced practice nursing services. Volume one: Medicare reimbursement.* Washington, DC: American Nurses Association.

Abood, S., & Keepnews, D. (2002). *Understanding payment for advanced practice nursing services. Volume two: Fraud and abuse.* Washington, DC: American Nurses Association.

American Academy of Nurse Practitioners. (2010). *Quality of nurse practitioner practice.* Retrieved May 4, 2011, from http://aanp.org/NR/rdonlyres/34E7FF57-E071-4014-B554-FF02B82FF2F2/0/QualityofNPPractice4pages.pdf.

American Academy of Nurse Practitioners. (2011). *Why choose a nurse practitioner as your healthcare provider?* Retrieved May 3, 2011, from http://npfinder.com/faq.pdf.

American Medical Association. (2011). *Physician consortium for performance improvement.* Retrieved April 30, 2011, from www.ama-assn.org/ama/pub/physician-resources/clinical-practice-improvement/clinical-quality/physician-consortium-performance-improvement/pcpi-measures.page?.

APRN Consensus Workgroup and the National Council of State Boards of Nursing APRN Advisory Committee. (2008). *Consensus model for APRN regulation: Licensure, accreditation, certification and education.* Washington, DC: Author.

Brown, D. J. (2007). Consumer perspectives on nurse practitioners and independent practice. *Journal of the American Academy of Nurse Practitioners, 19*(10), 523–529.

Buppert, C. (2008). How to fire a patient. *Journal for Nurse Practitioners, 4*(2), 97–99.

Bureau of Labor Statistics. (2012). *Occupational Outlook Handbook.* Retrieved August 15, 2012, from http://www.bls.gov/ooh/healthcare/registered-nurses.htm. Butler, R. N. (1995). Ten geriatric messages for managed care. *Managed Care and Aging, 2*(2), 1.

Caesar, N. B. (1995). How to negotiate before you sign the dotted line. *Physician's Managed Care Report, 3*(12), 142.

Centers for Medicare and Medicaid Services. (2012). *Quality improvement organizations: Overview.* Retrieved August 17, 2012, from www.cms.hhs.gov/QualityImprovementOrgs. Chaikind, H. R. (2003, March 6). *ERISA regulation of health plans: Fact sheet.* Washington, DC: Congressional Research Office, Library of Congress. Retrieved May 3, 2011, from http://www.allhealth.org/BriefingMaterials/ERISARegulationofHealthPlans-114.pdf.

Coalition for Patients' Rights. (2006). *Coalition for Patients' Rights™ fact sheet.* Retrieved May 3, 2011, from http://www.patientsrightscoalition.org/About-Us/Fact-Sheet.aspx.

Crosby, P. B. (1979). *Quality is free* (p. 20). New York: New American Library.

Dahle, K. L., Smith, J. S., & Wilson, J. R. (1998). Impact of a nurse practitioner on the cost of managing inpatients with heart failure. *American Journal of Cardiology, 82*(5), 686.

Department of Health and Human Services, Centers for Medicare & Medicaid Services (2011, May 6). Medicare program: Hospital inpatient value-based purchasing program. *Federal Register, 76*(88), 26490–26547.

Draper, D. A., Felland, L. E., Liebhaber, A., & Melichar, L. (2008). *The role of nurses in hospital quality improvement.* Retrieved May 3, 2011, from www.hschange.org/CONTENT/972/.

Dunton, N., Gajewski, B., Taunton, R. L., & Moore, J. (2004). Nurse staffing and patient falls on acute care hospital units. *Nursing Outlook, 52*(1), 53–59.

Gallagher, R. M. (2010). Quality is NOT an irreconcilable difference!!! *Nursing Management, 41*(8), 18–20.

Gallup Organization. (1993). *ANA-commissioned survey.* Princeton, NJ: Author.

Goolsby, M. J. (2008). *2008 AANP National NP compensation survey.* Retrieved May 4, 2011, from http://www.aanp.org/NR/rdonlyres/1F23310B-16FC-45F2-B935-A02C4C05F6ED/0/2008AANPNationalNPCompensationSurvey.pdf.

Hart, S., Bergquist, S., Gajewski, B., & Dunton, N. (2006). Reliability testing of the National Database of Nursing Quality Indicators' pressure ulcer indicator. *Journal of Nursing Care Quality, 21*(3), 256–265.

Hazzard, J. P. (2002). The invisible people. *Advance for Nurse Practitioners, 10*(7), 80.

Hibbard, J. H., Stockard, J., & Tusler, M. (2003). Does publicizing hospital performance stimulate quality improvement efforts? *Health Affairs, 22*(2), 84–94.

Hibbard, J. H., Stockard, J., & Tusler, M. (2005). Hospital performance reports: Impact on quality, market share, and reputation. *Health Affairs, 24*(4), 1150–1160.

Hill, C. (2007). *The Joint Commission awarded Robert Wood Johnson Foundation grant to test nursing-focused quality of care measures.* Oakbrook Terrace, IL: The Joint Commission.

Hill, D. T., Cohen, S. S., & Mason, D. J. (1999). Managed care for NPs: Focus groups reveal perils and promises of managed care for nurse practitioners. *Nurse Practitioner, 24*(2), 15–16.

Himali, U. (1995). Managed care: Does the promise meet the potential? *American Nurse, 27*(4), 14, 16.

Hugonnet, S., Uçkay, I., & Pittet, D. (2007). Staffing level: A determinant of late-onset ventilator-associated pneumonia. *Critical Care, 11*(4), R80.

Japsen, B. (2006, June 12). Rise of retail clinics giving doctors a chill: AMA to make push for more scrutiny of sites staffed by nurse practitioners. *Chicago Tribune.* Retrieved May 3, 2011, from www.acnpweb.org/files/public/ChicagoTrib_Retail_Clinics_AMA_June_2006.pdf.

Kmetik, K. (2007). PCPI: What you should know about Consortium performance measures. *Journal of Family Practice, 56*(10 suppl A), 8A–12A.

Kongstvedt, P. R. (2000). *The managed health care handbook.* Sudbury, MA: Jones & Bartlett.

Lachman, V. D. (1996). Positioning your business in the marketplace. *Advanced Practice Nursing Quarterly, 2*(1), 27–32.

Landon, B. E., Normand, S. L., Lessler, A., O'Malley, A. J., Schmaltz, S., Loeb, J. M., et al. (2006). Quality of care for the treatment of acute medical conditions in U.S. hospitals. *Archives of Internal Medicine, 166*(22), 2511–2517.

Leider, H. L., & Bard, M. A. (1993). Self-assessment and managed care. In D. B. Nash, *The physician's guide to managed care.* Gaithersburg, MD: Aspen.

Managed Care Fact Sheets. (2010). *Managed care national statistics.* Retrieved May 3, 2011, from www.mcareol.com/factshts/factnati.htm.

Mason, D. J., Alexander, J. M., Huffaker, J., Reilly, P. A., Sigmund, E. C., & Cohen, S. S. (1999). Nurse practitioners' experiences with managed care organizations in New York and Connecticut. *Nursing Outlook, 47*(5), 201–208.

May, C. A., Schraeder, C., & Britt, T. (1996). *Managed care and case management: Roles for professional nursing.* Washington, DC: American Nurses Association.

National Healthcare Safety Network. (2012). *Overview.* Retrieved August 19, 2012, from http://www.cdc.gov/nhsn/PDFs/pscManual/1PSC_OverviewCurrent.pdf.

National Library of Medicine. (2011). *Managed care.* Retrieved May 14, 2011, from http://www.ncbi.nlm.nih.gov/mesh?term=managed%20care.

National Quality Forum. (2002). *A comprehensive framework for hospital care performance evaluation.* Washington, DC: Author.

National Quality Forum. (2003). *National voluntary consensus standards for hospital care: An initial performance measure set.* Washington, DC: Author.

National Quality Forum (2004). *Nursing Sensitive Care.* Retrieved August 10, 2012, from http://www.qualityforum.org/Project_Details.aspx?id=1139National Quality Forum. (2007). *Tracking NQF-endorsed consensus standards for nursing-sensitive care: A 15-month study.* Washington, DC: Author.

National Quality Forum. (2009). *Nursing-sensitive maintenance 2009.* Retrieved May 3, 2011, from http://qualityforum.org/Search.aspx?keyword=nursing-sensitive&PageNo=2. National Quality Forum. (2011). *Mission.* Retrieved May 3, 2011, from http://www.qualityforum.org/About_NQF/Mission_and_Vision.aspx. NetMBA. (2008). *Marketing mix: The 4Ps of marketing.* Retrieved May 3, 2011, from www.netmba.com/marketing/mix/.

Office of Technology Assessment, Congress of the United States. (1986). *Nurse practitioners, physician assistants, and certified nurse-midwives: A policy analysis* (HCS 37). Washington, DC: U.S. Printing Office.

O'Grady, E. T. (2008). Advanced practice registered nurses: The impact on patient safety and quality. In *Patient safety and quality: An evidence-based handbook for nurses* (AHRQ Publication No. 08-0043). Rockville, MD: Agency for Healthcare Research and Quality. Retrieved May 3, 2011, from www.ahrq.gov/qual/nurseshdbk/.

PolitiFact. (2009). *There's rationing in health care now, and there still would be under reform bill.* Retrieved May 14, 2011, from http://www.politifact.com/truth-o-meter/statements/2009/aug/25/howard-dean/rationing-health-care-reform/.

Poll. (2002). 3 of 4 Americans never heard of NPs. *Advance for Nurse Practitioners, 10*(7), 14.

Physician Quality Reporting System (PQRS). Retrieved May 13, 2011, from http://www.acr.org/SecondaryMainMenuCategories/quality_safety/p4p/FeaturedCategories/P4PInitiatives/pqri.aspx.

Richards, F. (2010, October 1). *Managed care benefit administration functions.* Retrieved May 14, 2011, from http://www.ehow.com/list_7264458_managed-care-benefit-administration-functions.html.

Stahl, D. A. (1995). Managed care and subacute care: A partnership of choice. *Nursing Management, 26*(1), 17–19.

Stires, D. (2002, October 14). The coming crash in health care. *Fortune,* 205–212.

Stone, P. W., Mooney-Kane, C., Larson, E. L., Horan, T., Glance, L. G., Zwanziger, J., et al. (2007). Nurse working conditions and patient safety outcomes. *Medical Care, 45*(6), 571–578.

The Joint Commission. (2005). *Implementation guide for the NQF-endorsed nursing-sensitive care performance measures.* Oakbrook Terrace, IL: Author.

Tourangeau, A. E., Doran, D. M., McGillis Hall, L., O'Brien Pallas, L., Pringle, D., Tu, J. V., et al. (2005). Impact of hospital nursing care on 30-day mortality for acute medical patients. *Cancer, 104*(5), 975–984.

U.S. Department of Health and Human Services, Health Resources and Services Administration (HRSA). (2010, September). *The registered nurse population: Findings from the 2008 National Sample Survey of Registered Nurses.* Retrieved May 3, 2011, from http://bhpr.hrsa.gov/healthworkforce/rnsurvey/2008/nssrn2008.pdf.

U.S. Department of Health and Human Services. (2012) *Hospital compare.* Retrieved August 15, 2012, from http://www.hospitalcompare.hhs.gov.

Walker, C. (1996). Opening the door to managed care. *Subacute Care, 3*(2), 33.

Weisman, J. S. (2007). Hospital workload and adverse events. *Medical Care, 45*(5), 448–454.

11

Resource Management

*Eileen Flaherty**

INTRODUCTION

In any setting, the advanced practice nurse (APN) influences and is affected by the environment of an organization. The organization provides the structure in which the APN's clinical practice goals will be pursued.

The underlying assumption for any organization is that its reason for existing is to produce some product or service (output) that is of value. The corollary assumptions are that, because the output is of value, it will generate revenue, and that the revenue generated will both cover the costs of the resources expended (input) and provide some level of profit. Profit is necessary to ensure the continued viability of the organization, for example, to upgrade existing facilities, to replace outdated equipment, to expand services or to add new programs, and, in for-profit organizations, to provide a return for investors or owners and encourage continued investment. If this does not occur, the organization will not survive. To succeed in its mission, the organization must secure its financial viability through appropriate prioritization of outcomes and effective utilization of resources.

Organizational decisions can affect both the content and direction of the APN's practice or in fact determine to what extent APNs are able to practice within the organization. The absence of effective input from clinicians, either directly or through their advocates, can result in inappropriate or ineffective expectations of the clinician. Similarly, clinicians' decisions can generate unintended consequences that undermine the health and strength of the organization. Therefore, the APN needs to understand the business and financial structure and systems of the organization. For example, how does the APN's practice affect revenue generation and expenditure of resources? To what extent do business and fiscal policies enhance or constrain clinical practice?

STRUCTURE

In accomplishing its mission, an organization engages in a series of transactions that it tracks and manages through its financial system. These transactions are categorized according to the chart of accounts, a matrix structure that organizes the transactions. One axis of the matrix, the account codes, aggregates transactions according to type (e.g., patient care revenue, salaries, office supplies, maintenance contracts). The other axis, the cost center or revenue center or responsibility center, aggregates transactions according to function and may be identified by product line (cardiac center, cancer care center), physical location (patient care unit, outpatient clinic), or activity (blood bank, hemodialysis). The detailed designations in the chart of accounts are specific to each organization and, as such, not only aggregate transactions for better information and management but also

*Earlier versions of this chapter were authored by Christina Graf with Eileen Flaherty.

provide a picture of the organization and its internal structure. The aggregated transactions are summarized in a statement of operations called the profit and loss (P&L) or income and expense (I&E) statement that also quantifies the operating margin or the gain or loss (income minus expense) from operations. See **Figure 11-1.**

Most health-care organizations use accrual accounting in preparing financial statements. Accrual accounting specifies that revenues are recognized when services are provided and expenses are reported as resources are used. The matching principle requires that, when revenues are reported, the associated or matching expenses are reported. Thus, revenues reported for activities within a particular cost center are matched to the expenses generated in producing those revenues, and they reflect the activity and

PROFIT AND LOSS STATEMENT
FISCAL YEAR 2012
(In Thousands of Dollars)

	Actual	Budget	Variance	Variance Percent
Patient Services Revenue				
Inpatient	$515,994	$496,843	$19,151	3.9%
Outpatient	$341,769	$332,764	$9,005	2.7%
Total Patient Services Revenue (GPSR)	$857,763	$829,607	$28,156	3.4%
Deductions from Revenue				
Contractual Allowances	$498,732	$479,560	–$19,172	–4.0%
Charity Care	$23,760	$22,230	–$1,531	–6.9%
Net Patient Services Revenue	$335,272	$327,818	$7,454	2.3%
Indirect Research Revenue	$31,555	$30,951	$605	2.0%
Other Operating Revenue	$16,089	$15,126	$964	6.4%
Total Operating Revenue	$382, 916	$373,894	$9,022	2.4%
Expenses				
Salaries & Wages	$152,628	$151,908	–$720	–0.5%
Employee Benefits	$26,517	$26,726	$209	0.8%
Supplies	$58,682	$56,421	–$2,261	–4.0%
Utilities	$9,503	$10,187	$685	6.7%
Other	$81,249	$77,487	–$3,762	–4.9%
Depreciation	$27,300	$27,468	$168	0.6%
Provision for Bad Debt	$8,758	$10,126	$1,368	13.5%
Interest	$4,956	$5,485	$529	9.6%
Total Operating Expense	$369,592	$365,806	–$3,786	–1.0%
Income (Loss) from Operations	$13,324	$8,088	$5,237	n/a
Percent of Total Revenue	3.5%	2.2%		

NOTE: Positive variances are favorable to budget; negative variances are unfavorable to budget.

FIGURE 11-1 Sample profit and loss statement.

resource utilization that occurred in that reporting period, regardless of when actual monies for services are received or bills for resources are paid.

REVENUE

Revenue or income refers to the monies received for services provided and reflects the volume of output of the organization. Revenue is based on the price or charge allocated to each specific service, activity, or item. The organization's charge master is a list of the prices charged, which are intended to reflect the related costs plus some margin of profit. However, charges are usually discounted or bundled under a global fee for most payers, entirely waived for charitable care, or not collected from those who are expected to pay. Therefore, charges are not necessarily an accurate reflection of actual income from the service, activity, or item.

Revenue is generated primarily from the day-to-day activities of the organization and is termed *operating revenue.* In health-care organizations, the majority of the operating revenue is related to patient or client services rendered and may come from a variety of payers: the federal government (Medicare, military, and veterans benefit programs), state governments (Medicaid and other state programs), other third-party payers (Blue Cross/Blue Shield, health maintenance organizations, indemnity insurance plans), or the recipient of the service (self-pay).

Medicare revenues are determined not by charges or specific services but by a prospective payment system that allocates a fixed payment based on an episode of care. The payment is determined for inpatient episodes of care by the discharge diagnosis (diagnosis-related group [DRG]) and is adjusted for variations in regional cost of living, urban versus rural setting, and organizational involvement in medical education. Except for some small amount of adjustment for cost or length of stay outliers, the payment to an organization for each DRG is constant regardless of costs incurred. This prospective payment system is not applicable to psychiatric and rehabilitation units or hospitals, children's and cancer hospitals, or long-term care facilities, which are reimbursed on a reasonable cost basis, with some limits, for Medicare-eligible patients. For outpatients, Medicare has developed a similar prospective payment system using ambulatory payment classification groups (APCs), which aggregate services that are similar clinically and with respect to resource requirements. Medicare reimburses providers for services based on prior fixed rates for the APCs.

Medicaid and other state-sponsored payment programs reflect not only the intent of the program but also the economic and political environment of the state and thus vary widely from state to state. The state determines what will be covered and the level of reimbursement, and may limit payments through global or flat-rate fees for episodes of care, exclusion of certain services from coverage, discounting of specific charges, or targeted spending caps.

Many nongovernmental third-party payers negotiate contracts with health-care organizations, which may include DRG-like prospective payment systems, discounted or adjusted rates, risk-sharing agreements such as flat-rate payments per person per month for all defined care needs, prior authorization requirements, or other mechanisms that minimize the cost to the payer and distance the revenue from the charge. These payers, primarily managed care organizations, also include in their reimbursement systems co-pays, specified dollar amounts per episode of care, deductibles, and identified annual dollar amounts or deductibles that are paid directly by the consumer. Indemnity insurance payers typically reimburse based on charges, or more commonly on a negotiated percent of charges, but there also may be copayments or deductibles, payment ceilings, or service exclusions that shift the burden to the insured. In any case, indemnity insurance provides only a small percentage of the income of health-care organizations. Even smaller is the proportion of self-pay patients who are able to afford health care. The growing number of uninsured, who have no access to federal, state, or private coverage, generates a significant level of charitable care and bad debt for many health-care organizations.

In addition to the many reimbursement methods that exist, new payment mechanisms continue to emerge. For example, many payers have begun to link quality measures and outcomes with reimbursement incentives, also referred to as pay-for-performance programs. The intention of such programs is to encourage continuous improvement in the quality of care delivered in all health-care settings. In these arrangements, health-care organizations and their providers are held accountable to achieving defined quality standards to receive full payment for services.

In October 2008, the Centers for Medicare and Medicaid Services (CMS) implemented a reimbursement policy that denies Medicare reimbursement for 11 health-care-acquired conditions (HCAC) that were not present on admission: foreign object retained after surgery, air embolism, blood incompatibility, stage III and IV pressure ulcers, falls and trauma, catheter-associated urinary tract infection, vascular catheter–associated infection, surgical site infection after coronary artery bypass graft, surgical site infection following certain elective procedures (certain orthopedic surgeries and bariatric surgery), certain manifestations of poor blood sugar levels, and deep vein thrombosis or pulmonary embolism following total knee replacement and hip replacement. CMS named these medical errors "never events" because they should never occur for any patient. As health-care organizations are required to assume responsibility for the cost consequences of preventable complications, more emphasis is being placed on the leadership role nurses can play in reducing medical errors. More specifically, roughly half of all "never events" are nursing sensitive, such as pressure ulcers and patient falls, which further underscores the importance of high-quality nursing care in protecting patients and securing revenues. Intended to motivate hospitals to improve patient safety, CMS has encouraged state Medicaid programs to follow Medicare's lead. In addition, many commercial health plans are also seeking to implement payment plans that will hold hospitals financially accountable for preventable errors.

In addition to patient services revenue, organizations may generate other operating revenue, income from other day-to-day activities in areas such as the parking garage or the cafeteria, or indirect research revenue, the overhead received from research sponsors for providing facilities and administrative support for research projects. Total operating revenue is net patient services revenue plus other operating and research revenue, and reflects the total reimbursement in actual monies that the organization expects to receive from operations.

The organization may also generate nonoperating revenue that is not tied directly to the services or products provided and is managed and reported separately from operating revenue. Interest income may be generated on cash or investments. Gifts or donations may be given to a not-for-profit organization for a specific purpose or for the general purposes of the organization. If the gift is in the form of an endowment, the principle (the original amount of the gift) is invested and only the interest income on the investment may be used.

EXPENSE

Expenses are costs incurred in providing services or producing products. Wage and salary expenses are the costs of personnel, the labor costs required for production. Salaries are determined by the organization, subject to regulation regarding minimum wage and fair labor practices and, in some organizations, union contracts. They include base wages plus any differentials, premiums, bonuses, or other monetary rewards. Fringe benefits fall into two categories: those mandated by law, such as unemployment insurance and workers' compensation, and those specific to the organization, such as health insurance and pension benefits. Other benefits that incur costs are related to the organizations' personnel policies regarding sick, vacation, holiday, and other paid time off. In addition to the obvious salary cost for the worker on paid time off, there is an additional expense in the form of replacement cost (the cost to ensure that another worker is available) or the productivity cost (the cost of the output or associated revenue that is not realized). In a practice, if practitioners are functioning at efficient levels, the absence of one practitioner on a paid leave will result either in loss of revenue for patients not seen or increased costs for a temporary replacement for the practitioner. Note that this relates to paid absence. Unpaid absence leaves unspent wages available to support a temporary replacement or provides a cost offset to unrealized volume and associated revenue.

Nonsalary expenses are those nonpersonnel costs for consumable supplies, minor equipment, and related activities used in the delivery of service. Some are directly related to patient care activities, such as medical supplies, drugs, and blood products. Others are related to supports for the care process (office supplies, telephone charges), the environment (maintenance contracts, utilities), personnel (seminar registration, consultation fees), interest on loans, or bad debt.

Another type of expense is depreciation or the loss in value of capital assets. Capital expense refers to major investments in durable assets, such as facilities, equipment, and machinery. Capital assets are expected to have a value and useful life significantly greater than that of minor equipment. The threshold for determining what is capitalized is set by the organization and usually describes both a monetary value and an expected life span. For example, the threshold for capital might be equipment that costs more than $500 and has a useful life greater than 3 years. Under these guidelines, neither a $100 intravenous (IV) pole (monetary threshold) nor $1,000 worth of instructional videotapes (life span threshold) would be considered capital. Because capital assets are expected to be used over an extended period of time, their full purchase price does not appear as an operational expense at the time of purchase. Rather, in each reporting period for the duration of its useful life, the income and expense report reflects the capital depreciation or the loss in value of the capital asset as a result of use during the period. For example, if a capital purchase of $12,000 is expected to have a useful life of 10 years, one-tenth of its value is estimated to be used each year. Therefore, the financial statement would report depreciation of $1,200 per year or $100 per month.

COST CONCEPTS

A variety of cost concepts are relevant in understanding resource management.

Variable Versus Fixed Costs

Variable costs are those related to the volume of activity and fluctuate based on changes in volume. Fixed costs are those that remain constant regardless of fluctuations in volume. In personnel, the staff nurses may be considered variable—more are needed when the unit is at 90% occupancy than when it is at 75% occupancy—whereas the clinical specialist and nurse manager are fixed—one allocated to the unit regardless of the number of patients. Similarly, medical supply expense is variable based on patient volume and acuity whereas maintenance contract expenses may be fixed based on the terms of the contract and not driven by volume. Some expenses may be step-variable, that is, fixed over a short range and variable over a longer range. For example, one secretary may be sufficient for a practice with up to four clinicians, but a second secretary may be required if an additional clinician enters the practice. In that case, the number of secretaries is fixed at two unless the number of clinicians increases beyond eight. In general, all costs that are fixed in the short run are variable in the longer run. See **Figure 11-2.**

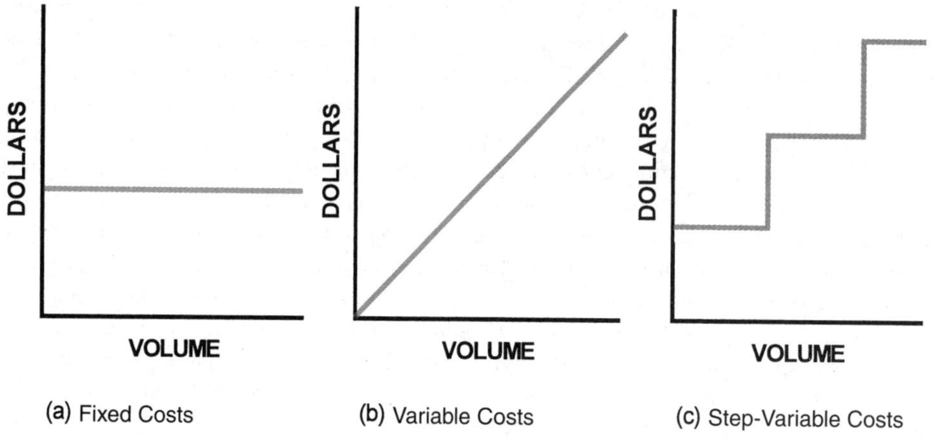

FIGURE 11-2 Fixed versus variable costs.

Direct Versus Indirect Costs

Direct costs are those related to the process of producing a product or service. Indirect costs are those incurred in supporting that process. In practice, the identification of expenses as direct or indirect depends on the context. In addressing an individual patient, caregivers—nurses, therapists, practitioners—would be considered direct whereas the leadership and support staff—secretaries, clinical specialist, or nurse manager—would be considered indirect. In considering patient populations aggregated by clinical care unit or practice, the entire staff of that unit or practice could be considered direct whereas support departments—human resources, environmental services, fiscal affairs—are identified as indirect.

Total Versus Unit Costs

Total cost is the aggregate cost incurred within a given time period for all volume of activity in that same time period. Unit cost is the cost of one unit of volume, calculated as the total cost divided by the total units of volume. Marginal cost is the additional cost required to produce one more unit of volume. Since the total cost includes both variable and fixed costs, it is possible to achieve economies of scale by increasing volume—and variable costs—on the unchanged fixed cost base. If a clinical care unit can increase its occupancy, it will expend more in variable direct care staff, but the cost per patient day will decrease because the fixed costs are spread over more patient days. Marginal cost for each additional patient day is equal to the cost of the variable staff and supplies for that patient day.

Incremental Versus Opportunity Costs

Incremental cost is the added cost incurred for an activity that would not be expensed if that activity did not occur. These costs may be variable or fixed, but they are essentially new costs and do not include current costs that may be redirected to the new activity. For example, if a clinical nurse specialist (CNS) proposes to teach a new series of classes on pediatric cardiac life support, incremental costs could include items such as demonstration mannequins, audiovisual aids, books, or other informational material and supplies for practical application. These would all be incremental costs because they would be incurred specifically for the purpose of the program. The participants' salaries are incremental if they are paid beyond their usual or regular hours to attend the program. If the program is to be given within the participants' regular working hours and it will be necessary to provide additional staff hours to cover those in class, these replacement costs are also included in the incremental costs. The CNS's time in preparation and teaching, and the facilities or space in which the classes are taught, would not be considered incremental costs because—if the classes were not given—the CNS's salary and the cost of maintaining the facilities would still be incurred. The incremental costs would be calculated for the number of students and programs presented over a given period of time.

Opportunity cost measures the loss of the effect of the next best alternative use of the resources allocated to a particular use. If the program described above is approved for implementation, what activity will the CNS forego to implement the program? If the participants are taking the course during their regular working hours and replacement is not required, what will they not be doing that might otherwise have been done? If the incremental resources were not allocated to this program, what would they be used for? The answers to these questions describe the opportunity costs. Identification and quantification of opportunity costs can provide important information in setting priorities and analyzing alternatives.

BUDGETING

Effective management presumes that an organization, in planning for its continuing existence, is able to describe and project the level of activity or production of services or products it will experience and anticipate the resources that will be required for that level of activity. The budget is the translation of that plan into quantities and dollars. The conceptual plan on which the budget is based may describe the projections for the entire organization or for some particular sector or activity and will determine the scope of the budget, including the time frame and the level of detail.

Types of Budget

Strategic planning is likely to be translated into a long-range budget that addresses the direction of the organization over the next 3 to 5 years or more. For this type of budget, the projections of volume and resources will be at a high level, with estimations of revenue and expense totals, but not at an extremely detailed level. The major drivers of volume and resources will be described and quantified, for example, anticipated changes in the patient mix, Medicare reimbursement rates, treatment protocols, or pharmaceutical expenditures. Other factors will be estimated in the aggregate based on current experience. The strategic plan and long-range budget are schematic representations of the direction of the organization rather than detailed blueprints. They need to be reviewed and refreshed at regular intervals to ensure that the organization continues to move in its preferred direction and to respond to significant changes in the health-care environment.

The operational budget, on the other hand, addresses the detailed, day-to-day activity of the organization. This type of budget looks in extensive detail at the projected volume and resources, and the associated revenue and expense, over a prescribed period of time. Usually the operating budget is constructed for the fiscal year, the organization's 12-month accounting cycle. The budget describes anticipated activity based on the specific operational goals and plans of the organization for that period of time and incorporates assumptions that will affect revenue and expense, for example, changes in reimbursement or inflationary increases in the cost of utilities or supplies. The budget is prepared at the detailed level of account within cost center. Actual experience is reported against the budget for each accounting cycle or month and cumulatively for the fiscal year to date, and is reported for each cost center and account code. However, each fiscal year's operating budget is independent of other years, that is, the positive or negative variance and the unspent budgeted monies from one fiscal year are not carried over into the next. The operating budget as a plan is valuable at the detailed level, the level at which the work occurs and at which the activity and resources must be managed. Aggregation of the budgeted and actual revenue and expense at the organizational level is also useful in providing overall direction and evaluation for the organization as a whole.

The capital budget reflects the projected expense for necessary facility improvement or acquisition of major durable equipment. Funding for the capital budget comes from the profit generated from operations, or from loans, which are also dependent on the organization's ability to generate a profit from operations. Although the capital budget may be prepared in yearly cycles, unlike the operating budget it is contained by the time frame of the project rather than of the budget year. Thus, capital funds may be allocated over several budget years for a particular remodeling project or equipment replacement proposal, and, unlike the operating budget, the funds will carry over from year to year until the project is completed. The capital budget is based on the plans and projections of the organization and will address the facilities and equipment needed to expand or upgrade services. These can generate the need for new or added clinical equipment such as cardiac monitors and ultrasound equipment; computer hardware (PCs, monitors, printers) and major software (electronic medical record, provider order entry system); and facilities improvement (renovation and remodeling). The capital budget also needs to address the maintenance needs of the organization, and therefore will also include such things as replacement of existing equipment, for example beds or ventilators that have reached the end of their useful life, or facilities maintenance such as the heating, ventilation, and air conditioning (HVAC) system. Finally, in preparing the capital budget, it is important to consider any additional nonsalary costs that will be incurred because of the use of the capital asset. For example, purchase of a monitoring system, clearly a capital expense, can also generate operating costs in the form of replacement leads or probes, batteries, or electrocardiogram (ECG) tracing paper, and potentially salary costs if additional personnel hours are required to monitor the monitors or file the tracings. These expenses must be identified and incorporated in the appropriate operating budget.

Frequently, organizations will consider initiating new activities or expanding or changing existing ones. The program budget is useful for this purpose. This type of budget isolates one activity or program from all other organizational activities to evaluate its effectiveness. The basis for the program budget is the conceptual plan of the program, or the program proposal, which also determines the time frame for the budget as well as the types of expenses to be included (e.g., total costs, incremental costs, opportunity costs). A plan to expand the hours of service for a medical urgent care clinic, using existing facilities and equipment, may be adequately described in a program budget that looks only at incremental volume, resources, revenue, and expense for the current fiscal year. Evaluation of the fiscal viability of the plan would consider the extent to which incremental revenue exceeds incremental expense. A plan to add a neonatal intensive care unit in a service that previously provided only routine and intermediate care would require a more extensive program budget. The quantification of activity would need to address potential volume—both numbers of neonates and clinical conditions—and probable income based on payer mix and reimbursement rates. Resource requirements would include both capital expenditures for facilities and major equipment and operational expenses for personnel, supplies, minor equipment, utilities, and overhead. Because of the time required to set up the program and the anticipated ramp-up from opening to full occupancy and utilization, the program plan would cover an extended period of time. Fiscal estimates would then need to be adjusted for the effect of inflation and reimbursement changes. Evaluation of the program would include a calculation of breakeven, that is, the point at which the average total revenue for an admission is equal to the average total cost. Before breakeven, the program generates a loss for each admission. After breakeven, the program generates net revenue for each admission. See **Figure 11-3.** Determination of the value of a program considers more than the fiscal benefit, for example, opportunity costs, social benefits and costs, or public relations value. These factors are difficult to quantify and are therefore not part of the program budget although they would be contained in the program proposal. When a program budget is approved and implemented, it becomes part of the operating budget for the implementation period and for all subsequent years. However, it is also useful to evaluate actual experience against the original program budget.

The projection of the cash budget is critical in the life of the organization. In the other types of budget, one of the guiding principles is matching revenue to expenses, that is, identifying the income for the activity that occurred in a particular time period and the expenses related to that activity that were incurred in that time period. Typically, however, the actual receipt of the revenue and the payment of the expenses do not occur in the same time period. Services are billed to third-party payers but the actual revenue is received weeks or even months later. Supplies are ordered, delivered, and used but the organization may be billed days or weeks later and the bills may be paid on a 30-or 60-or 90-day payment cycle. Thus, the revenue and expense projections for a particular accounting cycle in the operational budget, for example, do not reflect that cycle's cash flow, the actual cash coming into and going out of the organization. The cash budget projects this flow over the course of the fiscal year to ensure that there will be sufficient money in the organization

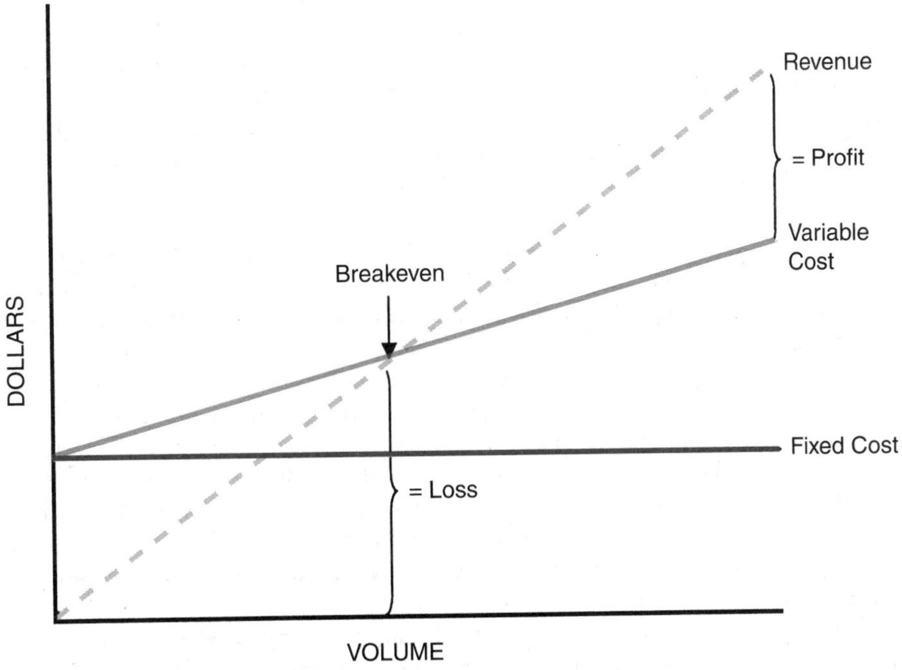

FIGURE 11-3 Breakeven.

to meet its obligations to its employees for payment of salaries, to its suppliers for payment of bills, and to its lenders for repayment of loans.

Budgeting Process

The budget process is based on the conceptual plan, goals, and objectives of the organization. The first step in this process is the identification of the activity that generates revenue and drives resource utilization. Within the health-care system, there are typical volume statistics that are used to quantify activity: admissions, discharges, patient days, patient visits, procedures, and tests. In the aggregate, however, these measures do not have the level of precision needed for accurate prediction of revenue and expenses. For purposes of predicting revenue, the volume needs to be further defined to reflect the basis of payment—by payer, by service, by product line, by DRG, or by test or procedure code.

For the purposes of predicting resource utilization, however, these categories may need to be further refined. DRG payments, for example, reflect medical condition and interventions but do not as clearly reflect nursing care needs of patients. As a result, patients in the same DRG—and generating the same revenue—may have different nursing care needs based on age, functional capabilities, communication issues, or learning needs and thus generate different levels of resource utilization. Payment systems may be based on global fees (e.g., for normal pregnancy and delivery) or on panels of patients (with the practice or organization receiving a per patient per month payment regardless of utilization of services) that are not reflective of the individual variability in care needs and resource requirements. It is necessary, therefore, to develop workload measures that identify both the resource drivers, that is, the significant activities that generate resource utilization, and the elements that account for individual variation within those drivers. For example, in the cancer infusion unit, the primary measure may be the patient visit or the therapeutic protocol. However, resource utilization may vary based on whether this is a new or returning patient, the length of the treatment, the patient's response to the therapy, or other issues or concerns that the patient raises in the course of the visit. Although it may not be possible to implement a workload measure that addresses this variability in minute detail, it is possible to develop measures that differentiate among patients and aggregate those with similar resource requirements. For patients with the same medical condition or undergoing the same therapeutic protocol, it may be possible to identify variations in resource utilization based on age, stage of treatment, functional level of activity, or other indicators. Using these indicators as well as the primary volume indicator of visit or protocol to describe patient populations, one can then generate a more accurate projection of required personnel and resources. The patients can be aggregated into groups with similar resource requirements and the groups can be weighted based on their average utilization relative to one another. For example, in a particular practice patients receiving a specific intervention may require 15 minutes of the clinician's time. However, a follow-up patient may only require 10 minutes and a new patient may require 40 minutes. All patients, however, may require 5 minutes for documentation and 5 minutes for follow-up. The intervention patient, therefore, will consume 25 minutes of time, and the others 20 minutes and 50 minutes, respectively. If the intervention patient is the benchmark and weighted at 1.0, the follow-up patient is weighted at 0.8 (20/25 (1.0) and the new patient at 2.0 (50/25 (1.0). Projecting visits by patient type and applying the appropriate weights will give a more accurate representation of the anticipated workload than projecting the visits alone.

Similarly, while there has been a current focus on considering mandated nurse–patient ratios as a way of ensuring adequate levels of care for patients, the ratios ignore the differences among patients in their need for nursing care. Identifying and measuring these nursing care requirements, often referred to as patient acuity, can be valuable information in managing and allocating nursing resources. To do so, many acute-care settings have implemented patient classification systems as a methodology for quantifying nursing workload. Such systems, which classify patients according to their needs for nursing care, enable organization to capture actual nursing workload and to measure productivity by looking at the relationship between nursing hours and workload over time. This approach can provide a new dimension for managing resources beyond the more simplistic but common measure of workload as patient days and nursing hours per patient day.

Variable personnel and material resource requirements are based on the projected workload volume. Using historical and current data, it is possible to construct a ratio of resources to volume—personnel hours per unit of work or supplies per unit of work. The personnel hours will include more than the direct care hours, as there is indirect time in the form of orientation for new staff, continuing education for current staff, practice or departmental meetings, teaching or precepting, or other organizational activities that are a necessary part of the working year. In addition, the personnel hours must reflect the impact of benefit time, as the individual on sick, holiday, or vacation time is not available to attend to the workload. Therefore, the personnel budget should be constructed first on the ratio of direct care hours to workload, that is, projected workload multiplied by the required hours per unit of work. Indirect time is added to this based either on a specific identification of the hours in the year that will be allocated to these activities or on a current ratio of indirect to direct care hours. For example, if clinicians are currently spending an average of 36 hours per week in direct patient activities and 4 hours per week in other organizational activities, the 11% (4/36) needs to be added to the calculated direct care hours to project the total worked time. In the same way, paid time off must be added, calculated as the number of paid absent days projected or, if there is variability, current paid absent days as a percent of total worked days.

Variable supplies can also be projected using a ratio of current utilization to workload and projecting that same ratio into the future. This approach assumes that future utilization rates will mirror current ones. Changes in procedures, practices, or products could affect this, however, and to the extent that those changes can be quantified, it is possible to adjust the ratio. Current utilization relevant to the change can be replaced with the anticipated utilization and the ratio recalculated. Personnel and materials that are not volume-driven are projected based on function and analysis of current utilization. It is important to remember that all fixed resources become variable over the long range, so it is important to look at the overall growth of volume and workload to determine whether the level of fixed resources continues to be sufficient.

When the projections of activity and resources have been completed, they are translated into dollars. The simple definition of total revenue is volume times price. However, this must be adjusted for the payer and contractual variations noted above. Personnel expenses are based on the salaries for the positions identified, including the cost of differentials, premiums, and fringe benefits. Nonsalary expenses will incorporate the existing cost for projected materials and supplies adjusted for anticipated price increases and general inflation. The revenues and expenses are totaled for the organization and the profit identified. If there is no profit—if the projected expense exceeds the projected revenue—or if the level of profit is not at the level needed to achieve its fiscal goals, the organization moves into the negotiation phase of the budget process. This is the most difficult phase of the process as the organization reviews its objectives and identifies steps to be taken to resolve the issue. If the conceptual plan, goals, and objectives for the budget were well thought out and clearly stated at the outset, and the activity and resources projected and quantified in relation to the plan, the negotiation phase is more likely to produce the budget plan that is most beneficial for the organization and its mission. Individual participants need to speak to the priorities and requirements of specific departments or programs but also evaluate them in relation to the requirements of other areas and of the total organization.

The final stage of budgeting, and the most important one, is implementation with evaluation. The plans developed and refined through the rest of the process—initiatives, practice changes, productivity improvements, and new or expanded programs—now move into the operational life of the organization.

Ongoing analysis identifies the extent to which actual experience matches budget projections. The organization can thus adjust as needed to unanticipated events that may affect overall outcomes. The analysis of actual to projected experience can be either fixed or flexible. Fixed budget analysis compares actual revenue and expense to the calculated budget. Variances may be favorable to budget—better than anticipated, that is, more revenue or less expense—or unfavorable to budget—not as good as anticipated, that is, less revenue or more expense. The limitation of this type of analysis is that it assumes that the budget is static, unaffected by events or activities that differ from budget assumptions related to outputs and inputs. Flexible budget analysis assumes a more dynamic budget, one in which the outputs and inputs can change but the relationship between the two remains constant. Thus, if a particular level of output drives an identified level of input, changes in the level of output will drive corresponding changes in the level of input.

If six intensive care patients require four nurses to care for them, a 3:2 patient-to-nurse ratio, nine patients will require six nurses. On a fixed budget analysis, the output—patients served—is favorable to the budget since there are more patients served, and presumably more revenue, than projected. The input, however, is unfavorable to the budget since there are more staff, and presumably more expense, than projected. On a flexible budget analysis, however, the 3:2 ration of output to input remains constant and the experience mirrors the budget. If the nine patients require only five staff, the ratio is 3:1.8 and the actual experience is favorable to the budget on a flexible budget analysis even though the output and expense is unfavorable to the budget on a fixed analysis.

Clearly, there is a place for both types of analysis in evaluating actual performance against projected. As noted in the discussion on cost concepts, although in the long run all costs are variable, in the short run some costs are variable and some are fixed. It is appropriate, therefore, to use a fixed budget analysis to evaluate fixed costs and a flexible budget analysis to evaluate variable costs.

MANAGING RESOURCES

The objective of financial management is to ensure that the organization generates a profit that is sufficient to maintain viability. The purpose of ongoing budget analysis is to determine the extent to which the organization is meeting its targets over a given period of time or for a particular program or activity, and to correct or improve its performance. Prudent management demands that the organization maximize revenue and contain costs to generate profit. Because both revenue and expenses are initially generated primarily by the clinicians who are providing services, it is important that all clinicians, including advanced practice nurses, understand and appreciate their contribution to the fiscal soundness of the organization. In this context, it is necessary to emphasize that fiscal considerations do not drive the activities of the organization. It is the mission, vision, and goals that determine direction and activities. However, the financial structure provides the framework for these activities and identifies at least one level of constraint and of opportunity.

Maximizing Revenue

Revenues are a composite of volume (the number of services provided) and price (income received for each service provided). Effective organizations ensure that they are generating as much income as possible. Fraudulent or deceptive practices such as billing for services not provided or providing unnecessary, expensive services clearly must be avoided. However, ethical strategies for maximizing revenues can be employed and can relate either to volume issues or price issues.

Once an organizational activity passes the breakeven point—that is, the point at which revenue equals expense—any additional volume will generate profit, all else being equal. It is not surprising, therefore, that there is so much emphasis, especially in practices, on how much volume and revenue the individual practitioner generates. In fact, in incentive practices within larger organizations, financial rewards to practitioners are based on volume and productivity. The measurement for identifying the individual practitioner's contribution to the organization most frequently is based on services billed. There is a desire, and in many situations even a demand, to demonstrate that the individual clinician is generating enough revenue to cover salary and to contribute to profit. This has driven the very appropriate efforts of nurse practitioners to secure billing privileges. (See Chapter 6 for a more extensive discussion of reimbursement issues.) However, this direct billing is not available in all settings or through all payers. Even where it is available, it may not be advantageous to the practice for the nurse practitioner to bill directly. Regardless, it is imperative to demonstrate the nurse practitioner's contribution to the practice and to develop other measures of volume and activity that can be used to evaluate the extent to which the nurse practitioner is generating revenue. These measures will be internal to the organization but need to be regularly reported and evaluated in relation to the overall success of the practice. Such measures will be required as well in other circumstances, where capitated or managed care payment systems do not accurately reflect through the billing system the volume of activity generated for the practice by the nurse practitioner.

In other organizational settings, volume may be measured by charges generated for particular procedures, tests, or services. This often leads clinicians to look for new ways of charging for various activities, assuming that this will maximize revenue and at the same time demonstrate their impact on revenue enhancement. With the decline of fee-for-service payment systems, however, increasing charges results in increased revenue potential from only the relatively small percentage of payers who have fee-for-service insurance or are self-pay. Even this potential may not be realized because of exclusions or payment maximums set by the insurer or because of the inability of the self-pay patient to pay all of the expenses for an episode of care. Unless there is significant revenue potential for an isolated activity, the income realized may not offset the cost of implementing and processing the charge.

Rather than focusing on charges, therefore, it is more effective for APNs to address issues with systems or practices that affect the volume of activity that is the basis for payment. Under Medicare's prospective payment system, for example, payment is based on the number of patients discharged within specific DRGs. If the length of stay per discharge can be reduced, a greater volume of patients can be admitted. What are the systems or practice issues that increase the length of stay without adding therapeutic value for the patient? What processes could occur before admission or subsequent to discharge that would reduce the length of stay? What services need to be provided that will attract patients to the facility? Consideration of these questions has led to a variety of approaches that ultimately result in increased volume, for example, preadmission testing and evaluation with same-day admission for surgical patients; telephone triage and follow-up or home visit programs for patients with early discharge; clinical pathways, case management, and early discharge planning programs; protocols to prevent, or promote early identification and treatment of, complications of hospitalization such as nosocomial infections or decubitus ulcers; or enhancing and expanding specific services such as cardiology or oncology. APNs in the inpatient setting are uniquely positioned to influence the efforts that affect volume. The APNs can identify approaches through study and analysis of existing systems and research on best practices. They can have significant input into the development of programs or protocols as part of the multidisciplinary team. They may support the implementation of changes through clinical evaluation, consultation, and education. Finally, the APNs may be the most appropriate clinicians to manage the particular program or activity.

In addition to adding volume, revenue can be increased by increasing reimbursement rates, the amount that the organization is actually paid for each product or service. However, this deceptively simple strategy is constrained by regulatory, contractual, and economic considerations. Actual reimbursement is determined by government regulation, contract negotiation, or organizational definition. Government-regulated reimbursement, such as for Medicare or Medicaid, is not organization specific and, although concerted lobbying efforts may have some impact, the potential for change is limited. Organizations may present evidence that they qualify for certain levels of reimbursement, for example, for direct medical education benefits, but otherwise will have little opportunity to affect payment levels. Reimbursement rates set through contract negotiations have greater potential for change, but only during the period of open contract negotiations. Because the negotiation outcome needs to be satisfactory to both parties, and because both parties as business organizations are interested in maximizing their profit, rate increases preferred by the one party may need to be tempered to be acceptable to the other party. Charges defined by the organization can easily be increased but the associated reimbursement rates cannot for many payers and, even with fee-for-service payers, may result in lower rather than increased revenue if the price increases result in a loss of volume to organizations with more competitive prices.

Strategies relating to the impact of price issues on maximizing revenue more successfully address systems to ensure that the organization receives all the revenue to which it is entitled under the existing regulations, contractual obligations, and pricing structure. Payment for services is contingent on the organization's demonstrating that it has in fact provided the relevant service or product. Different payers have varying requirements in the way that claims are processed, the forms that are used, and the specific data that are included. It is important, therefore, to understand what is required, where it needs to be recorded, and how it is presented to the payer.

All payers will require some level of detail on the services provided. This may be in the form of an itemized statement of all billable charges for an episode of care or the specification of relevant codes. Current Procedural Terminology (CPT) and Resource Based Relative Value Scales (RBRVS) are coding systems developed by the American Medical Association and adapted by government to identify and cost procedures and services provided by clinicians. The International Classification of Diseases, ninth modification (ICD-9) is developed by the World Health Organization and adapted for use in the United States by the federal government. It classifies diseases by system or category (e.g., blood disorders, neoplasms, infectious diseases) and may be used alone or in conjunction with other classification systems. DRGs and APCs as discussed earlier are used for Medicare claims for inpatient and outpatient hospital services and for selected nongovernmental payers.* Certain payers may also require evidence of preauthorization for specific procedures or treatments or referral authorization for specialty evaluation and management. Clinicians in many practices or in ambulatory settings may be more directly involved in identifying the appropriate code for the services rendered and must have a thorough understanding of the coding system and the relationship of codes to services provided. In other settings, coding may not be done by the clinicians, but the codes are determined based on

*Case mix classifications are used for reimbursement in other sectors of the health-care system by both governmental and private sector payers: Home Health Resource Groups (HHRGs) and the Outcome and Assessment Information Set (OASIS) in home care; the Minimum Data Set (MDS) and Resource Utilization Groups (RUGs) for long-term care.

information that the clinicians provide. The source document for information for coding and billing is the patient's medical record. Documentation in the medical record validates to the payer that the billed services were provided and justifies the organization's claim for payment. Inaccurate or incomplete documentation can lead to lost revenue opportunities if the coders are unable to identify all of the services that can appropriately be charged.

Reimbursement is negatively affected by payer denials and delays. Payers may deny reimbursement for services not covered (excluded from reimbursement based on the patient's policy or the contractual agreement with the organization) or for services not authorized (lacking required prior approval from the payer or from a designated clinician). Payment may also be denied for services deemed by the payer to be incompatible with the diagnosis, medically unnecessary, or not adequately validated. Payers who reimburse for hospital care on a per diem basis may carve out days for payment denial if delays in scheduling tests or consultations, or in initiating discharge planning and referrals, result in additional, otherwise avoidable inpatient days. Billing challenges by payers may also result in payment denials if supporting documentation does not appear in the medical record that the billed services were in fact rendered. Payers will audit records to validate that billed services have been provided even after payments have been made. If there is not adequate supporting documentation, the organization is at risk not only for repayments but also for additional financial penalties.

Inadequate documentation can lead to delays in billing if additional information needs to be accumulated before coding determinations can be made. Lack of compliance with payers' filing requirements may also result in denial of payment. Claims that are questioned initially may be resubmitted with additional evidence of the validity of the claim, but this involves rework and delays. In addition, most payers have a filing limit, a defined period of time in which a "clean" bill is presented in order for the organization to be reimbursed at all. Delays in processing and submitting bills and generating reimbursement, whether related to incomplete documentation or because of other systems issues, also result in lost opportunities for interest income. Money that the organization has received can earn significant investment interest even in the short term. Money in accounts receivable—that is, income that is anticipated but not yet received—does not generate any additional revenue for the organization.

The APN in a practice setting that bills directly or indirectly for the practitioner's clinical activity needs a clear understanding of the requirements and systems for billing—what can be billed, how it is processed, what documentation is required, and times frames for billing. By following through on these requirements, the APN is able to contribute directly to the timely and accurate generation of income. In other settings, the APN with an understanding of the systems for reimbursement to the organization contributes indirectly by providing and promoting accurate and complete clinical documentation, identifying systems issues that can generate delays in the billing cycle, and supporting practices that enhance the potential for maximizing revenue. For example, in the inpatient setting, an APN caring for a complex patient with multiple comorbidities may be able to increase reimbursement by assessing and documenting each of the patient problems and interventions. Addressing the patient's DRG alone may limit reimbursement and not acknowledge expenses generated from additional care needs.

Containing Costs

The volume of products or services produced drives the total expenses of an organization. These costs are a function both of intensity, or the extent of resources required for each unit of volume, and of price, or the cost to the organization of individual resource units. Cost containment focuses on identifying the least costly alternatives for supplying the personnel and materials to produce these services or products. In addressing cost containment, the organization evaluates the alternatives not only in terms of total expenditures but also in relation to potential impact on other aspects of the organization.

It is less costly to pay lower salaries, but if salaries are not competitive in the market, costly vacancies and turnover are likely to result. Inferior products that are less costly to purchase may generate additional expense in replacement, rework, decreased customer satisfaction, and loss of business. The desired alternative therefore is the least costly alternative that is consistent with the mission and goals of the organization.

Wage and salary expenses constitute a significant proportion of the costs in health-care organizations. Market forces, regulatory requirements, and ethical personnel management practices provide a framework for personnel expenditures. Within this framework, however, the organization has flexibility in controlling expenses related both to intensity and price of personnel resources used. Intensity addresses the number of personnel or staff hours required to manage a given patient population. The volume and type of patients and their particular care needs—the workload generated by that patient population—drive the personnel resources required. Measuring and managing workload variability can provide opportunities for cost containment. For example, scheduling staff in consideration of daily, weekly, or seasonal volume variations can minimize expensive "down time," as well as staff frustration resulting from inadequate staffing at busy times. This requires an ongoing analysis of workload patterns and trends to identify recurring variations. Unexpected variations may be addressed with the use of overtime or outside agency personnel. Both of these alternatives are more expensive than the normal personnel costs for the workload involved but are justifiable for unpredictable workload variations. A consistent increase in activity, however, requires a consistent plan for managing the workload. If a practice is increasingly seeing patients later than the usual scheduled hours and incurring overtime and other increased costs as a result, it is worthwhile to analyze the cause of the variation. System inefficiencies may be delaying patient throughput and thus generating additional unnecessary expenses that can be eliminated by addressing the inefficiencies. Patterns of patient scheduling may be changing, resulting in fewer visits scheduled earlier in the day with more down time, suggesting that scheduled staff hours need to be adjusted to accommodate patient preferences. However, the variation may be the result of a net increase in numbers of patients and visits. If this is so, an analysis of the fiscal impact of the increased revenue and increased expense may demonstrate that adding regular staff to cover the increased activity will be more cost-effective than continuing to use overtime.

Intensity of personnel resource utilization may also be related to inefficient clinical practices. Routines, procedures, and protocols that are based on tradition ("we've always done it this way") rather than on analysis or research-based evidence may include unnecessary and time-consuming activities that do not add value for desired outcomes. How are medication administration times determined? What are the indicators that determine the level of support for activities of daily living that each patient requires? How frequently is it necessary to monitor vital signs on postoperative patients? In what circumstances are isolation precautions instituted and under what circumstances can they be discontinued? How effective are the standard protocols for preparation for tests? Do the standard patient teaching tools and programs result in patient learning? Does the timing of drawing blood for laboratory tests make sense in relation to the timing of meals or medication administration or other treatments? It may be instructive to evaluate the care that patients with the same condition receive from different caregivers or in different settings to determine whether differences in practices result in differences in outcomes. In some circumstances it may become evident that practices in one setting are more resource intensive but do not add value and can be adapted or eliminated.

For personnel resources, price is generally equated with the cost of salaries and benefits. Containing costs by reducing salaries or benefits is not often possible given market conditions and the mobility of today's workforce. It is possible, however, to ensure that the least costly resources are used in any given situation. Overtime, for example, is a very expensive way to staff. It can be used effectively for the occasional unanticipated increase in workload, but extensive, continuous use of overtime requires identification of causes and alternative approaches. In addition to volume increases, variability in workload practices, or system inefficiencies, overtime may be related to the capabilities of the staff involved. For example, inexperienced staff may need assistance with particular patient issues or with development of organizational skills, or experienced staff may be struggling with unfamiliar procedures or patient conditions. For these staff, education and mentoring can promote developing competencies that also increase efficiency and ultimately reduce the overtime. The mix of staff may not be appropriate or the total numbers of staff may not be sufficient for the workload experienced. In these circumstances, it can be less costly to provide more skilled staff or more total staff at regular salaries than to continue with overtime.

One approach addresses the mix of personnel and the perceived advantages of reducing the numbers of professional staff and substituting less expensive unlicensed assistive personnel (UAP). In some circumstances, this may be effective; but, given the increasing acuity of patients, such substitution may be counterproductive. In acute-care settings, for example, patients are requiring more and more complex care, most of which cannot be delegated to unlicensed staff. In addition, unlicensed staff increase the workload of the professional staff because they assume the added responsibility of directing and supervising the UAP. For direct care, it may be less costly to have a higher percentage of licensed staff and fewer total numbers than to have a lower percentage of licensed staff and greater total numbers. However, if the professional staff are responsible for clerical or environmental tasks that can appropriately be delegated to less costly personnel, providing those supports can be an effective cost management approach.

Cost containment efforts can also address some of the hidden costs in personnel management. Turnover generates significant costs in recruiting, hiring, and orienting new personnel. Additional costs may be incurred before the new employee is available if vacancies need to be covered with overtime or more expensive outside agency personnel. Programs to promote staff retention can therefore be valuable in reducing turnover and its associated costs. Absenteeism can also be costly. Some level of unanticipated absenteeism due to illness is anticipated. However, staff dissatisfaction, unmanageable workloads, frequent excessive overtime requirements, or on-the-job injuries can also contribute to high levels of absenteeism. The cost is increased by the need for replacements, again often with overtime or agency personnel. In addition, costs to the organization for workers' compensation are directly related to the number of claims filed out of the organization. Cost can be lowered—and, potentially, staff satisfaction and efficiency increased—by identifying and addressing the factors contributing to absenteeism and on-the-job injuries.

Like wages and salaries, the costs for supplies and equipment are affected by market issues and regulatory requirements, as well as by the volume and type of services provided. Intensity in this context refers to the number and kind of materials used for these services. Cost containment looks at the least costly alternative to providing the services. This can be addressed on two levels. What are the specific supplies and equipment required for a particular procedure, protocol, or service? In addition, given that a specific item is required, which is the best product to select among the alternatives available? In relation to the first question, it is important to look at the work and how it is accomplished. Materials assumed to be necessary for the service provided may incorporate items that are no longer necessary, do not add value, or are useful only to a subset of the patients receiving the service.

With the materials necessary for a service identified, the focus moves to selection of specific items among those available. Product evaluation requires the involvement of clinicians and others in the organization. Inherent in the identification of an item as necessary for a particular service is the description of its purpose and how it is to be used. The primary concern in product evaluation is how well the different products under review meet these criteria. Other criteria also need to be considered, such as availability from the manufacturer and storage and maintenance requirements. A product that meets all clinical criteria, but cannot be produced and delivered on a timely basis or has high maintenance (and associated down time) potential, may not be preferable to a less exotic but more available and reliable product.

Prices for materials and supplies are negotiated with vendors. Organizations may identify cost containment opportunities in the course of these negotiations through volume discounts or as part of purchasing groups. This raises the issue of managing the tension between standardization and customization. Frequently, standardizing supplies and equipment across service areas has significant benefits in reducing the expense for purchasing, storing, distributing, and using specific products. Although this limits the range of products available to the clinician, it also limits the time needed to become familiar with the product, to develop ease in working with it, and to use it in a variety of settings. It may, however, generate some level of waste if, for example, a standardized pack of supplies for a particular procedure contains items that are used in most but not all situations. Customization, on the other hand, matches the products specifically to the individual patient, clinician, or situation. It can have advantages in being more effective in achieving the desired outcome or in reducing the potential for waste. However, customization sometimes is more a matter of individual clinicians' preferences than of value added for the patient. It is important, then, to evaluate the pros and cons of standardization or customization in specific circumstances to identify the least costly alternative. In general, for products and processes that are used in a variety of settings, standardization is preferable not only because of the cost and productivity benefits but also because it promotes consistency in providing services. Alternatives to standardization should be undertaken only after careful evaluation to ensure that the marginal benefit of customization—that is, the greater value that accrues from the alternative—outweighs the fiscal and operational benefits of standardization.

As the previous discussions suggest, the appropriateness of measures to contain costs cannot be evaluated in isolation from outcomes. Cost efficiency identifies the minimum expenditure necessary to achieve an outcome. Cost-effectiveness identifies the minimum expenditure necessary to achieve the outcome that is consistent with the organization's mission and goals. Cost-effectiveness, therefore, incorporates an element of quality that is not inherent in cost efficiency. Vacuum-assisted dressing for postsurgical wound healing is significantly more expensive than traditional dressings and would not be considered cost efficient in a simple analysis that only addressed the expense incurred for dressings until wound healing is achieved. However, because it accelerates wound healing, this intervention reduces the necessary length of hospitalization and extent of postsurgical follow-up. As such, it is certainly cost effective, with benefits for both the patient and the provider organization. In some circumstances quality measures are not sufficiently developed to allow precise measurement of cost-effectiveness but, to the extent that such measures are available or can be approximated, they should be incorporated into analysis.

Cost-effectiveness and cost efficiency are typically analyzed using productivity measures or cost-benefit analysis. Productivity is the relationship of inputs and outputs, of resources used and products or services produced. Productivity relationships are expressed as ratios and can focus either on the output or on the input. Focus on the output addresses the question, "What does it take to produce the output?" and is the ratio of input to output, or resources divided by products or services. Examples of productivity measures focusing on output include hours per patient day, cost per procedure, and visits per episode of care. Focus on input addresses the question, "How well are resources being used?" and is the ratio of output to input, or products or services divided by resources. Examples of productivity measures focusing on input include visits per full-time equivalent (FTE), tests per staff hour, and case hours per available room hour. Productivity improves when output remains constant and input decreases, or when output increases and input stays constant. Productivity declines when output remains constant and input increases, or when output decreases and input stays constant. Productivity ratios are of little value in isolation. Comparisons of productivity ratios to targets set during the budgeting process, to historical experience and trends, and to other internal or external benchmarks are valuable for analysis and identification of opportunities for increasing efficiency and effectiveness.

Cost-benefit analysis is frequently used to evaluate a particular program or project, or to compare programs, approaches, or activities competing for resource allocation. The analysis compares the revenues and expenses generated by the program to determine the net benefit (income minus expense) or the ratio of benefits to costs (income divided by expense). Determination of the value of the program to the organization, however, is not determined exclusively by analysis of the financial benefit. Benefits and costs that are difficult to quantify, such as social benefits and costs, opportunity costs, public relations value, and loss leader opportunities, may be of considerable importance to the organization and influence decisions to implement or continue specific projects and programs.

Productivity is often focused on personnel resource utilization, but the concept also applies to material resources and to the overall utilization of services. Length of stay or number of days per inpatient stay, for example, can be considered to be a productivity measurement that identifies the relationship between the episode of care (output) and the patient days, representing the aggregated resources required to provide for that episode (input). Comparisons are made among patients or groups of patients for a given time period or across multiple time periods, and against internal and external benchmarks. Productivity improves if the length of stay (and associated expense) decreases for the same level of activity.

Cost-benefit analysis can identify the impact of productivity improvements for the organization. Baseline analysis of the net benefit (revenue minus expense) identifies the profit margin. Productivity improvements are designed to increase the profit margin by reducing the cost (but maintaining consistent income) for each episode of care. Moreover, decreasing length of stay has the added opportunity of creating capacity for additional volume. That volume will generate additional income as well as additional expense. Assuming a consistent patient population, if the cost per episode of care remains the same, the total profit (income minus expense) will increase although the profit per case remains the same. However, the cost per episode of care may well decrease (as fixed costs are spread over more cases) and enhance both the total profit and the profit per case. Cost-benefit analysis can also identify potential negative aspects of productivity improvement efforts. Length-of-stay reductions must be consistent with good clinical practice. Early discharge of patients may be clinically premature and result in readmission of the patient for continuation of care. Obviously, for the patient this is an undesirable outcome and therefore could not be considered cost effective. It cannot even be considered cost efficient because many payers, particularly those who reimburse on a cost per case, identify a time period after discharge during which a readmission (for a condition related to the original hospital stay) will be bridged to the original admission. Additional expense will be incurred, but the merged admissions will be considered as one episode for the purposes of reimbursement and additional payment will be denied.

IMPLICATIONS

Reimbursement levels and the associated incentives to contain costs are to a large extent payer driven. Reimbursement systems structured as fee-for-service include little incentive for the provider organization to contain costs. Since reimbursement is generated by charges that are paid either in full or at some negotiated percentage, increased utilization results in increased revenue so long as costs do not exceed the level of reimbursement. The majority of payers, however, have built into their reimbursement systems some incentives for containing costs. Reimbursement at the per diem or per visit rate is an incentive to reduce resource utilization and increase efficiency for that day or visit. Reimbursement based on cases (DRG-based, for example) build in incentives to reduce the length of stay as well as the resource utilization during the stay. Capitated reimbursement systems create the additional incentive to reduce the number of episodes of care—admissions or visits. Individual payer variations on the systems add complexity for providers and consumers. Some, for example, may offer additional payments for achieving specific clinical quality outcomes with defined patient populations such as pediatric asthma patients or adult-onset diabetic patients. Others may have payment tiers for certain benefits, with different consumer copayments for different levels of services (generic versus brand pharmaceuticals, for example).

Clinicians, however, generally are not attuned to incorporating reimbursement variables into clinical decision making for individual patients and prefer to provide care that is "payer-blind." They do have a responsibility, however, to promote efficiency in the allocation and utilization of health-care resources, and not only for the viability of the organization within which they practice. As health-care costs escalate, insured patients increasingly are at risk for higher out-of-pocket costs, including deductibles into the thousands instead of the hundreds of dollars before the insurer assumes liability, and they are entitled to value for their expenditure. In addition, social justice demands that constrained resources be used judiciously to ensure the maximum availability of health care to all members of society. The most appropriate approach for clinicians, therefore, is to provide cost efficient and effective care for all patients regardless of payer.

Fortunately, in many circumstances, cost containment efforts developed to accommodate a given payment modality can be designed to benefit—or at least not disadvantage—patients of other payers as well. Programs to reduce length of stay, efforts to improve productivity, analyses to identify the most cost-effective products, and benchmarking to identify best practices may be initiated because of the structure of one payment methodology, but their beneficial effects need not be limited to patients of that insurer type. However, because resources are not unlimited, in different circumstances difficult choices need to be made. Organizations rarely can respond to all requests for resources and often are in the position of needing to select among competing priorities that may all be necessary and worthwhile. Should the organization expand the cardiac program or the pediatric program; replace the ventilators in the critical care units or the ultrasounds in the echocardiology lab; construct additional ambulatory facilities or additional inpatient facilities? The decisions will require compromise and consensus, and a clear understanding of the benefits not only for the organization but also for the staff and, most important, for the patient. Advanced practice nurses have the knowledge and expertise to provide the clinical input and to advocate for the patient. To have a credible voice in this decision-making process, they must also have a clear understanding of the business and fiscal issues that affect resource allocation and management.

12

Mediated Roles: Working Through Other People

Thomas D. Smith
Maria L. Vezina
Mary E. Samost

ADVANCED PRACTICE AND PARTNERSHIPS

The four established advanced practice roles—certified nurse practitioner (NP), clinical nurse specialist (CNS), certified nurse-midwife (CNM), and certified registered nurse anesthetist (CRNA)—reflect significant evolution of the nursing profession and nursing practice. The APRN Consensus Model addresses some of the issues of role definition and scope of practice for the four APRN roles (NCSBN, 2008).The implementation mechanism for the APRN Consensus Model is Licensure, Accreditation, Certification, and Education (LACE) (Stanley, 2009). The APRN Consensus Model/LACE serves the purpose of standardizing APRN scope of practice and increasing access to APRNs. It also serves to support one of the recommendations of the Institute of Medicine's (IOM's) report *The Future of Nursing: Leading Change, Advancing Health* (IOM, 2011) to remove scope of practice barriers (Stubenrauch, 2010). According to *Nursing's Social Policy Statement* (American Nurses Association, 2010), these roles involve specialization, expansion, advancement, and autonomy, suggesting the necessary skills of managing people, the organization, and the environment of care. According to the IOM (2011), "more than a quarter of a million nurses are APRNs who hold master's or doctoral degrees and pass national certification exams. APRNs deliver primary, acute and medical home care as well as other types of health-care services. For example, they teach and counsel patients to understand their health problems and what they can do to get better, they coordinate care and advocate for patients in the complex healthcare system, and they refer patients to physicians and other health-care providers" (p. 52). Specifically, the CNS (advanced practice registered nurse [APRN]) role centers on the synthesis, integration, transformation, and translation of best practices as articulated in the literature (National Association of Clinical Nurse Specialists [NACNS], 2007). Davies and Hughes (1995) note that "the term advanced nursing practice extends beyond roles. It is a way of thinking and viewing the world based on clinical knowledge, rather than a composition of roles" (p. 157). This view of the world is an interactive process that emphasizes direct and indirect partnerships with both patients and a diverse group of health-care providers. In addition to clinical competency, the varied aspects of advanced practice also require socialization and interpersonal skills to form the foundation for collaboration, consultation, and clinical leadership. Although advanced practice roles require autonomy and authority to be fully enacted, the ability to achieve patient and system outcomes is dependent on partnerships with others to manage interdependent and interdisciplinary relationships. In fact, the NACNS (2007) concluded that "the synergy of working with, leading and coordinating teams of professionals in a highly communicative, focused care environment regardless of setting, will continue to be the hallmark of practice into the future" (p. 8). According to Bleich (2011), APRNs, as either "master's or doctorally prepared clinical scholars, may not have the extent of formal education in advanced research methods and statistical techniques, but they are nonetheless critical to clinical inquiry at the point-of-care and evidence-driven decision making within the organizational context. Their clinical expertise and advanced knowledge of nursing practice can be used in partnership with nurse scientists. Inter-and intra-professional connectivity will optimize nursing's impact in advancing health via the synergy that bridges scientific knowledge generation with translational expertise at the point of care. This synergy may also serve to link nursing better with other health care professions, giving nurses a stronger voice in decision-making forums and at policy tables" (Bleich, 2011, pp. 169–170).

CORE COMPETENCIES

APRNs function as clinicians using evidence-based knowledge to provide direct care, diagnose and manage health-care problems, coordinate services, educate patients and families, advocate for patients, and manage the health-care system in all its dimensions. This approach to care supports the continued focus on prevention of disease, maintenance of health, and resolution of functional problems (IOM, 2004). In *The Future of Nursing: Leading Change and Advancing Health,* the IOM (2011) stated that "nurses are developing new competencies for the future to help bridge the gap between coverage and access, to coordinate increasingly complex care for a wider range of patients, to fulfill their potential as primary care providers to the full extent of their education and training, to implement system-wide changes that take into account the growing body of evidence linking nursing practice to fundamental improvements in patient safety and quality of care, and to capture the full economic value of their contributions across practice settings" (pp. 53–54).

Accordingly, six core competencies, as shown in **Figure 12-1,** further define advanced nursing practice. These competencies have consistently been identified as essential features of advanced practice (American Association of Colleges of Nursing, 1996; Davies & Hughes, 1995; NACNS, 2004; National Council of State Boards of Nursing, 2006):

1. Expert guidance and coaching of patients, families, and other care providers
2. Consultation
3. Research skills, including use, evaluation, and conduct
4. Clinical and professional leadership, which includes competence as a change agent
5. Collaboration
6. Ethical decision-making skills

Given this overview of core competencies, the theme of relationships within the health-care arena is evident. The ability to work with and through others is inherent within these competencies and consequently indicates a strong foundation for practice. Although not explicitly stated in definitions of advanced practice, there is an understanding within interprofessional teams that APNs must be skillful and cognizant of the key elements of their partnerships with patients and other health team members. Managing the interpersonal strategies of providing care is critical to success as an independent care provider in a competitive health-care environment. For example, care provided by APRNs in the complex, acute setting is transitioning into the community, thereby increasing the need for the APRN to assess his or her strengths to provide accountable practice while working successfully with other providers. According to the IOM (2004), the opportunities presented by the current practice environment can be met through a strong foundation of clinical practice, specialty expertise, and a rigorous graduate education.

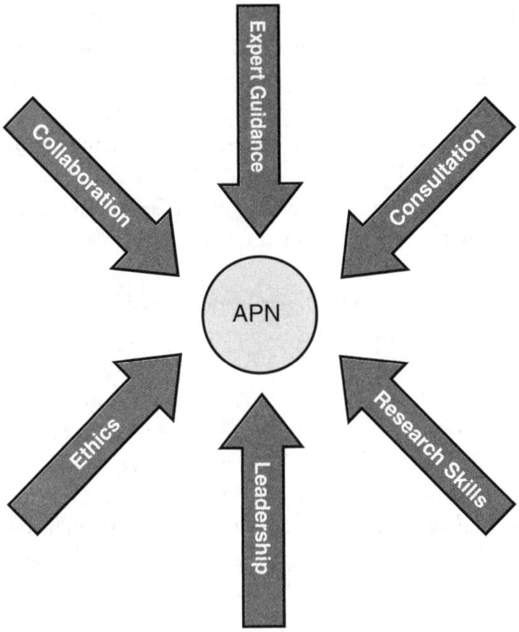

FIGURE 12-1 Core competencies of advanced nursing practice.

With reference to the six core competencies, several interpersonal themes emerge:

1. Expert guidance and coaching of patients, families, and other care providers reflect a mentor role, with expectations of others to either take the lead or share the pathway of care.
2. Consultation is the direct involvement of another practitioner, which denotes the need to confirm findings, diagnosis, and/or plan of care. The responsibility for care, however, rests with the primary practitioner. It can require an overlap within the same specialty for an added opinion or a discussion with a specialist for another view or preference of treatment. In either situation, the partnership is necessary for optimal patient care and a deliberate approach in the management of practice.
3. Research skills, including use, evaluation, and conduct, support the professional obligation to improve practice, often involving APRNs with other practitioners to evaluate methods of delivering care. Innovative change is possible when health-care professionals come together to redesign clinical practices. Efforts such as interdisciplinary or interprofessional education, research, performance improvement, and evaluation initiatives can have a significant effect on optimizing the system of health care.
4. Clinical and professional leadership can be powerful when approached in an interdisciplinary manner. Although the unique roles of distinct professions are useful within the framework of individual competencies, in patient care, the leadership of a team is a supportive experience for patients, especially for those with limited access to a health system and those with complex care needs. A focus on the specific patient and not on professional turf issues requires skill in leadership and change agency. In this realm, the blurring of roles is often helpful and not hurtful.
5. According to *Merriam-Webster's Collegiate Dictionary* (2003), collaboration means to work together, especially in a joint intellectual effort. The ANA (2010) *Nursing's Social Policy Statement* cites qualities of collaboration such as a common focus, recognition of another's expertise, and a collegial exchange of ideas and knowledge. Hamric, Spross, and Hanson (2005) refer to

collaboration as a "dynamic, interpersonal process in which two or more individuals make a commitment to each other to interact authentically and constructively to solve problems and to learn from each other in order to accomplish identified goals, purposes or outcomes" (p. 318). By definition, then, collaboration identifies relationships and involves an interpersonal process. The focus of the relationship needs to be positive and grounded in a problem-solving approach, creating interdependence as a mutually fulfilling experience between the involved parties. Although collaboration is a cornerstone of many APN roles, it eludes some clinicians. Consequently, models of collaboration have emerged to assist in structuring relationships and guiding the process of working partnerships.

6. Ethical decision-makings skills are a central component of effective advanced practice. According to Thompson and Thompson (1985), "To be professional is to be ethical, and to practice ethically requires an understanding of ethics, values and oneself." The goal of ethical practice is to do the right thing for the right reason (Thompson, Kershbaumer, & Krisman-Scott, 2001). Although grounded in one's values and presentation of self, the inclusion of the team in ethical decision making is key to the holistic care of patients. Ethical clinical practice requires an atmosphere of trust, mutual respect, and commitment to critical thinking and reasoning. To create this atmosphere, APNs, as the managers of care, need to work with others in an inclusive manner, so as to build a team whereby the ability to express values, feelings, beliefs, and knowledge can be encouraged and ensured as the ethical dimension of practice emerges.

MODELS OF COLLABORATION

The basis of collaboration is the belief that high-quality patient care is achieved by including the contributions of all care providers. In *The Future of Nursing: Leading Change, Advancing Health,* the IOM (2011) stated that "being a full partner transcends all levels of the nursing profession and requires leadership skills and competencies that must be applied within the profession and in collaboration with other health professionals" (p. 35). The Macy Foundation (2010) states that "mounting research shows that heath care delivered by nurses, doctors, and other health-care professionals working in teams not only improves quality, but also leads to better patient outcomes, greater patient satisfaction, improved efficiency and increased job satisfaction on the part of health professionals" (p. 2). Collaboration is often cited as the "key to success" for any initiative that extends beyond an individual's scope of activity. Collaboration is therefore the foundation of effective patient care. According to Arcongelo, Fitzgerald, Carroll, and Plumb (1996), a variety of interpersonal attributes are necessary for successful collaboration. These include trust, knowledge, shared responsibility, mutual respect, positive communication, cooperation, coordination, and optimism (p. 107). See **Figure 12-2.** The authors define these attributes as follows:

- *Trust* among all parties establishes a high-quality working relationship; it develops over time as the parties become more acquainted.
- *Knowledge* is a necessary component for the development of trust. Knowledge and trust remove the need for supervision.
- *Shared responsibility* suggests joint decision making for quality patient care and outcomes, as well as accountable practice, within the organization.
- *Mutual respect* for the expertise of all members of the team is the norm. This respect is communicated to the patient.
- *Communication* that is not hierarchical but rather two way ensures the sharing of patient information and knowledge. Questioning of the approach to care of either partner cannot be

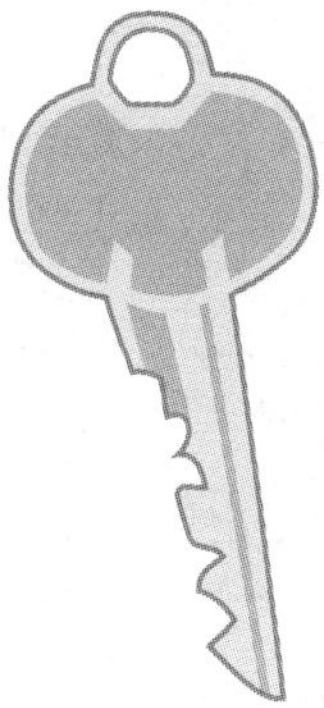
Collaboration is the Key to Success
Trust
Knowledge
Shared Responsibilities
Mutual Respect
Communication
Cooperation
Optimism

FIGURE 12-2 Collaboration attributes.

delivered in a manner that is construed as criticism, but as a method to enhance knowledge and improve patient care.

- *Cooperation* and *coordination* promote the use of the skills of all team members, prevent duplication, and enhance the productivity of practice.
- *Optimism* promotes success when the involved parties believe that collaboration is the more effective means of promoting high-quality care.

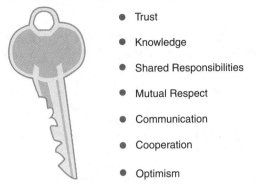

Although these attributes are key in any collaborative relationship, it is primarily the unique contribution of each member of the team that determines a successful outcome.

Although there are several models of collaborative practice, they often are distinguished by the response to two questions:

1. How is the expertise of each member of the team used to the fullest?
2. Who is responsible for decision making and patient care?

In **Table 12-1,** Strumpf and Whitney (1994) describe three practice models commonly used in primary care:

1. The parallel model
2. The sequential model
3. The shared model

In the parallel model, the APRN manages stable patients, and the physician cares for those who are more medically complex. In the sequential model, the APRN performs the intake assessment and the physician assumes responsibility for differential diagnosis and management, or the pattern may be reversed, with the physician screening all patients and delegating the care of patients identified as less complex to the APRN. In the shared model, the APRN and the physician care for an individual patient on an alternating schedule and based on patient needs. Arcongelo and colleagues (1996) identify a fourth model, the collaborative model, which involves the APRN as the primary care provider without regard for the complexity of the problem. The APRN collaborates as needed to provide safe, high-quality care but practices autonomously and independently. The communication in this model is ongoing, may transition to a comanagement arrangement during an unstable or complex period, but always involves the input of the two professionals in establishing the plan of care. One outcome of this style is the ability for the APRN to expand his or her knowledge and skills within the complex

TABLE 12-1

Models of Collaborative Practice

	Parallel Model	Sequential Model	Shared Model	Collaborative Model
APN role in patient care	Manage stable patients	Perform intake assessment	Manage patients identified by the physician to be less complex	Manage all levels of complexity
Physician role in patient care	Manage medically complex patients	Diagnosing and management of patients	Initial screening of patients Manage more complex patients	Comanage during unstable periods Collaboration between APN and physician in plan of care

realm of patient care and establish closer contacts with consulting team members while managing the complexity.

Regardless of the model of collaborative practice, the elements of trust and a positive working relationship are vital. Collaborative relationships are a "work in progress," not facilitated by inflexible expectations or boundaries. Over time, mutual expressions of expertise become grounded in an invisible pattern that is the glue of the successful relationship, reflective of growing skill, trust, and confidence among partners.

The advantages of collaboration often begin with negotiation by the involved roles regarding which patients and conditions are best managed by the APRN or the physician. This process may seem to be a hurdle to competent and successful APRNs, but armed with data, performance indicators (both financial and clinical), and the maturation of one's practice, the process of collaborative decision making promotes effectiveness of care. For example, in the management of chronic illness, APRNs tend to prescribe fewer drugs, order fewer tests, choose less expensive treatments, and spend more time with patients (Fitzgerald, Jones, Lazar, McHugh, & Wang, 1995). According to hospital salary surveys, the cost of an APRN is often 50% of the physician's or less. Subsequently, an effective collaborative APRN/physician practice would enable physicians to spend more time with patients with more complex health needs while APRNs focus on the care of more stable patients, as well as helping patients traverse the health-care continuum in managing their complex diseases.

In all health-care settings, it is becoming an increasing challenge to provide the ongoing surveillance and case management that can support sick and frail patients to function at their highest level possible. Naylor and colleagues (1994) found in a study of elders that CNPs were able to reduce posthospital complications and readmissions. The management of acute illness of established patients has also demonstrated a minimization of complications and cost while maximizing the quality of life for patients. Physicians are then available to deal with those situations that require the clinical decision making and intervention of specialized medical care. It is becoming increasingly apparent that future trends in health-care reform and public reporting will require greater collaboration and role recognition among all health-care providers as a strategy to relate effectively and efficiently with all patients.

Barriers to collaboration are rooted in the many traditions of the "Doctor-Nurse Game," which range from sex-role stereotypes to incongruent expectations of knowledge and skill acquisition. Intertwined within these concepts are those related to cultural, social, psychological, and financial complexities of the health-care system. Nonetheless, when patient-focused approaches to health care are endorsed, the critical aspects of collaborative relationships, skills, and practices are uncovered. The opportunities that patient-focused approaches fully engage among various health-care disciplines become self-evident over time. In other words, the dimensions of the physician-nurse relationship are fundamentally tied to the quality of patient care (Brandt, 2001). This observation alone provides the health-care system and clinicians with primary motivation to encourage effective relationships between professionals to identify opportunities for working through and with one other.

CLINICAL RELATIONSHIPS

The nature of advanced practice is such that most patient care can be managed because of the skill and knowledge of the practitioner within the role. However, each practitioner acknowledges the critical significance of consultation and referral when used in a timely and effective manner. Imbedded in these partnerships are the issues of relationships within the health-care team, communication styles, trust, and the ability to interact within these clinical relationships without a hierarchical framework. Although many APRNs have formal consultative relationships within their scope of practice, others do not. In addition, these formal structures vary among states and health-care institutions, with a range of directives from state boards, often from different disciplines. National efforts are underway to remove scope of practice barriers and allow for increased reimbursement for APRN services. Accordingly, these changes can result in significant savings and increase access, as well as performance improvement in patient safety and quality of care. With legislation and statute aside, the ability to work within a model of consultation and referral is necessary. Each member of the health-care team has knowledge and skill to offer the other and a partnership can often effect changes in practice and influence patient care outcomes that would not be possible if managed alone. Many consultative practices are also influenced by the environment whereby specialty and primary care is clearly differentiated. In these situations, consultative relationships are vital to improved care processes.

Often consultation and referral activities are confused with supervision, comanagement (the working together to manage a complex case), and direct oversight. In these situations, the accountability for practice may become lost, and roles are blurred. The limits of one's practice expertise or the need to receive advice should be viewed as complementary, not as a deficiency or "take over" approach. The professional interactions inherent in consultation and referral expand the APRN's ability to work with and through others, while maintaining autonomy over the situation until there is a mutually identified decision that a change in care is necessary. Although comanagement and referral (the relinquishing of care temporarily or permanently) may have different themes, the goal of care is still accomplished within a partnership mode. Hamric, Spross, and Hanson (2005) state that APRNs themselves are often confused about the differences. They refer to a more thoughtful definition of collaboration described as "a dynamic, interpersonal process in which two or more individuals make a commitment to each other to interact authentically and constructively to solve problems and to learn from each other in order to accomplish identified goals, purposes, or outcomes. The individuals recognize and articulate the shared values that make this commitment possible" (p. 318). Within this framework of collaboration, the varying processes of consultation, referral, or comanagement may assume the added dimension of a therapeutic, professional relationship acknowledging the role each member plays while supporting the complexities inherent in the delivery of high-quality patient care. Although knowledge, skill, and clinical expertise are all key factors in day-to-day practice, the elements of working with each other in this collaborative manner will determine and distinguish the best practices.

INTERPROFESSIONAL TEAMING

The importance of integrated health-care teams is fueled by a number of factors, including the increasing complexity of patient needs, especially among the growing population of elders; expansion in the continuum of care in various health-care delivery models; the sophistication of telecommunications and information networks; and changes in methods of health-care financing and reimbursement regulations. It is also evident that members of the interprofessional health-care team—physicians, APRNs, registered nurses (RNs), social workers, and other clinicians—often practice independently of one another, rendering care as if services for the same patient or groups of patients were unrelated. Interprofessional teaming differs from the multidisciplinary approach to care, which has been compared to the parallel play of children—with limited interactive and intersecting activity (Clark, 1994). See **Figure 12-3**. According to Cronenwett and Dzau (2010), interprofessional training and teaming are critical to meet the public's needs, provide the care they want, and control costs in health care.

Interdisciplinary teaming, currently referenced as interprofessional, was proposed as an alternative model of care decades ago (Pfeiffer, 1998). Interdisciplinary teaming requires that the members of the health-care team integrate their disciplines' work and create plans of care together, centering this plan on the patients' needs. This form of teamwork, interdisciplinary care, has been defined as a "special form of interactional interdependence between health care providers who merge different but complementary skills in the service of patients and in the solution of their health problems" (Tsukuda, 1990, p. 670). See **Figure 12-4**. The term *complementary* defines the team approach. However, a collection of like-minded individuals does not result in an interdisciplinary team. Because of the nature of this teaming, there must be a clearly defined purpose, goal, and approach to team activity, as well as the value and understanding that mutual accountability of each team member is crucial to the team's overall performance. The primary purpose of this type of team is collaborative decision making for patients. Decision making, in this model, occurs in a unified time line. Often, in a multidisciplinary team approach, a sequential time line is experienced as a dependent process in which the final decision is made by the "lead" member who pulls

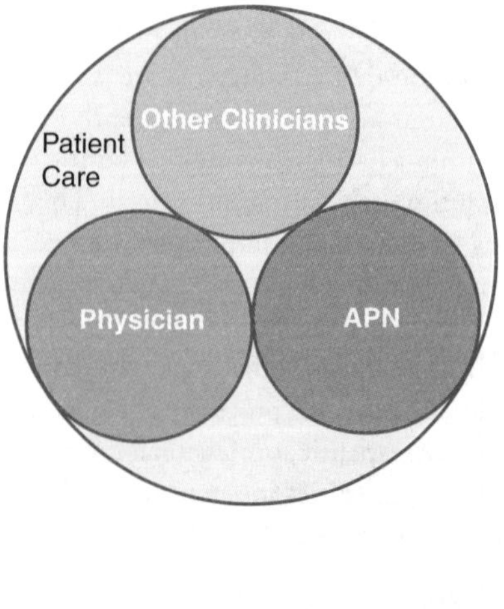

FIGURE 12-3 Multidisciplinary approach to patient care.

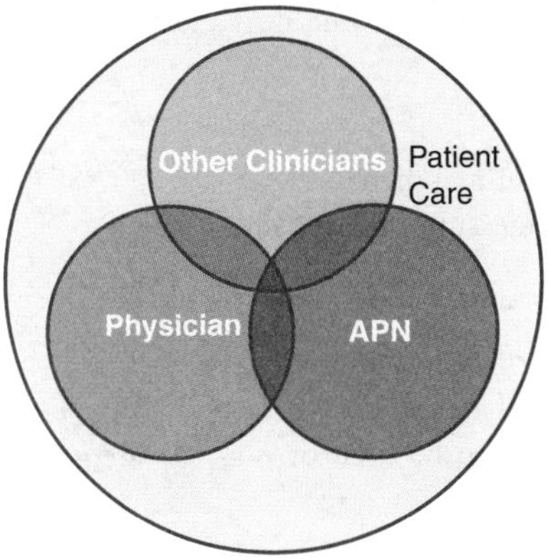

FIGURE 12-4 Interprofessional approach to patient care.

everything together. This type of decision making is limited, and potentially ineffective, when complementary activity is desired.

For the APRN, the influence of interdisciplinary teams is powerful. Creative teamwork can be achieved between at least two disciplines or expanded to include additional disciplines as well. Changing the norms of practice, however, may be necessary. Interdisciplinary teams are the epitome of working with and through others, while recognizing the importance of an individual's clinical expertise and today, even one's information technology proficiency.

There are a number of dimensions to consider when implementing interdisciplinary team relationships. According to Howe, Cassel, and Vezina (1998), these dimensions include the following:

1. Skills
   - Conflict resolution
   - Team interaction
   - Communication
   - Leadership
   - Outcomes-focused care
   - Performance improvement
2. Attitudes
   - Respect for other disciplines
   - Respect for patient and family input
   - Respect for patient management and patient-focused care
   - Awareness of outcomes-based practice
3. Knowledge
   - Roles, responsibilities, and scope of practice for each discipline
   - Role of the extended team
   - Group dynamics
   - Application of clinical concepts and quality measures among disciplines
   - Up-to-date knowledge of the health-care environment, policy, and technology

Inherent within this interdisciplinary framework, collaboration underpins the field of day-to-day practice within a team concept. According to Tsukuda and Stahelski (1990), collaboration takes on the dimension of cooperation with others, adding trust as an essential component of this interactional style, because patient outcomes are consistently dependent on the efforts of others. As a team member, one may ask the following questions:

- Are my own goals consistent with team goals?
- Do I advocate solutions for problems that will benefit team members?
- Do I work for consensus and focus on performance and measureable outcomes?
- Do I cooperate with other team members' activities?
- Do I do an equitable share of the group workload?
- Do I feel individual responsibility for the joint outcomes of the group members?
- Do I support the team in dealing with larger organizational and regulatory issues?
- Do I view my contributions as belonging to the group—to be used or not—as the group decides?
- Do I listen to team members in a positive and respectful manner?
- Do I actively participate in team meetings and assignments?

Advocates of interdisciplinary team approaches to care realize that there are many psychosocial influences on health and disease. This underscores the importance of relationship-centered care (Tresolini & The Pew-Fetzer Task Force, 1994) and patient-centered care (Coles, 1995), which are based on interpersonal communication techniques and a collaborative care model. A paradigm shift for all members of the health-care team may be necessary because new core competencies are required and need to be role modeled for the successful transition to occur. APRNs are often members of these teams and are positioned to initiate the transition to a more collaborative and patient-focused approach in their practice. APRNs often assume a mediator role to introduce these changes in the delivery of patient care and to assist the team in its growth and development in the core competencies of interdisciplinary team approaches.

APRNs may take a leadership role in influencing stages of team development. Their role is easily linked to the various members of the health-care team, allowing APRNs the advantage of connecting with each discipline, clearly expressing the similarities and the differences of each member's role and contribution. With this common ground set, the formation and development of a team can occur.

According to Tuckman (1965), four stages of team development are discussed:

- Forming
- Storming
- Norming
- Performing

As implied by the stages, the creation and maintenance of teams is personnel intensive, with professional adjustments required by every member of the team. Roles and relationships may be challenged, but they may also move to a new level whereby extraordinary achievements can occur. In this context, interdisciplinary teaming with its strong emphasis on relationship-centered care is the "best practice" for the 21st century.

PROFESSIONAL NURSING CONNECTIONS

Expanded roles for nurses span a century of growth and development, with the earliest days of clinical specialization in anesthesia, operating room, and obstetrical nursing. However, the knowledge and skills required in a basic nursing education lay the foundation for the advanced practice platform. Common ground skills and competencies include patient assessment, health promotion and maintenance, health education, advocacy, caring, accountability, continuity, and collaboration with other health team members. This overlap and sharing of skills create a bond of practice between RNs and

APRNs—forming professional nursing connections. How do these two groups move together in partnership? Hopefully, they join together with respect for the value of each role, intending to effectively use the expertise of each professional, while avoiding duplication of effort and promoting true collaborative relationships. Such connections can broaden the scope of health care and achieve professional satisfaction for both RNs and APRNs.

Regardless of the common ground, however, each advanced practice specialty has dealt with resistance from other nurses because advanced roles have often represented innovations in practice that shook the status quo of the nursing establishment and the overall health-care system (Bigbee & Amidi-Nouri, 2000). Rigid boundaries were often created and the struggle for recognition and acceptance followed. However, through organized and focused educational and political efforts, tensions were lessened and improved relationships flourished.

The roles of the RN and the APRN sometimes clash within the context of leadership for the delivery of patient care. Once an understanding of expertise and specialization is clearly reached and communicated, the contribution of each role can be qualified and recognized, and a complementary approach to health care defined. Evaluative research can also assist in this recognition and educational process—providing data to illustrate the effect of advanced practice nursing care on quality patient outcomes. Together, professional connections between the RN and APRN can be fortified and not diluted by professional conflict.

The common ground between RNs and APRNs creates a powerful force in health-care delivery. The professional bonding that exists between both groups reinforces the image of the RN and the APRN as coleaders of care. By practicing together, the RN–APRN team can design approaches to care that recognize each other's respective strengths and expertise—resulting in a dynamic practice arena free of hierarchy.

EXEMPLARS: ENACTING ADVANCED PRACTICE ROLES

The enactment of the advanced practice roles of the APRN, the CNS, CNM, and the CRNA are best detailed through the narratives set forth by the following exemplars. Using the standard set of interview questions listed, these enactments are related to existing practice settings. See **Boxes 12-1 through 12-5.**

Advanced Practice Nurse Interview Questions

To guide the interview process for chosen groups of APRNs, the following questions were used consistently for each group with the intent of assessing roles, expectations, and influences on practice.

1. How would you describe your role?
2. How would you describe your working relationship with physicians, other nurses, and other members of the health-care team?
3. What does *referral* mean to you?
4. What does *consultation* mean to you?
5. How open are members of other disciplines in taking direct referrals or consultation from you?
6. What degree of authority do you experience in these situations and in your role?
7. Do you observe that you bring about change and a higher order of knowledge to your practice area?
8. Can you discuss a situation that may exemplify your role, especially regarding your work through other people?

(text continues on page 238)

BOX 12-1

The Acute-Care Nurse Practitioner

This group of nurse practitioners (acute-care nurse practitioners [ACNPs]), situated within an oncology inpatient practice, describes their role as geared to management of their patient's experience of illness. The patient's diagnostic workup is often completed before admission in the ambulatory setting. Therefore, the patient's in-hospital experience focuses on the management of the acute phase of illness and treatment options as the goals of care. They describe their perspective as multidimensional. Using their registered nurse (RN) background, they always view the patient in a holistic manner. Advanced practice clinical competencies engage their ability to case manage and guide patients and families through the complexity of health care. Within this framework, the ACNP's relationships with the health-care team are key because they spend significant amounts of time discussing medical management and locating resources, managing symptoms, integrating feedback from other disciplines, and identifying alternatives to the health-care system when challenged by the limitations of third-party payers. Given their range of activities, this group of ACPNs consistently relate to a variety of other disciplines, primarily medicine, nursing, and social work.

This group describes their autonomy as follows: "We feel that our common ground is the care of the patient. Working with our team of physicians allows us many choices and flexibility.

"We decide the day-to-day care for our patients, and in acute or critical episodes, we often independently manage the process. Although critical incidents may be a time when the physician takes a more active role, this does not necessarily translate into the need to 'take over.' The goal is to work together—not to work around each other or without each other." The ACNP is usually the leader of care because of a number of factors, including the close relationship to the patient and family members, the advantages of consistency of care by the ACNP, and well-defined collaboration between physician and ACNP.

Regarding their relationships with RNs, the ACNPs state: "There is nothing better than working with a competent nurse. When this relationship occurs, there is such a strong bond that you firmly believe that there is absolutely nothing that can stand in the way of quality." On the other hand, ACNPs state that some nurses can become more passive about patient care when relating to an ACNP. Because the RN recognizes the "nurse" in the ACNP role, the RN may relinquish aspects of his or her responsibility for patient management or assessment to the ACNP. This transfer rarely occurs within the RN–physician relationship. NPs must therefore carefully assess the nature of the ACNP–RN relationship to avoid jeopardizing their ability to work through others while facilitating the advanced practice perspective.

Within the ACNP role, referrals are commonplace—ACNP to nutritionist, social worker, pharmacist, physical therapist, and home care services. Physicians often refer their patients to ACNPs, acknowledging their specialization, expertise, and consistency of care. Consultations are more informal within the inpatient setting. When acute patient situations occur, however, clinical consultation is common. ACNPs state: "Not a day goes by that I am not involved in a clinical consultation primarily focused on symptom management, such as pain control, the side effects of chemotherapy, nausea, vomiting, constipation, or palliative care." This type of consultation is almost always verbal for, it seems, "physicians want to maintain control of the written consultation process within the hospital experience." ACNPs consult other ACNPs as well, often involving clinical specialization expertise—usually within a verbal, face-to-face framework.

The degree of authority within the discipline of nursing is explained by acute care ACNPs in a variety of ways. ACNPs are integral in the decision making about their patients and have significant influence on the nursing care being delivered. Using a specialization approach, ACNPs take advantage of opportunities to teach about clinical sequelae and implications. One ACNP states: "I often teach at the bedside about what is going on with the patient, and I am watchful

BOX 12-1
The Acute-Care Nurse Practitioner—cont'd

for the types of questions the nurses have. This helps me observe the growth of the staff and assess their advancing competency. It is really a very rewarding experience for me." Through rounding with staff nurses, ACNPs also have the opportunity to clarify the patient story and often act as a facilitator of communication about patients among team members. ACNPs state their role as "performing the editing role"—distinguishing the critical elements of the patient story and routing the necessary data in a more concise and relevant way to obtain what is necessary for their patients. As one ACNP stated, "Our role within the interdisciplinary team is one of monitor of the communication patterns and the perspective at hand. We often translate what is going on into a relevant, concise language that evokes a rapid, clear understanding by those team members who need to hear the information."

According to this group, the design of the ACNP embraces many relationships within the health-care team and consists of these major components:

1. Gatekeeper
2. Decoder of the complexity of the situation
3. Director of care, delineating roles and responses
4. Problem solver, often suggesting alternatives when barriers arise
5. Provider of a secure environment for staff nurses to ask questions and learn
6. Guide for directing the patient care experience, providing the driving force behind what needs to be done, when, and why

Integral to these components is the ability to work with others, to recognize the many roles inherent within the heath-care team, to value the team's input and contribution, and to recognize that influencing others should be always focused on the unified goal of high-quality patient care.

BOX 12-2
The Clinical Nurse Specialist

The clinical nurse specialists (CNSs) describe their role as multifunctional, defining their framework of practice as more focused within a nursing model rather than medicine. CNSs categorize their role into two primary domains: clinical and professional. Clinically, this CNS group describes their role as including a major teaching component and direct clinical practice to facilitate and influence care of complex patients. These functions are often intertwined because they routinely bring about change and a higher order of knowledge by role modeling, mentoring, and coaching staff to perform at "the next level." CNSs also intervene within the health-care team to make clinical recommendations to change the course of action or resolve conflicts for optimal patient care. Professionally, the CNS also assumes major responsibilities for the development of policies, procedures, protocols, and standards of care. Within this context, the education of patients in health promotion and maintenance is key. Standards of care are holistic in nature, spanning the physical, psychosocial, and spiritual needs of patients. The needs of nurses are also critical. The CNS encourages the professional growth of staff, often provides career counseling, and directs the building of expertise among nurses in a specific, individualized manner.

Continued

BOX 12-2
The Clinical Nurse Specialist—cont'd

The CNSs describe their role with physicians as collegial with a defined focus on specialty patient care management, often receiving referrals for a specific patient population (e.g., diabetes) or an occurrence such as death/dying and bereavement. CNSs are consistent in their view of the "big picture," focusing not just on disease and pathophysiology but on the patient's response to the disease. With other nurses, CNSs describe their role as an enabler—one of camaraderie focused on patient care. CNSs also provide clinical, professional, and legal clarification regarding issues of care to ensure a safe patient environment.

When asked about autonomy, this CNS group cited self-direction and motivation as key elements in working with others. Several strategies are used to engage others in change and ultimately provide state-of-the-art, valid, and effective approaches to care:

1. Use benchmark data and national standards to energize staff to change or modify practices.
2. Develop and educate staff so they can question their patient care environment and relate to a higher level of performance through evidence-based practice and scholarly query.
3. Involve staff in various levels of patient care projects, moving forward together in change.
4. Ground all projects in the literature and best practices so as to base decisions on evidence and promote confidence in the process.

The CNS role engages an inclusive approach within these strategies, which guarantees a successful and lasting outcome over time.

Referrals are routine in complex cases. The CNS is often the originator of referrals to other members of the health-care team but integral to bringing team members together to problem solve. Inclusiveness is again a key element of the CNSs' practice domain and a hallmark of their effectiveness in patient care through their ability to relate to others.

Consultation, on the other hand, is associated with the level of the CNS's clinical expertise and is often initiated by other members of the health-care team—physicians, nurses, and social workers. As an inductive thinker, the CNS has a clearly articulated interest in the patient experience of care. Using these tenets of practice and change—standards, safety, and ethics—the CNS is able to define a plan for care, engaging caregivers to undertake the plan and empowering others to assume an appropriate trajectory for the patient.

As the integrator of care, the CNS exemplifies how positive interdisciplinary relationships ensure positive outcomes for patients. CNSs are teachers, clinical experts, care providers, case finders, role models, mentors, patient advocates, coaches, team members, policy makers, project leaders, innovators, case managers, career counselors, and change agents. With a vision of best practices as their foundation for care, the CNSs hold the value of expertise and dynamic working relationships within the health-care team as critical elements to the success of their role.

BOX 12-3
The Midwife

Midwives, in a combined ambulatory and inpatient setting, describe their advanced practice role as primary caregiver of women along the life cycle with a focus on low-risk obstetrical and gynecological care, health promotion, wellness, family-centered care, risk assessment, and management of common illnesses and acute conditions. Clinically, this group views their role as centered on direct care with a strong emphasis on patient education and health promotion. Their relationships with other members of the health-care team revolve around this focus.

BOX 12-3
The Midwife—cont'd

Midwives independently care for a patient caseload, often comanaging more acute conditions with physicians or employing the physician as consultant.

Regarding referral, midwives in this practice describe the process as formalized and often interchangeable with consultation. They define many of their referrals as transfers to the care of a physician because of a specialized need of the patient over time. Ongoing referrals to other disciplines are also common, usually engaging the services of social work and home care. In these instances, the midwife maintains the primary care responsibility for the patient. With consultation, the process is also formal. Using written communication, consultations are often provided through the required practice protocols that identify the consulting physician and the decision guidelines for the consultation. Within this collaborative relationship, the midwife is able to transition the care of the patient when a condition warrants. This can be accomplished in a comanaged arrangement or by a referral of the care responsibility to another caregiver. However, the midwife has an expectation to be involved in the communication of the plan of care and the ultimate follow-up of the patient being referred. The midwife explains that the "relationships with physicians in my practice are necessary and denote many shared responsibilities. I find this relationship to be within an interdependent framework since we both need to work together to manage the patient safely in given situations. I have a consulting agreement with a primary physician for immediate feedback and intervention as well as with other physicians who are colleagues and can be employed for a less acute need. But I also have the need to maintain my primary care role for my patients."

Working with the nursing staff involves interdependence. The need for the registered nurse (RN) to facilitate a plan of care and become integral in the assessment and the education of patients is key. One midwife states, "I find that once my role is accepted and understood, positive relationships follow and communication about patients is facilitated. I admit that I need nurses to ultimately deliver good patient care. I cannot do everything myself." Nurses and other health team members who seek out the midwife as primary caregiver ultimately improve the patient experience because the model of working together and understanding the role is achieved. One midwife states that over the past decade this recognition of the midwife role has improved tremendously, especially because of updated scope of practice legislation and changes in third-party reimbursement.

When asked about autonomy and authority over practice, midwives strongly identify that their influence over care processes is recognized by others. The primary reason for this influence is the public respect, acceptance, and demand for their roles and services. They add that this authority is stronger and more flexible in an ambulatory setting and can be less autonomous in a hospital-based birthing unit, especially when associated with a medical residency program. Interdisciplinary competition in these settings can affect the perceived authority and working relationships of the midwife with other clinicians, as well as patients.

When discussing their relationships with nurses, midwives were clear that within the specialty of women's health, RNs do not abdicate components of their roles to midwives. RNs often question an approach to care, exchange ideas to complement care, and practice as team members. The specialty of women's health is often not characterized as illness-focused but within a health promotion/health maintenance framework, enabling the team approach to flourish. Respect for the team's contribution to the varied aspects of the needs of patients enables the nurse-midwives to work effectively with and through others. As one nurse-midwife summarized her role: "Being on the same page in our plans for care is easily delineated within this advanced practice role. Thus collaboration is a natural outcome. Respect is key, and once earned, paves the way to collaborative practice."

BOX 12-4

The Primary Care Nurse Practitioner

This group of primary care nurse practitioners (NPs) view their role as provider of a comprehensive holistic health-care experience for their patients. With independence and autonomy, the primary care NP has a threefold responsibility to assess, diagnose, and manage a variety of common and chronic illnesses within all the dimensions of the physical, psychosocial, and financial elements of care. "My caseload of patients" is a common reference point, delineating the accountability of this group of NPs for their patients over time—not limited to a hospital experience but to the continuum of care. In primary care, the NP possesses a leadership role in the practice generally by providing a surveillance function—a "third eye"—always watchful of the effectiveness of day-to-day patient care delivery. The need to evaluate systems and clinical outcomes is essential to the role.

The team approach in this type of practice is fundamental and involves a strong interdisciplinary, participative approach to care. Patients are independently managed, comanaged with physicians, or referred within their continuum of care. The need to relate effectively with all members of the health-care team is constant. Multidisciplinary options coexist within an interdisciplinary framework—creating many opportunities for therapeutic relationships among staff, patients, and family members.

Within the primary care practice, RNs are the "heart" of any clinical operation. The RN complements the APN role, especially in the areas of patient teaching, patient monitoring, and data gathering. Although roles are often strongly delineated, sharing clinical activity among health-care team members is consistent and necessary.

As a result of the primary care focus, referrals to specialists are commonplace. But as one NP explained, "Losing the primary relationship with a patient to a specialist is a concern." The information and insight the specialist provides will enhance the care the patient receives from his or her primary care provider. There are also instances when a specialist and primary care provider work collaboratively on the health-care management of a patient over the longer term. Feedback on the means to best manage the patient is the expected outcome. One NP stated: "We expect to have our patients return to us for their care and to benefit from the expertise and evaluation by the specialist."

Consultations, on the other hand, are frequently engaged by other caregivers. Within a mature primary care practice, a multidisciplinary team approach is often developed. Formal consultations usually occur within the practice. The opportunity to have "curbside" or "hallway" consultations with these same specialists or experts exists as well. This type of consultation is often informal. The NPs from this practice cited that the key criteria for successful and effective consultations of any type include the development of positive relationships, a clear direction of the plan of care, and a model of inclusivity among team members.

Primary care NPs describe their authority as an essential part of their potential for success in their role, while maintaining autonomy and a knowledge base to provide sufficient holistic primary care to patients. Practicing side-by-side with physicians and other NPs creates opportunities for sharing advice or consultation. Leading patient care in this practice setting is very satisfying and empowering to this group of advanced practice nurses (APNs). At the same time, however, this sense of control and satisfaction occurs only when interdisciplinary teamwork is achieved by doing the following:

1. Listening to others
2. Teaching others
3. Demonstrating the APN role in positive, creative ways
4. Communicating openly
5. Demonstrating expertise

BOX 12-4
The Primary Care Nurse Practitioner—cont'd

Respect from other members of the team enables the primary care NP to facilitate and lead care effectively. When sharing the same mission, within this framework of practice, advancement of learning and change occurs. By empowering and educating staff at all levels, the barrier of the "task" is removed and has been replaced with a "connection" to the patient's illness experience. Assisting staff to understand the rationale for care is a definitive way to initiate change and a higher level of performance. In addition, the primary care NP often exhibits his or her own clinical specialization and expertise, which may provide a different perspective of care, adding to the knowledge base of the staff. As educator, the NP is capable of working through other people, engaging the staff's interest in the mission and work at hand. Knowledge is power, and this power translates into effective practice.

BOX 12-5
The Nurse Anesthetist

The role of the certified registered nurse anesthetist (CRNA), within a hospital practice, is described as an advanced practice specialty with a strong and eventful history that has provided many benchmarks for nurses seeking expanded roles. As an anesthesia provider, the goal of the CRNA is to provide safe and comfortable anesthesia for all types of surgical procedures in multiple settings across the care continuum for patients of all ages spanning the American Society of Anesthesiologists (ASA) classifications of "healthy" to "gravely ill/impending death." In discussing this broad role definition, the concept of independence is also clearly expressed especially because the CRNA often is able to administer anesthesia without the direct supervision of a physician, depending on state regulations and the requirements of the employing health-care institution. For example, this CRNA stated that in her practice an anesthesiologist is required to practice in specified ratios with the CRNA and that an anesthesiologist must be present in the room at the start of general anesthesia induction.

The clinical relationship between the CRNA and the anesthesiologist is clearly described as one of a collegial and trusting nature, with open communication. However, outside of the clinical arena, the political tension between the two disciplines is present and with a long history of debate and interprofessional struggle and competition. With the demonstration of expertise, however, positive communication patterns and relationships have developed around the patient and quality care in institutional settings. The day-to-day operational framework has thereby demonstrated advancement over time in terms of professional acceptance and colleagueship.

Within the operating room, the surgical team assumes a vibrant interdependent structure. This CRNA stated: "Teamwork is the expectation in the operating room setting. The involvement with RNs, surgeons, and surgical technologists is intense and very focused on the individual patient and the procedure at hand and can sometimes be described as somewhat of an isolating relationship because of this directed focus." Regarding the relationship between the CRNA and RN, it is described as important but less influential in affecting the role of the CRNA when compared with the other team members such as the surgeon or technologist. The relationship with surgeons is described as one of respect for the specialization of anesthesia and sometimes dependent during the course of surgery because the CRNA often leads patient stabilization efforts when a critical change in condition occurs.

Continued

BOX 12-5
The Nurse Anesthetist—cont'd

In the specialty of anesthesia, the CRNA usually does not make referrals but is the recipient of referrals from other providers. With the exception of some specialized services such as pain management, CRNAs do not have their own patient caseload because the patients have a primary relationship with their surgeon. Consultations, on the other hand, comprise a major component of anesthesia practice. Consultations reflect clinical, legal, and medical aspects of the plan of care. Surgeons frequently request a consultation from a CRNA, respecting the expertise of this specialization to assess the risks of surgery. In this endeavor, the surgeon is dependent on the expertise of the anesthesia specialist. Within this activity, the CRNA attains primary patient and family contact, subsequently establishing the patient-family relationship.

Authority in practice is significant within the specialty of anesthesia. "Many other disciplines do not share a common ground in this specialty: thus my role is unique within patient care." The CRNA in this practice comments that she also identifies that through her unique expertise, the independence and influence of her role takes hold. "Other members of the health-care team recognize my competence, which directly affects my sense of autonomy and authority. I am called on to assist others in their clinical assessment of patients, as well as the advancement of professional knowledge and skills of residents and nurse anesthesia students. With this broad range of influence, my sense of authority is promoted."

The ability of the CRNA to influence change and a higher order of knowledge in the arenas of perioperative and perianesthesia practice is strongly affected by teaching by example, demonstrating competence, and role-modeling professional behaviors to all members of the health-care team. Using this framework, the CRNA in this practice identifies that she is able to influence change and advance knowledge by relying on a clinical approach rather than an academic approach. In many practices, however, CRNAs also assume formal faculty roles within various levels of educational programs throughout the country.

Although working through other people is an expectation of any health-care professional role, interdisciplinary exposure is often more limited for CRNAs and can potentially contribute to isolation. Interdisciplinary relationships are strongest within the perioperative team of the surgeon, anesthesiologist, nurse, and technologist. Extending this relationship to other clinical staff and family members is challenging. In addition, CRNAs are often placed within a separate administrative structure within the health-care facility or practice, contributing to the isolation, especially from other professional nurse colleagues.

Within the context of advanced practice, the goal of the CRNA is to promote nursing, advance health care, and ensure a safe and high-quality patient care experience. As the earliest advanced practice role, CRNAs have successfully built a strong presence in health care.

CONCLUSION

The dynamic interplay of partnerships and interdependence between advanced practice and other team roles in health care is a professional opportunity. Working with and through others is the cornerstone of the successful engagement of the health-care team and endorses the presence of advanced practice over time.

REFERENCES

American Association of Colleges of Nursing. (1996). *The essentials of master's education for advanced practice nursing.* Washington, DC: Author.

American Nurses Association. (2010). *Nursing's social policy statement: The essence of the profession.* Washington, DC: Author.

Arcongelo, V., Fitzgerald, M., Carroll, D., & Plumb, J. (1996). Collaborative care between nurse practitioners and primary care physicians. *Primary Care, 23*(1), 103–113.

Bigbee, J., & Amidi-Nouri, A. (2000). History and evolution of advanced nursing practice. In A. B. Hamric, J. A. Spross, & C. M. Hanson (Eds.), *Advanced nursing practice: An integrative approach* (2nd ed.). Philadelphia: WB Saunders.

Bleich, M. R. (2011). IOM report. The future of nursing: leading change, advancing health: milestones and challenges in expanding nursing science. *Research in Nursing and Health, 34*(3), 169–170. DOI: 10.1002/nur.20433.

Brandt, A. (2001). The nurse-physician relationship in historical context. In M. Hager (Ed.), *Enhancing interactions between nursing and medicine.* New York: Josiah Macy Jr. Foundation.

Clark, P. (1994). Learning on interdisciplinary gerontological teams: Instructional concepts and methods. *Educational Gerontology, 20*(2), 349–364.

Coles, C. (1995). Educating the health care team. *Patient Education and Counseling 26*(5), 239–244.

Cronenwett, L., & Dzau, V. (2010). Co chairs' summary of the conference. In B. Culliton & S. Russell (Eds.), *Who will provide primary care and how will they be trained?* (Preface, p. 6). New York: Josiah Macy, Jr, Foundation.

Davies, B., & Hughes, A. M. (1995). Clarification of advanced nursing practice: Characteristics and competencies. *Clinical Nurse Specialist, 9*(3), 156–160.

Fitzgerald, M. A., Jones, P. E., Lazar, B., McHugh, M., & Wang, C. (1995). The midlevel provider: Colleague or competitor. *Patient Care, 29*(1), 20–37.

Hamric, A. B., Spross, J. A., & Hanson, C. M. (2005). *Advanced nursing practice: An integrative approach* (3rd ed.). Philadelphia: WB Saunders.

Howe, J., Cassel, C., & Vezina, M. (1998). Structuring the GITT didactic experience. In E. Siegler, K. Hyer, T. Fulmer, & M. Mezey (Eds.), *Geriatric interdisciplinary team training* (p. 90). New York: Springer.

Institute of Medicine. (2004). Quality chasm series: Patient safety—*Achieving a new standard for care.* Washington, DC: National Academy Press.

Institute of Medicine. (2011). *The future of nursing: Leading change, advancing health.* Washington, DC: The National Academies Press.

Macy Foundation. (2010). *Educating nurses and physicians: Toward new horizons.* (2010, June). Retrieved July 10, 2012, from http://www.macyfoundation.org/docs/macy_pubs/JMF_Carnegie_Summary, Web Version (3), pdf, p. 2.

Merriam-Webster's Collegiate Dictionary (11th ed.). (2003). Springfield, MA: Merriam-Webster, Inc.

National Association of Clinical Nurse Specialists. (2004). *Statement on clinical nurse specialist practice and education* (2nd ed.). Harrisburg, PA: Author.

National Association of Clinical Nurse Specialists. (2007). *Competency validation survey.* Harrisburg, PA: The Association.

National Council of State Boards of Nursing Advanced Practice Registered Nurses Task Force. (2006). *Draft: A vision of the future of advanced practice regulation.* Chicago: Author.

Naylor, M., Brooten, D., Jones, R., Lavizzo-Mourey, R., Mezey, M., & Pauly, M. (1994). Comprehensive discharge planning for the hospitalized elderly: A randomized clinical trial. *Annals of Internal Medicine, 120*(12), 999–1006.

NCSBN Board of Directors Endorses the Consensus Model for APRN Regulation: Licensure, Accreditation, and Certification. (2008, July 7). Retrieved August 21, 2012, from https://www.ncsbn.org/7_23_08_Consensue_APRN_Final.pdf

Pfeiffer, E. (1998). Why teams? In E. Siegler, K. Hyer, T. Fulmer, & M. Mezey (Eds.), *Geriatric interdisciplinary team training* (p. 16). New York: Springer.

Stanley, Joan. (2009). Reaching consensus on a regulatory model: What does this mean for APRNs? *Journal for Nurse Practitioners, 5*(2), 99–104.

Strumpf, N., & Whitney, F. (1994).Teaching collaborative skills to nurse practitioner students. In E. Siegler & F. Whitney (Eds.), *Nurse-physician collaboration.* New York: Springer.

Stubenrauch, J. M. (2010). AJN reports. Report on the future of nursing: Recommendations aim to transform nursing education and practice. *American Journal of Nursing, 110*(12), 21–22. DOI: 10.1097/01.NAJ.0000391228.48071.be.

Thompson, J. E., Kershbaumer, R., & Krisman-Scott, M. (2001). *Educating advanced practice nurses and midwives: From practice to teaching.* New York: Springer.

Thompson, J. E., & Thompson, H. O. (1985). *Bioethical decision making for nurses.* Norwalk, CT: Appleton Century Fox.

Tresolini, C. P., & The Pew-Fetzer Task Force. (1994). *Health professional education and relationship-centered care.* San Francisco: Pew Health Professions Commission.

Tsukuda, R. A. (1990). Interdisciplinary collaboration: Teamwork in geriatrics. In C. K. Cassel, D. E. Riesenberg, L. B. Sorensen, & J. R. Walsh (Eds.), *Geriatric medicine* (2nd ed., pp. 668–675). New York: Springer-Verlag.

Tsukuda, R. A., & Stahelski, A. J. (1990). Guide to team skills: Predictors of cooperation in health care teams. *Small Group Research, 21*(2), 220–233.

Tuckman, B. W. (1965). Developmental sequences in small groups. *Psychological Bulletin, 63*(1), 384–399.

UNIT 3

Competency in Advanced Practice

13 Evidence-Based Practice

Deborah C. Messecar
Christine A. Tanner

INTRODUCTION

Translating evidence into practice is a key skill for advanced practice nurses (APNs). The increasing interest in knowledge translation, the process of moving research into practice and putting knowledge into action, coincides with the growing engagement in the evidence-based practice (EBP) approach, in which practitioners make practice decisions based on the integration of the research evidence with clinical expertise and the patient's unique values and circumstances (Straus, Glasziou, Richardson, & Haynes, 2011). Evidence-based practice builds on the process of using knowledge gleaned from systematic reviews and the results of individual studies, but includes much more, such as evidence from opinion leaders, the products of reasoning, clinical knowledge from practice experience, and patient preferences, to name a few (Melnyk & Fineout-Overholt, 2010). The importance of teaching critical appraisal of evidence and knowledge translation skills has only intensified in APN programs, for several reasons. First, the use of research for practice continues to be lacking as patients often fail to receive recommended standards of care or are receiving potentially harmful or unproven treatment (McGlynn, Asch, & Adams, 2003; Sung, Crowley, Genel, et al., 2003). A second major impetus for the movement to evidence-based practice is the growth of scientific evidence supporting health care and the development of methods for integrating the available evidence expeditiously into guidelines for practice (Arnoff, 2011). Information technology has greatly augmented our abilities to access this information. A third factor is that media dissemination of information has made patients increasingly savvy about different available treatments, enabling them to ask more informed questions about their illnesses and care (Cohen & Adams, 2011). Fourth, the urgency of using evidence to improve clinical care has been highlighted by the Institute of Medicine (IOM) reports on knowing what works in health care (IOM, 2008) as well as prior reports on quality and safety (IOM, 2001, 2004). Robust evidence-based practice skills applied with expert clinical judgment can help APNs narrow the gap between research and practice, and improve the quality and safety of care.

The objective of this chapter is to present a view of clinical judgment and the different patterns of clinical reasoning, and their relationship to translating evidence into practice. The importance of fostering clinical judgment and critical thinking in APN education was emphasized in the recent Carnegie report (Benner, Sutphen, Leonard, & Day, 2010). The emphasis on clinical judgment in APN education is consistent with recognizing that knowledge translation should include the complex process of applying the general facts derived from research in a particular situation, given the patient's circumstances and preferences (Tanner, 2009). Research on clinical judgment is presented to illustrate how nurses use reasoning patterns as they assess patients, selectively attend to clinical cues, interpret these data, and respond or intervene, and how evidence translation fits into this process. The role of context, the knowledge and experience background of the nurse, and the effect of knowing the patient on these reasoning processes is also described. A research-based model of clinical judgment (Benner,

Tanner, & Chesla, 2009; Tanner, 2006) is presented to provide a framework for understanding how the APN can draw on clinical decision-making skills developed over time in practice along with new skills in accessing and evaluating evidence to continuously improve the methods of care he or she is employing. This model helps guide judgments about what scientific literature is relevant for the questions at hand and whether the evidence the APN has to support the assessments, interpretations, and actions should be applied. In addition, tips on how to access and evaluate research evidence to improve the quality of the APN's clinical judgments are provided.

EVOLUTION OF EVIDENCE-BASED PRACTICE AND KNOWLEDGE TRANSLATION

Historically, evidence-based practice was presented as a new paradigm in health professions practice (Tanner, 1999). This approach devalued intuition, the use of clinical opinion based on experience, and basic scientific rationale as sufficient grounds for clinical decision making, and instead stressed the examination of evidence solely from clinical research (Bergus & Hamm, 1995). The aim of evidence-based practice defined in this manner is to reduce wider variations in individual clinician's practices, eliminating worst practices and enhancing best practices, thereby reducing costs and improving quality. This goal and the assumptions underlying what counts as evidence were troubling to many clinicians (Dearlove, Rogers, & Sharples, 1996; Mitchell, 1999; Smith, 1996). Their concern was that expert clinical judgment would be replaced by a cookbook approach to decision making. In response to this criticism, the definition of evidence-based medicine was revised to be more comprehensive in its view of what counts as evidence and what should figure into decisions regarding patient care. Evidence-based medicine is the use of the best research evidence in making decisions about the care of individual patients. To practice evidence-based medicine, clinicians must integrate their personal clinical expertise with the best available evidence from systematic research and apply this within the context of their patient's unique values and circumstances (Sackett, Rosenberg, Gray, Haynes, and Richardson, 1996; Straus, Glasziou, Richardson, & Haynes, 2011).

This revised and updated view recognized individual clinical expertise, which is defined as the proficiency and judgment that individual clinicians acquire through clinical experience and clinical practice, as a valid source of evidence. Increased expertise not only includes more effective and efficient diagnosis, but also more thoughtful identification and compassionate use of individual patients' predicaments, rights, and preferences in making clinical decisions about their care (Sackett et al., 1996; Straus et al., 2011). Best available external clinical evidence was defined as clinically relevant research, which may include basic sciences research, but was preferentially from patient-centered clinical research that focuses on the accuracy and precision of diagnostic tests (including the clinical examination), the power of prognostic markers, and the efficacy and safety of interventions. Use of external clinical evidence should invalidate previously accepted diagnostic tests and treatments, and replace them with new ones that are more powerful, more accurate, more efficacious, and safer. External clinical evidence can inform, but can never replace, individual clinical expertise, and it is this expertise that decides whether the external evidence applies to the individual patient at all, and if so, how it should be integrated into a clinical decision. In contrast, internal evidence is typically generated through practice initiatives, such as outcomes management or quality improvement projects undertaken for the purpose of improving clinical care in the setting in which it is produced.

The terms *evidence-based practice* and *knowledge translation* are related, and sometimes used interchangeably. Knowledge translation is defined as a process that includes knowledge synthesis and the tailored dissemination of knowledge inquiry to improve health and provide more efficient and effective health services (Straus, Tetroe, & Graham, 2009). Knowledge translation is a larger, more inclusive concept than evidence-based practice and includes all steps between the creation of new knowledge and its application. It includes evaluating practice-based evidence, facilitating evidence-based practice, and engaging in collaborative practice inquiry. The discussion of evidence-based practice in this chapter is focused on the search for, synthesis of, and implementation of research findings in practice and how this links with use of the APN's clinical judgment. Evidence-based practice in this view includes decision making about and implementation of care practices based on several kinds of evidence, such as findings from the literature, local practice data, national standards or opinions of recognized experts, and information on patient preferences. APNs are expected to integrate their clinical experience with conscientious, explicit, and judicious use of research evidence to inform their clinical judgment and make decisions that maximize the well-being of their patients.

RESEARCH ON CLINICAL JUDGMENT AND THE RELATIONSHIP TO EVIDENCE-BASED PRACTICE

What is clinical judgment? Almost all health professionals view clinical judgment as an essential skill. In nursing, the terms *clinical decision making* or *problem solving* and more recently *critical thinking* have been used interchangeably to refer to the same phenomenon, which has been viewed as a disengaged, analytical, and objective process, directed toward resolution of problems and achievement of clearly defined ends. However, research on expert practice suggests that clinical judgment is far more complex (Benner, Tanner, & Chesla, 2009; Tanner, 2006) and incorporates skills that look more like engaged practical reasoning. Engaged practical reasoning occurs when the nurse recognizes a pattern by being attuned to subtle changes in the patient's clinical state and other salient information, and then forms an intuitive clinical grasp of the situation without evident forethought (Benner, Tanner, & Chesla, 2009; Tanner, Benner, Chesla, & Gordon, 1993). This flexible and nuanced ability to read the clinical situation is key to interpreting what is going on and responding appropriately. Knowledge of the illness experience for both the patient and the family as well as their physical, social, and emotional strengths and weaknesses are just as important as clinical features of the disease.

Clinical judgment is thus defined as an understanding or inference about a patient's needs, concerns, or health problems, followed by the decision to act (or not act), to use or modify standard approaches, or to improvise new ones as deemed appropriate by the patient's response (Benner, Tanner, & Chesla, 2009; Tanner, 2006). *Clinical reasoning,* in contrast to clinical judgment, is the thinking process by which clinicians make their judgments and includes the process of generating alternatives, weighing them against the evidence, and choosing the most appropriate course of action (Benner, Tanner, & Chesla, 2009; Tanner, 2006).

Clinical judgment has been studied from different theoretical perspectives (Benner, Tanner, & Chesla, 2009; Brannon & Carson, 2003; Kosowski & Roberts, 2003; Ritter, 2003; Simmons, Lanuza, Fonteyn, Hicks, & Holm, 2003; White, 2003), with different clinical foci (McCarthy, 2003), and with different research methods (Benner et al., 2009; Kosowski & Roberts, 2003; McDonald, Frakes, Apostolidis, Armstrong, Goldblatt, & Bernardo, 2003; Ritter, 2003; Simmons et al., 2003; White, 2003). From this growing body of literature on clinical judgment, several general conclusions can be drawn.

The Clinician's Background Is More Influential on Clinical Judgment Than Objective Data

The clinician's background influences his or her clinical judgment in a given clinical situation more than the objective data at hand. Clinical judgment requires knowledge, which is abstract, generalizable, and applicable in many situations. Knowledge required for clinical judgment is derived from science and theory, and grows with experience as scientific abstractions are filled out in practice. This knowledge is often tacit and is an important factor in aiding clinicians to recognize clinical states instantaneously.

The clinician's background includes experiential learning, particularly that gleaned from personal clinical experience. Three types of knowledge play a part in how the clinician perceives a given situation. Theoretical knowledge, which is acquired through understanding of scientifically derived knowledge and theory, is used in a particular situation as a specific application of an abstract rule or principle. The description of techniques for examining the thorax and lungs in a physical assessment text is an example of theoretical knowledge that may be applied by the clinician to individual patients. Practical knowledge is acquired through working with many patients. So, adapting or revising one's examination of the thorax and lung techniques for a patient who cannot sit up based on one's past experience or the experience of others is an example of practical knowledge. Knowledge, both theoretical and practical, often determines what stands out as important in a particular situation. Research-based knowledge can contribute to the clinician's overall knowledge base for assessing risks. Knowledge helps the clinician observe selectively. Research directed toward describing phenomena of concern to the nurse helps provide information about what cues are highly associated with particular problems. This allows the nurse, using this knowledge base, to select data relevant to determining the problems the patient may be experiencing. Knowledge also guides action and contributes to the clinician's repertoire of interventions.

An additional essential component of the knowledge required for clinical judgment is the importance of knowing the individual patient and being able to draw on this understanding to better predict and anticipate individual patient responses (Benner et al., 2009; Peden-McAlpine & Clark, 2002). Clinicians come to clinical situations with their own perspectives on what is good and right, and these values profoundly influence what they attend to, the options they consider using, and ultimately what they decide to do (Benner et al., 2009; Ellefsen, 2004). The clinician's outlook is not determined by individual notions of right and wrong, but rather is developed through interaction with others in the practice discipline. For example, the ethic for disclosure to patients and families or the importance of comfort in the face of impending death sets up what will be noticed in a given clinical exchange and will shape the way in which the clinician responds. Stereotypes and biases also affect perception.

Good Clinical Judgment Requires Knowing the Patient and Responding to His or Her Concerns

In addition to theoretical and practical knowledge, knowledge of the particular patient, both knowing the patient's typical responses and knowing the patient as a person, is central to good clinical judgment (Haynes, Sackett, Guyatt, & Tugwell, 2006; Tanner et al., 1993). When the clinician knows the typical patterns of responses, certain aspects of the situation stand out as salient and others recede in importance. Comparing the current picture to the patient's typical picture allows the clinician to make important qualitative distinctions about how a patient's condition has or has not changed. Knowing the patient facilitates the provision of individualized care.

Knowing patients is defined as a taken-for-granted understanding of patients that comes from working with them, listening to their accounts of their experiences with illness, watching them closely, and understanding how they typically respond (Tanner et al., 1993). This tacit knowledge, which the clinician may not be able to fully describe to an outside observer, is more than what can be obtained in formal assessments. Knowing the typical pattern of responses, certain aspects of a patient's situation stand out as salient, and other aspects of that same patient situation may recede in importance.

Understanding how this patient responds under these circumstances forms the basis for the individualized care called for by the IOM's report (2001) on quality.

The level of involvement with the patient influences the way the clinician engages in problem solving, the outcome of the process, and the sense of satisfaction on the part of the clinician (Benner et al., 2009). Central to sound clinical decision making is a concern for revealing and responding to patients as persons, respecting their dignity, and caring for them in ways that preserve their personhood. Developing a sense about the right level of involvement is a skill learned through experience. The skilled clinician has a good clinical grasp, recognizing both familiar and individual patterns. The patient's responses to the nurse's actions are observed, and the nurse's reactions are then modified according to how the patient is responding (Benner et al., 2009; Tanner, 2006). Clinical grasp and clinical response are therefore inextricably linked.

Clinical Judgment Is Influenced by the Context in Which Care Occurs

Neither context nor emotions have typically been accounted for in most models of rational decision making. Models of decision making that ignore context, emotion, and the individual's experience eliminate the possibility of seeing these as important in clinical judgment. However, from the work of Benner and colleagues (2009), we know that judgment occurs in the context of a particular situation, when the nurse is emotionally attuned to the situation, meaningful aspects simply stand out as important, and the choice of responses is guided by the nurse's interpretation of the particular situation. The context for practice that influences decisions to test and treat can include political and social milieu (Benner et al., 2009; Tanner, 2006), as well as patient factors such as socioeconomic status (Scott, Schiell, & King, 1996). Another view is that social judgment or moral evaluation of patients is socially embedded, independent of patient characteristics, and as much a function of the pervasive norms and attitudes of the clinicians in a given setting (McDonald et al., 2003).

For clinician providers, health care is increasingly practiced in a context of heightened accountability (Klardie, Johnson, McNaughton, & Meyers, 2004). APNs are expected to demonstrate that they can provide care that is both clinically and cost effective (DeBourgh, 2001; Younglut & Brooten, 2001). The struggle for the APN in this environment is to deliver high-quality cost-effective care while still incorporating the needs and preferences of the individual patient (Klardie et al., 2004).

Clinicians Use a Variety of Clinical Reasoning Patterns Alone or in Combination

Work in the art of medical decision making has illustrated that the essence of clinical reasoning continues to elude understanding (Sox, Blatt, Higgins, & Marton, 2007). In studies conducted with nurses during the past 20 years, evidence suggests that nurses use a variety of reasoning patterns alone or in combination (Benner et al., 2009; Tanner, 2006). The pattern of reasoning that the clinician uses depends on the demands of the situation, the goals of the practice, the clinician's experience with similar situations, and the perception of what makes excellent practice. The reasoning patterns used are influenced by the nurse's knowledge, biases, and values; the relationship with the patient; and other factors in the clinical situation.

Analytic Processes

An analytic reasoning pattern is characteristic of a beginner's performance or a more experienced clinician when stumped. Analytic reasoning is characterized by deliberate, rational thought that includes the generation of alternatives, weighing against evidence, and evaluating possible courses of action. Analytic reasoning can be influenced by biases and stereotypes. Diagnostic reasoning is an example of analytic thinking. This is a process in which the clinician attends to presenting signs and symptoms (cues), generates alternative explanations for the cues (diagnostic hypotheses), collects additional data to help rule in or rule out possible explanations, systematically evaluates each explanation in light of the data, and arrives at a diagnosis, or inference, about the patient's health status. Once sufficient data are gathered, the process of evaluating hypotheses begins.

Intuition

Intuition is characterized by immediate grasping of a clinical situation and is a function of familiarity with similar experiences (Benner et al., 2009). Intuition is a judgment without a rationale. Researchers speculate that intuition is a form of pattern recognition in which the practitioner picks up on cues that are perceived as a whole and are not arrived at through conscious, or linear analytic processes. Experienced clinicians develop a sense of salience, in which important aspects of a given clinical situation stand out because of past experience with similar situations. Rational calculation is not required to make use of this form of reasoning; however, deliberative rationality may be used to check out the soundness of conclusions derived from intuition. The role and desirability of intuitive reasoning patterns continues to be controversial within the nursing literature. Intuition has been decried as a poor substitute for science. In this view, intuition is minimized as nothing more than a special case of inference, drawing on rational processes that are unconscious and inaccessible (Crow & Spicer, 1995; English, 1993). Recent studies in primary care and the application of evidence-based practice indicate, however, that intuition is a highly valued form of reasoning and plays a vital role in clinical decision making (Tracy, Dantos, & Upshur, 2003).

Narrative Thinking

Evidence suggests that narratives are an important part of clinical reasoning (Bruner, 1986; Kleinman, 1988). Patient narratives provide us with access to understanding the experience of health and illness. Bruner claims that human motives, intents, and meanings are understood through narrative thinking, which he contrasts with paradigmatic thinking that conforms to the rules of logic. Paradigmatic thinking is thinking through propositional argument. Narrative thinking is thinking through telling and interpreting stories. The difference between these two types of thinking involves how humans make sense of and explain what they see. Propositional argument is making sense of a particular by seeing it as an instance of a general type. Narrative thinking is trying to understand the particular case. Kleinman has identified the importance of understanding the narrative component of illness, claiming that patient narratives may help clinicians direct their attention not only to the biological world of disease, but also to the human world of meanings, values, and concerns.

Hence, patient narratives help clinicians to focus their attention not only on the patient's disease problems, but also on the meaning of that illness for the particular patient and on the affect that disease will have on the patient's lifestyle and ways of coping. Hearing the account of an experience with an illness not only improves the understanding of the patient's overall situation, it helps identify problem-solving priorities that cannot be made explicit through disengaged analytical reasoning. Studies of physicians (Borges & Waitzkin, 1995; Hunter, 1991) and nurses (Benner et al., 2009; Zerwekh, 1992) suggest that narrative reasoning creates deep background understanding of the patient as a person; consequently, clinicians' judgments can be understood only against this background.

Clinical narratives are a way of teaching and learning from other care providers and a way of reflecting on and understanding one's own practice. By dialoguing with others who may have different vantage points, knowledge about clinical situations is produced that helps to limit tunnel vision and snap judgments. Using narrative as a way of communicating with other health providers leads to learning how to better identify signs and symptoms in particular patient populations, knowing specific patients and learning to recognize how these patients respond, and identifying clinical experts with whom you can consult (Benner et al., 2009). Discussing your observations and data with more experienced clinicians enhances clinical judgment. Even as an experienced nurse, you consult with colleagues, draw on their perspectives, and benefit from the pooled experience of other clinicians. Clinical narratives and the multiple perspectives of skilled clinicians work together with science and technology to create knowledge that is both cumulative and reliable.

Clinical reasoning can also include processes that might be characterized as engaged practical reasoning. Engaged practical reasoning includes recognition of a pattern, an intuitive clinical grasp, or a response without evident forethought. Conditions of uncertainty are what prompt the seeking, appraising, and implementation of new knowledge by clinicians. Uncertainty occurs when the best course of action to take, or best decision, is not readily apparent. The openness to accept that there may be different, and possibly more effective, methods of care other than those that are currently employed acts as the impetus to weighing evidence against expectations, norms, or standards.

Reflection on Practice Is Often Triggered by a Breakdown in Clinical Judgment

Reflection is defined as a process of thinking about and exploring an issue of concern triggered by an experience. For example, clinicians are often troubled by a patient encounter that did not go well. Reflecting on the meaning of an experience, making sense of it, and incorporating it into one's view of self and the world is part of everyday life. Reflection prompts the clinician to identify new information or alternative perspectives that can be helpful in future encounters. To engage in reflection, the clinician has to be able to connect the patient's response and outcomes with specific clinical actions. Narrative is an important tool of reflection; having and telling stories of one's experience as a clinician helps turn experience into practical knowledge (Aström, Norberg, Hallberg, & Jansson, 1995; Benner et al., 2009). Use of reflection is a habit and a skill that can be cultivated and developed over time. Through the introspective process of connecting one's actions to patient outcomes, reflection has the potential for generating new knowledge (Kuiper & Pesut, 2004; Ruth-Sahd, 2003).

Model of Clinical Judgment

A research-based model of clinical judgment developed by Tanner in 1998 and revised in 2006 is presented in **Figure 13-1.** There are four key phases in the model. The first is "noticing," in which the clinician develops a perceptual grasp of the situation at hand. In this phase, the clinician's expectations of the situation are formed as a result of his or her knowledge of the patient; clinical or practical knowledge of similar patients; and textbook and research-based knowledge. The context of the clinical situation will further influence the initial grasp of the situation. The second phase depicted in the model is "interpreting." In this phase the clinician forms an understanding of the situation by using one or more reasoning patterns. Assessments and additional data collection may be conducted to rule out hypotheses until the clinician reaches an interpretation that supports an appropriate response. During the "responding" phase, the clinician may act or choose not to act depending on the situation. "Reflecting" occurs when the clinician observes the patient's responses to the action taken. *Reflection-in-action* refers to the clinician's ability to see how the patient is responding to the action—and adjust the treatment based on that assessment. Much of this reflection-in-action is tacit and not obvious.

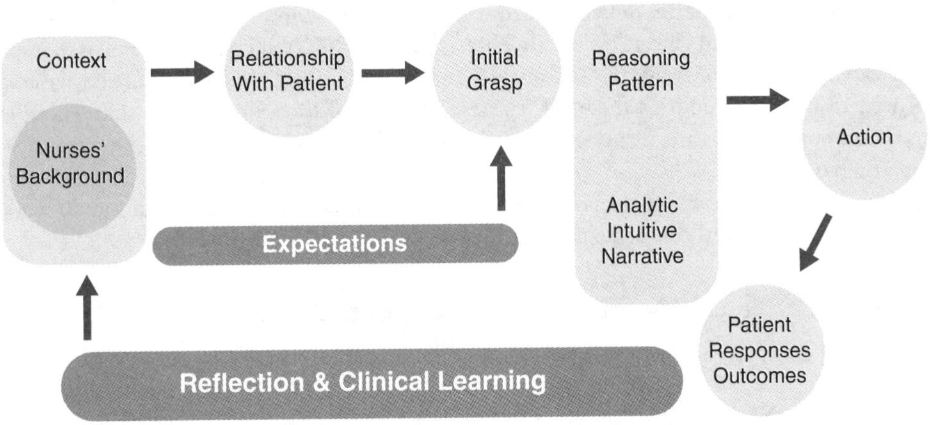

FIGURE 13-1 A model of clinical judgment.

Reflection-in-action with its subsequent clinical learning completes the cycle, showing that what clinicians gain from their experience contributes to their ongoing clinical knowledge development and their capacity for clinical judgment in future situations.

Summary

The model of clinical judgment presented provides a framework for improving the quality of the clinical judgment used by the APN. First, the model illustrates where in the process of clinical reasoning the knowledge that might be obtained by external evidence can be applied. Second, the model recognizes the value of clinical expertise initially not accounted for by the original proponents of evidence-based practice. Third, because the model recognizes a broader range of contextual factors that could affect the patient's responses, it is more inclusive in the types of research that are viewed as valid. Fourth, because the model incorporates the value of knowing the patient in the clinical reasoning process, it supports a model of patient-centered care (IOM, 2001).

ACCESSING AND EVALUATING RESEARCH EVIDENCE TO IMPROVE CLINICAL JUDGMENTS

Several problems exist with using the research literature for evidence-based primary care and hospital practice (Gorman, 2001; Melynyk & Fineout-Overholt, 2010; Shapiro, 2007, 2010). Clinicians are under increasing pressure to keep up to date and to base their practice more firmly on evidence, but few have the necessary time or skills to do this (Melnyk & Fineout-Overholt, 2010).

Historically, only a small fraction of the total research literature included efficacy studies of clinical practice that form the basis for evidence-based medicine (Haynes, 1993; Shapiro, 2010). Few if any studies addressed appropriateness, meaningfulness, and feasibility of health-care innovations (Sharpiro, 2010). This has contributed to the complaint of many clinicians that the research literature has limited applicability to clinical practice (Greer, 1988; McAlister, Graham, Karr, & Laupacis, 1999).

In the past, most clinicians considered the research literature to be unmanageable (Gorman, 2001; Melynyk & Fineout-Overholt, 2010; Shapiro, 2007, 2010; Williamson, German, Weiss, Skinner, &

Bowes III, 1989). On top of this difficulty, many clinicians do not know how to interpret the statistical results of the studies they do locate (Windish, Huot, & Green, 2007). If clinical research is to improve clinical care, it must be relevant, of high quality, and accessible, and clinicians must have the skills they need to use it. To address these difficulties, APNs need to build skills in sharpening their focus on the outcomes of care, forming clear and researchable questions, accessing the literature, and interpreting its relevance.

To access the best possible evidence at the point of clinical contact, the clinician should work on the development of several competencies that support evidence-based practice.

Competencies That Support Evidence-Based Practice

Focusing on Outcomes and Context

Evidence-based medicine has been widely promoted as a means of improving clinical outcomes. To focus on outcomes in medical decision making, Bergus and Hamm (1995) and Sox and colleagues (2007) suggest that clinicians use the following four-step process. First, the clinician forms an internal mental framework for the decision task, sketching out the potential treatment options and outcomes. Next, the variations among the different outcomes are estimated. In collaboration with the patient and family, the values of the potential outcomes are considered. The course of action that, on average, will result in the best outcome is then chosen. The scientific evidence—base rate information, sensitivity, specificity, positive predictive value of a positive test results, and proportion of the population positively affected by certain interventions—is the information needed for estimating the likelihood of achieving different outcomes with different courses of action.

Straus, Glasziou, Richardson, and Haynes (2011), in their guidebook on the practice and teaching of evidence-based medicine, define the best research evidence as patient-centered clinical research into the accuracy and precision of diagnostic tests, prognostic markers, and interventions. These elements of evidence used for predicting outcomes are defined and described in **Table 13-1.** Several practical implications can be drawn from review of the definitions of the core concepts in the table. For example, to determine the predictive value of a test, clinicians need good estimates of the prevalence or probability of disease in a patient.

A limitation of this approach to best evidence is nursing's interest in questions beyond diagnostic tests and interventions (Jennings, 2000) to include important issues surrounding the context of care. Although evidence from qualitative exploratory studies is not usually included in texts on evidence-based medicine, these studies are helpful for guiding advanced practice decision making. Appropriateness and meaningfulness, according to Evans (2003) and the Joanna Briggs Institute (2008), addresses the psychosocial aspects of care, relating to the patients' experiences, their understanding of health and illness, and the outcomes they hope to achieve from their health-care encounter. These dimensions of care are best addressed with nonexperimental research designs, including both quantitative and qualitative methods (Shapiro, 2010). Change in health-care delivery environments is difficult, and evidence of effectiveness and appropriateness may not be enough to overcome problems that surface with change. In addition to the usual sources of high-level evidence, such as randomized controlled trials (RCTs), systematic reviews, observational studies, and interpretive studies, may yield good evidence, especially related to aspects of organizational culture that could both affect the ease of acceptance of the new practice and help determine how best to implement it (Evans, 2003). These studies inform our decision making by helping us better understand patient responses. Understanding patient responses is a critical condition for using reflection to engage in clinical learning.

TABLE 13-1

Information Needed for Estimating the Likelihood of Achieving Different Outcomes with Different Courses of Action

Core Concept	Definition	Features
Base rate information: prevalence	The proportion of persons in a given population who have a particular disease at a point or interval of time	Useful for health services planning. May be the only rates available. Prevalence studies are particularly useful in guiding decisions about diagnosis and treatment. Knowing that a patient has a given probability of having a disease influences the use and interpretation of diagnostic tests.
Base rate information: incidence	New cases in a specified period	Use incidence rates when (a) you are comparing the development of disease in different population groups; (b) you are attempting to determine whether a relationship exists between a possible causal factor and a disease. Allows you to determine whether the probability of developing a disease differs in different populations or periods in relationship to specific causal factors.
Sensitivity	Proportion of people with the disease who have a positive test	Determines the ability of the test to identify correctly those who have the disease. The more sensitive a test, the more certain you can be that a negative test rules out disease.
Specificity	Proportion of people without the disease who have a negative test	Determines the ability of the test to identify correctly those who do not have the disease. The more specific a test, the more certain you can be that a positive test rules in disease.
Positive predictive value of positive tests	Probability of disease, given the results of a positive test	Sensitivity and specificity are characteristics of the test itself; however, predictive values are influenced by how common the disease is. For diseases of low prevalence, the predictive value of a positive test goes down sharply.
Absolute risk reduction	Difference in adverse event rates between the control and experimental group	Is used to help determine the clinical significance of a treatment—needed to calculate NNT*.
Number needed to treat	Number of patients needed to treat to prevent one additional bad outcome	Calculated by dividing 1 by the absolute risk reduction. NNT indicates clinical impact of a treatment.

Continued

TABLE 13-1

Information Needed for Estimating the Likelihood of Achieving Different Outcomes with Different Courses of Action—cont'd

Core Concept	Definition	Features
Confidence interval	Range of values on either side	A 99% confidence interval is interpreted of an estimate as the range of values within which one can be 99% sure that the population value lies.
P value	Measure of statistical significance	Specifies the strength of the evidence.

NNT, number needed to treat.

Asking Answerable Questions

The inability to ask a focused and precise clinical question can be a major impediment to evidence-based practice. To build skill in asking focused clinical questions, it helps to categorize questions according to their level of specificity and according to whom the question applies, the intervention being considered, and the outcomes of interest.

Clinical questions can be categorized into needs for background and foreground knowledge (Melnyk & Fineout-Overholt, 2010; Straus et al., 2011). Background knowledge is needed when our experience with a condition or problem is limited. Background questions ask *who, what, for whom, why, where, when,* and *how well?* Framing a background question is relatively easy because the question is usually asking in general about a disorder. Finding information to answer background questions is also relatively easy. Sources of information likely to provide answers to these questions include textbooks, drug guides or other reference books, and narrative review articles—summaries of an area or topic written by an expert in the field (McKibbon & Marks, 2001).

As clinicians grow in experience, they have increasing numbers of questions about the foreground of managing patients. Foreground questions are prompted by a precise need for information about a specific clinical situation. This skill of framing foreground questions can be improved by breaking the question down into its component parts. Think about the subjects or groups involved, what intervention is being used, and what the outcomes of interest are. The four key elements of foreground questions are the patient or problem, the intervention or treatment, the comparison intervention or treatment, and the outcome of interest (Melnyk & Fineout-Overholt, 2010; Straus et al., 2011). Foreground questions typically require more information sources to adequately supply the answers (McKibbon & Marks, 2001). For example, questions about treatment effectiveness are best addressed by evidence from an RCT design, whereas questions about patients' feelings and perceptions about their illness experiences are better addressed in studies that use a qualitative design.

Using the Clinical Literature

The clinical literature can be used for regular surveillance or keeping up to date and for problem-oriented searches. To conduct searchers on a regular basis, clinicians need effective searching skills and easy access to bibliographic databases. After the answerable question has been identified, use the population/problem, intervention, comparison, outcome, time (PICOT) format to help frame the literature search **Box 13-1.** The PICOT format is a particularly useful framework to help novice searchers organize their electronic database searches (Craig & Smyth, 2007; Melnyk & Fineout-Overholt, 2010; Shapiro, 2007, 2010; Shapiro & Donaldson, 2008).

Two types of electronic databases are available. The first type is bibliographic and permits users to identify relevant citations in the clinical literature. MEDLINE and the *Cumulative Index to Nursing and Allied Health Literature* are examples of this first sort of database. Google Scholar (http://scholar.google.com) is a new database that is also becoming more popular. The second type of database takes the user directly to primary or secondary publications of the relevant clinical evidence. Examples of this second type of database include the *Cochrane Database of Systematic Reviews* and the American College of Physicians (ACP) Journal Club, a publication of the American College of Physicians–American Society of Internal Medicine, which abstracts articles on diagnosis, prognosis, treatment, quality of care, and medical economics. The ACP database has recently been "repurposed" and formatted to make clinician searching for answers to clinical questions easier (Haynes, 2008). These databases are available online from libraries and from the organizations themselves via the Internet.

Appraising Evidence from Studies

After evidence has been retrieved, the next step is to evaluate, or appraise, the evidence for its validity and clinical usefulness. Appraisal is crucial because it lets the clinician decide whether the retrieved research literature is reliable enough to give useful guidance. Because a number of published reports lack sufficient methodological rigor to be reliable enough for answering clinical questions, guidelines for evaluating literature have been developed to assist clinicians without extensive research expertise to evaluate clinical articles.

Box 13-2 shows a typical set of critical appraisal questions for evaluating articles about therapy. These questions were synthesized from a number of sources (EBP HealthLinks and CEBM Web site; Badenoch & Heneghan, 2006; Straus et al., 2011). Although the questions seem to reflect common sense, they are not entirely self-explanatory. Some assistance is required to help clinicians apply them to specific articles and individual patients. The *Evidence-Based Medicine Toolkit* (Badenoch & Heneghan, 2006) provides guidance on how to answer the appraisal questions that they specifically recommend. For example, on the question, "Were research participants 'blinded'?" the text gives the clinician a definition of the term *blinding,* and then might provide an example that would help clinicians decide whether the studies they were evaluating met this criteria. In addition to providing a guide for evaluating therapy articles, the *Evidence-Based Medicine Toolkit* has questions for appraising articles on diagnosis, prognosis, and harm (risks for certain diseases or conditions). The *Evidence-Based Medicine Toolkit* is a great resource for beginners. As with any other skill, expertise and speed come with practice. The evidence does not automatically dictate patient care, but it does provide the factual basis on which decisions can be made.

BOX 13-1
PICOT Format

P Population or problem of interest
I Intervention or practice of interest
C Comparison intervention or practice—usually what is currently done
O Outcome of the intervention or practice
T Time frame in which outcome is expected

BOX 13-2
Appraising Therapy Articles

Critical appraisal questions used to evaluate a therapy article:
Is the study valid?
Was there a clearly defined research question?
Was the assignment of patients to treatments randomized and was the randomization list concealed?
Were all patients accounted for at its conclusion? Was there an "intention-to-treat" analysis?
Were research participants "blinded"?
Were the groups treated equally throughout?
Did randomization produce comparable groups at the start of the trial?
Are the results important?
How large is the treatment effect?
How precise is the finding from the trial?

As APNs begin to build their literature critical appraisal skills, several Web sites can be accessed to further refine these skills. The HealthLinks site (http://healthlinks.washington.edu/ebp) at the University of Washington includes an evidence-based practice section that contains numerous resources for finding, evaluating, and rating the literature. In addition to this site, the Center for Evidence-Based Medicine (CEBM) has the CATmaker critical appraisal tool (http://www.cebm.net/index.aspx?o=1157), which can be downloaded to help the APN create Critically Appraised Topics (CATs) for the key articles they encounter about therapy, diagnosis, prognosis, etiology/harm, and systematic reviews of therapy.

Sources of Primary Clinical and Research Literature

MEDLINE is provided free on the Internet from many sites, and at least one of these, PubMed (http://www.ncbi.nlm.nih.gov/pubmed), also includes restored search strategies that are designed to select studies most likely to be relevant and valid for clinical practice. MEDLINE is produced by the National Library of Medicine in Bethesda, Maryland, and is the best-known bibliographic database of indexed medical literature. MEDLINE is searchable by medical subject headings and subheadings, as well as by author, journal, title, and keyword. The journals covered by MEDLINE are noted for their overall reliability and quality; however, the articles still must be scrutinized carefully for their validity and quality as evidence. A hand search of current journals is still one of the best ways to find newly published information. However, this is one of the most time-consuming and labor-intensive approaches to retrieving evidence.

Using Appraising Summaries

Meta-analysis uses statistical techniques to combine results across studies. Integrative reviews rely on summaries, logical synthesis, and narrative to characterize findings. Research-based guidelines center on care of a particular patient population and specify processes of care associated with good outcomes. Both HealthLinks and the CEBM Web sites have links to several sources of summaries.

Meta-Analysis

Meta-analysis requires enough studies with sufficient commonality to provide a valid conclusion. In other words, studies have to be looking more or less at the same outcome and the same intervention. Meta-analysis is often used when several studies have been conducted but findings were inconclusive. Meta-analyses combine the statistical results from several studies into one statistic that can be used to gauge the size of the treatment's impact on the outcome of interest. To do this, first an effect size is calculated for each finding of interest in the studies being reviewed. Then a pooled effect size is calculated for all findings together.

There is controversy about the statistical techniques and assumptions of meta-analysis. Bias in the combined analysis is possible if the selection of studies was flawed or the elimination of methodologically poor studies was not done using an objective process. There are also inherent problems with data pooling, especially if the studies are not similar enough in design, sample size, outcome types, and forms of the independent variables used. Identifying weaknesses in this kind of systematic review can be done by using the guidelines in the *Evidence-Based Medicine Toolkit* (Badenoch & Heneghan, 2006) or by using a similar guide on the HealthLinks or CEBM sites. Once you have examined the major components of the review, you can make a judgment about whether you think it is a high-quality review and whether the findings are valid.

Integrative Research Review

Integrative research reviews do not use statistical techniques to summarize results across studies. Rather, they rely on the logical comparison and synthesis of the reviewer. The integrative research review method is the research synthesis approach that most review articles in clinical care journals use. The quality of these reviews and their resulting conclusions are even more dependent on the reviewer's skill in critical appraisal. High-quality reviews make explicit how studies were selected for review and the rules that were used to judge the overall evidence. The reviewer should state whether some studies were weighted more heavily than others and should provide a rationale for doing so. If some studies were discounted, this also should be described. At present, integrative research review is the only mechanism available for looking at qualitative studies that address the same topic.

Practice Guidelines

Practice guidelines can include formal clinical protocols put forth by a professional organization, clinical paths formed by a practice group, and research-based recommendations that translate conclusions of a meta-analysis or an integrative research review into clinical practice conclusions. A practice guideline should clearly state what the guideline does and does not cover, what patient group it was designed for, the options at each decision point, the actions recommended, and the outcomes associated with each course of action. There should be a clear description of the supporting evidence and how it was gathered and evaluated. Because the literature is always evolving, practice guidelines should be explicit about how current they are. The comprehensiveness of the guideline should also be described. On the HealthLinks site, there is a link to the EBM toolkit that has a practice guidelines appraisal tool.

Locating Sources of Summaries

Ovid (www.ovid.com) has released an integrated literature service called Evidence-Based Medicine Reviews (EBMR). This Web-based service includes the *Cochrane Database of Systematic Reviews, Best Evidence,* MEDLINE, and full-text journals. This resource contains full-text reviews of clinically relevant articles from throughout the medical literature published in EBMR and ACP Journal Club, and full-text topic overviews published in the *Cochrane Database of Systematic Reviews,* published by the Cochrane Collaboration. Links between the Ovid databases and EBMR allow users to link from a citation to a review to the full text of that reviewed article, and then to other readings referenced in the article.

The *British Medical Journal* (BMJ) publishing group and the American College of Physicians–American Society of Internal Medicine have created *Clinical Evidence,* the first major attempt to provide an up-to-date, evidence-based textbook (www.clinicalevidence.com). Subscribers can choose between receiving the service online, via a handbook titled the *Clinical Evidence Handbook,* or a combination of the handbook plus online, as well as via PDA resources. A free trial is permitted to allow potential users the opportunity to explore the usefulness of the service.

The Agency for Healthcare Research and Quality (AHRQ) National Guidelines Clearinghouse provides evidence-based information on health-care outcomes; quality; and cost, use, and access. In examining what works and does not work in health care, AHRQ's mission includes both translating research findings into better patient care and providing policy makers and other health-care leaders with information needed to make critical health-care decisions. Reports compiled by evidence-based practice centers are available on a range of topics and can cover a number of therapies for a given condition. By using your browser's "Find" feature, you can quickly locate a given topic.

The Cochrane Collaboration produces a structured database of high-quality systematic reviews of RCTs. Originally established in Britain, it is presently composed of numerous centers in several countries. Reviews involve exhaustive searches for all RCTs, both published and unpublished, on a particular topic. One limitation of the database is that the reviews focus mainly on therapies, although an increasing number of reviews on diagnostic topics are being developed. The studies are analyzed using standardized methodology and meta-analysis. The Cochrane Library, now managed by Wiley, contains high-quality, independent evidence to inform health-care decision making. It includes reliable evidence from Cochrane and other systematic reviews, clinical trials, and more. Cochrane reviews bring you the combined results of the world's best medical research studies and are recognized as the gold standard in evidence-based health care.

Nursing-specific resources for evidence reviews have also been developed. The Joanna Briggs Institute (JBI; at www.joannabriggs.edu.au), based in Australia, is committed to evidence translation and use worldwide. JBI produces evidence summaries and provides guidelines on evidence application to practice. The *Online Journal of Knowledge Synthesis for Nursing* is a peer-reviewed online journal dedicated to the scientific advancement of evidence-based practice in health care. The journal presents current scientific evidence to inform clinical decisions and ongoing discussions on issues, methods, clinical practice, and teaching strategies for evidenced-based practice. Each article is written as a synthesis of research studies on a single topic and concludes with practice implications.

Clinical Significance and Appraisal Process

Having identified evidence that is both valid and relevant, the next step in using the evidence is to make a judgment about applying the evidence with your patient, in your setting. **Box 13-3** provides a list of questions that clinicians can use to make a judgment about the clinical application of the research findings. You must determine whether your patient is sufficiently similar to the study participants for the results to be applicable. Critical factors that can affect generalizability include demographics such as race, age, and gender. Other factors to consider relate to the feasibility of implementation of the proposed intervention, diagnostic test, and so on. Once the clinician has weighed the clinical use of the evidence and determined that implementation is feasible or desirable, he or she can either implement it directly in a patient's care or use it to develop protocols and guidelines.

BOX 13-3
Clinical Significance Appraisal Process: Questions to Guide Thinking

To determine applicability to practice, answer the following questions:
Were the subjects similar to patients for whom you might provide care now or in the future?
Could you base an intervention on the findings of this external evidence?
Would any intervention you might identify be within your scope of practice?
What does the body of evidence say about the general question that motivated the inquiry?
What actions does the body of evidence warrant?

EVIDENCE-BASED PRACTICE AND ATTITUDE

This chapter has not been developed as a stand-alone resource for learning the principles of evidence-based practice. It is almost impossible to learn how to search effectively and appraise efficiently without the help of others and without good resources. Working in groups is the best method to master these skills. Share the task of searching and appraising with others. Use secondary publications such as the *Best Evidence* text developed by the BMJ publishing group. Develop a system for storing work and sharing it with others. Electronic information storage and retrieval systems are evolving rapidly, so continued updates in the available technology are necessary. When evidence is used to inform clinical judgment, the APN can take advantage of new knowledge developments so that care can be more individualized, effective, streamlined, and dynamic.

REFERENCES

Arnoff, S. C. (2011). *Translational research and clinical practice.* New York: Oxford University Press.

Aström, G., Norberg, A., Hallberg, I. R., & Jansson, J. (1995). Experienced and skilled nurses' narratives of situations where caring action made a difference to the patient. *Scholarly Inquiry for Nursing Practice, 7*(3), 183–193.

Badenoch, D., & Heneghan, C. (2006). *Evidence-based medicine toolkit* (2nd ed.). London: BMJ Books.

Benner, P., Sutphen, M., Leonard, V., & Day, L. (2010). *Educating nurses: A call for radical transformation.* San Francisco: Jossey-Bass.

Benner, P., Tanner, C. A., & Chesla, C. A. (2009). *Expertise in nursing practice: Caring, clinical judgment, and ethics* (2nd ed.). New York: Springer.

Bergus, G. R., & Hamm, R. M. (1995). Clinical practice. How physicians make medical decisions and why medical decision making can help. *Primary Care: Clinics in Office Practice, 22*(2), 167–180.

Borges, S., & Waitzkin, H. (1995). Women's narratives in primary care medical encounters. *Women and Health, 23*(1), 29–56.

Brannon, L. A., & Carson, K. L. (2003). The representativeness heuristic: Influence on nurses' decision making. *Applied Nursing Research, 16*(3), 201–204.

Bruner, J. (1986). *Actual minds, possible worlds.* Cambridge, MA: Harvard University.

Cohen, R. A., & Adams, P. F. (2011). Use of the Internet for health information: United States 2009. NCHS data brief, no. 66. Hyattsville, MD: National Center for Health Statistics.

Craig, J. V., & Smyth, R. L. (2007). *The evidence-based practice manual for nurses* (2nd ed.). Edinburgh: Churchill Livingston Elsevier.

Crow, R., & Spicer, J. (1995). Categorisation of the patient's medical condition—An analysis of nursing judgment. *International Journal of Nursing Studies, 32*(5), 413–422.

Dearlove, O. R., Rogers, J., & Sharples, A. (1996). Evidence-based medicine. Authors' redefinition is better but not perfect [letter; comment]. *BMJ, 313,* 170–171.

DeBourgh, G. A. (2001). Champions for evidence-based practice: A critical role for advanced practice nurses. *AACN Clinical Issues: Advanced Practice in Acute and Critical Care, 12*(4), 491–508.

Ellefsen, B. (2004). Frames and perspectives in clinical nursing practice: A study of Norwegian nurses in acute care settings. *Research and Theory in Nursing Practice, 18*(1), 95–109.

English, I. (1993). Intuition as a function of the expert nurse: A critique of Benner's novice to expert model. *Journal of Advanced Nursing, 18*(3), 387–393.

Evans, D. (2003). Hierarchy of evidence: A framework for ranking evidence evaluating healthcare interventions. *Journal of Clinical Nursing, 12,* 77–84.

Gorman, P. (2001). Information needs in primary care: A survey of rural and nonrural primary care physicians. *Medinfo, 10*(pt 1), 338–342.

Greer, A. L. (1988). The state of the art versus the state of the science. The diffusion of new medical technologies into practice. *International Journal of Technology Assessment in Health Care, 4*(1), 5–26.

Haynes, R. B. (1993). Where's the meat in clinical journals? *ACP Journal Club, 119,* A16.

Haynes, R. B. (2008). ACP Journal Club is dead . . . long live ACP Journal Club. *ACP Journal Club, 148*(2), A8.

Haynes, R. B., Sackett, D. L., Guyatt, G. H., & Tugwell, P. (2006). *Clinical epidemiology: How to do clinical practice research* (3rd ed.). New York: Lippincott Williams & Wilkins.

Hunter, K. M. (1991). *Doctor's stories: The narrative structure of medical knowledge.* Princeton, NJ: Princeton University.

Institute of Medicine. (2001). *Crossing the quality chasm: A new health system for the 21st century.* Committee on Quality of Health Care in America. Washington, DC: Author.

Institute of Medicine. (2004). *Keeping patients safe: Transforming the work environment of nurses.* Washington, DC: The National Academies Press.

Institute of Medicine. (2008). *Knowing what works in health care: A roadmap for the nation.* Washington, DC: The National Academies Press.

Jennings, B. M. (2000). Evidence-based practice: The road best traveled? *Research in Nursing and Health, 23*(5), 343–345.

Joanna Briggs Institute. (2008). The JBI approach to evidence-based practice. Retrieved September 6, 2011, from http://latrobe.libguides.com/JoannaBriggs.

Klardie, K. A., Johnson, J., McNaughton, M., & Meyers, W. (2004). Integrating the principles of evidence-based practice into clinical practice. *Journal of the American Academy of Nurse Practitioners, 16*(3), 98–105.

Kleinman, A. (1988). *Illness narratives: Suffering, healing and the human condition.* New York: Basic Books.

Kosowski, M. M., & Roberts, V. W. (2003). When protocols are not enough: Intuitive decision making by novice nurse practitioners. *Journal of Holistic Nursing, 21*(1), 52–72.

Kuiper, R. A., & Pesut, D. J. (2004). Promoting cognitive and metacognitive reflective reasoning skills in nursing practice: Self-regulated learning theory. *Journal of Advanced Nursing, 45*(4), 381–391.

McAlister, F. A., Graham, I., Karr, G. W., & Laupacis, A. (1999). Evidence-based medicine and the practicing clinician. *Journal of General Internal Medicine, 14*(4), 236–242.

McCarthy, M. C. (2003). Situated clinical reasoning: Distinguishing acute confusion from dementia in hospitalized older adults. *Research in Nursing and Health, 26*(2), 90–101.

McDonald, D. D., Frakes, M., Apostolidis, B., Armstrong, B., Goldblatt, S., & Bernardo, D. (2003). Effect of a psychiatric diagnosis on nursing care for nonpsychiatric problems. *Research in Nursing and Health, 26*(2), 225–232.

McGlynn, E. A., Asch, S. M., & Adams, J. (2003). The quality of health care delivered to adults in the United States. *New England Journal of Medicine, 348,* 2635–2645.

McKibbon, K. A., & Marks, S. (2001). Posing clinical questions: Framing the question for scientific inquiry. *AACN Clinical Issues, 12*(4), 477–481.

Melnyk, B. M., & Fineout-Overholt, E. (2010). *Evidence-based practice in nursing and healthcare* (2nd ed.). Philadelphia: Lippincott Williams & Wilkins.

Mitchell, G. J. (1999). Practice applications. Evidence-based practice: Critique and alternative view. *Nursing Science Quarterly, 12*(1), 30–35.

Peden-McAlpine, C., & Clark, N. (2002). Early recognition of client status changes: The importance of time. *Dimensions of Critical Care Nursing, 21*(4), 144–151.

Ritter, B. J. (2003). An analysis of expert nurse practitioners' diagnostic reasoning. *Journal of the American Academy of Nurse Practitioners, 15*(3), 137–141.

Ruth-Sahd, L. A. (2003). Reflective practice: A critical analysis of data-based studies and implications for nursing education. *Journal of Nursing Education, 42*(11), 488–497.

Sackett, D. L., Rosenberg, W. M., Gray, J. A., Haynes, R. B., & Richardson, W. S. (1996). Evidence-based medicine: What it is and what it isn't. *British Medical Journal, 312*(7023), 71–72.

Scott, P., Shiell, A., & King, M. (1996). Is general practitioner decision-making associated with patient socio-economic status? *Social Science and Medicine, 42*(1), 35–46.

Shapiro, S. E. (2007). Evidence-based practice for advanced practice emergency nurses. *Advanced Emergency Nursing Journal, 29*(4), 331–338.

Shapiro, S. E. (2010). Grading evidence for practice. *Advanced Emergency Nursing Journal, 32*(1), 59–67.

Shapiro, S. E., & Donaldson, N. E. (2008). Evidence-based practice for advanced practice emergency nurses, part II. Critically appraising the literature. *Advanced Emergency Nursing Journal, 30,* 139–147.

Simmons, B., Lanuza, D., Fonteyn, M., Hicks, F., & Holm, K. (2003). Clinical reasoning in experienced nurses. *Western Journal of Nursing Research, 25*(6), 701–719; [discussion] 720–724.

Smith, B. H. (1996). Evidence-based medicine. Rich sources of evidence are ignored. *British Medical Journal, 313*(7050), 169–171.

Sox, H. C., Blatt, M. A., Higgins, M. C., & Marton, K. I. (2007). *Medical decision making.* Philadelphia: American College of Physicians.

Straus, S. E., Glasziou, P., Richardson, W. S., & Haynes, R. B. (2011). *Evidence-based medicine: How to practice and teach EBM* (4th ed.). Churchill Livingstone: Edinburgh.

Straus, S. E., Tetroe, J., & Graham, I. D. (2009). *Knowledge translation in health care: Moving from evidence to practice.* Oxford: Wiley-Blackwell.

Sung, N. S., Crowley, W. F. Jr., Genel, M., et al. (2003). Central challenges facing the national clinical research enterprise. *Journal of the American Medical Association, 289,* 1278–1287.

Tanner, C. A. (1998). Clinical judgment and evidence-based practice: Conclusions and controversies. *Communicating Nursing Research, 31*(2), 19–35.

Tanner, C. A. (1999). Evidence-based practice: Research and critical thinking. *Journal of Nursing Education, 38*(3), 99.

Tanner, C. A. (2006). Thinking like a nurse: A research-based model of clinical judgment in nursing. *Journal of Nursing Education, 45*(6), 204–211.

Tanner, C. A. (2009). The case for cases: A pedagogy for developing habits of thought. *Journal of Nursing Education, 48*(6), 299–230.

Tanner, C. A., Benner, P., Chesla, C., & Gordon, D. R. (1993). The phenomenology of knowing the patient. *Image: The Journal of Nursing Scholarship, 25*(4), 273–280.

Tracy, C. S., Dantas, C. C., & Upshur, R. E. (2003). Evidence-based medicine in primary care: Qualitative study of family physicians. *BMC Family Practice. Retrieved August 15, 2012,* from http://www.biomedcentral.com/1471-2296/4/6.

White, A. H. (2003). Clinical decision making among fourth-year nursing students: An interpretive study. *Journal of Nursing Education, 42*(3), 113–120.

Williamson, J. W., German, P. S., Weiss, R., Skinner, E. A., & Bowes III, F. (1989). Health science information management and continuing education of physicians. A survey of U.S. primary care practitioners and their opinion leaders. *Annals of Internal Medicine, 110*(2), 151–160.

Windish, D. M., Huot, S. J., & Green, M. L. (2007). Medical residents' understanding of the biostatistics and results in the medical literature. *Journal of the American Medical Association, 298*(9), 1010–1022.

Youngblut, J. M., & Brooten, D. (2001). Evidence-based nursing practice: Why is it important? *AACN Clinical Issues: Advanced Practice in Acute and Critical Care, 12*(4), 468–476.

Zerwekh, J. V. (1992). The practice of empowerment and coercion by expert public health nurses. *Image: The Journal of Nursing Scholarship, 24*(2), 101–105.

14 Advocacy and the Advanced Practice Nurse

Karen Piren

INTRODUCTION

The health-care delivery system is a complicated maze of services with many gates and gatekeepers. Not surprisingly, many consumers need help navigating their way through this intimidating maze. The advanced practice nurse (APN) is in a good position to advocate for individual consumers and families who confront barriers to getting the health-care services that they need. Nurses can also advocate for systemic changes to remove the barriers. It takes education, sophistication, and determination to advocate at both of these levels. This chapter examines the roots of advocacy in nursing and the skills needed for this practice role. Through case examples, we highlight several opportunities and issues to stimulate dialogue and action.

ROOTS OF ADVOCACY IN NURSING

Nursing leaders such as Florence Nightingale, Sojourner Truth, Lillian Wald, and Margaret Sanger are testaments to the nursing profession's historic roots in championing improved health care, especially for the most vulnerable among us (Mason, Leavitt, & Chafee, 2012). These pioneers advanced human rights, compassionate care, and lasting societal changes. Given this impressive legacy, it is interesting that the patient advocate role is seen as an innovation in nursing in the past 25 years, and it is still only in the early stages of acceptance (Mallik & Rafferty, 2000).

Nurse scholars provide support that patient advocacy is an important part of the practice of expert nurses (Segesten, 1993). Indeed, the American Nurses Association (ANA) *Guide to the Code of Ethics for Nurses* (2008) calls on nurses to collaborate with other health professionals and consumers to promote community and national efforts to meet the health needs of the public. Given the complexities of today's health-care environment, nurse advocates are needed more than ever. The International Council of Nurses (ICN) also includes advocacy as an essential nursing activity. However, the presumption that nurses advocate for patients in all practice settings is based on little evidence (Milette, 1993), and there is scant literature describing how nurses learn how to advocate (Foley, Minick, & Kee, 2002a). It appears that nurses value advocacy, know that they should advocate, and often do so in their daily work. However, the profession does not consistently address advocacy in its body of knowledge and methods for transferring that body of knowledge to entrants into the discipline. In many ways, advocacy is an ambiguous role component for APNs.

Evidence Base for Advocacy

One reason for this ambiguity is that advocacy means many things to many people, and there is no well-accepted, evidenced-based advocacy model for nursing practice. That does not mean that patient advocacy is lacking. It means that it is not well articulated, researched, or taught. Mitchell and Bournes (2000) suggest that "advocacy is a concept that conceals more than it reveals" (p. 209) and that an explicit theoretical foundation for this activity would enhance its value to the nursing profession. Because the profession purports that advocacy is a social mandate for nurses, the need for theoretical explication and nursing research is compelling.

The evidence base for the advocacy role or effectiveness of advocacy interventions is limited. Mallick and Rafferty (2000) examined the growth and diffusion of nurses' claim to patient advocacy in the nursing literature of the United States and the United Kingdom over 20 years (1976–1995). Most of the published manuscripts have come out of the United States and their focus on specialty areas in nursing; other than that, there are few studies. Given the early stages of the empirical exploration of this area, most of the work is exploratory, the methodology is qualitative, and samples are small. However, several studies explored the concept of advocacy in relation to nursing.

Negarandeh, Oskouie, Ahmadi, Nikravesh, and Hallberg (2006) conducted a grounded theory study of 24 nurses and identified barriers and facilitators influencing the role of advocacy in Iranian nurses. Semistructured interviews were used for data collection. Through data analysis, several main themes emerged that hindered or facilitated patient advocacy. Powerlessness, lack of support, law, lack of motivation, limited communication, physicians leading, risks of advocacy, and insufficient time were themes identified as hindrances to patient advocacy. Facilitators identified were the nurse–patient relationship, recognizing patients' needs, nurses' responsibility, physician as colleague, and nurses' knowledge and skills. Barriers identified by Hanks (2007) in a concept analysis include lack of institutional support and power, lack of education, and lack of time. Millette (1993) studied the nurse's view of client advocacy and how this concept might affect practice. Surveying 222 nurses and interviewing a subset of 24 of these subjects, this investigator found that the concept of client advocacy has much appeal to practicing nurses but that they need a high level of moral development to implement this advocacy role in bureaucratic settings. Geoffrey's (1998) study of nine nurses caring for dying patients also addresses the environments in which nurses practice. Using grounded theory to explore advocacy as a means of empowering these dying patients, Geoffrey describes the effects of rituals on the practice of advocacy. Adhering to routines such as getting morning care for assigned patients completed before noon keeps the nurse busy enough to avoid talking to patients, determining barriers to recovery, and acting to remove those barriers. Advocacy requires an individualized approach and an openness to challenge power structures. The focus on completing tasks can distance the nurse from patients and lead to poor advocacy skills.

Two other studies explore advocacy among practicing nurses. In a British study, Snowball (1996) used a semistructured interview with 15 medical-surgical nurses to explore their understanding of advocacy. These nurses viewed the therapeutic relationship as the key to advocacy at both the proactive and reactive levels. Foley, Minick, and Kee (2002b) used hermeneutic interpretive methods of stories to study the development of skills in advocating for patients in Army nurses in Bosnia. They found that developing advocacy skills was largely haphazard, not based on what these nurses were taught. But when the nurses found themselves in situations that called for advocacy, they often rose to the occasion, and they developed skills along the way.

These studies document that despite the limited empirical basis for advocacy in nursing, the concept and the practice are evolving in ways that are consistent with the values of the nursing profession. Nurse leaders, researchers, and educators elucidate philosophical foundations for advocacy (Curtain, 1979), required skills (Connolly, 1999), and curricula (Jones, 1982). Advocacy is not always included in descriptions of the advanced practice nursing role (Hamric, Spross, & Hanson, 2009; Mezey & McGivern, 1999). However, several authors suggest that advocacy is highly desirable, an indicator of excellence in practice, a domain in advanced practice nursing, and an essential component of the primary mental health-care and community support system models (Benner, 1984; Gadow, 1980; Haber & Billings, 1995; Millette, 1993; U.S. Department of Health and Human Services [DHHS], 1987).

Nurses occupy a middle ground between the consumer and the health-care system, an optimal place to mediate (Bishop & Scudder, 1990; Stein, Watts, & Howell, 1990). Although there is a critical need for research and development of the advocacy role, there is some guidance for APNs.

Definitions of Advocacy

What is advocacy? Snowball (1996) suggests that advocacy suffers from conceptual ambiguity. Advocacy is derived from the Latin *advocatus,* which means one who summons to give evidence (Gates, 1995). *Advocate* is a noun and a verb—to act for, speak for, plead for, or defend. *Advocacy* is the function of these verbs and has been described as informing, advising, or counseling (Gadow, 1980, 1989; Kohnke, 1982; Mitchell & Bournes, 2000).

Historically, advocacy has been linked to the potential powerlessness of a patient, although the rising power of the consumer affects our definitions of advocacy (Hewitt, 2002). Shroeder and Gadow (2000) distinguish advocacy from paternalism and consumerism. Paternalism is the commitment to making decisions for the client because the professional is obligated to impose expertise on behalf of the person in need; a person in need is presumed to be incapable of rational judgment. In contrast, consumerism is the commitment to remain uninvolved in client decisions; persons in need are nonetheless capable of rational judgment, and their right to self-determination must be respected. This author provides a view of advocacy as a practical partnership between a professional who has expertise to offer and the client who is experiencing the inherent ambiguity associated with significant health concerns.

Most people confronting a serious health problem require "reorientation" so that they can define the situation, reflect on their values, and make decisions. In this view, advocacy is a partnership in which the person confronting a health issue and the professional offering assistance develop a mutually satisfying interpretation of the situation. In the partnership, they reach a meaning they can both affirm. The meaning can be considered a narrative or interpretation that coherently connects all the elements of the situation. Essentially, "advocacy becomes participation with clients in co-authorship of a health narrative" (Schroeder & Gadow, 2000, p. 85).

Levels of Advocacy

Definitions of advocacy tend to be client- or systems-focused, suggesting two levels of advocacy for APNs. Client-focused definitions of advocacy emphasize enhancing client autonomy and assisting clients in voicing their values (Connolly, 1999). At this individual/family client level, the APN uses a set of skills to help people identify their needs and obtain services, and provides support to meet those needs. Systems-focused definitions of advocacy refer to influencing providers to improve existing services and develop new ones (Stuart & Laraia, 2001). At this systems level of advocacy, the APN uses many of the same skills needed at the individual/family level—and some new ones—to advocate for changes in the health-care delivery system itself.

Advocacy at the Individual and Family Levels

The client-focused definition of advocacy speaks to patient advocacy, the most common type of advocacy in nursing practiced at both the individual and family levels. The most dominant model for patient advocacy comes from the counseling paradigm. Burgeoning during the civil rights and women's movements of the 1960s and 1970s, nurses were moving past previous modes of subservience to physicians and institutions to a direct relationship with the patient. Inherent in that relationship is the recognition that the nurse has the authority that comes with claim to a scientific body of knowledge that is not fully accessible to the lay person (Abbott, 1988). The nurse's ethical responsibility is to transfer as much of that knowledge as possible to the patient and support that person in making informed choices. Patient advocacy becomes teaching, nonjudgmental support of the person's choices, and assistance in acting on those choices (Hanks, 2010).

This counseling model is the mainstay of advanced practice nursing at the individual and family levels. The more contemporary "consumer empowerment" model reminds us that people do not want or need continual counseling by professionals; they may not be seeking professionals' "noninvolvement," but consumers would prefer consultation rather than counseling. They seek a reduction in the medical model orientation that health professionals know what is best to "protect" patients. Nurses who define advocacy primarily as protecting patients (Foley et al., 2002a) may have difficulty with the contemporary principles of consumer self-advocacy. Consumer advocates do not seek paternalistic protection. They do seek professionals who can help them navigate the system, a high priority for consumers and families who define advocacy as "a go-between who knows the system and will advise you" (Connolly, 1999, p. 390).

There are many ways that APNs can advocate at the individual and family level. The following case example provides one exemplar.

Advocacy Exemplar: Individual and Family Level

The complex issues of removing children from their families and placing them with adoption services while negotiating a difficult, fragmented child protection system provides fertile ground and many opportunities for APNs to demonstrate their role as advocates. The overburdened, disjointed systems make it difficult for members of a care team to understand the complexities of an individual seeking to regain custody of his or her children. In many ways, the individual is alone, pitted against a group of professionals representing the children—professionals who barely have time to communicate. Negotiating the system is a complex, difficult endeavor.

Individual and family advocacy can be valuable to individuals attempting to navigate these systems. Vulnerable populations, such as the poor and uninsured, victims of abuse, single mothers, and individuals with developmental disabilities or mental illness, are in particular need of advocacy services. Schroeder and Gadow (2000) describe a tradition of service delivery in the United States that effectively prohibits many of these individuals from participating in decisions regarding health care. They describe a system in which professionals identify themselves as the expert authority, thereby disempowering the individuals and destroying the possibility of an equal (or mutual) relationship between an individual and professional. Nurse advocates can counter the effects of this paternalistic system by enhancing personal autonomy and participating with individuals in determining their needs (Shroeder & Gadow, 2000).

The Case of Maria

This case describes Maria and her involvement in the family court system. It illustrates how an APN can identify barriers within a multifaceted system; plan, coordinate, and monitor services; and follow up with other advocates within the system.

Maria is a 30-year-old, single, bilingual mother of four who was born in the United States to parents of Hispanic origin. Her involvement with the court began several years ago when her estranged husband abused their oldest daughter. Maria herself had also been the victim of his abuse. Although she left her husband shortly after her daughter's abuse, three of her four children were placed in foster care. The fourth resided with Maria's mother, and Maria participated fully in this daughter's daily life. Maria enjoyed a close and loving relationship with her intact family, which included a sister.

Maria was referred to an APN in psychiatric–mental health nursing for case management services. She was referred by an urban family court as part of a child welfare mediation process of planning for the future of the three children in foster care. Concurrently, the APN collaborated with a university law school, a court-appointed mediator, various child protection case managers, and Maria's attorney. The nurse provided strength-based case management services (Sullivan, 1991), counseling, and support to Maria during court-mediated meetings, as well as links to services identified by the client and nurse.

In addition to attending monthly mediation hearings over a 6-month period, the APN met with Maria weekly. Maria was a quiet, shy young woman who exhibited developmental and speech delays. Her affect was depressed, and she expressed feelings of hopelessness and despair. The legal system had, in fact, determined that three children would be placed for adoption. Maria, on the other hand, expressed a strong desire to be reunited with her family. In particular, Maria wanted to regain custody of her oldest daughter.

The APN made an initial assessment based on the strengths-based case management model (Sullivan, 1991). Maria had several strengths. She was young, relatively healthy, and able to identify solid family supports. She expressed a fervent desire to care for her children and demonstrated a willingness to discuss difficult, painful issues. She expressed a strong desire to follow the recommendations of the court, although she sometimes found it difficult to do so. In addition to reuniting her family, her personal goals were to obtain a high school diploma and get a driver's license and a car. The ocean was less than an hour away, and she dreamed of driving to the beach with her children to see the ocean for the first time.

Initially, Maria did not make eye contact with the APN, and answered questions only after careful thought. The nurse construed this to mean that Maria was searching for the answer she thought the nurse wanted to hear. Her feelings of powerlessness and hopelessness were highlighted during the first mediation meeting, when the nurse noted that no one in the room spoke to her. They spoke about and around her. For her part, Maria sat quietly listening to the discussion about the future of her family.

Shea, Mahoney, and Lacey (1997) describe the importance of empowerment and advocacy to victims of abuse. According to these authors, creating and sustaining a therapeutic caring relationship, encouraging self-determination, and supporting patient decisions promote empowerment and advocacy. The APN needs to communicate a sense of hope while establishing realistic expectations for success to promote empowerment and independence.

In addition, Shea and colleagues (1997) recognize that to break the coercive control that abusers have over their victims, nurses need to avoid using interventions that represent further control of the victim, thereby perpetuating the cycle of abuse. Advocates must be wary and avoid paternalistic relationships, exercising care in understanding the needs and desires of those in need of their services (Mitchell & Bournes, 2000).

The primary issue preventing Maria from regaining custody of her children was their safety. Maria's estranged husband had continued to contact her, despite the fact that there was a restraining order against all contact with her or the children. Maria felt powerless and clearly did not know how to react when this occurred. The nurse and university law school advocates readily discovered that Maria had never been provided with a copy of the restraining order. The university law school advocates obtained a copy of the order and gave Maria clear, concise instructions regarding implementation. In addition, they arranged for Maria to receive a free cell phone from a battered women's shelter, enabling her to call 911 in the event of an emergency. For additional security, the nurse and Maria located a safe house and developed an escape plan.

Several other issues were apparent to the nurse and university law school advocates in this case. A few are discussed here. First, before the nurse and law school involvement, Maria's only advocate throughout the process had been a very caring but overburdened court-appointed attorney. Although he did everything he could to assist Maria, time constraints and the inability to assess Maria's cognitive deficits limited his ability to assist her. On the other hand, the children had individual case managers, the Department of Youth and Family Services, the Assistant Attorney General, child advocates, individual therapists, and numerous others working on their behalf. It was easy to understand why the court and mediation process were intimidating to Maria and how they contributed to her feelings of hopelessness and powerlessness. A second issue that affected Maria's need for advocacy was that many individuals involved in her case scheduled her appointments at overlapping times without consideration for the time or money required to keep them. In addition, Maria had difficulty reading, a fact that was unknown to any of the individuals involved in her case.

The APN needed to help overcome all of these barriers. Reinforcing her strengths, she helped Maria find hope tempered with realistic expectations. In addition to arming her with the restraining order, cell phone, and escape plan, the APN helped her obtain a city bus pass and a color-coded calendar she could read to help her keep her appointments. She also helped her enroll in high school general equivalency diploma classes. This set of advocacy interventions helped set in motion immediate and long-term forces of self-empowerment for Maria.

In the end, the court changed its position and granted Maria custody of her oldest daughter. The two younger children were placed for adoption in the foster home they had resided in for a number of years. Although Maria was distraught over the loss, she was able to meet the family, who invited her to remain involved in the children's lives.

Issues and Discussion

In this case example, the APN used Sullivan's strength-based case management model to guide her advocacy efforts. She identified strengths, as well as gaps in the system, and applied practical solutions to overlooked troubles. The interventions built on Maria's strengths, supported her autonomy, and ultimately enhanced her self-esteem. Collaborating with child protective services and others involved in the case created an environment wherein the advocates identified an opportunity to propose meaningful interventions and broaden the range of options to Maria, which had long been overlooked by the team.

Connolly (1999) describes skills and competencies needed by the APN patient advocate. These skills include empathetic listening, self-confidence, assertiveness, negotiation, collaboration, communication, physical assessment, mental status assessment, crisis intervention, case management, change agency, and teaching. Snowball (1996) found the therapeutic relationship "key to advocacy" (p. 73). Clearly, all of these skills are within the scope and education of APNs. However, paramount to the success of the patient advocate is a philosophical foundation that individuals, particularly those who are vulnerable and suffer from any disease or impairment, are unique human beings who deserve and require respect, dignity, and the right to make decisions concerning their lives. Application of the science that nurses learn, coupled with a desire to improve the lives of other human beings, make "human advocacy" a fundamental part of the nursing process.

Systems-Level Advocacy

Systems-level advocacy is nursing practice at the community level. Public health nurses think of it as "upstream thinking." For example, one can treat the child with lead poisoning and help navigate the child and his family through the clinics and lead abatement programs case by case. However, a more upstream advocacy approach would be to prevent lead poisoning through strict preventive policies and programs for abating all houses with lead paint, especially in cities. Consumers need both levels. APNs can be engaged in both levels, with different intensity. Although not all APNs desire a policy-level advocacy role, they can support policies and programs that their nursing colleagues are advancing on behalf of consumers.

The advocacy skills that APNs need to successfully advocate for individuals and families are foundational for systems-level advocacy. Advocacy at this level usually involves developing new policies and programs, or at least changing the old way of doing things enough to make a difference for the people that nurses serve. Communication skills are crucial. Active listening skills are as important as verbal skills; indeed, more insight is gained from listening than from speaking. Insight into the problem leads to more creative problem solving and ideas for negotiating system solutions. Negotiation is more complex at the systems level than at the individual and family levels because generally there are more stakeholders involved when advocating policies and programs. The APN needs to be assertive enough to overcome resistance to change and collaborative enough to create or join with others who can help advance the advocacy goal.

To be most effective at the systems level, APNs need to understand program and policy development. Hanley (2002) describes several models regarding public policy that can guide APNs. For example, the stage-sequential model details a series of stages, beginning with identifying a policy problem and getting that problem placed on the policy discussion and action agendas in the appropriate forum (i.e., state or federal legislature, administrative agencies, funding organizations, and the like). Developing policy options with supporting budgets and infrastructures for implementation (i.e., staffing, regulations, and so on) follows. Program implementation and evaluation are the final stages. Moving through these stages requires an understanding of the change process in general, with skill development in creating and sustaining a vision for change, anticipating and dealing with resistance to change, developing a broad base of support, and understanding the art of compromise.

Advocacy Exemplar: Freeing People from Nursing Homes

Americans are fiercely proud of their freedom to live their lives as they choose. Many older adults and people with disabilities are in danger of losing that freedom when they have difficulty managing daily living tasks and the challenges of chronic health conditions. The forces driving frail elders and the disabled into institutional care are well documented (Kane, Kane, & Ladd, 1998). Once placed in a nursing home, institutionalized people often find it difficult to return home or to another community-based setting such as assisted living. The "system" works against it. The institutional bias in our federal and state long-term care payment policies is a serious impediment to consumers who want to leave nursing homes. Many states invest most of their dollars in nursing home care as opposed to home care. Professionals often assume that people who enter a nursing home really need that level of care and cannot be returned to their communities. The idea that the older adult's condition might improve, or that there may be other alternatives outside of a nursing home, are foreign concepts to many professionals and state policy makers. Even some who consider themselves to be advocates for the elderly believe that a nursing home is the "safest place" for those who have crossed the institutional threshold. Crossing back seems unthinkable. Navigating the crossing is extremely difficult.

Systems advocacy is needed to change this thinking that is embedded in our policies and programs. We can offer institutionalized elders and people with disabilities more choices, and they can return to the community with help from nurses and others to navigate the way back home.

The Case of Community Choice Counseling

One example of systems advocacy led by an APN is a state program developed as part of a set of "senior initiatives" in New Jersey to offer older adults independence, dignity, and choice (Reinhard, 1999). Known as "Community Choice Counseling," this program has been evaluated by researchers at Rutgers Center for State Health Policy (Howell-White, 2003). The goals and social change strategies used to create this program are offered as an exemplar for systems advocacy.

In 1994, an APN in community health nursing was appointed to serve the New Jersey Commissioner of Health as the Director of Policy and Research. Interested in developing policies and programs to support people with chronic conditions who want to live in their communities, this nurse director investigated the range of community-based options for long-term care available for older adults and people with disabilities. Like most states at the time, New Jersey had few options, and 97% of the public dollars in long-term care were spent on nursing home care (Reinhard, 1999). Despite this dismal record, New Jersey was approximately average among the states (Ladd, 1999). National data document that institutional bias is rampant in this country.

At least three things are needed to change this institutionalization bias. First, more long-term care alternatives must be created by developing programs and obtaining the funding to support them. Second, ways to inform consumers and professionals about these alternatives before people are unnecessarily institutionalized must be developed. Third, strategies to continually assess those who enter nursing homes to see if they still need and prefer that residential care option must be created. The overall goal is to help consumers and professionals understand that people can move in and out of these various long-term care options—it is not a unidirectional, linear movement. People can and should be able to move from nursing homes to their homes, and any other long-term care option.

The most important way to begin this systems advocacy is to develop and communicate a shared vision for change. Indeed, an advocate's most critical driving force for change is the strength and integrity of the vision energizing the goals for change. In this case, it was the vision of "freeing people" from unnecessary and unwanted institutionalization. It is advancing nursing's view that aging is not a period of inevitable decline. The nursing model holds that people of all ages can enter periods of disability, and they can regain health. The assumption that an older adult or a person with a disability can never attain or regain function is anathema to the nursing paradigm. Independence, dignity, choice: these principles helped the new director to bring together a coalition of advocates and policy makers interested in seeking the policy changes needed to fuel the evolution to the nonlinear, noninstitutional thinking that is consistent with the nursing philosophy of attaining, maintaining, and regaining health and independence.

To achieve this vision, several system changes were needed. First, the governor consolidated all senior programs into one department and appointed the nurse advocate as the deputy commissioner in charge of redesigning long-term care in the state. After considerable negotiation with the governor's office, the state budgeted $60 million in state and federal dollars to develop more consumer-directed home-care options and more respite care for family caregivers (Reinhard, 1999). The state also created a locally based information and assistance system so older adults and their families could learn about their options and navigate the system (Reinhard & Scala, 2001). The state also initiated a counseling program to make sure that people in nursing homes are also able to find out about these choices. That program was named "Community Choice Counseling (CCC)" (Lagnado, 2001).

This program began with energetic nurses in the new New Jersey Department of Health and Senior Services (NJDHSS). Starting with two registered nurses, 300 nursing home residents were helped to return to their homes and communities within 4 months. Telephone follow-up of 10% of these former nursing home residents found positive outcomes, including high consumer satisfaction, few reinstitutionalizations, and low costs to the consumer and state for community placement. Staff found that many of these older adults and persons with disabilities had "gotten stuck." For some, the admission to the nursing home was intended to be for a few months for recovery from an illness or accident. However, without help from a person outside the nursing home who could provide specific direction to get back to the community, their length of stay turned into 6 months, a year, or more. Based on these initial findings, the nurse leaders obtained the support of the governor to continue and expand the program.

Armed with pilot data, the nurse advocate began to develop a coalition to advocate for change. As nurses learn in their study of the change process, analyzing the driving and restraining forces to change is the starting point. In this case, the restraining forces to changing the institutional bias of long-term care are those who would be most threatened by altering the status quo. Nursing homes worry about the state emptying out their residents. The state's Office of Management and Budget worries not about emptying out the nursing homes but about hiring 40 nurses and social workers in the effort to do so. The directors of the county Office on Aging worry that they will have more resource-intense people living in the community if the state "deinstitutionalizes" older adults. Senior advocates who do want more home-care options also worry that the state will not deliver on the home-care side but will simply try to save money by taking people out of nursing homes. All of these concerns are legitimate. Resistance to change can be an advocate's greatest strategy for change because it helps sharpen one's thinking and adjust policies and programs to respond to the concerns raised.

Empirical evidence to support a vision is a strong driving force for change. Skills in conducting research and translating it in a meaningful way are crucial in systems advocacy. In this case, the pilot data were helpful in exploding the myth that people who leave nursing homes require an intensive level of care that will "suck the community dry." The evidence shed light on the reality that many people in nursing homes do not need a lot of care. They need supportive services in the community, not necessarily intensive care. The $120 per day spent in a nursing home can go far in the community for many institutionalized persons. For example, some people in the pilot only needed meals on wheels.

Advocates also need to advance a plan for change that addresses the concerns of the resistors. For example, the nurse advocate worked with the department's nurse leaders to initially target particular people in nursing homes to approach for counseling about their choices in the community. The CCC protocol calls for a state-employed nurse to talk with people who have been in the nursing home for approximately 3 to 6 months, a time when they might have recovered from their initial health problems that led to the nursing home admission. These people have exhausted their Medicare benefits and are well on their way to becoming Medicaid beneficiaries. If they are not helped at this point, they will begin to lose their homes and informal supports. Return to the community becomes even more difficult later.

Resistance to change will continue, especially during the early stages of implementation. Systems advocacy is needed most during this stage because one failure will make it harder to initiate a similar change in the future. The attitude often becomes, "We tried that once and it failed." In this case, CCC staff members reported initial resistance from nursing home staff. In more than one case, nursing home discharge planners stated that they feared dismissal from their jobs if they cooperated with the CCC counselors (Lagnado, 2001). Most felt they needed constantly updated information about community resources and materials to help them explain various nursing home alternatives. The nurse advocate and her staff sought and obtained a grant from the Centers for Medicare and Medicaid Services to help develop those materials.

Issues and Discussion

Advocacy can help move an idea into action. Stabilizing that new policy or program is the only way to make systems advocacy a success. Legislation is one way to make sure that the idea will continue because it becomes illegal to return to the old way of doing things. Another way is to provide evidence that the new way is working and incorporate the new way into the culture of the organization (in this case the state).

To obtain an objective, formative evaluation of this expanded program, NJDHSS contracted with the Rutgers Center for State Health Policy (CSHP) in 1999 to design and implement an evaluation of the CCC program. Initial findings were encouraging (Silberberg & Howell-White, 2000). The most recent findings continue to support a continuation of the program (Howell-White, 2003). What began with a group of spirited nurses in New Jersey has resulted in critical change for the delivery of services to senior citizens. New Jersey has more than doubled the percent of long-term care funds spent on home-and community-based care for older adults. In fact, from its initiation in 1998 to 2004, more than 5,000 persons were transferred from nursing homes to community living (Medstat, 2005).

The CCC program is based on the belief that people want to exercise their choice. No one would be forced to leave a nursing home but would be given information and help to move to their preferred living situation. The CSHP evaluation focused on how satisfied people are with their choice to leave the nursing home and their quality of life in their current living situation. They also examined the dependency needs of these former nursing home residents and the extent to which those needs are being met. The CCC program evaluation resulted in several salient research findings (Howell-White, 2003). Most former nursing home residents are now living in a home-based setting and are very satisfied with their current living situation. Their quality of life improved. Most are able to do things that make life more enjoyable, such as visiting with family and friends.

Most are able to perform almost all activities of daily living (i.e., bathing, dressing, eating) and about half of the instrumental activities of daily living (i.e., shopping, cooking, taking prescribed medications). Although former nursing home residents are living fairly independently, receiving only a little help with activities of daily living, many are receiving assistance with the instrumental activities of daily living.

These findings indicate that most former nursing home residents are very satisfied when they are helped to leave a nursing home and return to the community. For the most part, they are receiving the services they need and have an improved quality of life. Moreover, the CCC counselors (and the program in general) seem to support and help in the nursing home residents' return to the community. Based in part on these findings, the state is continuing the program with the staffing and budget needed to continue it.

This case study exemplifies several simultaneous systems changes. It emphasizes change-agent skills as the most critical advocacy skills needed by the nurses who created and advanced these ideas. Few APNs will choose to lead this kind of systems advocacy. But many will choose to support or resist it. At a minimum, APNs need to understand systems advocacy. Systems advocacy involves citizenship and a call for participation in the decisions that affect our lives and the lives of those we serve (Joel, 1998; Paquin, 2011).

Consumer-Driven Systems-Level Advocacy

Nurses can lead systems advocacy efforts both as professionals and as consumers. One case example comes from the mental health arena. The consumer movement in mental health is a strong model for the influence of consumers. Consumers provide the unique perspective of their experience with mental illness (Solomon, 2001). There is no consumer health-care group more powerful than the National Alliance for the Mentally Ill (NAMI). The consumer movement in mental health and the work of NAMI is reflected in the landmark report, *Mental Health: A Report of the Surgeon General* (U.S. DHHS, 1999). Following this report, The President's New Freedom Commission Report *Achieving the Promise: Transforming Mental Health Care in America* (U.S. DHHS, 2003) calls for a transformation of the mental health system with consumer involvement in shifting the mental health system to a system of individually defined recovery. The following describes another exemplar of systems advocacy; this exemplar is driven by consumers, particularly a nurse.

Advocacy Exemplar: A Nurse Consumer in Suicide Prevention

Advocacy is one role consumers may assume. Many health professionals are family member consumers affected by suicide. In fact, the National Strategy for Suicide Prevention (U.S. DHHS, 2001) is directly related to a grassroots movement started by a couple, Elsie and Jerry Weyrauch, who are parent survivors of suicide. Suicide survivors are family members, significant others, or acquaintances who have experienced the loss of a loved one as a result of suicide.

The Case of Elsie

Elsie Weyrauch is a retired psychiatric nurse. Her husband Jerry is a retired navy officer. Elsie and Jerry lost their daughter Terri Ann, a physician, to suicide 15 years ago. Since then, they have worked tirelessly for suicide prevention. They founded the Suicide Prevention Advocacy Network, Inc. (SPAN), a grassroots advocacy organization, in 1996 in Marietta, Georgia.

SPAN links the energy of those bereaved by suicide with the expertise of leaders in education, religion, science, business, government, and public service to significantly reduce suicide. It is a nonprofit organization dedicated to the creation and implementation of national, state, and local suicide prevention strategies (SPAN, 2002). SPAN includes suicide survivors, suicide attempt survivors, and community activists. SPAN activities have included holding awareness events; visiting and writing letters to legislators, advocating for the passage of congressional resolutions related to suicide; participating in public hearings; hosting suicide awareness events in Washington, DC; cosponsoring a national strategy meeting; and sitting on federal advisory groups.

The story of SPAN (as described in the national strategy) over 6 years is an inspiring testimonial to the role of consumers as advocates and the nurse-consumer as an advocate. SPAN championed guidelines developed by the United Nations and the World Health Organization (1996) as a way to encourage development of a national suicide prevention strategy for the United States. Their work to marshal social will for suicide prevention generated congressional resolutions recognizing suicide as a national problem and suicide prevention as a national priority. These resolutions provided further impetus to develop a national suicide prevention strategy (U.S. DHHS, 2001).

SPAN propelled the creation of an innovative public-private partnership to jointly sponsor a National Suicide Prevention Conference, convened in Reno, Nevada, in October 1998 (also known as the Reno Conference). Participating agencies within the U.S. Department of Health and Human Services (DHHS) were the Centers for Disease Control and Prevention (CDC), the National Institutes of Health (NIH), the Office of the Surgeon General, the Substance Abuse and Mental Health Services Administration, the Health Resources and Services Administration, the Indian Health Service, and the Public Health Service Regional Health Administrators. Conference participants, including researchers, mental health and substance abuse clinicians, policy makers, suicide survivors, consumers of mental health services, school staff, and community activists and leaders, discussed eight background papers that were commissioned to summarize the evidence base for suicide prevention (Silverman, Davidson, & Potter, 2001). Working in interdisciplinary groups, participants at the Reno Conference offered many recommendations for action that were shaped into a list of 81 by an expert panel.

Surgeon General David Satcher then issued the Call to Action to Prevent Suicide, a blueprint for addressing suicide that succeeded through awareness, intervention, and methodology based on the highest-ranked 81 Reno Conference recommendations (U.S. Public Health Service [PHS], 1999). A National Strategy Leadership Consultants Group was formed and four public hearings were held. A federal steering group drafted the national strategy. The surgeon general released the *National Strategy for Suicide Prevention: Goals and Objectives for Action* 2 years after the Reno Conference (U.S. DHHS, 2001). The national strategy is now informing funding priorities, research, and state and local plans. Despite this tremendous progress in suicide prevention, the Weyrauchs continue to urge local, state, federal, and international communities to never let up. Now in their seventies, they exclaim, "We can't wait. We're too old."

Issues and Discussion

Often consumers serve not only as advocates but also as activists who assertively and unrelentingly assault the barriers to their cause. The Weyrauchs have been able to dialogue with every level of government and industry, and with mental health professionals and researchers, survivors, and suicidal individuals. For example, legislators who are themselves survivors have come forward as spokespersons for the survivor experience and the need for suicide prevention. From what started in a small operation in their own home, the Weyrauchs have inspired a movement that has spurred increased awareness, legislative activity, partnerships, funding, and collaboration on a state, national, and international level. In fact, they have accomplished what mental health professionals and suicidologists only dreamed about. They have served as a bridge for groups to begin dialogue and to take assertive action.

They have also pushed the barrier of stigma. The stigma associated with mental illness, substance abuse, and suicide is the most formidable obstacle to future progress in the arena of mental health, contributing to failure to seek help, low reimbursement for mental health services, and inadequate funding for prevention (U.S. DHHS, 1999). In a SPAN-sponsored event, quilts from many states were displayed on the Capitol steps to bring the faces to the stories of the survivors. Elsie and Jerry always have time to comfort a new survivor at an event and welcome them to the community embrace of survivors, and when they are ready, give them a task.

Clearly one of the contributing factors to their success, in addition to their determination, commitment to their daughter's memory, and tremendous family talent, is combining the forces of their training and experience in military and nursing leadership. They have collaborated with willing partners, such as legislators, who are also suicide survivors and—probably most important—with the former Surgeon General Satcher. Surgeon General Satcher was the first surgeon general to focus on mental health and suicide prevention.

APNs, including Virginia Trotter Betts and Beverly Malone, past presidents of the American Nurses Association, and Janet Grossman (one of the original authors of this chapter), have collaborated with the Weyrauchs in activities such as fundraising, leading the national strategy meeting, serving on conference planning committees, and preparing the national strategy. Nurses have much to learn by listening to the consumer perspective and trying unconventional ways to address critical public health issues such as suicide. Through partnerships, APNs can learn to join forces with consumers and work under their leadership.

To borrow from the view described by Schroeder and Gadow (2000), the Weyrauchs established a partnership in which consumers, professionals, and politicians composed a mutually satisfying interpretation of the urgency of suicide prevention. In the partnership they reached a meaning ("suicide prevention can't wait," and "we don't have much time") that they all affirmed. The meaning was an interpretation that coherently connected all the elements of the situation in co-authorship of a health narrative (Schroeder & Gadow, 2000). The National Strategy for Suicide Prevention is that health narrative.

This exemplar illustrates several of the themes in the literature on advocacy, including the following:

- Advocacy is an activity that is not owned by one sector of health care.
- The consumer is an expert.
- Advocacy is a partnership between consumers and professionals.
- Advocacy calls for the development of creative strategies.

HOW NURSES LEARN ADVOCACY

Whether advocating for individuals and families or advocating for system changes that will support them better, APNs need to develop many skills. We emphasize those skills in the case examples. Developing these skills takes practice. Benner (1991) emphasizes that the expert nurse learns the advocacy role through regular dialogue with other members of the nursing community, the patient, the patient's family, and other clinicians. Foley and colleagues (2002a) suggest that nurses new to the field need nurturing and administrative support to take on this role.

Fundamental to nursing is the understanding of each individual as a unique human being and of the needs created by their illness or condition. This knowledge is acquired through the nurse–patient relationship and therefore is distinctly nursing knowledge. Recognition that it is the individual, not the professional, who can make decisions for himself or herself calls for a synthesis of this knowledge and an understanding that "freedom, respect and integrity are essential to our full development as a person" (Foley et al., 2002a, p. 3).

Application of this philosophy may be more deeply rooted in a value system than in a learning process (Foley et al., 2002a). In their study, Foley and colleagues found that advocating for others was a natural and important aspect of practice rather than a learned process. The value of advocacy stems from family and community experience, and is integral to their (nurse's) being as persons. Although the value of advocacy cannot be taught, faculty "may need to define advocacy in relationship to patient care" (Foley et al., 2002a, p. 185).

Some nurses learn how to advocate by watching other nurses interact with patients and by working with mentors (Foley et al., 2002a). Role modeling and dialogue provide opportunities for positive learning experiences. Expert nurses and clinicians are positioned to provide examples and dialogue necessary to developing advocacy. This finding corresponds to Benner's (1991) belief that advocating is learned as part of the nursing community when the notion of good is enacted and discussed daily. Foley and colleagues (2002a) state, "Dialogue is essential in a practice such as nursing, in which knowledge is both scientific and historical, and therefore is dependent upon shared understandings among clinicians, patients, and families" (p. 181). However, nurses must experience the concepts of caring, suffering, hope, and recovery to internalize them (Benner, 1991).

Throughout the process of role modeling and mentoring, validation and a supportive environment are necessary if nurses are to gain the confidence required to advocate for patients (Foley et al., 2002a). Experienced nurses who recognize the risk that new nurses take in revealing their knowledge deficits create positive learning experiences and support a foundation for the development of advocacy practice. New nurses require corroboration that their practice and judgment are correct. Foley and colleagues (2002a) found that "experienced nurses can consciously help new nurses learn advocacy through preceptorships or one-to-one-mentoring" (p. 185).

Graduate programs in advanced practice nursing do not typically prepare graduates in the advocacy role. Sarah Lawrence College offers the only master's degree in the growing field of health advocacy, describing the role as promoting patients' rights in an increasingly complex health-care system. Resources available to the APN include Web sites (such as www.nursingworld.org) and documents such as the *Guide to Grassroots Activism,* available on the American Association of Colleges of Nursing Web site (www.aacn.nche.edu). These references can provide information on important issues that need nurses' advocacy and guidance in preparing correspondence or approaching legislators.

CONCLUSION

Advocacy is not an evidenced-based role, but it is a historic role. APNs need to develop practice skills to advocate at both the individual/family and systems levels. The profession needs to conduct more empirical studies to guide this practice, and we need to strengthen our education and diffusion strategies to advance this practice role. APNs can contribute to all these efforts. Nurses need to make visible stories of advocacy practice for their colleagues. Advocacy activities of nurses need to be more systematically analyzed and the effect of the activities documented.

REFERENCES

Abbot, A. (1988). *The system of professions: Essays on the division of expert labor.* Chicago: University Press of Chicago.

American Nurses Association. (2008). *Guide to the Code of Ethics for Nurses.* Silver Springs, MD: American Nurses Publishing.

Benner, P. (1984). *From novice to expert: Excellence and power in clinical nursing practice.* Menlo Park, CA: Addison-Wesley.

Benner, P. (1991). The role of experience, narrative and community in skilled ethical comportment. *Advances in Nursing Science, 14*(2), 1.

Bishop, A., & Scudder, J. (1990). *The practical and moral and personal sense of nursing: A phenomenological philosophy of practice.* Albany: State University of New York.

Connolly, P. M. (1999). Consumer advocacy. In C. A. Shea, L. R. Pelletier, E. C. Poster, G. W. Stuart, & M. P. Verhey (Eds.), *Advanced practice nursing in psychiatric and mental health care* (p. 387). St. Louis: Mosby.

Curtain, L. L. (1979). The nurse as advocate: A philosophical foundation for nursing. *Advances in Nursing Science,* 1(3), 1-10.

Foley, B. J., Minick, M. P., & Kee, C. C. (2002a). How nurses learn advocacy. *Journal of Nursing Scholarship, 34*(2), 181–187.

Foley, B. J., Minick, M. P., & Kee, C. C. (2002b). Nursing advocacy during a military operation. *Western Journal of Nursing Research, 22*(4), 492–498.

Gadow, S. (1980). Existential advocacy: Philosophical foundation of nursing. In S. F. Spicker & S. Gadow (Eds.), *Nursing: Images and ideals* (p. 79). New York: Springer.

Gadow, S. (1989). Clinical subjectivity. Advocacy for silent patients. *Nursing Clinics of North America, 24*(2), 535–541.

Gates, B. (1995). Whose best interest? *Nursing Times, 91*(4), 31–32.

Geoffrey, M. (1998). Ritual action and its effect on the role of the nurse as advocate. *Journal of Advanced Nursing, 27*(1), 189–194.

Haber, J., & Billings, C. (1995). Primary mental health care: A model of psychiatric–mental health nursing. *Journal of the American Psychiatric Nurses Association, 1*(5), 154.

Hamric, A., Spross, J., & Hanson, C. (Eds.). (2009). *Advanced practice nursing* (4th ed.). St. Louis: Elsevier/Mosby/Saunders.

Hanks, R. G. (2007). Barriers to nursing advocacy. *Nursing Forum, 42*(4), 171–177.

Hanks. R. G. (2010). The medical-surgical nurse perspective of advocate role. *Nursing Forum, 45*(2), 97–107.

Hanley, B. (2002). Policy development and analysis. In D. J. Mason, J. K. Leavitt, & M. W. Chafee (Eds.), *Policy and politics in nursing and health care* (4th ed.). Philadelphia: WB Saunders.

Hewitt, J. A. (2002). Critical review of the arguments debating the role of the nurse advocate. *Journal of Advanced Nursing, 37*(5), 439–445.

Howell-White, S. (2003). *Current living situation and service needs of former nursing home residents: An evaluation of New Jersey's nursing home transition program.* New Brunswick, NJ: Rutgers Center for State Health Policy.

Joel, L. (1998). On citizenship in a great profession. *American Journal of Nursing, 98*(4), 7.

Jones, E. (1982). Advocacy—A tool for radical nursing curriculum planners. *Journal of Nurse Education, 21*(1), 40–45.

Kane, R., Kane, R., & Ladd, R. (1998). *The heart of long-term care.* New York: Oxford University Press.

Kohnke, M. F. (1982). *Advocacy: Risk and reality.* St. Louis: Mosby.

Ladd, R. (1999). *State LTC profiles report, 1996. Balancing long-term care.* Minneapolis, MN: Division of Health Services Research and Policy, School of Public Health.

Lagnado, L. (2001, February 21). Living and dying: An innovative New Jersey program offers what may be a more humane alternative to nursing homes. *Wall Street Journal,* p. R11.

Mallik, M., & Rafferty, A. M. (2000). Diffusion of the concept of patient advocacy. *Journal of Nursing Scholarship, 32*(4), 399–404.

Mason, D. J., Leavitt, J. K., & Chafee, M, W. (Eds.). (2012). *Policy and politics in nursing and health care* (6th ed.). St. Louis: Elsevier/Mosby/Saunders.

Medstat. (2005). *New Jersey—Community choice initiative.* Washington, DC: Promising Practices in Home and Community-Based Services.

Mezey, M., & McGivern, D. (Eds.). (1999). *Nurses, nurse, and practitioners: Evolution to advanced practice.* New York: Springer.

Milette, B. (1993). Client advocacy and the moral orientation of nurses. *Western Journal of Nursing Research, 15*(5), 607–618.

Mitchell, G., & Bournes, D. (2000). Nurse as patient advocate? In search of straight thinking. *Nursing Science Quarterly, 13*(3), 204–209.

Negarandeh, R., Oskouie, F., Ahmadi, F., Nikravesh, M., & Hallberg, I. R. (2006). Patient advocacy: Barriers and facilitators. *BMC Nursing, 5,* 3. Retrieved August 20, 2012, from http://www.biomedicalcentral.com/1472-6955/5/3/.

Paquin, S. O. (2011). Social justice advocacy in nursing. *Creative Nursing, 17*(2), 63–67.

Reinhard, S. (1999, April 27). Testimony before the Senate Appropriations Committee. Trenton, New Jersey.

Reinhard, S., & Scala, M. (2001). *Navigating the long-term care maze: New approaches to information and assistance in three states.* Washington, DC: AARP Public Policy Institute.

Schroeder, C., & Gadow, G. (2000). An advocacy approach to ethics and community health. In E. Anderson & J. McFarlane (Eds.), *Community as partner: Theory and practice in nursing* (3rd ed., p. 78). Philadelphia: Lippincott Williams & Wilkins.

Segesten, K. (1993). Patient advocacy: An important part of the daily work of the expert nurse. *Scholarly Inquiry for Nursing Practice, 7*(2), 129–135.

Shea, C., Mahoney, M., & Lacey, J. (1997). Breaking through the barriers to domestic violence intervention. *American Journal of Nursing, 97*(6), 26–33.

Silberberg, M., & Howell-White, S. (2000). *Transitions to the community: A survey of former nursing home residents discharged after community choice counseling.* New Brunswick, NJ: Rutgers Center for State Health Policy.

Silverman, M., Davidson, L., & Potter, L. (Eds). (2001). National suicide prevention conference background papers. *Suicide and Life-Threatening Behavior, 31*(1, suppl).

Snowball, J. (1996). Asking nurses about advocating for patients: "Reactive" and "proactive" accounts. *Journal of Advanced Nursing, 24*(1), 67–75.

Solomon, A. (2001). *The noonday demon: An atlas of depression.* New York: Scribner.

Stein, L., Watts, D., & Howell, T. (1990). The doctor-nurse game revisited. *New England Journal of Medicine, 322*(8), 546–549.

Stuart, G. W., & Laraia, M. T. (2001). *Principles and practice of psychiatric nursing* (7th ed.). St. Louis: Mosby.

Suicide Prevention Advocacy Network USA. (March 2002). Newsletter.

Sullivan, W. P. (1991). *Case management in alcohol and drug treatment: Conceptual issues and practical applications.* Springfield, MO: Southwest Missouri Center for Social Research.

World Health Organization. (1996). *Prevention of suicide: Guidelines for the formulation and implementation of national strategies (ST/ESA/245).* Geneva: World Health Organization.

U.S. Department of Health and Human Services. (1987). *Toward a model plan for a comprehensive community-based mental health system.* Rockville, MD: Author.

U.S. Department of Health and Human Services. (1999). *Mental health: A report of the Surgeon General.* Rockville, MD: US Department of Health and Human Services, Substance Abuse and Mental Health Services Administration, Center for Mental Health Services, National Institutes of Health, National Institute of Mental Health.

U.S. Department of Health and Human Services. (2001). *National strategy for suicide prevention: Goals and objectives for action.* Rockville, MD: U.S. Department of Health and Human Services, Public Health Service.

U.S. Department of Health and Human Services. (2003). *Achieving the promise: Transforming mental health care in America.* Rockville, MD: U.S. Department of Health and Human Services, New Freedom Commission on Mental Health.

U.S. Public Health Service. (1999). *The Surgeon General's call to action to prevent suicide.* Washington, DC: U.S. Public Health Service.

15

Case Management and Advanced Practice Nursing

Denise Fessler
Patricia M. Haynor
Irene McEachen
Marylou Yam

HISTORICAL BACKGROUND

Case management and advanced practice nursing share a long history in the United States. Although these concepts have only been coined in nursing literature for the last two decades (Tahan, 1998), their roots can be found in nursing history as early as the 1860s (Kersbergen, 1996). Reading between the lines of health-care and nursing history, it is possible to witness the evolution of the process of nurses with expert clinical knowledge who manage care. With the passage of the Patient Protection and Affordable Care Act of 2010, the evolution continues, and at a more accelerated pace.

The case management process was used in the 1860s in early settlement houses for immigrants and the poor. Information was collected on family needs, required services were identified and delivered, and a system of follow-up was designed to ensure appropriateness and continuity (Reynolds & Smeltzer, 1997). In 1901, Mary Richmond, a social services pioneer, published a model of case coordination with the client as the core concern. Richmond's concern for her clients revolved around the lack of communication and coordination that frequently resulted in the duplication of services as clients moved through the system (Weil & Karls, 1985).

U.S. public health nursing was founded toward the end of the 19th century by Lillian Wald (Dock, 1937). The work of the public health nurse was to respond to the needs of the populations at greatest risk in our society (i.e., new immigrants living in tenement housing) and to provide ways to reduce illness and promote health (Wald, 1915). Wald was considered a visionary not only for her pioneering work in public health, but also for the establishment of a nationwide system of insurance for home-based care and the recognition of the independence and accomplishments of public health nurses. Interestingly, the public health nurses in the early 1900s were not subject to physician orders and established themselves as health educators and promoters of wellness (Frachel, 1988). The following quote from an editorial in *The Public Health Nurse,* although written in 1919 about public health nurses, could easily appear in today's literature referring to the advanced practice nurse (APN) (Profession of promoting health, 1919, p. 12):

> *Why not come boldly forth, one and all, and claim the right to exercise the promotion of health as a profession? The best-educated nurses spend as many years in training to exercise their profession as physicians to prepare themselves for the care and scientific prevention of disease.*

These public health nurses were perceived as the elite in nursing because they practiced autonomously and creatively (Reverby, 1987). The clinical expertise of these nurses is explained historically by the presentation of practice stories using an approach that seeks to understand the narrative without preconceived expectations or judgment (Palmer, 1969). Several competencies of the public health nurse were readily elicited from historical anecdotes: public health nurses' activities included "making inquiries, shrewd identification of evidence, steady plodding, helping others to help themselves, teaching, explanation and demonstration, and organizing a household to knit the family" (Zerwekh, 1992, p. 85). In short, this could be a description of today's APN. Wald's (1915) early experiments in community-based care left a rich legacy that is still pertinent in today's health-care environment. Her work suggested that we (a) create a mix of public and private programs that link effectively with health-care institutions as "value-added" or complementary to client needs, (b) use evidence-based practice as a counterbalance to document cost versus effectiveness, (c) institute sufficient control over practice to produce desired outcomes, and (d) have expert practitioners with sufficient education and abilities to manage complex care (Buhler-Wilkerson, 1993).

Wald's legacy is similar to the interdisciplinary definition of case management that was developed by the Case Management Society of America (CMSA), defining case management as "a collaborative process of assessment, planning, facilitation and advocacy for options and services to meet an individual's health needs through communication and available resources to promote quality cost effective outcomes" (CMSA, 1995, p.8) . The historical anecdotes of Wald's public health nurses demonstrated the work of an expert nurse who managed care for individuals and populations. These nurses practiced the core functions of case management: assessment, planning, linking, monitoring, advocacy, and outreach.

In the early 1900s, as an expansion of the role of the community-based public health nurse caring for individuals, the federal government mandated the United States Public Health Service to develop a system of case management with the community as the client. Their initial charge was to coordinate larger environmental problems such as sanitation and the prevention and control of epidemics. The thrust to address individual needs through the United States Public Health Service did not occur until passage of the Social Security Act in 1935, which provided funds to support these activities (Shonick, 1988). The 1920s saw the development of the Community Chest Movement and other social planning agencies (excluding nursing) to deal with coordinating care for families in distress and abused children. Within this same period, child guidance centers were created that experimented with multidisciplinary team planning (including nursing) to avoid duplication or fragmentation of services (Kersbergen, 1996).

After World War II, the Veterans Administration established a center in Los Angeles for veterans' benefits, which was its first model for "one-stop" health care. This was the inception of its ongoing model for a continuum of care (Weil & Karls, 1985).

The 1960s and 1970s witnessed a proliferation of human services as a result of the Civil Rights Movement and President Johnson's "War on Poverty" (Weil & Karls, 1985). This proliferation of newly developed programs resulted in fragmented, duplicative, and uncoordinated services that were difficult for the public to navigate. Case management enabled the consumer to become an active participant in services provided. Additional programs for the mentally ill and mentally challenged, and legislation for health services to the military, continued to encourage integration of services and the development of a continuum of care. Demonstration projects in the 1970s created the role of "systems agent," a person charged with coordinating system resources for clients and accountability for success of this movement (Intagliata, 1982). In the 1980s, case management services moved beyond public health and the mentally ill and veterans' administration services into the acute-care hospitals with the initiation of the prospective payment system. At the same time health insurance companies also initiated case management to shorten hospital stays and coordinate and manage services for participants with high costs or catastrophic illnesses (Brault & Kissinger, 1991; Mollica & Gillespie, 2003). The entrance of health maintenance organizations (HMOs) and preferred provider organizations (PPOs) as insurance products for prepaid health-care delivery added to the frenzy to control costs while delivering quality care. The efforts to coordinate services and control costs affected the majority of health-care consumers by the late 1980s, as prepaid or per case payment systems became the norm in both private and public sectors. At the start of the 21st century we see HMOs and PPOs giving way to accountable care organizations (ACOs) and medical homes (Watson, 2011). Controlling costs remains the mainstay for fiscal viability, and nurse case management continues to play a pivotal role in this arena.

On March 23, 2010, President Obama signed into law the Patient Protection and Affordable Care Act (PPACA, 2010). The intent of this act is to ensure access to high-quality, affordable health-care coverage for 93% of all Americans. Its goal is to contain costs while delivering this comprehensive care. The act is complex and has been constitutionally challenged by several states. On June 28 of 2012, the United States Supreme Court released its ruling, finding PPACA to be constitutional. In the majority opinion, the constitutionality of the individual mandate section of the Patient Protection and Affordable Care Act (PPACA)—the centerpiece of the case—was upheld. This individual mandate requires all Americans to buy insurance or pay a fine. The concept of a fine was seen as unconstitutional and subsequently redefined as a tax that the government has the constitutional power to impose, and PPACA survived on that basis. Political attention has now turned to the presidential election of November 2012. Should a new president be elected who is not supportive of PPACA, repealing this legislation could be a possibility, if the new Congress also aligns itself with such presidential sentiments (New York Times, 2012).

Within the Centers for Medicare and Medicaid Services (CMS), provisions of the PPACA create ACO. An ACO is a network of professional care providers and settings for care, including hospitals. Each network will address the needs of a minimum of 5,000 patients . It is not a place but a concept contained within a corporate structure. ACO professionals include physicians, nurse practitioners, physician assistances, and clinical nurse specialists (HealthCare.gov, 2012).

An example of PPACA impacting the role of NPs is contained in Section 5501 (PPACA, 2010, p. 534), which "provides a 10 percent (10%) bonus payment under Medicare for fiscal years 2011 through 2016 to primary care practitioners (including nurse practitioners, clinical nurse specialists, and physicians assistants) and general surgeons practicing in health professional shortage areas." The act also turns the spotlight on medical homes. The concept of a medical home grew from a 2002 Future of Family Medicine project that recommended that every American have a "personal medical home" through which to receive comprehensive health-care services.

DIFFERENTIATING THE LEVELS OF NURSE CASE MANAGEMENT PRACTICE

Historically, discussion has been centered on the use of nurse case managers prepared at the baccalaureate versus the advanced practice level (Bower, 1992; Cesta & Tahan, 2003; Connors, 1993; Mahn & Spross, 1996). The American Nurses Association (ANA, 1992) asserts that minimum preparation for a nurse case manager is a bachelor's degree with 3 years of relevant experience. However, in practice, nurses functioning in case management positions have differing clinical and educational backgrounds, including, in some settings, registered nurses (RNs) without a master's degree or even a bachelor of science in nursing (BSN). Their roles and responsibilities are also quite varied and defined in different ways, depending on the clinical site. The Tahan and Huber study (2006) provides an analysis of changes that occurred in the practice of case management over the 5-year period between the mid-1990s and early 2000s, and highlights the activities, relationships, knowledge, and skills most required in recent years.

Connors (1993) suggested that because case managers serve clients with varying levels of care across the continuum, not every client who is case managed is complex or catastrophic. He pointed out that even though the nurses with master's degrees may be best suited to fill case management positions, this may not be possible given the practice demands. One approach would be to have baccalaureate-prepared nurses manage most clients and have APNs manage those cases with more complex needs. In other words, the nurse's expertise "should be matched with the complexity of the situation and amount of autonomy required to fulfill the role" (Connors, 1993, p. 196).

Support for the APN case management role, particularly with high-risk or high-cost client populations, has been documented in the literature (Connors, 1993; Cronin & Maklebust, 1989; Hamric, 1992; Krichbaum, 1999; Naylor, Brooten, Campbell, Jacobsen, Mezey, & Pauly, 2010). The APN has expert knowledge regarding the clinical population for which standards and pathways are written, and sees the whole client and understands his or her needs on a continuum-of-care basis. Moreover, the APN has the additional requirement of outcome accountability (Krichbaum, 1999).

An expanding use of APNs is noticed in the case management of patients with chronic diseases. As a result of their education and clinical skills, APNs are able to focus on the multidimensional nature of chronic illness. A group of hospital-based clinics called on APNs to join a team effort that successfully improved clinical outcomes for patients with diabetes (Boville, Saran, Salem, & Clough, 2007).

Similarly, Mahn and Zazworsky (2000) pointed out that APNs are well suited to perform case management for complex client populations because of their advanced education, autonomy, ability to conduct extensive assessments, and ability to initiate and modify treatment regimens. These authors cited the work of Connors (1993), Hamric (1992), Lamb (1992), and Mahn and Spross (1996) to describe how the competencies of the APN role mirror those of the nurse case manager. Umbrell (2006) and Curtis, Lien, Chan, Grove, and Morris (2002) demonstrated the effectiveness of the APN in trauma management. The APN possesses specialized knowledge in providing "direct care, consultation, research utilization/continuous quality improvement, collaboration, data analysis and information management, change agency, ethical decision making and expert guidance and coaching" for a specific client population (Mahn & Zazworsky, 2000, p. 568). Such competencies are all congruent to those of nurse case managers. To a lesser extent, arguments have also been presented for separate graduate programs in case management versus increasing case management content in existing advanced practice master's programs (Falter, Cesta, Concert, & Mason, 1999; Sowell & Young, 1997). One argument is that nurse practitioners (NPs) and clinical nurse specialists (CNSs) who are prepared at the master's level have the advanced clinical knowledge needed to care for clients with complex health-care needs and these nurses can effectively work with high-risk clinical populations. On the other hand, graduates who are master's prepared in case management have in-depth knowledge and skill in case management models, systems, and tools, health-care financing, reimbursement, and community resource use. These nurses can provide case management services and provide the leadership to design systems of care coordination and quality management in health-care organizations. Graduates from both types of master's programs can make a significant contribution to case management practice, administration, education, and research (Cesta & Tahan, 2003). More research demonstrating the effectiveness of nurses who have baccalaureate and master's degrees needs to be conducted. Moreover, it is important that a distinction be made among nurses prepared at the baccalaureate, master's–advanced practice (NP or CNS), and master's–case management levels. See **Box 15-1** for a description of the levels of nurse case management practice.

NURSE CASE MANAGEMENT MODELS

A review of the literature provides many types of case management models and differentiates the contributions each makes within a designated field. The common aspects of these models are advocacy, services brokering, risk management, care coordination, and a process designed to accomplish these objectives (Huber, 2000). Knollmueller (1989) identified seven models of case management: (a) social, (b) primary care, (c) medical/social, (d) HMO, (e) independent, (f) insurance, and (g) in-house. Stempel, Doerge, Van Mie, and Combs (1997) describe four types of nurse case management: (a) clinical case management, (b) payer-based case management, (c) program case management, and (d) community case management. More recently Daniels and Ramsey (2005) proposed the use of five main models of case management that they have observed: (a) clinical case management, (b) collaborative practice models, (c) populations models, (d) functional models, and (e) clinical resource management models. In commenting on these models, Zander (2008) noted that some hospitals are incorporating APNs to fill the case management functions alone or working with other case management personnel. A multidisciplinary team at the Johns Hopkins Bloomberg School of Public Health designed the Guided Care Model for the better care of older people with chronic conditions. In this model, a primary care registered nurse prepared in chronic care works with two to five physicians and

BOX 15-1

Differentiating Between the Nurse Case Manager with a Baccalaureate Degree or Master's Degree as an APN, and a Nurse with Specific Master's Preparation in Case Management

Levels of case management:

Baccalaureate registered nurse (RN) case managers have foundational theoretical and clinical knowledge in nursing. These nurses are able to manage the care of patients who are less complex and more predictable, often with the assistance of critical paths. These nurses may work in collaboration with an advanced practice nurse (APN) case manager prepared at the master's level or a nurse case manager prepared at the master's level.

Master's–APN case managers have clinical expertise and advanced knowledge in health and wellness promotion and illness intervention models for specific patient populations. These nurses can manage patients with complex health needs, such as those in high-risk, vulnerable populations, and those who require high resource consumption. In addition, these nurses are expected to conduct research related to case management practice, disease management, and clinical outcomes.

Nurses with master's level preparation specifically for the functional role of case manager possess expert knowledge and skill in case management models, processes and tools, healthcare financing, reimbursement, outcome monitoring, and measurement. These nurses are able to design and monitor systems of care coordination and deliver case management services, and are expected to conduct research related to case management practice and clinical outcomes.

members of the care team to provide patient-centered, coordinated, and cost-effective care. Their research demonstrated that the Guided Care Model improved the self-reports of chronic health care for multiple-morbid older persons (Boyd et al., 2009).

The literature on nurse case manager practice within the different models reflects some dilemmas regarding the purpose, scope, and functions of the nurse case manager role. Although there is a large body of anecdotal stories, research in the field is still working to control the effect of extraneous variables in studies and developing nursing-sensitive outcomes. Qualitative descriptions of nurse case management practice have pointed to some common themes across all nurse case management practice. They include (a) working with individuals, families, and populations at risk; (b) applying the nursing process to enhance quality and cost outcomes; (c) accessing individuals and families in more than one setting; and (d) coordination and advocacy integrated throughout (Lamb, 1995).

Hellwig, Yam, and DiGiulio (2003) proposed an advocacy model for nurse case management practice. In the authors' qualitative study, hospital-based nurse case managers described that their advocacy was based on the needs of the patient and the patient's family, payer issues, and obstacles and opportunities for advocacy. Participants indicated the obstacles included time constraints and examples of opportunities were physician support, rapport with insurance companies, and use of a team approach (Hellwig et al., 2003).

The nurse case management models used in practice today are as rich and diverse as the individuals, families, and populations they serve. Current practice within hospital-based models in many organizations has moved from a primarily clinical case manager role to one of an intense discharge planning model. Conversely, the hospital-to-community-based and community-based models have experienced an increasing need for a high level of clinical expertise in their case managers, as well as the traditional knowledge of community resources and health-care reimbursement methodologies. Historically, nursing case management moved into the foreground with public health nursing at the beginning of the 20th century. As models continue to evolve in response to practice needs and environmental changes, the models for the 21st century must continue to include and enhance the role APNs can and do play in community-based practice models. According to Zander (2008), case management models that are reviewed at the executive level in hospitals are considered very expensive. In light of this we need more cost-benefit research on case management efforts and models.

CASE MANAGER RESPONSIBILITIES AND SKILLS

Quality of care and efficient use of limited resources have been a hallmarks of case management since the 1860s, with the intervening influence of early settlement houses, public health nursing, federal and state legislation, and managed care. Regardless of who drives the process (e.g., insurance company, employer, federal government, or private entrepreneur), the outcome expectations are similar. The definitions of quality and efficiency may differ by source, but all models require a skill and knowledge set of their case managers. The setting in which the case manager practices, the model design, and the patient population dictate the overall knowledge base and clinical expertise required. The national quality agenda will be supported by the involvement of nurse case managers. Case managers in all settings are alert to the importance of evaluation of quality and the appropriateness of care delivered to patients (White, 2004).

Successful nurse case management mandates a wide variety of both management and clinical skills. Some of the most typical management skills include delegation, conflict resolution, collaboration, crisis intervention, coordination, direction, consultation, and fiscal accountability. Clinical skill requirements vary from model to model and may include nurses educated from the diploma/associate degree to master's level. The suggested practice areas for differing levels of education (baccalaureate to master's) are also discussed in this chapter. Nurses educated at the diploma/associate degree level frequently find themselves in positions in nurse case management similar to the baccalaureate RN case manager described in Box 15-1. A summary of the most common skills and competencies of nurse case managers is found in **Table 15-1.** This table is not meant to be an exhaustive listing of skills and competencies, but rather a snapshot view of what is needed by nurse case managers in varying situations.

Nurse case management continues to be a hybrid within nursing and has led many to examine the issue of "clinical expertise" as listed in the job descriptions of case managers. Calkin (1984), in attempting to differentiate between the expertise of a nurse case manager and an APN case manager,

TABLE 15-1

Skills and Competencies of the Nurse Case Manager

Skill/Competency	Goal
Patient advocacy	Assist patient in achieving autonomy and self-determination
Guardian of confidentiality	Preserve dignity and privacy
Case selection expert	Identify recipients of case management
Care coordinator	Procure and broker services; seamless continuum
Assessment and reassessment	Problem identification/resolution; monitor outcomes
Discharge planner	Facilitate movement in care continuum
Follow-through	Optimum care within resources available
Use management	Use resources appropriately
Knowledge of insurance structures/ benefits	Interpret resources available to patient
Cost-benefit analysis (fiscal advocacy)	Demonstrate case management effect on care, usually monetary
Negotiation	Procure what patient requires for health purposes
Clinical expertise*	Intervene appropriately, improve outcomes
Critical thinking	Think out of the box to find creative solutions and increase case manager autonomy
Competent professional (includes accountability, knowledge of standards of practice, legal issues, and research ability)	Do the right thing at the right time for the right reason
Outcomes management	Evaluate and manage outcomes
Interpersonal (communication, assertiveness, collaboration, and tact/diplomacy)	Gather information and channel to appropriate sources
Organizational (time management, marketing/networking, prioritization, and report writer)	Use time and people resources wisely

*Depends on case management model and setting.

Sources: Powell, S. K. (2000). *Case management: A practice guide to success in managed care.* Philadelphia: Lippincott Williams & Wilkins; and More, P. K., & Mandell, S. (1997). *Nursing case management: An evolving practice.* New York: McGraw-Hill.

defined the former as experts by experience and the latter as prepared by a combination of clinical experience and education. The advanced practice case managers retain their use of experience-based intuition, but use their additional academic and clinical preparation to manage more highly complex and unpredictable individuals and populations. Although the focus of advanced practice case managers is still on providing direct patient care, they also make significant contributions toward coordination of multidisciplinary care. This advanced practitioner in a case manager role can continue to monitor, advocate, and coordinate care for patients across the continuum and can develop programs and systems to support both community-based and private-practice-based care (Erickson, 1997).

Not all case managers practice the duties and responsibilities of managing patient care at the same advanced level. As nurse case managers become involved in more complex cases, the need for advanced education becomes apparent. This growth in complexity has resulted in the need for APNs to join the ranks of case managers (Stanton, Swanson, Sherrod, & Packa, 2005).

TOOLS AND STRATEGIES

Through the development of clinical expertise, knowledge of research processes, communication skills, critical thinking, decision making, and leadership skills, the APN is uniquely qualified to influence case management and chronic care management in a variety of health-care environments. The strategic use of APNs in the case management role to improve communication and collaboration with the treatment team is an effective tool, given the importance of primary care practitioner involvement in the success of case and chronic care management interventions. Evidence-based interventions and standardized outcome measures are important strategies used in chronic care management programs to improve the quality of health-care services. In an effort to assist case managers and program designers to identify effective tools and evidence-based guidelines for case management, and to standardize the evaluation of the outcomes of case management interventions, the Case Management Society of America (CMSA) created the Council for Case Management Accountability (CCMA) in 1996 (CMSA, 2002). Through the use of expert case management researchers and practitioners, the CCMA has identified five care domains and outcomes in which case management has been shown or believed to have an effect:

- *Patient knowledge:* Case management patients need adequate knowledge on a number of fronts, including knowledge about health benefits and services, knowledge about their health conditions, and knowledge about their treatment plans. Successful case management results in improved patient knowledge.
- *Patient involvement in care:* Health care is a cooperative endeavor; patients play a key role in high-quality, cost-effective care. Successful case management involves clients in the decisions and actions of self-care.
- *Patient empowerment:* Case management should help patients build a sense of self-efficacy regarding their ability to manage their own health, as well as an ability to negotiate the care system successfully.
- *Patient adherence:* Cost-effective health care is predicated on patients' consistent adherence to their treatment programs. Successful case management results in higher rates of patient adherence.
- *Coordination of care:* Case managers provide consistency of care across the continuum while eliminating redundancy and waste (CMSA, 2002).

The CCMA's goal was to publish state-of-the-science "white papers" in each of these domains, with the goal of providing case managers with the latest evidence-based intervention strategies and tools along with standardized outcome measures. Through the use of these tools, case managers increase the likelihood of successful case management interventions and form a basis for consistent research and comparison of case management results. The work of the CCMA also helps to focus program development in the domains in which case management is thought to have an impact on health outcomes of individuals and at-risk populations.

Little is known to date regarding the amount or type of nursing (or "dose of nursing") needed to affect patient outcomes. This knowledge is necessary in applying case and chronic care management interventions (Brooten & Naylor, 1995). For example, there have been a number of published studies highlighting the effectiveness of APNs as case managers for Medicare-aged members with heart failure. The question becomes, is it necessary for the APN to have direct patient interaction or contact at the primary care office or clinic or in the home, or is it just as effective to use telemedicine approaches with this population? Should the use of the APN be applied to high-risk chronic care management, or should APNs be included in health education and promotion strategies? What interventions provide the most effective health and financial outcomes? Similar to the work of the CMSA-CCMA project, the University of Iowa College of Nursing has been involved since 1995 in research supported by the National Institute of Nursing entitled "The Iowa Nursing Intervention and Outcomes Projects—NIC [Nursing Interventions Classifications] & NOC [Nursing Outcomes Classification]." The NIC is a comprehensive standardized language used to describe evidence-based nursing interventions and provide the documented literature and research on which each is based. Each intervention reflects current clinical practice and research. All interventions are accompanied by a list of background readings that support the development of the intervention; all interventions have been reviewed by experts in clinical practice and by relevant clinical practice specialty organizations; a feedback process to receive suggested changes has been developed (Iowa Interventions and Outcomes Project, 2002).

The NOC is standardized language that describes patient outcomes sensitive to the nursing interventions noted in NIC. When tied to the work of the CCMA (focusing on those interventions and outcomes linked to the five core domains of case management), NIC and NOC can assist case managers in using evidence-based nursing interventions for care planning and the identification of appropriate outcome measures. This work is comprehensive, readily available, and updated on a regular basis. In addition, NIC and NOC are available on CD-ROM, which allows for easy access by case managers. Although few case managers and administrators are aware of the work of the CCMA or of NIC and NOC, researchers have begun to evaluate the use of the classification system in practice settings (Solari-Twadell & Hackbarth, 2010; Wong, 2008).

Another strategy used to ensure high-quality, effective case management processes and outcomes is the development of electronic medical records and/or database systems with care management assessment, planning, and outcomes tracking capabilities. Systems that alert the treatment team to gaps in care, for example, abnormal biometric data, and non–evidence-based treatment regimens, improve patient outcomes as well.

In the absence of existing outcomes data, those who routinely evaluate the quality of programs consider the following equation as an indicator of the potential for good outcomes: good structure + good processes = good outcomes (Donabedian, 1980).

Finally, and most important, tools used to identify those individuals who can most benefit from exceptional case management services and interventions that focus on communication and relationship building are critical. Predictive models and algorithms that produce registries of the chronically ill high-risk patients have become important tools in identifying the 5% of the population that can account for 50% of the medical costs—these are the individuals who can most benefit from case management services (Forman & Kelliher, 1999). Additional training and development in techniques such as motivational interviewing and intrinsic coaching increases the case manager's ability to improve a person's ability to make choices and to seek relevance and value in making health changes that directly relate to his or her life goals (Miller & Rollnick, 2002).

CHRONIC CARE MANAGEMENT AND THE ROLE OF THE ADVANCED PRACTICE NURSE

APNs have played an active role in both case and chronic care management, particularly as a case manager within the acute and community care settings. Research has found many benefits of using APNs in the case management role, in particular, qualities such as clinical expertise and improved access and communication with treating physicians in the community. This improved access and communication, along with the expert clinical knowledge regarding a particular disease state, can result in observable improved outcomes for individual patients receiving treatment for these targeted conditions within disease management programs.

According to Watts and colleagues (2009), the skills of the APN in case management led multidisciplinary teams to achieve significant gains in patient self-management, decision support, and delivery system design. Because APNs are trained to think holistically, to foster team building (a factor in implementing planned care), and to educate and motivate patients, they are particularly needed in multidisciplinary/group-based practices that strive to address the needs of chronically ill members, such as the patient-centered medical home or the ACO (Dancer & Courtney, 2010; Naylor & Kurtzman, 2010; Watts et al., 2009).

Some research has been conducted on the cost-effectiveness of APN management of patients with chronic illness. Paez and Allen (2006) evaluated the cost-effectiveness of APN case management to lower blood lipids in patients with coronary heart disease. Their findings "suggest that case management by an APN is a cost-efficient and therapeutically effective strategy in managed care, to improve the care of patients with cardiovascular disease" (p. 439) (Boville et al., 2007).

THE ADVANCED PRACTICE NURSE: CHRONIC CARE MANAGEMENT EXAMPLES

Example 1: The Advanced Practice Nurse in the Program Development Role in a Managed Care Setting

K is a typical APN care manager within the managed care setting. She has a strong clinical background in oncology. As part of her role in the medical management department, K was recently asked to participate in the strategic planning for the development of a new care management program.

Expert clinical knowledge and an ability to apply this knowledge are critical in the development of successful care management interventions for managed care. Knowledge of a particular disease process is essential to identify the applicability of disease management interventions. For example, many conditions are considered to be potential targets for disease management primarily because of a high prevalence or high costs of preventable complications associated with the particular disease. However, not all diseases can effectively be managed using disease management program principles. The hallmark of these programs is coordination of health-care services and improving self-care measures. The APNs' expert clinical knowledge of a particular disease state and their knowledge of the care provided within the health-care system can identify critical junctures at which disease management interventions can be the most effective.

K used both of these skills in her evaluation of cancer as a potential target for disease management. Although cancer is prevalent among commercial populations and is also a high-cost disease state, it is considered to be a difficult disease to manage. K noted that many individuals with cancer are admitted to the hospital as a result of the side effects of chemotherapeutic agents. With education and improved self-care measures, could these admissions be avoided? Could this be the critical juncture in managing avoidable costs? She then proceeded to recommend the design of an education packet and telephonic outreach protocol focusing on prehydration for members undergoing chemotherapy to prevent dehydration admissions, and dietary considerations in the prevention of anemia. She designed an educational packet to include reputable Web sites for lay review of the national cancer treatment protocols and a number of community resources and support groups. Through her knowledge of the disease process and an opportunity for improved care, K identified a key juncture for focused disease management intervention. The rate of admissions for the complications of chemotherapy—specifically dehydration and anemia—are the clinical outcome measures that will determine the success of this program.

In addition, collaboration with the treating oncologist to support the physician's treatment plan and encourage patient participation in the program is critical. The APN, working with the health plan's medical director, can assist in meeting this goal.

Example 2: The Advanced Practice Nurse's Role in Continuous Quality Improvement

M is an APN with extensive experience in hospice care. Many cancer patients are successfully treated; however, many other cancers result in terminal conditions. Few terminal cases receive the benefits of hospice care. M, as a case manager in the managed care setting, has noted this trend and has suggested that there be an evaluation of end-of-life care for disease management. Improvements in the quality of care provided in these circumstances may result in the reduction of acute service admissions and improved quality of life, particularly through pain management and support of individuals and families through death and dying. This example demonstrates the need to have APNs in the managed care setting consistently in search of areas for improvement and disease management intervention. With frequent review of the literature and observation of trends, the APN frequently identifies, plans, and implements care management solutions. Rather than reacting to market forces and trends, the APN, as a member of the managed care team, consistently seeks areas for continued improvement and service to clients. The health plan that uses this intellectual capital is provided with managed care solutions that not only provide value to its customers facing escalating health-care costs and the challenges of variability in the quality of care received, but also can differentiate itself from reactionary competitors.

REIMBURSEMENT AND MARKETING OF CASE MANAGEMENT PRACTICE

Physicians' current procedural terminology (CPT) codes are available for the reimbursement of case management services in a fee-for-service environment. Therefore, clinicians who normally bill for services using the CPT coding system, such as physicians and APNs, can bill for time used to deliver case management services in the outpatient setting. Managed care organizations have also begun to pay for improvement to establish accountable care arrangements (ACAs) with primary care practices providing shared savings and/or pay for improvement opportunities focusing on quality of chronic care management, transitions in care, patient access, and cost-effectiveness.

As more physician groups enter shared-savings ACAs and pay-for-performance arrangements, predictive modeling and case management services have become the solution to managing the health risk of the small percentage of individuals who drive the large percentage of health-care expenditures. In addition, it is not uncommon for case management to be a revenue-generating option/service line for hospitals and managed care organizations affected/motivated by health-care reform and new reimbursement models. Case management services and the systems/tools used to support these activities are in high demand. Consequently, APNs with exceptional case management skills and experience are valuable.

EDUCATION FOR NURSE CASE MANAGEMENT PRACTICE

Outside academic settings, education on case management can occur via continuing education courses, institutes, and on-the-job training. Within academic settings, case management concepts may be integrated into baccalaureate- and master's-level curricula or taught in required or elective courses. Also, at the graduate level there are master's programs in case management. Another model is to offer case management as a concentration in which students take a required number of courses in addition to training in a clinical specialty or administration.

On-the-job training or short training courses are not likely to be adequate because offering content solely as an elective course cannot expose all nurses to essential knowledge bases necessary to assume case management functions. To best prepare nurses for case management practice within a managed care environment, it is recommended that educators adopt a systematic approach to the integration of case management in nursing curricula. Approaches to incorporating such content are described elsewhere (Mundt, 1996; Powell & Tahan, 2008; Sinnen & Schifalaqua, 1996; Sowell & Young, 1997).

Overall, at the baccalaureate level, case management should be considered a core curriculum concept and threaded throughout the undergraduate program. At the graduate level, in addition to core graduate and specialty content, advanced practice curricula should contain theory and clinical experiences related to case management, care coordination across the continuum, community resource use, and managed care concepts including reimbursement and health-care financing. Because nurse case managers look to the skills of other health-care professionals in their care planning, an interdisciplinary course would also prove invaluable.

The curriculum sponsored by the CMSA notes that there are essential elements of study. These include managed care, use management, and legal and ethical issues, among others. It is also noted that change is constant and case managers must keep up with the changes in the health-care system (Powell & Ignatavicius, 2001).

Finally, there is a need for graduate programs to prepare nurse case management specialists. Master's programs in case management should include core graduate content, as well as specialized content related to case management models, strategies, tools, quality management, health-care financing and reimbursement systems, managed care, health-care outcomes, client education, community resources, clinical practice in case management, and role development. Course work and clinical experiences with specific aggregate populations is highly recommended. Moreover, such curricula need to prepare graduates who can practice case management in both inpatient and outpatient settings and organizational venues, such as insurance companies. Offering master's programs in case management and integrating case management content at the master's level for APNs will produce practitioners who can deliver nursing case management services, create systems of care coordination, and institute policy that will reflect quality outcomes.

The newer terminal degree offering for APNs, the doctor of nursing practice, offers many new avenues of knowledge and skills to further enhance the case management role of the APN. The integration of nursing science with advanced levels of systems thinking and accountability in designing, delivering, and evaluating evidence-based practice to improve quality, safety, and outcomes should add significantly to the patient experience and decrease cost. New leadership skills directed at the development and implementation of patient-driven health policy and effective collaboration with nursing and other disciplines to promote cultural competence in response to health-care needs has the potential to engage patients as active participants in improving their health status.

CONCLUSION

This chapter has explored the historical roots of the case manager role; levels of practice for nurse case managers; various case management models; case management roles and skills; tools and strategies, including chronic care management for APNs; and issues such as reimbursement, marketing, and education for practice. This is an exciting and challenging time to be an APN within a case management practice environment. Those who successfully grasp the role and function will be the pacesetters for tomorrow's health-care challenges. This will also ensure a place at the table for nursing as it grows and develops and provides the nation with innovative care models.

REFERENCES

American Nurses Association. (1992). *Case management by nurses.* Kansas City, MO: American Nurses Association.

Boville, D., Saran, M., Salem, J. K., & Clough, L. (2007). An innovative role for nurse practitioners in managing chronic disease. *Nursing Economic$, 25*(6), 359–364.

Bower, K. S. (1992). *Case management by nurses* (2nd ed., pp. 13–15). Kansas City, MO: American Nurses Association.

Boyd, C. M., Reider, L., Frey, K., Scharfstein, D., Leff, B., Wolff, J., et al. (2009). The effects of guided care on the perceived quality of health care for multi-morbid older persons: 18 month outcomes from a cluster-randomized controlled trial. *Journal of General Internal Medicine, 25*(3), 235–242.

Brault, G. L., & Kissinger, L. D. (1991). Case management: Ambiguous at best. *Journal of Pediatric Health Care, 5*(4), 179–183.

Brooten, D., & Naylor, M. D. (1995). Nurses' effect on changing patient outcomes. *Image, 27*(2), 95–99.

Buhler-Wilkerson, K. (1993). Public health then and now: Bringing care to the people. *American Journal of Public Health, 83*(12), 1778–1786.

Calkin, J. (1984). A model for advanced nursing practice. *Journal of Nursing Administration, 14*(1), 24–30.

Case Management Society of America. (1995). *Standards of practice for case management.* Little Rock, AR: Case Management Society of America. Case Management Society of America. (2002). Center for Case Management Accountability. Retrieved September 9, 2002, from http:// www.CMSA.org/ccma-main.

Cesta, T., Tahan, H.A. (2003). *The case manager's survival guide,* 2nd edition. St. Louis, MO: Mosby.

Connors, H. R. (1993). Impact of care management modalities on curricula. In K. Kelly & M. Maas (Eds.), *Managing nursing care* (pp. 190–207). St. Louis: Mosby.

Cronin, C. J., & Maklebust, J. (1989). Case-managed care: Capitalizing on the CNS. *Nursing Management, 20*(3), 38–47.

Curtis, K., Lien, D., Chan, A., Grove, P., & Morris, R. (2002). The impact of trauma case management on patient outcomes. *Journal of Trauma: Injury, Infection and Critical Care, 53*(3), 477–482.

Dancer, S., & Courtney, M. (2010). Improving diabetes patient outcomes: Framing research into the chronic care model. *Journal of the American Academy of Nurse Practitioners, 22,* 580–585.

Daniels, S., & Ramey, M. (2005). *The leaders guide to hospital case management.* Sudbury, MA: Jones & Bartlett.

Dock, L. (1937). Whence the term "public health nursing"? *Public Health Nursing, 29*(12), 712–714.

Donabedian, A. (1980). *Explorations in quality assessment and monitoring: The definition of quality and approaches to its assessment.* Ann Arbor, MI: Health Administration.

Erickson, S. M. (1997). Managing case management across the continuum: An organized response to managed care. *Seminars for Nurse Managers, 5*(3), 124–128.

Falter, E. J., Cesta, T. G., Concert, C., & Mason, D. J. (1999). Development of a graduate program in case management. *Journal of Care Management, 5*(3), 50–56, 72, 74, 76–78.

Forman, S., & Kelliher, M. (1999). *StatusOne: Breakthroughs in high risk population health management.* San Francisco: Jossey-Bass.

Frachel, R. R. (1988). A new profession: The evolution of public health nursing. *Public Health Nursing, 5*(2), 86–90.

Hamric, A. B. (1992). Creating our future: Challenges and opportunities for the clinical nurse specialist. *Oncology Nursing Forum, 19*(1 suppl), 11–15.

HealthCare.gov. (2012, August 20). *Accountable Care Organizations: Improving Care Coordination for People with Medicare.* Retrieved August 20, 2012, from http://www.healthcare.gov/news/factsheets/2011/03/accountablecare03312011a.html.

Hellwig, S. D., Yam, M., & DiGiulio, M. (2003). Nurse case managers' perceptions of advocacy. *Lippincott's Case Management, 8*(2), 53–63.

Huber, D. L. (2000). The diversity of case management models. *Case Management, 5*(6), 248–255.

Intagliata, J. (1982). Improving the quality of community care for the chronically mentally disabled: The role of case management. *Schizophrenia Bulletin, 8*(4), 655–674.

Iowa Interventions and Outcomes Project. (2002). *Nursing interventions classification.* Retrieved August 10, 2002, from www.nursing.uiowa.edu/centers/cncce/nic/nicquestions.htm.

Kersbergen, A. L. (1996). Case management: A rich history of coordinating care to control costs. *Nursing Outlook, 44*(4), 169–172.

Knollmueller, R. N. (1989). Case management: What's in a name? *Nursing Management, 20*(10), 38–42.

Krichbaum, K. (1999). Advanced practice nurse case managers and care pathways. In M. Snyder & M. P. Mirr (Eds.), *Advanced practice nursing: A guide to professional development* (2nd ed., pp. 99–116). New York: Springer.

Lamb, G. S. (1992). Conceptual and methodological issues: Nursing case management research. *Advances in Nursing Science, 15*(2), 16–24. Lamb, G. S. (1995). Case management. *Annual Review of Nursing Research, 13,* 117–136.

Mahn, V. A., & Spross, J. A. (1996). Nurse case management as an advanced practice role. In A. B. Hamric, J. A. Spross, & C. M. Hanson (Eds.), *Advanced nursing practice: An integrative approach* (pp. 445–465). Philadelphia: WB Saunders.

Mahn, V. A., & Zazworsky, D. (2000). Nurse case management as an advanced practice role. In A. B. Hamric, J. A. Spross, & C. M. Hanson (Eds.), *The advanced practice nurse case manager: An integrative approach* (2nd ed., pp. 549–606). Philadelphia: WB Saunders.

Miller, W. R., & Rollnick, S. (2002). *Motivational interviewing—Preparing people for change* (2nd ed.). New York: Guilford Press. Retrieved April 1, 2008, from www.totallycoached.com/en/aboutus/intrinsiccoaching/.

Mollica, R. L., & Gillespie, J. (2003). *Care coordination for people with chronic conditions: Partnership for solutions.* Retrieved May 17, 2011, from http://partnershipforsolutions.org/DMS/files/carecoordination/pdf.

More, P. K., & Mandell, S. (1997). *Nursing case management: An evolving practice.* New York: McGraw-Hill.

Mundt, M. H. (1996). Key elements of nurse case management in curricula. In E. L. Cohen (Ed.), *Nurse case management in the 21st century* (pp. 48–54). St. Louis: Mosby.

Naylor, M., Brooten, D., Campbell, R., Jacobsen, B. S., Mezey, M. D., Pauly, M., et al. (2010). Comprehensive discharge planning and home follow-up of hospitalized elders. *Journal of the American Medical Association, 28*(7), 613–620.

Naylor, M., & Kurtzman, E. (1999). The role of nurse practitioners in reinventing primary care. *Health Affairs, 29*(5), 893–899.

New York Times. (June 29, 2012). Health care reform and the Supreme Court (Affordable Care Act). Retrieved August 20, 2012 from http://topics.nytimes.com/top/reference/timestopics/organizations/s/supreme_court/affordable_care_act/ index.html.

Paez, K. A., & Allen, J. K. (2006). Cost effectiveness of nurse practitioner management of hypercholesterolemia following coronary revascularization. *Journal of the American Academy of Nurse Practitioners, 18*(9), 436–445.

Palmer, R. E. (1969). *Hermeneutics.* Evanston, IL: Northwestern University.

Powell, S. K. (2000). *Case management: A practice guide to success in managed care.* Philadelphia: Lippincott Williams & Wilkins.

Powell, S. K., & Ignatavicius, D. (2001). *Core curriculum for case management.* Philadelphia: Lippincott Williams & Wilkins.

Powell, S. K., & Tahan, H. A. (2008). CMS core curriculum for case management (2nd ed.) Philadelphia: Wolters Kluwer/Lippincott Williams & Wilkins. Profession of promoting health. (1919). *Public Health Nurse, 11*(1), 10–12.

Reverby, S. M. (1987). *Ordered to care: The dilemma of American nursing, 1850–1945.* New York: Cambridge University.

Reynolds, C. G., & Smeltzer, C. H. (1997). Case management: Past, present, future—The drivers for change. *Journal of Nursing Care Quality, 12*(1), 9–19.

Shonick, W. (1988). Public health services: Background and present status. In S. J. Williams & P. R. Torrens (Eds.), *Introduction to health services* (3rd ed., pp. 85–123). New York: Delmar.

Sinnen, M., & Schifalaqua, M. (1996). The education of nurses: Nurse case managers' view. In E. L. Cohen (Ed.), *Nurse case management in the 21st century* (pp. 55–62). St. Louis: Mosby.

Solari-Twadell, P. A., & Hackbarth, D. (2010). Evidence for a new paradigm of the ministry of parish nursing practice using the nursing intervention classification system. *Nursing Outlook, 58*(2), 69–75.

Sowell, R. L., & Young, S. W. (1997). Case management in nursing curriculum. *Nursing Care Management, 2*(4), 173–176.

Stanton, M. P., Swanson, M., Sherrod, R. A., & Packa, D. R. (2005). Case management evolution: From basic to advanced practice role. *Lippincott's Case Management, 10*(6), 274–284.

Stempel, J., Doerge, J., Van Mie, K., & Combs, J. (1997). Nurse case management. In B. Case (Ed.), *Career planning for nurses* (pp. 133–160). Albany, NY: Delmar.

Tahan, H. A. (1998). Case management: A heritage more than a century old. *Nursing Case Management, 3*(2), 55–60.

Tahan, H. A., & Huber, D. L. (2006). The CCMC's national study of case manager job descriptions. *Lippincott's Case Management, 11*(3), 127–144.

Umbrell, C. E. (2006). Trauma case management: A role for the advanced practice nurse. *Journal of Trauma Nursing, 13*(2), 70–73.

Wald, L. D. (1915). *The house on Henry Street.* New York: Henry Holt & Co.

Watson, A. C. (March/April 2011). Finding common ground in case management: New titles and terminology along the healthcare continuum. *Professional Case Management,* 16(2), 52-54. Watts, S. A., Gee, J., O'Day, M. E., Schaub, K., Lawrence, R., Aron, D., et al. (2009). Nurse practitioner–led multidisciplinary teams to improve chronic illness care: The unique strengths of nurse practitioners applied to shared medical appointments/group visits. *Journal of the American Academy of Nurse Practitioners, 21,* 167–172.

Weil, M., & Karls, J. (1985). Historical origins and recent developments in case management. In Weil, M. (Ed.), *Case management in human service practice.* San Francisco: Jossey-Bass.

White, A. B. (2004). Case management and the national quality agenda: Partnering to improve the quality of care. *Lippincott's Case Management, 9*(3), 132–140.

Wong, E. (2008, October 24). Coining and defining novel nursing terminology. Part 2: Critical incident nursing intervention. *International Journal of Nursing Terminologies and Classifications, 19*(4), 132–139. Zander, K. (2008). *Hospital case management models.* Danvers, MA: HCPro, Inc.

Zerwekh, J. V. (1992). Public health nursing legacy: Historical practical wisdom. *Nursing and Health Care, 13*(2), 84–91.

16 The Advanced Practice Nurse and Research

Suzanne M. Burns
Beth Quatrara

INTRODUCTION

The advanced practice nurse (APN) is a consumer, facilitator, collaborator, and leader in research conduction. The APN develops a research attitude in others and fosters evidence-based practice through the integration of research findings into clinical practice. The APN applies the scientific method to clinical problem solving and provides leadership in the use and conduct of research. Although for many years the concept of "conducting research" was not considered to be a dominant APN competency, this has changed. This chapter discusses APN research competencies and behaviors, and practical methods to successfully integrate research activities into practice. Buy-in and barriers to the APN research role are discussed in addition to strategies for success. Most important, how the APN develops a practice milieu that embraces evidence and considers research "part of what we do every day" is covered.

RESEARCH AS AN APN ROLE COMPONENT

The APN, a practice-based clinician with graduate education, is educated to contribute to nursing knowledge. APNs' education and clinical expertise contribute to their unique potential to be consumers of research while understanding the nuances of applying the new knowledge to patient-specific situations and unique practice settings. They translate research into practice and pragmatically implement the findings to provide high-quality care. By promoting evidence-based practice (EBP), APNs help narrow the theory-research-practice gap that plagues the clinical environment (Hanberg & Brown, 2006).

Research is a long-standing core competency of the APN role that continues to be emphasized as a central component regardless of the practice setting or specific role function (American Association of Colleges of Nursing [AACN], 1995, 2011; American Nurses Association [ANA], 1995; Hamric, 2009). It is not limited to a few clinicians practicing in a defined area. Today, the role of the APN as a researcher is stressed as a particularly essential element of APN education and practice. The new *Essentials of Master's Education in Nursing* requires that APNs graduate with the knowledge and skill to translate and integrate scholarship into practice (AACN, 2011). Schools of nursing that graduate master's-prepared nurses are required to demonstrate that APNs are trained to apply research outcomes within practice settings, resolve practice problems, work as change agents, and disseminate results (AACN, 2011). Similarly, the doctorate of nursing practice degree (DNP), a doctoral program for APN clinicians, emphasizes that the APN is expected to maintain a scholarly practice by focusing on practice improvement and innovation as well as testing care delivery models (AACN, 2006). The

APN role in research is further endorsed in the ANA's *Scope and Standards of Practice* (2004), noting that APNs integrate research findings into practice in addition to demonstrating competency behaviors that require APNs to "contribute to nursing knowledge by conducting or synthesizing research that discovers, examines and evaluates knowledge, theories, criteria, and creative approaches to improve healthcare practice" and to "formally disseminate research findings through activities such as presentations, publications, consultations and journal clubs" (ANA, 2004, p. 40). These educational requirements and practice statements clarify and reinforce the APN practice role in research. APNs' unique contributions as consumers of and contributors to research are recognized on many levels.

APN RESEARCH COMPETENCIES

Similar to other APN core competencies, research is a skill that builds and strengthens over time (Hamric, 2009). As the APN advances in the research role, she or he moves through three competency phases (De Palma, 2009). In the first, the APN focuses on interpreting and implementing research outcomes (De Palma, 2009). During this time, the APN gains research confidence and proficiency by introducing EBP. The APN facilitates the application of research by introducing both clinicians, including registered nurses, and administrators to EBP. When responding to clinical questions, the APN directs others to the literature and teaches them how to critique research and adapt their practice as appropriate to the findings. Effectively integrating research into practice is a key attribute that the APN brings to the practice setting. Taking into consideration readiness for change, resource requirements, and educational needs, the APN uses training, experience, and clinical authority to lead EBP changes and influence quality care. The APN uses a variety of forums to demonstrate this competency, including role-modeling, journal clubs, grand rounds, and clinical practice meetings.

In the second research competency phase, the APN begins to evaluate practice (De Palma, 2009). Using outcomes research, the clinician examines the effect of applying EBP guidelines to patient care or explores the impact of using research findings to improve quality indicators (De Palma, 2009). At this competency level, the APN begins to define measurement criteria and evaluate interventions in terms of documented outcomes. Measuring outcomes to determine the effectiveness of change is essential to the research role. Outcome results are used to make a final decision about sustaining the change versus placing the intervention on hold and reevaluating the process. Defining outcome measures before implementing change is required to obtain maximum effectiveness. Determining specific measurements, the method of data collection, and the party responsible for the data collection facilitates the evaluation process. Evaluation points, although specific to the exact intervention, can include a variety of indices such as clinical outcomes, satisfaction, time, and money. Several outcome tools already exist, and resources such as the *APN Data Collection Toolkit* may assist clinicians in the evaluation process (Vohra & Bryant-Lukosius, 2009).

In addition to clinical practice evaluation, APNs are also obligated to examine their own practice by evaluating the effect of their role. APN-specific outcomes, which can be similar to practice outcomes, are measured to showcase role efficacy, demonstrate research role competency, and validate APNs' unique contributions to patient care. Collecting APN role-specific outcome measures is an important aspect of practice that cannot be overlooked.

The third research competency incorporates the collaborative generation of new knowledge (De Palma, 2009). At this final stage of research competency, APNs are working with multidisciplinary team members to design and implement studies that have implications for nursing practice. The benefits of collaborative APN research include shared expertise, academic influence, access to clinical populations, efficient data collection, improved research relevance, and the creation of an environment that promotes the application of scholarship in patient care (Burman, Hart, & McCabe, 2005; Mercer, 2008; Schramp, Holtcamp, Phillips, Johnson, & Hoff, 2010).

There are also benefits to collaborative research with APN peers. For example, a collaborative APN research network founded by six university schools of nursing (APRNet) is facilitating and conducting research among primary care practice APNs (Deshefy-Longhi, Swartz, & Grey, 2002). Through this network, APNs across participating states are sharing data and designing studies to meet their clinical needs and enhance nursing knowledge. Since 2002, this APN practice-based research network has contributed to the development of several APN practice-focused studies (Deshefy-Longhi, Swartz, & Grey, 2008; McCloskey, Grey, Deshefy-Longhi, & Grey, 2003; Olsen, Dixon, Grey, Deshefy-Longhi, & Demarest, 2005). APNs benefit from collaboration in the research process and dissemination efforts such as publication and presentations (Christenbery, 2011). Partnering with colleagues to build skills in manuscript preparation and response to editor requests contributes to the APN's professional growth in the research role. Working with peer groups provides support and encouragement.

De Palma (2009) suggests that APNs operationalize the three research competencies at two levels. At the fundamental level, the APN learns and applies these skills in graduate school. At the expanded level, the APN builds on these skills through actual research involvement. It is undoubtedly difficult for the beginning APN to readily implement classroom research skills, but practical investigative experience can be achieved through a variety of activities such as clinical problem solving, presenting research findings, participating in quality improvement projects, conducting product evaluations, and examining practice protocols for evidence of needed change. As the APN progresses from a facilitator of research to a conductor of research, the APN's competency in this role component is developed. Early research experience as a team member helps to build skills as a team leader. Acquiring skills in the research process, including protocol testing and publication writing, result from active participation, mentored guidance, and teamwork.

FROM APPLICATION TO CONDUCTION OF RESEARCH: STEPS ALONG THE WAY

As described, the APN's academic preparation includes how to evaluate and conduct research, yet few practicing APNs feel adequately prepared to lead a research project in their practice arena following graduation. Clinicians may find that many of the principles learned in school fall short when applied to clinical practice. However, there are practical steps for successful integration of APN research competencies. For the research gap to narrow so that an evidence-based scientific approach to care is embraced by nursing staff, the APN's ability to develop a milieu that promotes such a philosophy is essential (Burns, 2002; Kleinpell, 2008). To successfully engineer a scientific milieu in a clinical setting, selected APN behaviors such as problem solving, change agency, mentoring, leadership, and working with a multidisciplinary team are required.

Problem Solving and Applying the Evidence to Practice

The APN is often called on to propose solutions for clinical problems. The imperative for success is improving outcomes. Oddly enough, even when strong evidence exists, practice changes may occur slowly or not at all. An example is the ubiquitous practice of instilling normal saline into endotracheal tubes before suctioning. Though evidence continues to strongly suggest that the practice is both ineffective and potentially harmful, it continues to be a common practice in critical care units (Hanberg & Brown, 2006). Thus, the ability to use a logical yet creative approach to applying evidence or conducting clinical research serves to support the reality that research is an integral and important part of everyday practice.

The APN begins by helping staff nurses to understand the meaning of EBP. The term means that the clinician is aware of the evidence that exists for a practice and the strength of the evidence. Professional and regulatory agencies often perform systematic reviews to determine the existing evidence for selected practices, especially high-risk procedures or practices. Practice guidelines are developed from these reviews and generally identify the level of scientific evidence for each recommendation from the lowest (i.e., consensus statements by professional organizations) to the highest (i.e., meta-analyses of randomized controlled trials [RCTs]). The decision to implement the guidelines is made by considering the relevancy of the practice change to the specific population of interest and by considering the potential for "unintended consequences" that may ensue. EBP changes may also be required by regulatory agencies, in which case the hospital must comply. APNs are often the individuals charged with implementation. An example is the use of restraints. Health-care agencies must ensure that they are appropriately applied and that use is rigorously monitored. Another example is the implementation of a technique that could potentially affect the rate of intravenous line infections and subsequent development of sepsis. Because of the high potential risk associated with such a change, rigorous follow-up evaluation or outcomes tracking following implementation is required. In contrast, implementation of a low-risk intervention such as the use of "bagged baths" in the place of traditional options may require only periodic audits of clinicians using the products and oversight by institutional wound, ostomy, and continence nurses.

When authoritative guidelines do not exist to help with EBP changes, consensus statements by professional organizations may be available and are quite helpful. These statements are based on systematic reviews of the available evidence. Similar to guidelines, the statements help the user understand the level of evidence so that careful application may occur. Other similar resources that may also be referenced are practice alerts. These tend to be published by professional organizations and are generally narrowly focused on a specific practice such as avoiding the use of blue food coloring in tube feedings. Finally, a literature review on the topic of interest will help the APN guide clinicians in determining the need for a practice change or for a clinical study to answer the question.

Although some EBP changes may be initiated using existing research, the vast majority of practice traditions that exist have little science to validate their efficacy. For example, although the Centers for Disease Control and Prevention (CDC) and the Infusion Nursing Society both recommend specific timing related to the use of selected site dressings used to cover and secure central venous (CV) catheter lines, they do not help the clinician decide among many commercially available products. Related questions, such as how long the methods adhere, which are best for the skin, and which methods work best with specific catheters, remain unanswered. In these cases the design and conduct of a clinical study to determine the answer is a reasonable and expected part of the APN's role.

APNs integrate evidence from many realms and also blend experiential knowledge of the culture and support systems to shape recommendations for clinical practice changes (Profetto-McGrath et al., 2007). If the APN determines that a clinical study is necessary to answer a practice question, it is essential to determine the project feasibility. A well-thought-out, narrowly focused, well-designed study is essential for clinician buy-in. In fact, selection of projects, especially first-time projects, should be carefully done to ensure a "quick win." More difficult projects can follow as clinicians and the APN become more sophisticated in the conduct of clinical studies and more confident in each other's capabilities. The following questions are helpful to determine the potential feasibility and subsequent success of conducting a clinical study:

1. *Is the proposed study a topic of interest to the clinicians?* Without clinician interest in the topic, the study is unlikely to move forward. In fact, it may be seen as the "APN's project" versus one owned by the unit or clinicians.

2. *Can it be done in a reasonable amount of time?* This is especially important for first-time projects. The project should be able to be completed in a couple of months or interest and enthusiasm will diminish. In a study by Winfield, Davis, Schwaner, Conaway, and Burns (2007), clinicians in a postanesthesia care unit questioned the best method for securing peripheral intravenous (PIV) lines. Because they were able to estimate the number of PIVs placed in a month, they were able to complete their study in approximately 3 months. Interest in the study stayed high throughout the study period.
3. *Can the data be collected in the course of a clinical day?* Although qualitative studies are important to practice and are attractive to nurses, they are time consuming and difficult to accomplish in a clinical setting. Quantitative studies, on the other hand, are easier to accomplish. Nurses are used to collecting data. If the study is focused on a clinical problem, such as the PIV study noted previously, much of the data collection can be accomplished in the course of providing patient care. In addition, data that are routinely collected may also contribute to evaluating nursing interventions, and when aggregated and analyzed, can help establish best practices (Resnick, 2006).
4. *Will the study require informed consent?* Studies that measure the effect of an intervention or practice or that challenge a "policy" or established practice standard require informed consent. From a practical perspective, it is desirable, especially for beginning clinical researchers, to design studies that do not require consent. The time that practicing clinicians must spend to obtain consent is often beyond that reasonably taken from normal care responsibilities and may be especially complicated if the patient is unable to give consent and the family must be approached.

   Studies that do not require informed consent are relatively common and are better choices for beginning researchers. For example, in the PIV study noted previously, four different PIV-securing methods were compared and assigned randomly. Consent was waived because no standard of care was breached (there was no existing standard securing method).
5. *Will the study require funding?* Many clinical projects such as the PIV example do not require a funding source. Supplies are often those used in the course of patient care and complex analyses are rarely necessary. However, some may require financial support and this should be considered before beginning. If an institutional or unit budget is not available for such support, other avenues may be explored.

   Small amounts of money are fairly easy to obtain, but they require time and energy to acquire. Examples include funding sources such as institutional quality assurance grants or small project monies ($100 to $500) provided by professional organizations. Another source may be unit funds; the manager or administrator should be consulted ahead of time to determine if this is a viable solution. Another option is to collaborate with an academic colleague or a statistician from the beginning so they are part of the project team. Regardless, to be feasible, funding sources for selected elements of the project should be considered early in the development and design of the project. It is desirable to have an infrastructure in place that ensures support for statistical analyses, so that each project does not require a unique solution.
6. *Are there barriers to evidence use?* Some cultures resist the APN's efforts to implement practice changes. It may be useful to develop a strategy for delivering the findings in a less formal manner. Staff members often prefer one-on-one coaching, inservices, staff meetings, and learning methods that are not intimidating. Involving others from the start helps reinforce the premise that the work does not belong solely to the APN. Regardless, everyone is not successful implementing research findings. The process requires strong critical thinking and facilitation skills. APNs can enhance the growth of clinicians in these areas by meeting their learning needs early

on, exchanging expertise, and stimulating participation throughout the study (Burns, 2008; Ferguson, Milner, & Snelgrove-Clarke, 2004; Kennel, Burns, & Horn, 2009). These and other successful strategies are discussed later in this chapter.

Mentoring and Leadership

To encourage staff to accept the philosophy that research is a necessary part of what they do every day, the APN's ability to mentor them in the process goes a long way. Although this statement seems somewhat obvious, it is far from being so. Many individuals are good at envisioning projects, and some may even inspire others to participate. Unfortunately, a less appreciated behavior linked with success is the APN's ability to ensure that all steps of the project are completed. This is hard work and often requires dogged determination to support, lead, and mentor others throughout the course of the project. Past performance speaks to this ability, and it is essential that the APN be able to realistically assess his or her previous experience in completing projects and mentoring others. An APN who is working with clinicians on a clinical or service line quality improvement project, for example, should not assume that participating individuals can independently accomplish the assigned tasks. Clinicians working on the project may have selected a project to learn how to do clinical research; experience in some of the steps of the process, however, such as how to accomplish a literature review, may be lacking. The APN needs to anticipate this and help the individual accomplish the review. This one-on-one teaching is important to demystify the process, eliminate barriers, move the process along, and ensure success. The support and teaching provided by the APN also helps with his or her credibility and ensures the development of others.

The APN's enthusiastic leadership goes a long way to making others excited about the process. This leadership extends to all aspects of the clinical project, from problem identification to application. Most important, the projects should be fun. As noted previously, many bedside clinicians feel that research is for others (e.g., those with doctorates), and they are fearful of embarking on any project that remotely looks like a study. A sense of humor, as in all aspects of nursing practice, goes a long way toward eliminating the fear of doing research and making it fun to accomplish.

Change Agency and a Systems Approach

Perhaps one of the most important behaviors of the APN is the ability to navigate the environment in which he or she practices. This understanding of the system is essential if appropriate changes are to be implemented. The APN must be able to identify the need to change an existing practice and the effect of this practice change. The APN's clinical knowledge and understanding of how to get something done in a clinical environment helps ensure that high-quality is maintained. To that end, the APN has a responsibility to the institution to evaluate clinical and system-focused initiatives. In fact, these initiatives may be another way of demonstrating that "research is part of what we do" and are essential to the development of a widespread scientific approach to practice. An example might be an initiative to implement a specific care protocol derived from a published RCT. The protocol may well be evidence-based and warranted; however, implementation without careful consideration of existing processes of care and barriers to change could result in negative unanticipated outcomes. The APN's knowledge of the processes of care and understanding of how best to apply and monitor adherence to the new protocol is essential to evaluate its effect on the outcome of interest. This kind of scientific approach to the problem proactively avoids variations in practice that negatively affect clinical and financial metrics.

In some cases, data do not exist to guide system changes. The role of the APN is to help evaluate the outcomes associated with the system change so that the initiatives can be adapted as needed or to maintain and sustain positive outcomes. These kinds of projects often fall under the title of quality improvement (QI). Although slightly different from research studies in that they are rarely as rigorous in design or methods for conduction, they can be popular projects for clinician participation. An example is a project in a medical intensive care unit (MICU) designed to determine the effect of an outcomes management approach to the care of long-term mechanically ventilated patients, using APNs to manage and monitor the patients, a clinical multidisciplinary pathway, and weaning and sedation guidelines (Burns et al., 1998; Burns & Earven, 2002). The project was a popular one for the clinicians involved in it, and the institution was especially interested because both clinical and financial outcomes for this patient population required improvement. The favorable results of the project (shorter weaning times and length of stay) coupled with improved financial outcomes were the stimulus to replicate the model in all adult intensive care units system-wide (Burns et al., 2003).

The behaviors discussed previously, in addition to the attributes of the APN, determine the effectiveness of the APN in making research come to life in a clinical setting. However, barriers to success do exist (Carroll et al., 1997). The most commonly cited barriers to the development of a research milieu include clinical access to patient populations, "buy-in" from clinicians, administrative support, attaining resources (i.e., time and money), and completing and publishing the results. Barriers and potential solutions are addressed in the following section.

Removing Barriers to APN Research Activities

Although the application of evidence to practice has been an expectation of the APN role in the past, the actual conduction of clinical research has not been strongly emphasized. This is changing as regulatory agencies, such as The Joint Commission, and professional groups that reward hospitals for demonstrating an evidence-based nursing practice, such as the American Nurses Credentialing Center (ANCC) Magnet Recognition and the American Association of Critical-Care Nurses (AACN) Beacon awards, include the conduction of research as part of their expectation for recognition. These organizations have identified that clinical outcomes improve when nursing care is evidence-based (AACN, 2011; ANCC, 2011; Steele-Moses, 2010). In addition, the presence of an active formal nursing research program demonstrates the hospital's commitment and support.

Clinical research and APN involvement is critical to the profession. To that end a variety of methods are necessary to remove barriers and facilitate the role of the APN in conducting clinically relevant research activities.

Clinical Access and Clinician Buy-In

Selecting a patient population to study is not generally difficult; the choice is driven by the question and the practice or service setting in which the APN works. It is important to remember that for clinical research to become a useful and real part of everyday practice, the research must be relevant. Greater buy-in is achieved when there is harmony or mutual interest of the involved participants. APNs can foster a spirit of inquiry and reinforce the idea that research is a journey. The culture of inquiry can evolve one question at a time (Pepler et al., 2006; Rivers, Cohen, & Counsell, 2006). The APN acts as a clinical intermediary to influence practice changes by sharing evidence through clinical rounds, in staff education, and by demonstrating practice changes. In this way APNs can bridge the gap between theory and clinical practice (Ferguson et al., 2004; Weeks, 2005).

Clinical access may be denied (or even covertly discouraged) if the research is not seen as important to the clinical practice. When clinicians are involved, and buy-in is high, access to patients is rarely an issue. Unfortunately, APNs who seek to pursue only their own research interests will quickly find that clinicians may not be supportive.

Strategies that have been suggested to encourage a research philosophy and buy-in include traditional solutions such as the establishment of journal clubs. In reality, journal clubs tend to last only for a few meetings, may be poorly attended because they are often held away from the clinical setting, and are often less than inspiring. Although they may be one way of infusing a research focus into practice, they are rarely the complete answer. Instead, the evaluation of scientific articles may be more acceptable and interesting if used in conjunction with a clinical question that emerges from a practice committee meeting or clinical dilemma.

As previously noted, clinicians are interested in research that has direct application to their practice (Chulay, 2006). In a series of taped interviews with MICU nurses who had been engaged in unit-based research, participants stated that the choice of project was important to the clinicians' belief that research is a necessary part of practice (Burns, 2002). In these unit-based studies, data collection was integrated, whenever possible, into the regular patient care day. In addition, the clinicians all noted the importance of how the research was used to change practice routines. And finally, clinicians also noted the importance of having a research mentor to guide them through each step of the process.

Administrative Support

Administrative support for clinical projects (especially those requiring clinician time or money) heavily hinges on the APN's previous accomplishments. Generally, many of the same attributes (e.g., perseverance, follow-through, and attention to detail) are required for any project to be successful. In addition, communication is essential for a true partnership built on trust and mutual respect between the administrator and the APN. Updates on the project progress, identification of barriers to the process, and plans for dissemination of the results help ensure administrative understanding and future support.

It is helpful for the APN and administrator to have a discussion about goals for developing a research-based practice early in the partnership. Through the conversation a logical and sequential set of steps can be designed to ensure the APN's success. It is important as well that the APN and administrator agree on the program philosophy and define the boundaries for the program (e.g., support of various aspects such as meeting times, statistical analyses, and financial or educational support for clinicians who present study results outside of the institution).

Fueled in part by the growth in the Magnet Recognition Program, more organizations are establishing dedicated clinical nursing research roles. A more formal framework for research enhances the APN's opportunity to lead or participate in some aspect of clinical research. This may also take the form of including research as an element in the performance appraisal for staff at designated points in a clinical ladder.

Time and Money

In today's practice environment, it is sometimes difficult to believe that there is also time to do research or even to evaluate existing research in an effort to determine whether practice changes should be implemented. The refrains "we're too busy" or "we'll do it when we have more time" are common.

The APN's ability to demonstrate how research activities can be accomplished as part of a normal clinical day is essential to ensuring success. In fact, as discussed previously, when considering the feasibility of a research project or EBP change, a realistic assessment of the clinical environment should be accomplished first. Feasibility includes the cost of the project and potential financial outcomes associated with it. Both feasibility and financial solutions were addressed previously in this chapter.

COMPLETING THE RESEARCH ("CLOSING THE LOOP"): ADVANCED PRACTICE NURSE SCHOLARSHIP

A mark of true scholarship is to "close the loop" by presenting the outcomes of the research project to key stakeholders. In some cases this means providing an update in the form of a study summary at the unit level, or if generalizable, to other patient care areas. The outcomes may also be presented at local or national meetings and may be published as well. Unfortunately, many APNs accomplish wonderful research-based practice changes or research studies, but they do not disseminate the results.

Learning how to present the material is an important skill and improves with practice. Initially, the APN should seek a mentor who is experienced in presenting and publishing. Although writing and presenting skills may be difficult for the beginning APN, the importance of working to improve the skills cannot be understated. Institutions interested in presentation and publication of APN-related research activities are wise to consider built-in supports such as individuals who have publication experience to help the clinicians learn how to present and publish their work. This specific kind of mentoring is helpful to teach APNs these scholarly activities. In addition, such a supportive commitment is a practical means of ensuring that the work is disseminated and that the APN and institution are recognized for these contributions to nursing knowledge.

AN APPROACH TO CLINICAL RESEARCH: THE EXPERIENCE OF ONE INSTITUTION

As discussed throughout this chapter, the APN's level of development largely determines the scope of the clinical research that is attempted. It is essential to start slow and small; the unit level is appropriate at the early stages. Subsequent projects may be attempted at a service line level or with more than one unit. Finally, institutional research projects can be initiated. Regardless of the level, the support of the institution is essential and good communication and a team approach are required. One institution's experience is described to illustrate key components of a successful clinical research program.

A Professional Nursing Staff Organization Research Program

Our Professional Nursing Staff Organization (PNSO) set a goal of establishing a program of clinical nursing research that is productive, widely disseminated within the hospital, and sustainable. To accomplish this goal, the PNSO sought the help of one of the hospital's APNs who had a background in clinical unit-based research (Burns, 2010).

The philosophy of the program is that clinical research is a necessary part of nursing practice and clinicians at all levels should be included. To that end the infusion of an institution-wide research milieu is essential. A formal institutional research program designed for professional nurses is a key component.

To ensure that the PNSO research program is successful and sustainable, the focus of the program is the development of bedside clinician researchers. The program director's role is to teach research, one step at a time, to selected clinicians. This oversight is time and effort intensive because the director provides formal classes to teach aspects of research and subsequently helps the clinicians as needed to develop studies with their teams.

The clinician researchers are carefully selected. They are called research mentors (RMs) for two reasons. First, the clinicians are taught by the director how to guide and mentor their teams through all aspects of conducting a project. The mentoring skills that the RMs learn are transferable to other aspects of leadership and are at the core of the APN role. Second, one of the major objectives of the program is to develop a *sustainable* program. Following the completion of the RMs' first study, the expectation is that they develop second-generation projects with *less* need for intensive oversight and guidance from the director. The research mentor program is one of the best ways to build research capacity and create a sustainable structure for the organization and conduct of research.

This successful model is popular, and over 400 bedside clinicians are currently involved in research projects of some type (Burns, 2010). The study topics vary widely, but all are fairly narrowly focused to ensure completion. Three examples are described in the following sections to illustrate this concept.

Temperature Changes with Oral Fluid Intake

Clinicians on a surgical acute-care unit questioned the timing related to oral temperature measurement following hot or cold liquid ingestion. Although most nursing textbooks note that between 15 and 30 minutes should elapse following oral intake, a literature review demonstrated that previous studies had been done with mercury thermometers and mostly in men. The clinician researchers believed a study testing the practice with digital thermometers (now the dominant technology) would be valuable. To that end they designed their study (Quatrara et al., 2007).

The study was done testing the effect of cold and hot beverages on health-care volunteers' temperatures over time. All liquid temperatures were strictly controlled, as was the room temperature and the length of time the liquids were in the mouth. The researchers learned that waiting 30 minutes before temperature measurement yielded more accurate readings. The study resulted in a change in practice within the hospital and was published so that others might also make appropriate practice changes.

Blood Pressure Measurement in an Ambulatory Cardiology Clinic

Clinicians in an ambulatory cardiology clinic had noted that the method used to measure blood pressure (BP) in their clinic varied greatly among clinicians. They were concerned because they were aware that the American Heart Association (AHA) had published guidelines stating that the patient should be in a chair with feet on the ground and with arms supported. In addition, the guidelines recommended that the heath-care provider wait for a few minutes before measurement.

Despite the existence of the guidelines, the clinicians noted that buy-in to changing the practice did not exist and that variation in BP measurement technique was the norm throughout the ambulatory clinics at the institution. They believed that a study to test the effect of using the AHA guidelines on their clinic patients would be a useful method to teach the value of research, confirm the AHA recommendations, and help convince others that EBP changes were essential to quality care. They designed a study that randomly assigned the patients to different positions and wait times. Their findings supported the AHA recommendations, and in addition demonstrated that an average differential of 14 points may be noted with improper technique (Turner et al., 2008). As a result of their study, BP measurement technique was changed in their clinic and other departments throughout the institution followed suit. They presented the content at a number of national meetings, and a manuscript on the study is in press.

Peripheral Intravenous and Central Venous Line Securement Methods

Two different unit teams lead by RMs in the postanesthesia care unit (PACU) and acute-care medicine units questioned the efficacy of the current methods used to dress and secure PIV and CV lines. Both designed studies comparing methods approved by the CDC to their existing methods (Trotter, Brock, Schwaner, Conaway, & Burns, 2008; Winfield et al., 2007). The two groups found that the methods commonly used in their practice were inferior to other tested methods. The results were used to change and standardize PIV and CV catheter dressing and securement practices throughout the institution. In addition to the positive effect on practice that resulted from the work, the changes also resulted in an institutional cost savings. The results were presented at a variety of professional forums and were published in clinical journals.

Research Program Outcomes

The clinical research program has accomplished the goals set for the first 5 years of program development (Burns, 2010). Selected examples are listed below by program objective:

- *To develop a research-based nursing* ***culture*** *by training selected clinicians.* More than 52 clinicians have been trained and over 400 nurses from 32 practice units or settings are involved in team projects lead by the program clinician researchers. The program accepts new applicants yearly via a competitive process, and interest and enthusiasm are high.
- *Development of an* ***infrastructure*** *that supports the evolution and growth of a nursing research program and nurses who do clinical research.* Our PNSO research program director and assistant are on the organizational chart, and their roles are clear and visible. Administrative and clerical support is present and financial support for research activities is available.
- *To improve nursing practice by* ***disseminating the results*** *of the studies.* Application of study findings occurs as appropriate within the institution via our nursing institutional practice committee mechanism. Many presentations have been given locally, regionally, and/or nationally. Sixteen manuscripts are published or in press (many more have been submitted and are in review).
- ***To recognize and celebrate*** *the accomplishments of the nursing research.* The program and program outcomes have been recognized both directly and indirectly via mechanisms such as the Magnet and Beacon awards, and media recognition (local TV station video pieces on the nursing studies, Web postings, and even news articles [e.g., *New York Times*]). Plus the program outcomes and the research projects are recognized at our annual Evidence-Based Practice Day and with internal awards for the projects.

CONCLUSIONS

Excellence in advanced practice depends on creating sustainable and active evidence-based practice. For the APN to guide and shape practice, research must be integrated. Whether we serve as consumers of research by reading and applying results of scientific reports or actually conduct studies to determine the answer to a clinical question, research must be evident as an important element of everyday practice. The role of the APN as a research mentor and leader is essential to ensure that EBP is integrated and widespread. Only then will research truly be "part of what we do."

REFERENCES

American Association of Colleges of Nursing. (1995). *The essentials of master's education for advanced practice nursing.* Washington, DC: American Association of Colleges of Nursing.

American Association of Colleges of Nursing. (2006). *The essentials of doctoral education for advanced practice nursing.* Retrieved May 2, 2011, from http://www.aacn.nche.edu/DNP/pdf/Essentials.pdf.

American Association of Colleges of Nursing. (2011). *The essentials of master's education in nursing.* Retrieved May 2, 2011, from http://www.aacn.nche.edu/Education/pdf/Master'sEssentials11.pdf.

American Association of Critical-Care Nurses Beacon Award for Excellence. (2011). Retrieved June 1, 2011, from http://www.aacn.org/wd/beaconapps/content/mainpage.pcms?menu=beaconapps.

American Nurses Association. (1995). *Nursing's social policy statement.* Washington, DC: American Nurses Association.

American Nurses Association. (2004). *Nursing: Scope and standards of practice.* Washington, DC: Author.

American Nurses Credentialing Center Magnet Recognition Program. (2011). Retrieved June 1, 2011, from http://nursecredentialing.org/Magnet.aspx.

Burman, M. E., Hart, A. M., & McCabe, S. M. (2005). Doctorate of nursing practice: Opportunity amidst chaos. *American Journal of Critical Care, 14*(6), 463–464.

Burns, S. M. (2002). Clinical research is part of what we do! The experience of one medical intensive care unit. *Critical Care Nurse, 22*(2), 100–113.

Burns, S. M. (2008). From research to bedside: Desire a successful and sustainable clinical research program? UVA Health System implemented a clinical research mentor model. *Advance for Nursing, 10,* 14–16.

Burns, S. M. (2010, May 1). A journey to make research part of what we do: From inception to success. *HCPro's Advisor to the ANCC Magnet Recognition Program, 6*(5).

Burns, S. M., Earven, D., Fisher, C., Lewis, R., Merrel, P., Schubart, J., et al. (2003). Implementation of an institutional program to improve clinical and financial outcomes of patients requiring mechanical ventilation: One year outcomes and lessons learned. *Critical Care Medicine, 31*(12), 2752–2763.

Burns, S. M., & Earven, S. (2002). Improving outcomes for mechanically ventilated medical intensive care patients using advanced practice nurses: A six-year experience. *Critical Care Nursing Clinics of North America, 14*(3), 231–243.

Burns, S. M., Marshall, M., Burns, J. E., Ryan, B., Wilmoth, D., Carpenter, R., et al. (1998). Design, testing and outcomes of an outcomes managed approach to patients requiring prolonged ventilation. *American Journal of Critical Care, 7*(1), 45–57.

Carroll, D. L., Greenwood, R., Lynch K. E., Sullivan, J. K., Ready, C. H., & Fitzmaurice, J. B. (1997). Barriers and facilitators to the utilization of nursing research. *Clinical Nurse Specialist, 11*(5), 207–212.

Christenbery, T. L. (2011). Manuscript peer review: A guide for advanced practice nurses. *Journal of the American Academy of Nurse Practitioners, 23*(1), 15–22.

Chulay, M. (2006). Good research ideas for clinicians. *AACN Advanced Critical Care, 17,* 253–265.

De Palma, J. A. (2009). Research. In A. B. Hamric, J. A. Spross, & C. M. Hanson (Eds.), *Advanced nursing practice: An integrative approach, 4th ed., pp. 217–248.* St. Louis: Saunders.

Deshefy-Longhi, T., Swartz, M. K., & Grey, M. (2002). Establishing a practice-based research network of advanced practice registered nurses in southern New England. *Nursing Outlook, 50*(3), 127–132.

Deshefy-Longhi, T., Swartz, M. K., Grey, M. (2008). Characterizing nurse practitioner practice by sampling patient encounters: An APRNet study. *Journal of the American Academy of Nurse Practitioners, 20*(5), 281–287.

Ferguson, L., Milner, M., & Snelgrove-Clarke, E. (2004). The role of intermediaries, getting evidence into practice. *Journal of Wound, Ostomy and Continence Nursing, 31*(6), 325–332.

Hamric, A. B. (2009). A definition of advanced practice nursing. In A. B. Hamric, J. A. Spross, & C. M. Hanson (Eds.), *Advanced nursing practice: An integrative approach, 4th ed., pp. 75–93.* St. Louis: Saunders.

Hanberg, A., & Brown, S. C. (2006). Bridging the theory-practice gap with evidence-based practice. *Journal of Continuing Education in Nursing, 37*(6), 248–249.

Kennel, S., Burns, S. M., & Horn, H. (2009). Stimulating student interest in nursing research: A program pairing students with practicing clinician researchers. *Journal of Nursing Education, 48,* 209–211.

Kleinpell, R. M. (2008). Promoting research in clinical practice: Strategies for implementing research initiatives. *AACN Advanced Critical Care, 19,* 155–163.

McCloskey, B., Grey, M., Deshefy-Longhi, T., & Grey, L. J. (2003). APRN practice patterns in primary care. *Nurse Practitioner, 28*(4), 39–44.

Mercer, T. A. (2008). Research settings, regional consortium provides much-needed resource, networking opportunity for nurse researchers. *Advance for Nurses, 10*(4), 23.

Olsen, D. P., Dixon, J. K., Grey, M., Deshefy-Longhi, T., & Demarest, J. C. (2005). Privacy concerns of patients and nurse practitioners in primary care: An APRNet study. *Journal of the American Academy of Nurse Practitioners, 17*(12), 527–534.

Pepler, C. J., Frisch, S., Rennick, J., Swidzinski, M., White, C., Brown, T., et al. (2006). Strategies to increase research-based practice. *Clinical Nurse Specialist, 20*(1), 23–31.

Profetto-McGrath, J., Smith, K. B., Hugo, K., Taylor, M., & El-Hajj, H. (2007). Clinical nurse specialist use of evidence in practice: A pilot study. *Worldviews on Evidence-Based Nursing, 4*(2), 86–96.

Quatrara, B., Coffman, J., Jenkins, T., Mann, K., McGough, K., Conaway, M., et al. (2007). The effect of respiratory rate and ingestion of hot and cold beverages on the accuracy of oral temperatures measured by electronic thermometers. *Medsurg Nursing, 16*(2), 105–108.

Resnick, B. (2006). Outcomes research: You do have the time! *Journal of the American Academy of Nurse Practitioners, 18*(11), 505–509.

Rivers, R., Cohen, L., & Counsell, C. (2006). Science critical to patient care. *Nurse Leader, 4*(3), 40–44.

Schramp, L. C., Holtcamp, M., Phillips, S. A., Johnson, T. P., & Hoff, J. (2010). Advanced practice nurses facilitating clinical translational research. *Clinical Medicine and Research, 8*(3/4), 131–134.

Steele-Moses, S. K. (2010). The journey to Magnet: Establishing a research infrastructure. *Clinical Journal of Oncology Nursing, 14,* 237–239.

Trotter, B., Brock, J., Schwaner, S., Conaway, M. R., & Burns, S. M. (2008). Central venous catheter dressings put to the test. *American Nurse Today, 3,* 43–44.

Turner, M., Chaney, C., Dame, M., Parks, C., Staggers, S., Stell, M., et al. (2008). Measuring blood pressure accurately in an ambulatory cardiology clinic setting—Does patient position and timing really matter? *Journal of Medical Surgical Nursing, 17*(2), 93–98.

Vohra, J. U., & Bryant-Lukosius, D. (2009). The advanced practice nursing data collection toolkit: A compendium of research tools. *Topics in Advanced Practice Nursing, 9*(4). Retrieved August 15, 2012, from http://www.slideworld.org/viewslides.aspx/Topics-in-Advanced-Practice-Nursing-eJournal-ppt-84061.

Weeks, S. K., & Satusky, M. J. (2005). Demystify nursing research. *Nursing Management, 36,* 42–47.

Winfield, C., Davis, S., Schwaner, S., Conaway, M., & Burns, S. M. (2007). Evidence: The first word in safe I.V. practice. *American Nurse Today, 2,* 31–33.

17

The Advanced Practice Nurse and Complementary Therapies

Rothlyn P. Zahourek

INTRODUCTION

Interest in "natural remedies" and Eastern and indigenous healing has grown in the last 30 years as consumers become more knowledgeable in accessing health and illness information from the Internet. The field of what used to be called *alternative medicine* has evolved and is now called *complementary-alternative medicine (CAM)* or *integrative* care. That term may again change to *complementary-integrative (CI)* or simply to *holistic care*. Each term has a slightly different meaning. See **Table 17-1.** For advanced nursing, *CI* and *holistic* are preferable terms because both imply a philosophical framework that is greater than the modality. Much of the data presented in this chapter will use the term *CAM* because the practice and research literature still uses that term. CAM, however, implies an emphasis on modality, rather than on a philosophical approach. In this chapter the terms *CAM, CI,* and *holism* will reflect "the integrative nature of nursing practice rather than . . . an alternative method of health care" (Sparber, 2001, p. 2).

Historically, nurses have been at the forefront of developing holistic care and CI modalities. Florence Nightingale's (1859/1969) early statistical and clinical work taught the health-care community about the importance of environment and spirituality on health and healing. Nightingale believed that nurses put the patients in the best condition for nature to act on them, and that all disease is essentially a "reparative process." She argued for a comprehensive approach that emphasized cleanliness, fresh air, color, fresh food, and the presence of pets to aid healing in the sick and injured. She also emphasized spirituality.

The holistic, bio-psycho-social-spiritual-cultural model is introduced in fundamental nursing texts. Nurses value the role of the interpersonal relationship in their healing work, and they incorporate the role of environmental influences and culture. Nursing has pioneered in the integration of comfort-enhancing mind-body therapies such as prepared childbirth education, preparation for surgery programs, and the use of gentle massage. Relaxation, imagery, fostering a therapeutic relationship and communication, and the development of Therapeutic Touch (TT) and Healing Touch (HT) have been part of our nursing lexicon for decades. Reiki, another "subtle energy" therapy, is now practiced by nurses in many hospitals and outpatient settings to promote comfort and enhance healing. However, a holistic nursing foundation has waxed and waned throughout our development as a profession. As the nurse practitioner (NP) movement developed in the late 1960s, nurses became more "medicalized" and specialized in both focus and practice. Consequently, many nurses may be marginally prepared or unprepared to meet their patients' holistic needs. Advanced practice

TABLE 17-1

Terms Associated with Complementary Integrative Therapies and Holistic Nursing

Term	Definition	Source
Holism	(a) Identifying the interrelationships of the bio-psycho-social-spiritual dimensions of the person, that is, recognizing that the whole is greater than the sum of its parts; and (b) understanding the individual as a unitary whole in mutual process with the environment.	American Holistic Nurses Association
Complementary and alternative medicine	Practices that include various medical and health-care systems and practices, and products that are not presently considered to be part of conventional medicine.	National Center for Contemporary and Alternative Medicine at the National Institutes of Health
Conventional allopathic medical and nursing practice	Practices that have been well accepted, have some research support, and are taught in standard educational programs, and for which some degree of understanding exists for the mechanism of action. This mechanism of action is in question for many of our treatments particularly in psychiatry.	
Alternative therapies	Used in place of conventional medicine. An example of an alternative therapy is Bach flower remedies for diabetes.	
Complementary therapies	A diverse group of health-care systems and not necessarily proven therapies that are used in conjunction with conventional medicine/nursing. An example is encouraging exercise, meditation, and massage to manage hypertension.	National Center for Contemporary and Alternative Medicine
Integrative medicine (nursing)	"Healing-oriented medicine that takes account of the whole person (body, mind, and spirit), including all aspects of lifestyle. It emphasizes the therapeutic relationship and makes use of all appropriate therapies, both conventional and alternative."	Rakel, 2007, p. 7

nurses (APNs), aware that they are focusing exclusively on the medical aspects of their practice, may rediscover the richness of more holistic approaches that promote more job satisfaction and less burnout.

As nurse practitioners became more specialized, developing group-specific knowledge and skills (i.e., children, women, and mental health clients), they became preoccupied with *parts* of the person or group but not the integral whole (Erickson, 2007). In response, Kubsch and colleagues (2007) advocated for a paradigm shift from a reductionist frame of reference (i.e., characteristic of our current allopathic health-care system and some NP programs) to one that reflects a holistic philosophy that includes complementary approaches. In such a shift health is synonymous with well-being. Tension, however, continues to exist between physicians, nurses, and consumers as this paradigm shift is occurring. The tension is further accentuated in the attempt to balance client satisfaction with the demands for cost containment and institutional practitioner productivity quotas.

Holism and Holistic Nursing

Many nurses who identify themselves as "holistic" incorporate CAM approaches. According to the American Holistic Nurses Association (AHNA), holistic nurses recognize two views of holism: (a) identifying the interrelationships of the bio-psycho-social-spiritual dimensions of the person, that is, recognizing that the whole is greater than the sum of its parts; and (b) understanding the individual as a unitary whole in mutual process with the environment. Both views are valued, and the goals of nursing can be achieved within either framework (AHNA, 2004). Either holistic philosophy is congruent with the theoretical base for advanced nursing practice of CAM modalities and a holistic integral nursing practice. This holistic emphasis is the framework for this chapter. A modality (complementary or conventional), therefore, is less important than the holistic intent of the practitioner. A danger for APNs lies in placing too great an emphasis on the modality rather than the theoretical and philosophical foundations for practice.

Healing is basic to nursing practice and is a term often used in conjunction with holistic nursing and CI modalities. It is a process rather than an endpoint. It may include cure, but it implies recovery from a state of feeling shattered or fragmented into one of new or restored wholeness. The person becomes aware of a shift in his or her perception of a life experience, finds new meaning, and often develops new behaviors (Zahourek, 2009).

At the First American Samueli Symposium, a panel that included six nurse leaders grappled with issues of definition and research in healing. Quinn, Smith, Ritenbaugh, Swanson, and Watson's paper (2003) discusses the process and potential outcomes of a "healing relationship" as the basis for both research and practice. This relationship is the "quality and characteristics of interactions between healer and healee that facilitate healing" and includes "empathy, caring, love, warmth, trust, confidence, credibility, honesty, expectation, courtesy, respect, and communication" (Dossey, 2003, p. A11). Donnelly (2006) explains that "holistic nursing interventions have always originated from the perspective of the person, community or family" (p. 215) and suggests that holistic nursing can help transform today's health-care system. Holistic nursing is "all nursing practice that has healing the whole person as its goal" (AHNA, 1998). Holistic nurses become "therapeutic partners" to strengthen human responses by facilitating the healing process and promoting wholeness (Mariano, 2007, p. 166).

A Nursing Summit on Integrative Care

In 2002, a select group of nurse leaders met at the Minnesota Center for Spirituality and Healing and formalized a plan for nurses in integrative care (Eliopoulos, 2002). They emphasized that nurses' practice of CAM should be grounded on a holistic model such as that developed by AHNA. State boards of nursing (BON) need to become better informed about CAM. Nurses should participate in developing research agendas and be included on panels and multidisciplinary projects. Nurses should clarify and articulate their values about healing and avoid the disease-based medical model when describing and implementing CI therapies.

The American Nurses Association (ANA), in collaboration with the AHNA, updated the holistic nursing scope and standards for practice of holistic nursing and added a section on advanced practice (Mariano, 2007). As a specialty, holistic nursing is based on "a philosophy, a body of knowledge, and an advanced set of nursing skills applied to practice that recognize the totality of the human being, the interconnectedness of body, mind, spirit, energy, social/cultural relationship context, and environment. Philosophically it is a world view, and not just a modality" (Mariano, 2007, p. 166). Practice is drawn from various healing systems, incorporates CAM modalities, and through "unconditional presence and intention" creates healing environments; self-care and self-responsibility are essential components. Holistic nursing approaches may be integrated into any conventional practice.

For decades, nurses have used holistic interventions that are defined by National Center for Complementary and Alternative Medicine (NCCAM) as CAM (Snyder, 1985). Some of these include relaxation, art, guided imagery, movement, massage, meditation, music, sound therapy, and prayer. Nurses incorporate subtle energy therapies such as TT, HT, aromatherapy, and Reiki in their work in various clinical settings (Dossey & Keegan, 2012).

MILESTONES IN THE DEVELOPMENT OF COMPLEMENTARY-INTEGRATIVE HOLISTIC PRACTICE

The research base for CAM continues to grow. NCCAM was founded at the National Institutes for Health (NIH) in 1999 as an outgrowth of the Office of Alternative Medicine (NCCAM, 2010). The most current (2007) National Health Interview Survey (NHIS) and continuing studies support that approximately 38% of adult Americans use CAM (NCCAM, 2007). NCCAM now funds research in more than 260 institutions and supplies information for practitioners, researchers, and consumers, including Internet-accessible information sheets and up-to-date research compilations on modalities and supplements.

NCCAM recently (2010) changed its categorizes of CAM modalities from four "domains"—*biologically based practices, energy medicine, manipulative and body-based practices,* and *mind-body medicine*—to the 2010 categories of *natural products, mind-body approaches, manipulative body-based practices, whole system approaches,* and *other*. Many nurses who practice Therapeutic Touch, Healing Touch, or Reiki have protested the change of *energy therapies* categorized in a section under "other". See **Box 17-1.**

According to the NCCAM Web site, "some CAM practices involve manipulation of various *energy* fields to affect health. Such fields may be characterized as veritable (measurable) or putative (yet to be measured)." Practices based on veritable forms of energy include those involving electromagnetic fields (e.g., *magnet therapy* and *light therapy*). Practices based on putative energy fields (also called biofields) generally reflect the concept that human beings are infused with subtle forms of energy (NCCAM, 2011). Such interventions include Qigong, Reiki, Therapeutic Touch, and Healing Touch. In these modalities practitioners use intent in transmitting a universal energy to a person, either from a distance or by placing their hands on or near that person.

Many CAM practices involve personal or self-care activities (e.g., exercise, meditation, and prayer), natural and herbal products (e.g., over-the-counter nonregulated dietary supplements, herbs, megavitamins, and probiotics), or treatments given by specialized practitioners (e.g., acupuncturists, chiropractors, and doctors of oriental medicine). Some practices are grounded in culture and tradition (Auyurveda) and others are original nursing interventions (TT and HT). Modalities considered to be CAM continue to change as a specific practice becomes more standardized because the research supports its mechanism, efficacy, or safety. Acupuncture, acupressure, aromatherapy, biofeedback, chiropractic care, diet, exercise, guided imagery, some herbal medicine, some homeopathy, humor,

BOX 17-1
National Center for Contemporary and Alternative Medicine's Classification System: Contemporary and Alternative Medicine Domains with Examples

- Natural products: substances found in nature; herbs, special diets, amino acids, probiotics, and vitamins in doses in excess of standard practice
- Mind-body approaches: use techniques to enhance the mind's ability to affect bodily functions (e.g., yoga, meditation, acupuncture, relaxation, imagery, hypnosis, biofeedback, and spiritual practices such as prayer)
- Manipulative and body-based practices: manipulation of body parts (e.g., massage, reflexology, or chiropractic)
- Whole system approaches: traditional Chinese medicine, Ayurvedic, homeopathy, naturopathy
- Other: includes movement therapies, traditional healers, and energy therapies or use of energy fields: (a) magnetic energy, which can be measured (i.e., magnets for pain) and (b) biofields, which are not currently measurable, and believed to surround and penetrate the body like auras (i.e., Reiki, Therapeutic Touch, and Healing Touch)

Adapted from National Center for Contemporary and Alternative Medicine Web site. Retrieved August 26, 2011.

hypnosis, magnets, massage, meditation, music, prayer, and relaxation techniques all currently enjoy a substantial research base; reports of these modalities can be found on the NCCAM Web site (http://nccam.nih.gov/health). See **Box 17-2** for the variety of materials available through NCCAM.

NCCAM 2011 Strategic Plan

On February 4, 2011, NCCAM released its third strategic plan, *Exploring the Science of Complementary and Alternative Medicine: Third Strategic Plan 2011–2015*. The plan outlines goals

BOX 17-2
National Center for Contemporary and Alternative Medicine

The NCCAM Web site includes new and updated fact sheets; these are in the public domain and duplication is encouraged:

- Ten things to know about evaluating medical resources on the Web
- What is complementary and alternative medicine (CAM)?
- CAM use and children
- Who uses CAM? Statistics
- Domains
- About clinical trials and CAM
- Most frequent health topics: acupuncture, arthritis, black cohosh, cancer, chelations, chiropractic, dietary supplements, depression, echinacea, ephedra, gingko, ginseng, glucosamine, homeopathy, herbs at a glance, meditation, menopause, and St. John's wort

Continued

BOX 17-2
National Center for Contemporary and Alternative Medicine—cont'd

- Links to valuable reports by the National Center for Contemporary and Alternative Medicine (NCCAM) can be found on DavisPlus.

For information about NCCAM or any aspect of CAM, contact the Clearinghouse at 1-888-644-6226, fax at 1-866-464-3616, or e-mail info@nccam.nih.gov. Send written requests to NCCAM Clearinghouse, P.O. Box 7923, Gaithersburg, MD, 20898-7923.

NCCAM publications:

- *Complementary and Alternative Medicine at NIH* is a quarterly publication by NCCAM, highlighting current research, research funding opportunities, calendars of activities, and clearinghouse information. Available by mail, on NCCAM's Web site, or via e-mail by contacting the NCCAM Clearinghouse. The publication is not copyrighted.
- Treatment information: by treatment or therapy and disease or condition, available at http://nccam.nih.gov/health/bytreatment.htm.
- National Institutes of Health consensus development program. Available at http://consensus.nih.gov.
- Live help, video lectures, CAM on PubMed, and research results.

National Center for Contemporary and Alternative Medicine Web site: http://nccam.nih.gov.

and objectives to determine priorities for future research in complementary and alternative medicine. (Plan is available at http://nccam.nih.gov/about/plans/2011/introduction.htm; accessed July 2, 2011.)

Within the strategic plan are three goals and five strategic objectives. The three overarching goals have relevance for advanced practice nurses:

1. Advance the science and practice of symptom management.
2. Develop effective, practical, personalized strategies for promoting health and well-being.
3. Enable better evidence-based decision making regarding CAM use and its integration into health care and health promotion.

Goal 1: Advance the Science and Practice of Symptom Management

People commonly use CAM to manage symptoms of diseases and conditions that are difficult to treat such as back or neck pain, arthritic or other musculoskeletal pain, and insomnia. Recent evidence suggests that some CAM approaches help to mitigate these symptoms and, in some cases, they engage innate biological processes involved in pain and emotion management. More research is needed to understand whether and how such interventions augment existing approaches and to identify the related biological mechanisms.

Goal 2: Develop Effective, Practical, Personalized Strategies for Promoting Health and Well-being

Many CAM and integrative practitioners use interventions such as meditation, relaxation, movement therapies, or yoga to help motivate people to adopt and sustain healthier lifestyles. Dietary supplements and/or herbs are also used to promote better health. Recent evidence suggests that those who use CAM may have better health-seeking behaviors.

Goal 3: Enable Better Evidence-Based Decision Making Regarding CAM Use and Its Integration Into Health Care and Health Promotion

NCCAM continues to support research that addresses this need and provide evidence-based information on the CAM practices for the professional and lay public. An emphasis in the current plan is for research that is applicable to and is generated from the "real world" of clinical practice. While basic research to study biological processes associated with CAM will continue, outcomes research and effectiveness of CAM in practice will be an addition.

HEALTH CARE REFORM (2011)

Although the implementation of President Obama's health-care reform (the Affordable Care Act) is still in process, many provisions have implications for advanced practice nurses including an emphasis on health maintenance, prevention, and better management of chronic disease and related symptoms. Combating the high percentage of obese Americans, particularly in children, provides opportunities for APRNs using a variety of approaches including CAM. Often such health-care challenges respond well to complementary modalities.

THE 2010 INSTITUTE OF MEDICINE REPORT ON THE FUTURE OF NURSING

According to the Institute of Medicine (IOM) report on the future of nursing (2010), the United States is transforming its health-care system to provide high-quality care leading to improved health outcomes, and nurses can and should play a significant role. Although the APN's expanded role has been under scrutiny, this role in primary care is important in providing wellness and prevention services, as well as diagnosis and management of many uncomplicated common illnesses and the management of chronic illness. The current conflicts between what APNs can do based on their education and training and what they may do according to state and federal regulations must be resolved so that they are better able to provide seamless, affordable, and high-quality care (Fairman, J. A., Rowe, J., Hassmiller, S., & Shalala, D., 2011). Scope-of-practice regulations in all states should reflect the full extent not only of nurse's but of each profession's education and training. Elimination of barriers for all professions with a focus on collaborative teamwork will maximize and improve care throughout the nation.

The IOM report, NCCAM's 2010 strategic plan, and the tenets of health-care reform all contend that prevention, management of chronic illness, and the promotion of comfort at all stages of life are goals to which our society must aspire. These resonate with many CAM modalities that focus on noninvasive, more natural interventions to promote healthy lifestyles and the management of chronic conditions that do not seem to respond well to conventional medical practices.

THE COACHING MOVEMENT

The health, wellness, and life coaching roles have been growing in numbers across disciplines in the last few years. Part of health-care reform is to establish a *medical home.* The term was originally used for primary care physicians in 1967 by the Academy of Pediatrics. The medical home will be "home base" for health care. Currently, it is conceived to be a multidisciplinary team whose emphasis is prevention of illness and wellness maintenance in primary care. The health coach is considered part of wellness initiatives (Jonas, 2009). Recently the International Council of Nurses with Sigma Theta

Tau created the document "Coaching in Nursing" (Donner & Wheeler, 2009), which established standards and described a relationship between health and wellness coaching and nursing.

Hess (2011) defines *holistic* coaching as "skilled professional purposeful results-oriented and structured relationship-centered interactions with clients by registered nurses for the purpose of promoting the health and well-being of the whole person" (p. 16). It is not therapy or counseling. The goal is creating healthy behaviors and lifestyle changes, and the relationship offers the opportunity to use numerous CAM approaches, if appropriate.

RESEARCH ON CONTEMPORARY AND ALTERNATIVE MEDICINE USE

A consistent pattern of increased CAM use has been demonstrated through numerous national surveys over the last 20 years. The most recent survey by NCCAM, released in December 2008, shows that about 38% of U.S. adults aged 18 years and above and 12% of children use some form of CAM (NCCAM, 2008). The first landmark utilization survey (Eisenberg et al., 1993) found that approximately 33% of individuals in the United States had used one or more unconventional therapies during the preceding year. In a follow-up study, Eisenberg and colleagues (1998) found an increased use—42.1% of Americans had used one or more CAM therapies. The NCCAM report released in May 2004 of the largest survey of Americans to date was conducted with the National Center for Health Statistics (NCHS) in the Centers for Disease Control and Prevention (CDC). The study surveyed 31,044 adults and found that 55% believed CAM was beneficial particularly when combined with conventional approaches; 36% used some form of CAM, and when prayer was included as a modality, up to 62% used CAM. When prayer was included, the mind-body domain was most commonly used; when prayer was excluded, biologically based therapies (22%) were most common (mind-body therapies: 17%). Prayer and seeking spiritual guidance continued to be the most commonly used modality for specific health problems. According to all the epidemiological studies, in addition to prayer, the most commonly used modalities include mind-body interventions, herbs, supplements, homeopathy, acupuncture, massage, chiropractic, stress management procedures, and energy work such as Reiki and TT (NCCAM, 2008).

In this most recent survey (2008), more CAM users are women, people with higher education, people who have been hospitalized in the last year, and former smokers. Participants used CAM for diverse problems: pain (back, neck, and joint pain); colds; anxiety and depression; insomnia; and gastrointestinal problems. Most often people used CAM (55%) to improve their health and in combination with conventional medicine. Another 50% were simply interested in trying CAM; others believed conventional medicine would not help. For some, their conventional provider suggested CAM or the person felt conventional treatments were too expensive. The 2004 survey did not query the amount of money people spent on CAM. The previous report (Eisenberg et al., 1998) estimated that the U.S. public spent $36 to $46 billion on CAM; between $12 billion and $20 billion was spent out of pocket, $5 billion of which was spent on herbal products. The common emphasis on "natural" products and remedies in everything from shampoo to hormone replacement therapy reflects this trend. Continued research may show that the reasons and purposes for CAM use are as diverse as the consumers who use them.

Consumers incorporate complementary therapies in designing their own integrative health plans. Success of these plans is demonstrated by the findings that 79% of respondents using both CAM therapies and traditional medicine "perceived the combination to be superior to either one alone" (Eisenberg et al., 2001, p. 1). Jonas (1997) concluded that consumers' complementary therapy use does not always mean dissatisfaction with conventional medicine (p. 34). One might speculate, however, from simply listening to the evening news, that in the 15 years since his article, dissatisfaction with health-care accessibility, expense, and quality has continued. Newer statistics on CAM use are not currently available.

An important finding from all the surveys is that more than half of the respondents do *not* share their use of CAM practices with their health-care provider. Reasons for nondisclosure included feeling that it was not important for the provider to know; the provider did not ask; the patient thought it was none of the provider's business; or the provider would not understand. It is important to note that primary care providers were mandated in 1998 to question patients about the use of complementary practices and record the information in their permanent records (United States Department of Health and Human Services [USDHHS], 1998).

National Center for Contemporary and Alternative Medicine as a Resource

NCCAM is a vitally important link for health-care professionals and consumers in providing information about the research status of CAM therapies (see Box 17-2). A regular free newsletter is available that contains listings and abstracts of recent research results, as well as more substantial articles on such topics as placebo response or prayer and spirituality.

Consumers are engaging in CI health-care practices whether the health-care professional guides them or not. Health-care providers must be knowledgeable about the safety and efficacy of complementary therapies to help clients choose the best modalities.

COMPLEMENTARY-INTEGRATIVE MODALITIES AND ADVANCED HOLISTIC NURSING PRACTICE

The role of the APN is to support patients in their choice of holistic-integrative practices, make recommendations, and deliver safe and effective complementary therapies when appropriate.

Examples of Complementary-Integrative Holistic Practice Modalities

Several years before the landmark Eisenberg and colleagues study (1993), nurses were practicing and publishing about CAM modalities. Snyder (1985) completed a book titled *Independent Nursing Interventions* that included CAM approaches (e.g., relaxation, imagery, massage). Clark published *Wellness Nursing* (1986), and *Holistic Nursing: A Handbook for Practice* was first published in 1988 (and is now in its sixth edition [Dossey & Keegan, 2012]). Clements and Martin published *Nursing and Holistic Wellness* (1990). Zahourek published early papers on the use of hypnosis with pain (1982a, 1982b) and two clinically based books: *Clinical Hypnosis and Therapeutic Suggestion in Nursing* (1985) and *Relaxation and Imagery* for nurses (1988). Delmar has published *The Nurse as Healer,* a series of small books edited by Lynn Keegan on such topics as *Creative Imagery in Nursing* (Shames, 1996) and *Awareness in Healing* (Rew, 1996). It is also paradoxical that McCloskey and Bulechek (1992) classified several of these same therapies as nursing interventions in the year before Eisenberg's report (1993). Their 7-year research project funded by the National Institute of Nursing culminated in the publication of the *Nursing Interventions Classification* (NIC). This comprehensive standardized classification of research-based nursing interventions (McCloskey & Bulechek, 2000) included "simple guided imagery" (p. 595), "simple massage" (p. 596), and "simple relaxation therapy" (p. 598). The literature since then has blossomed and articles now appear with some regularity on holistic approaches and nurses' involvement with CAM. General practice journals such as *American Nurse* and *American Journal of Nursing,* as well as specialty journals (e.g., *Journal of the American Psychiatric Nurses Association*), theoretical journals such as *Nursing Science Quarterly,* and research journals such as *Nursing Research,* all publish articles related to CAM practice. The sixth edition of *Holistic Nursing: A Handbook for Practice* was published in 2012 by Barbara Dossey and Lynn Keegan. These texts have been valuable resources for holistic nursing theory development and for providing resources on numerous CAM modalities practiced by holistic nurses.

Mind-Body Therapies and Advanced Nursing Practice

Relaxation, imagery, and therapeutic suggestion (hypnosis) have become standard practices to help relieve pain. Kitko (2007) describes rhythmic breathing as an easy way to learn intervention for reducing pain. The nurse helps the patient focus on an activity (e.g., purposeful breath), enhancing the relaxation response. Good and colleagues (2010) used a set relaxation process of jaw and mouth relaxation, slow breathing and stopping thinking in words compared to music, and music combined with these relaxation techniques in patients following abdominal surgery. Both groups were compared to a control group. Immediate effects of reduction of pain day one and day two were found with the relaxing music group. Similar results were obtained by Sand-Jecklin and Emerson (2010) in their exploratory study on the impact of live music with patients who had an unplanned/emergent admission to an acute-care hospital. These patients it was assumed would have a high level of muscle tension, pain, and anxiety. Participants in this study reported significant reduction in pain, anxiety, and muscle tension and rated the live music as highly helpful with these symptoms. There were also significant reductions in systolic blood pressure and respirations but not in the diastolic or pulse rate.

NCCAM reviewed studies on mind-body interventions with cancer patients and found that evidence exists that these interventions aid in improving mood, coping, and quality of life, as well as ameliorating chemotherapy-induced nausea and vomiting and pain. According to this report, strong evidence exists that these techniques also are effective in the treatment of coronary artery disease and enhance cardiac rehabilitation. Several systematic reviews are available through the Internet site Google Scholar (http://scholar.google.com/). Most of these reviews were completed before 2008 and most are for specific conditions such as fibromyalgia, cancer pain, and lifestyle change and management.

The *placebo effect* is an unexpected beneficial mind-body response that results from a person's anticipation that an intervention—pill, procedure, or injection—will help. A clinician's style in interacting, certain symbols such as the stethoscope, and certain rituals also may bring about a positive response that is independent of any specific treatment and are easily and consciously used during an interaction. A major report on the mechanism and value of the placebo as a mind-body response can be found in the *CAM at the NIH* newsletter (2007). In this newsletter, the placebo effect is treated as a potentially positive therapeutic tool rather than a research problem. Using positive suggestions, no matter what the modality, has greater chance of success than if communication is negative or fosters a poor response to an intervention. Saying "this will hurt" (negative), or "this may cause some brief discomfort but is so powerful we know it can make you better" (positive), may both set off a "placebo" response but in opposite directions. According to a study by Kaptchuk and colleagues (2010), placebos given without deception improved symptoms of irritable bowel syndrome (IBS).

Guided Imagery

Human imagery is a holistic phenomenon described as a "multidimensional mental representation of reality and fantasy that includes not only visual pictures but also remembrance of situations and experiences such as sound, smell, touch, movement and taste" (Zahourek, 2002, p. 113). There are many different forms of imagery, including imagery for behavioral rehearsal, impromptu imagery, biologically based imagery, and symbolic and metaphoric imagery (Schaub & Dossey, 2009). Ashen (1977) developed a still relevant theory of imagery: images are stored in the mind as an experiential unit that includes the image, somatic response, and its meaning. In this context, imagery is used as a therapeutic tool for aiding anxiety and pain and behavioral rehearsal for change.

Imagery is used in healing trauma and posttraumatic stress disorder, often combined with cognitive-behavioral therapy. It is used to treat numerous acute problems such as preparation for childbirth and for surgery, and augmenting and minimizing side effects from medications and treatments. Grief resolution is, in part, an imagery process because people can be guided to imagine their loss and themselves as strong and coping, and subsequently find meaning in their experience. Reed (2007) describes several uses of imagery in clinical practice in which the study groups who received the imagery intervention had significantly more pain relief and required less pain medication. Eslinger (2000a, 2000b) encourages nurse anesthetists to incorporate some of the techniques to "greatly enhance patient comfort and satisfaction" (2000a, p. 159). Eslinger (2000b) also presents case studies of hypnosis combined with guided imagery to help patients with hemophilia and migraine headaches. Recent studies from Belgium (Macrae, 2011) have documented the positive effects of hypnosis on women with breast cancer recovering from surgery.

Energy Therapies and Holistic Complementary-Integrative Nursing Practice

A "disruption in the flow of energy surrounding a person's being that results in disharmony of body, mind and/or spirit" is a nursing diagnosis (North American Nursing Diagnosis Association [NANDA], 2005). Energy therapies include both nontouching and hands-on therapies that work in the person's biofield of energy that, so far, cannot be consistently measured. Those energy therapies most often used by nurses, Therapeutic Touch, Healing Touch, and Reiki, are purported to facilitate a person's bodily as well as energetic balance, and thus reduce symptoms of disease and the disease itself. These are currently taught in continuing education and in holistic nursing programs and courses. Denner (2009) discusses the science of energy therapies as "communication networks," relating them to concepts from quantum physics, as well as ancient Eastern and Shamanic healing practices. Being centered, focused, meditative, and intentional are foundations for these practices. Generally, the practitioner holds an intention for the greatest good for the person rather than for a specific outcome. The practitioners' qualitative sensations of energy flow and balance are the cornerstones of these therapies.

Research on energetic modalities has been difficult in both nursing and in CAM. Engebretson and Wardell (2007) discuss in detail the methodological issues and problems for this modality that apply to research on many of these therapies. Research continues to support that these energetic approaches produce comfort and relaxation, and do not cause harm unless an important conventional treatment is avoided.

Anderson and Taylor (2011) discuss biofield therapies on cardiovascular disease management and review studies on Healing Touch, Therapeutic Touch, and Reiki. They conclude that the primary benefit is using these interventions as adjuncts to standard treatment since they enhance relaxation and enhance the body's own healing capacity. They also recommend continued rigorous study of these interventions with specific populations.

Therapeutic Touch (TT), Healing Touch (HT), and Reiki

In the early 1970s, nurse Dolores Krieger and healer Dora Kunz developed TT to help people with comfort and healing. According to meta-analyses of studies on the effects of TT (including quantitative, qualitative, and mixed-methods research), TT is useful in decreasing anxiety and promoting comfort (Peters, 1999; Winstead-Fry & Wijeck, 1999). Some studies have also been conducted on its effect on wound healing, but these effects have been inconsistent.

Healing Touch, a biofield energy modality, evolved from TT in the early 1980s and was more extensively developed as a training program by Janet Mentgen in 2002. Similar to TT, HT incorporates other theories and practices and is based on the idea that the body is a complex energy system that can be influenced by another's intention for healing and well-being. In a review of over 30 studies on HT, Wardell and Weymouth (2004) found that although the studies reported positive results in reducing stress, anxiety, and pain, and enhancing healing time and quality of life, the quality of the research was such that generalizable results could not be determined. Wardell has compiled an annotated bibliography that is available on the Healing Touch International Web site (http://healingtouch.net).

Originally practiced outside of conventional health care, the Japanese spiritual practice of Reiki is an increasingly popular modality. Reiki is an energy-based therapy in which the practitioner's vibrational energy is connected to a universal source (e.g., chi, qi, prana) and is transferred to a recipient for healing (Miles & True, 2003). Additional nursing reports discuss reducing anxiety and pain after abdominal hysterectomy (Vitale & O'Conner, 2006), self-care for nurses (Vitale, 2009), and orthopedic pain (DiNucci, 2005).

Reiki is similar to HT and TT, but these modalities have had substantially more research and are grounded in nursing theory and practice. Recently, Baldwin and colleagues (2010) assembled three teams to collect and systematically review the research on Reiki. In meta-analysis, 26 Reiki articles have been reviewed for strengths and weaknesses. Their results and a database that continues to grow are accessible on the Web site www.centerforreikiresearch.org. Only 12 articles were based on robust experimental design and used adequate outcome measures.

In a recent review (Janin & Mills, 2010) researchers used a best evidence synthesis approach to evaluate 66 studies on Therapeutic Touch, Qigong, Reiki, Healing Touch, Johire, and others using a specific critical review checklist. Most of the studies were of average to minimum quality for randomization, use of control, and statistical methods. The outcome measures were pain related. Strong evidence was found that pain intensity was reduced and general functioning increased. Related disorders of anxiety and depression and long-term benefits were equivocal. Fazzino and colleagues (2010) completed another review of literature on energy healing and pain from 1980 to 2008. Reiki, HT, and TT were included. While they made recommendations for future research on these modalities, they concluded that studies that included anxiety and pain found some reduction, and that the amount and frequency of pain medication were reduced.

Biological Remedies

Biologically based practices according to NCCAM include, but are not limited to, botanicals, animal-derived extracts, vitamins, minerals, fatty acids, amino acids, proteins, prebiotics and probiotics, whole diets, and functional foods. Although these products have not been regulated, the Food and Drug Administration (FDA) is currently developing good manufacturing practices (GMPs) for dietary supplements. Newly marketed products are not subject to premarket approval or surveillance. Americans use supplements and herbs to promote overall health, to improve performance and energy, to treat depression, and to treat and prevent such illnesses as colds and flu. People with multiple illnesses and those who have a specific illness, consume large amounts of alcohol, or are obese tend to be frequent users (NCCAM, 2008). Because new research changes our knowledge base, readers are referred to the NCCAM and Cochrane review Web sites where updated research results from large national studies and systematic reviews on herbs and supplements can be found: www.http://nccam.nih.gov/; http://nccam.nih.gov/health/herbsataglance.htm; and http://www2.cochrane.org/reviews/.

The journal *Holistic Nursing Practice* has a regular column on herbs and supplements. Regular articles in *Holistic Nursing Practice* by Stephanie Ross include Arnica Gel for osteoarthritis (2008) and herbal medicine in women's health (2011) (reviews cranberry for urinary tract infections, chocolate for cardiovascular health, valerian for sleep, and St John's wort for mild to moderate depression). The *American Nurse Today* (Fitzgerald, 2007) did a continuing education article on the use of herbs that included descriptions of six herbs (feverfew, gingko biloba, red yeast rice, saw palmetto, St. John's wort, and valerian) and their potential drug-herb interaction. Rosenfeld (2008), in a popular magazine, *Parade,* reviews the safety and effectiveness of ginseng, garlic, echinacea, chamomile, St. John's wort, ginkgo biloba, valerian, ginger, saw palmetto, hawthorn, black cohosh, and feverfew. His information coincides with the office of dietary supplements fact sheets, which review the research, uses, and side effects of these and other herbs and supplements. Currently, more studies are being conducted on black cohosh for menopausal symptoms and vitamin D for bone health. Health effects of omega-3 fatty acids for people with depression and B vitamins and berries in age-related neurodegenerative diseases are also being reported on the NCCAM and Cochrane review Web sites. NCCAM has several Web pages devoted to herbs and supplements. The page "Herbs at a Glance" lists 42 popular herbs that can be accessed, including black cohosh, cranberry, ephedra, ginger, gingko biloba, kava, milk thistle, and green tea. Consult the NCCAM Web site for the most current information on their effectiveness, as well as drug-herb-supplement interactions.

Because many patients may use supplements without knowledge of their dosages, effects, or potential side effects, APNs, and particularly those with prescriptive authority, need to know how to access accurate information on herbal remedies and supplements. Used for centuries and in many cultures, herbs can be as effective as our manufactured medications; therefore, some of the same cautions and precautions exist. Cautions for herbs and supplements listed by NCCAM include being aware of the following:

- If a person has substituted an herb or supplement for a conventional medication
- What impact the supplement might have on the client's overall condition
- What interactions might occur between the supplement or herb and other medications
- Particular risks for people with diabetes, hypertension, or mental health problems such as depression and for people facing invasive procedures
- If a woman is pregnant or if treating children

Since many studies indicate that patients do not tell their health-care providers what supplements or herbs they are taking, it is vital to ask patients what they taking, even if the substances are "over the counter," are "natural," or seem benign. A practitioner well educated in supplements and herbs can be a useful resource.

Aromatherapy

Another popular nursing intervention grounded in a holistic philosophy is aromatherapy (Smith & Kyle, 2008), which was developed by nurse Jane Buckle (2005). Essential oils derived from plants (common herbs) are either placed on cotton near a person or in a steam distiller. Aromatherapy is often used in conjunction with conventional therapies for pain, anxiety, spasms, insomnia, and infection. Scientific evidence is growing about its efficacy. Many anecdotal reports describe positive effects in nursing homes, hospitals, and emergency rooms (Buckle, 2005; Garner, 2007). As with herbs and supplements, the practitioner needs to be aware of potential side effects and interactions. These oils should never be used internally because they are many times stronger than the herb itself.

Spirituality

One of the most frequently reported uses of CAM is prayer and spirituality. Because the efficacy studies on prayer are contradictory, the controversy most likely will continue. However, dealing with patients' spiritual needs, and our own, is important. For many, coping with this rapidly changing, and increasingly technological world is causing existential crises of disconnectedness and a sense of alienation. Threats of devastation from global warming, wars, and financial crises dominate the news, compounding the anxiety with futility. When illness or injury occurs, or when a loved one dies, the need for solace and a sense of connection, purpose, and meaning become even greater.

The North American Nursing Diagnosis Association (NANDA) recognizes spiritual distress as a diagnosis, and the ANA's Code of Ethics states that nurses must consider a person's value system and religious beliefs. Burkhardt and Nagai-Jacobsen (2002) did early work on spirituality in nursing. Spirituality is different from religion; it is the "essence of our being . . . it permeates our living in relationships and infuses our unfolding awareness of who and what we are, our purpose in being, and our inner resources" (Burkhardt & Nagai-Jacobsen, 2009, p. 617).

In practice, spirituality is related to active intentional listening and presence. It may involve helping others to find meaning in suffering. Being present with a patient, creating a healing environment, and "inviting reflections" as stories from patients may ameliorate suffering (Deal, 2011). Elders, for example, derive a sense of meaning from reminiscing and telling their life story to someone who is genuinely interested. Spiritual practices, such as mindful meditation, centering, practicing yoga, and developing the capacity to be present, are useful for nurses themselves to prevent burnout and create a sense of purpose and meaning in busy and demanding practices.

Baldacchino and Draper (2001) reviewed the literature from 1975 related to spiritual coping (187 articles) and concluded that illness often rendered feelings of a loss of control. Support of spiritual coping strategies in holistic care seemed to enhance self-empowerment, leading to a sense of purpose and meaning. Nurses need to know how to address patients' spiritual needs as they arise. Eldridge (2007) lists nine spiritual interventions: be there; listen actively; use touch; reflect and remember; laugh; share the experience; pray or encourage the patient to pray; use inspirational words or music; and evaluate spiritual needs. Nurses do not force their own beliefs on others, and they need to remember the difference between spirituality and religion, and respect the religious beliefs and practices, or lack thereof, in those for whom they care.

Nurses must nurture their own spirits by pausing and reflecting about what is going on around them. Pausing to remember one's intention and to breathe as one washes hands between patients may be one way to relax and prevent burnout, as well as focus attention more completely on the patient and/or tasks at hand. This seems a challenge in our demanding health-care environment, which does not often promote its caregivers' healing.

Creating a Healing Environment

Modern health-care facilities are more aware of the need to create healing environments. Newer hospitals have largely private rooms that are bright with pleasant views. More space is provided in patient rooms to allow for families. The impact of noise and aromas are considered. The old locker room for the staff is being replaced in some forward-thinking institutions with stress reducing, peaceful spaces with recliners, soft lighting, and music where staff can rest.

Healing gardens, meditation areas, animals and fish tanks, and attention to color and use of space to create calm and rest is becoming the norm. McCaffery (2007, 2010) compared the effect on mildly depressed older adults of participation in different environmental strategies: walking in a beautiful

Japanese garden, a walk with guided imagery, and art therapy. Using focus groups, she determined that all three groups' symptoms improved. Cole and Gawlinski (2000) reported a pilot study that explored the effects of animal-assisted therapy (using an aquarium with fish) on the stress levels of patients awaiting orthotopic heart transplantation in a cardiac care unit. Both patients and nurses were satisfied with the program.

PRACTICE ISSUES FOR THE ADVANCED PRACTICE NURSE AND COMPLEMENTARY-INTEGRATIVE THERAPIES

The APN's responsibility to society's changing health-care needs can be interpreted through the ANA's *Social Policy Statement* (2010). In this document, *expansion* "refers to the acquisition of new practice knowledge and skills and legitimizing role autonomy within areas of practice that overlap traditional boundaries of medical practice." Expansion includes "both specialization and expansion and is characterized by the integration of theoretical, research-based, and practical knowledge (as part of graduate education)" (p. 4). New practice knowledge and skills related to complementary therapies for APNs may include CAM science, nursing science, research-based nursing interventions, and guidelines for integrative or holistic practice.

Activities for the registered nurse and for APNs are outlined in the *Holistic Nursing Scope and Standards of Practice* (ANA/AHNA, 2007; currently being revised). Specific APN roles include consultation and prescriptive authority. Within that standard, the APN "uses advanced knowledge of pharmacology, psychoneuroimmunology, nutritional supplements, herbal and homeopathic remedies" and is cognizant of and evaluates potential effects, side effects, and interactions (Mariano, 2007, p. 183).

Educational Considerations for Complementary-Integrative and Holistic Nursing

Preparing APNs with the education and experiences to support patients in their plans to use CAM and to deliver safe and effective CI nursing interventions is a challenge for nurse educators, continuing education providers, administrators, and accrediting agencies. CAM has been included in medical education and is now more often discussed in nursing undergraduate and graduate programs. The inclusion of complementary and alternative therapies in graduate and undergraduate nursing curricula is vital for all nurses to be current and knowledgeable in their practice. According to Burman (2003), most NP programs include some CAM education. Sok, Erlen, and Kim (2004) evaluated the integration of CAM material into nursing education and advanced practice programs, and suggest that graduate programs develop a recognized course of CAM study. They propose a 2-year program for NPs that includes content on the basics of CAM the first year followed by a second year of intensive specialization. Fenton and Morris (2003) completed an electronic Web survey of deans of schools of nursing to determine the degree of integration of CAM into their curricula. They concluded from a sample of 125 schools that 60% used the definition of holistic nursing practice in their curricula and 84.8% included complementary modalities. Several graduate-level programs have been developed to foster the specialty of holistic nursing. New York University has developed a holistic nurse practitioner program and Florida Atlantic, Christine E. Lynn College of Nursing has developed a graduate clinical nurse specialist program in holistic nursing. This program is based on the philosophy of "understanding the wholeness of persons connected with others and the environment through caring" (Purnell & Lange, 2011, p. 140).

For more than two decades members of AHNA have been committed to developing resources for nurses seeking to expand their practice. The AHNA has an active and well-developed education committee that addresses curriculum development in formal education, as well as monitors and endorses continuing education programs in CAM and holistic nursing (Hanley et al., 2010). See **Box 17-3.**

Educational opportunities and online modules are available on the AHNA Web site, as well as resources for accessing the scope of knowledge and research in holistic nursing. See **Box 17-4.**

Guidelines for curriculum development, advanced practice, and certification are available in the form of *Standards of Advanced Holistic Nursing Practice for Graduate-Prepared Nurses* (AHNA, 2002b; ANA/ANHA, 2007). The American Holistic Nursing Credentialing Center (AHNCC) now certifies holistic nurses at basic (HNC) and advanced (AHN-BC) levels. They endorse several basic and graduate programs. See **Table 17-2.** Most graduate and many certificate programs are now taught online.

Complementary-Integrative Therapies in Regulated Nursing Practice

Requirements for education and training, licensure, and reimbursement for CAM practitioners and advanced practice nurses are regulated by states. Understanding the qualifications and practice domains of nurses and other practitioners is the foundation for integrative practice. Sparber (2001) surveyed state boards of nursing to identify policies regarding registered nurses' (RNs') use of complementary therapies. At that time "forty-seven percent of the BONs had taken positions that permitted nurses to practice a range of complementary therapies; thirteen percent were in the process of discussing this matter; and forty percent, although they had not formally addressed the topic, did not necessarily discourage these practices" (p. 1). In 1991, the Arizona BON was one of the first to issue a formal advisory on CAM. Kentucky, Massachusetts, and Pennsylvania followed by recognizing energy therapies of TT, HT, and massage therapies (now recognized in 25 states and an additional 7 are considering). Sparber's 2001 report has not been updated, but more recently, Denner (2007) and Radzyminski (2007) reviewed the legal status of nurses and CI modalities. See **Box 17-5.** The AHNA is in the process of surveying BONs to determine their policies on CAM and holistic nursing practice.

BOX 17-3
Certificate Programs from American Holistic Nurses Association

- Certificate Program in Integrative Aromatherapy
- Healing Touch Certification Program
- Integrative reflexology
- Whole Health Education Certificate
- Holistic Stress Management Instructor Certification Workshop
- Integrative Healing Arts
- Great River Craniosacral Therapy Institute training program
- Aromatherapy for Health Professionals
- Certificate of Integrative Health and Certificate in Spirituality, Health, and Healing
- AsOne Holistic Coaching Training Program

Updated August 2011.

BOX 17-4
Examples of Resources from American Holistic Nurses Association

- *Holistic Nursing: Scope and Standards of Practice* (American Nurses Association & American Holistic Nurses Association, 2007)
- *Holistic Nursing: A Handbook for Practice* (Dossey & Keegan, 2012)
- *Core Curriculum for Holistic Nursing* (Dossey, 1997)
- *Journal of Holistic Nursing,* the official Journal of American Holistic Nurses Association (AHNA), published by Sage publications
- *Beginnings,* the newsletter published by AHNA
- AHNA Web site: www.ahna.org
- Certificate continuing education programs endorsed by the AHNA

TABLE 17-2
Programs Endorsed by the American Holistic Nurses' Certification Corporation

Department	Location	Program(s)
Xavier University Department of Nursing	Cincinnati, OH	BSN
Capitol University, Department of Nursing	Columbus, OH	Accelerated program BS, MS
Metropolitan State University School of Nursing	St. Paul, MN	BSN
Humboldt State University, School of Nursing	Arcata, CA	BSN
Western Michigan University, Bronson School of Nursing	Kalamazoo, MI	BSN
University of Colorado at Colorado Springs	Colorado Springs, CO	BSN and MSN
New York University, Department of Nursing	New York, NY	APN
Indiana University School of Nursing, South Bend	South Bend, IN	BSN
West Virginia University School of Nursing	Morgantown, WV	BSN
University of Texas Medical Branch at Galveston, School of Nursing	Galveston, TX	BSN, generic and flexible option tracks
University of Texas at Tyler, School of Nursing	Tyler, TX	BSN
Dominican University of California, School of Arts and Science	San Rafael, CA	BSN and MSN
University of Colorado—Colorado Springs, CO	Colorado Springs, CO	BSN and MSN
University of Texas at Brownsville and Texas Southmost College	Brownsville, TX	BSN

Continued

TABLE 17-2

Programs Endorsed by the American Holistic Nurses' Certification Corporation—cont'd

Department	Location	Program(s)
Tennessee State University	Nashville, TN	BSN and MSN
Eastern University	St. Davids, PA	RN-BSN
Florida Atlantic University	Boca Raton, FL	BS, MS in Holistic Nursing
Bronson School of Nursing	Kalamazoo, MI	BSN

APN, advanced nurse practitioner program; *BSN,* baccalaureate program; *MSN,* master's program.

These are the endorsed programs as of August 2011. American Holistic Nurses' Certification Corporation endorsement indicates that the school of nursing provides a program of study based on the standards of practice for holistic nursing.

The Advanced Practice Nurse and Holistic Nursing Research and Complementary Therapies

The holistic and CI nursing research base has grown substantially in recent years. Graduate nursing programs have supported research focused on both theory development and the evaluation of modalities. Enzham-Hagedorn and Zahourek (2007) provide both a theoretical model and an extensive chart of studies on all aspects of holistic nursing. It is imperative that APNs become aware of the evidence and precautions derived from various research approaches to make informed choices about using any modality or encouraging their clients to do the same. The AHNA Web site has a research section that includes articles, a Web library, a glossary of terms, and many other resources for those wishing to do holistic nursing research (www.AHNA.org/research). (For specific case studies, refer to the bibliography located on DavisPlus.)

BOX 17-5
Legal Cautions

1. Is the modality within the scope of practicing nursing, or is it practicing medicine without a license? This is a particular problem as APN practice begins to look more like medical practice with overlapping roles and functions. Here a firm grounding in nursing theory and diagnosis will add clarity.
2. Standards of care for contemporary and alternative medicine (CAM) may be less clear than for conventional practice. Consider risk management guidelines of the institution and state nurse practice acts.
3. Is the practice in concert with the guidelines of the nurse practice act in the state in which the nurse practices?
4. Has the practice or modality been limited to another discipline? Some disciplines have their own licensure (e.g., chiropractic might limit the nurse's practice of craniosacral therapy).
5. Nurses traditionally counsel clients regarding nutrition and supplements. Does the state in which the nurse practices limit that counseling or prohibit prescribing over-the-counter herbs and supplements? Most often APNs with prescriptive authority are the only nurses qualified to prescribe such substances.

Role Development and Avenues and Models for Advanced Practice Nurses as Complementary-Integrative Practitioners

Nontraditional, holistic interventions are common APN practices. More nurses are becoming independent CI or holistic practitioners. Health coaching has become a role with a scope and standards of practice for the holistic nurse. An entire issue of *Beginnings,* published by AHNA (Holistic nurse coaching, 2011), is devoted to the role function of coaching. A 2006 issue of *Beginnings* is devoted to holistic nurses developing private practices. Nurses describe practices that include HT, massage, counseling, a radio show, work in cardiology, and aromatherapy. A 2008 issue described various practice settings including an herbal practice, home care and hospice, providing bedside music, aromatherapy, palliative care, and private practice. Numerous reports exist about nurses integrating relaxation, imagery, music, aromatherapy, and Healing Touch and Reiki into conventional practice in hospitals, offices, and community settings. APNs interested in developing complementary therapy practices or delivering holistic nursing interventions must take responsibility for obtaining the necessary education, experience, and (when appropriate) certification.

APNs may be involved in CI practice in which patients have a choice between a conventional and an alternative practitioner. If APNs may recommend complementary therapies they need to be informed about which therapies are safe and effective for a specific patient's plan of care, being cognizant about the patient's condition. **Box 17-6** contains questions that APNs can use as a guide to recommending CI therapies. Many interventions are elective and can be integrated into conventional care to help patient and family increase comfort and a sense of mastery over their situation.

BOX 17-6

Question Guide for Advanced Practice Nurses Recommending Complementary-Integrative Therapies

- Has the therapy been used to manage the symptom or initial treatment?
- Is there research evidence that the therapy is safe and effective?
- Is the therapy appropriate for the patient?
- Does the patient want or expect the therapy to work?
- Are there providers who are skilled in providing the therapy?
- Has the patient had prior or current experience with complementary therapies?
- What modality does the patient's cultural group tend to use most frequently?
- When you refer a patient to a complementary-integrative health-care provider, do you know the provider's credentials and licensing requirements, the qualifications of the practitioner, and some evidence of competence?
- Counseling patients in their decision to use complementary therapies also includes consideration for the cost of the treatments. Although insurance companies cover some complementary modalities (e.g., chiropractic, hypnosis, and massage), most modalities are paid for out of pocket and are often quite expensive.
- Counsel patients about access to herbs and supplements on the Internet. Which are legitimate and is the cost reasonable?

The NCCAM home page offers guidance for recommending therapies on the section "Be an informed consumer." This includes such issues as selecting a CAM practitioner, paying for CAM, and 10 things to know about evaluating medical resources on the Web. In bold letters is the statement **"Tell your doctor about your CAM use."** NCCAM and the Office of Dietary Supplements continue to be valuable resources for updated reviews and meta-analyses of research. Sufficient understanding of both the patient's disease process and the specific therapy are mandatory requirements before referral to a specific CI practitioner is made. Communication and collaboration with the CI practitioner is useful in providing comprehensive care.

Ethical Considerations

The APN has the obligation to foster patients' choices about the care they receive and must function within the *ANA Code of Ethics for Nurses with Interpretative Statement* (2001). According to Mariano (2007), the ethical stance of the holistic nurse is as an "option giver," a partner, and a "co-prescriber." "The relationship is a copiloting of the individual's health experience whereby one respects the person's decision about his or her own health. It is a process of engagement, rather than compliance" (p. 169).

The ethical principles of autonomy, nonmalfeasance, beneficence, and justice must be considered when advising or referring patients who use or consider using complementary therapies that are beyond advanced nursing practice. Patients have the right to choose treatments consistent with their own values and culture. The APN's ethical obligation "involves not only respecting patient decisions but also fully informing the patient about the potential risks and benefits of CAM therapies" (Kaler & Ravella, 2002). The constructs of nonmalfeasance, beneficence, and autonomy in three holistic organizations were studied by Wardell and Engebretson (2001, p. 333) who concluded that

> *by appreciating the value of diverse healing modalities and sharing the decision making with clients, clinicians preserve patient autonomy and honor the principle of beneficence. Providers risk malfeasance if they ridicule, trivialize, or discourage patients' access to therapies from which they could benefit.*

Ensuring that all patients have equal access to complementary therapies requires monitoring changes in insurance coverage and community resources.

CONCLUSION

It is a holistic philosophy and evidence-based nursing science that facilitates the development of an integrative practice rather than a fragmented approach of adding optional therapies. That philosophy recognizes the integrative wholeness of each individual as the individual interacts with and reacts to his or her personal and larger environments. The challenge in our hurried world is to keep that focus for both the patient and ourselves. Maintaining healthy wholeness for ourselves is part of that holistic equation. As role models for other nurses and health-care professionals, APNs can affect the entire health-care system. Because of nurses' legacy in holistic philosophy, APNs have much to offer in the field of CAM, CI, and holistic nursing. Although modalities are important, they become more powerful for patients' and our own well-being if that practice is grounded in a strong commitment to holism, no matter what the modality. With this commitment to practice we can participate in creating a future that enriches ourselves, our patients, and society at large. See **Box 17-7.**

BOX 17-7
Expanding and Advancing Contemporary and Alternative Medicine

To integrate contemporary and alternative medicine (CAM) into conventional health care and enable clients to benefit from the best of all treatments available, the advanced practice nurse (APN) will need to do all of the following:

- Acquire and maintain current knowledge and competency in holistic nursing practice, including CAM therapies and practices integrated within that practice.
- Provide care and guidance to persons through nursing interventions and therapies consistent with research findings and other sound evidence.
- Adhere to a professional code of ethics and healing that seeks to preserve wholeness and dignity of self and others.
- Recognize each person as a whole: body-mind-spirit.
- Assess patients holistically, using appropriate traditional and holistic methods.
- Create a plan of care in collaboration with the patients and their significant others, if they wish, consistent with cultural background, health beliefs, sexual orientation, values, and preferences, that focuses on health promotion, recovery or restoration, or peaceful dying so that the person is as independent as possible.

Based on American Holistic Nurses Association. (2002a). *AHNA: Position on the role of nurses in the practice of complementary and alternative therapies.* Retrieved July 15, 2002, from www.ahna.org/limited/cam.rtf.

REFERENCES

American Holistic Nurses Association. (1998). *Description of holistic nursing.* Flagstaff, AZ: Author.

American Holistic Nurses Association. (2002a). *AHNA: Position on the role of nurses in the practice of complementary and alternative therapies.* Retrieved July 15, 2002, from www.ahna.org/limited/cam.rtf.

American Holistic Nurses Association. (2002b). *AHNA standards of advanced holistic nursing practice for graduate-prepared nurses.* Flagstaff, AZ: Author.

American Holistic Nurses Association. (2004). What is holistic nursing? Retrieved June 10, 2012, from www.ahna.org.

American Nurses Association. (2001). *Code of ethics for nursing with interpretative statements.* Washington, DC: Author.

American Nurses Association. (2010). *Nursing's social policy statement: The essence of the profession. Revised.* Silver Springs, MD: Author.

American Nurses Association, American Holistic Nurses Association. (2007). *Holistic nursing: Scope and standards of practice.* Washington, DC: Author.

Anderson, J. G., & Taylor, A. G. (2011). Biofield therapies in cardiovascular disease management. *Holistic Nursing Practice, 25*(4), 199–204.

Ashen, A. (Spring 1977). Eidetics: An overview. *Journal of Mental Imagery 1,* 5–38.

Baldacchino, D., & Draper, P. (2001). Spiritual coping strategies: A review of the nursing research literature. *Journal of Advanced Nursing, 34*(6), 833–841.

Baldwin, A. L., Vitale, A., Brownell, E., Scicinski, J., Kearns, M., & Rand, W. (2010). The touchstone process: An ongoing critical evaluation of Reiki in the scientific literature. *Holistic Nursing Practice, 24*(5), 260–276.

Buckle, J. (2005). Aromatherapy. In B. Dossey, L. Keegan, & K. Guzetta (Eds.), *Holistic nursing: A handbook for practice* (4th ed., pp. 829–848). Sudbury, MA: Jones & Bartlett.

Burman, M. E. (2003). Complementary and alternative medicine: Core competencies for family nurse practitioners. *Journal of Nursing Education,* 42(1), 28–34.

Burkhardt, M. A., & Nagai-Jacobsen, M. G. (2002). *Spirituality: Living our connectedness.* Albany, NY: Delmar Thompson Learning.

Burkhardt, M. A., & Nagai-Jacobsen, M. G. (2009). Spirituality and health. In B. Dossey, L. Keegan, & L. Keegan (Eds.), *Holistic nursing: A handbook for practice* (5th ed., pp. 617–642). Sudbury, MA: Jones & Bartlett.

CAM at the NIH Newsletter. (2007). *The placebo effect as a therapeutic tool.* Retrieved December 15, 2008, from http://nccam.nih.gov/news/newsletter/.

Clark, C. C. (1986). *Wellness nursing: Concepts, theory, research and practice.* New York: Springer.

Clements, I., & Martin, E. J. (1990). *Nursing and holistic wellness: A new beginning.* Dubuque, IA: Kendall/Hunt Publishing.

Cole, K. M., & Gawlinski, A. (2000). Animal-assisted therapy: The human-animal bond. *AACN Clinical Issues, 11*(1), 139–149.

Deal, B. (2011) Finding meaning in suffering. *Holistic Nursing Practice, 25*(4), 205–210.

Denner, S. S. (2007). The advanced practice nurse and integration of complementary and alternative medicine. *Holistic Nursing Practice, 21*(3), 152–159.

Denner, S. S. (2009). The science of energy therapies and contemplative practice. *Holistic Nursing Practice, 23*(6), 315–334.

DiNucci, E. M. (2005). Energy healing: A complementary treatment for orthopaedic and other conditions. *Orthopaedic Nursing, 24*(4), 259–269.

Donnelly, G. F. (2006). From the editor: The transformation of healthcare: A wicked problem. *Holistic Nursing Practice, 20*(5), 215–216.

Donner, G., &Wheeler, M. (2009). *Coaching in nursing: An introduction.* Indianapolis, IN: International Council of Nursing and Sigma Theta Tau. Retrieved July 9, 2011, from http://www.icn.ch/es/pillarsprograms/coaching-in-nursing-an-introduction/.

Dossey, B. M. (1997). *Core curriculum for holistic nursing.* Boston: Jones & Bartlett.

Dossey, B. M., & Keegan, L. (2012). *Holistic nursing: A handbook for practice* (6th ed.). Sudbury, MA: Jones & Bartlett.

Dossey, L. (2003). Samueli conference on definitions and standards in healing research: Working definitions and terms. Definitions and standards in healing research: The first American Samueli symposium (Ed.), W. Jonas & R. A. Chez. A supplement to *Alternative Therapies in Health and Medicine, 9*(3), A10–A12.

Eisenberg, D. M., Davis, R., Ettner, S. L., Appel, S., Wilkey, S., VonRompay, M., et al. (1998). Trends in alternative medicine use in the United States, 1990–1997. *Journal of the American Medical Association, 280*(18), 1569–1575.

Eisenberg, D. M., Kessler, R. C., Foster, C., Norlock, F. E., Calkins, D. R., & Delbanco, T. L. (1993). Unconventional medicine in the United States: Prevalence, costs, and patterns of use. *New England Journal of Medicine, 328*(4), 246–252.

Eisenberg, D. M., Kessler, R. C., Van Rompay, M. I., Kaptchuk, T. J., Wilkey, S. A., Appel, C., et al. (2001). Perceptions about complementary therapies relative to conventional therapies among adults who use both: Results from a national survey. *Annals of Internal Medicine, 135*(5), 344–351.

Eldridge, C. R. (2007). Meeting your patients' spiritual needs. *American Nurse Today, 2*(10), 51–52.

Eliopoulos,C. (2002). Leading the way to integration. *Integrative Nursing,* 1(1), 1.

Engebretson, J., & Wardell, D. W. (2007). Energy-based modalities. *Nursing Clinics of North America, 41*(2), 243–260.

Enzham-Hagedorn, M., & Zahourek, R. P. (2007). Research paradigms and models for investigating holistic nursing concerns. *Nursing Clinics of North America, 41*(2), 335–353.

Erickson, H. L. (2007). Philosophy and theory of holism. *Nursing Clinics of North America, 41*(2), 139–163.

Eslinger, M. R. (Ed.). (2000a). Complementary therapies in anesthesia [Special Issue]. *CRNA: The Clinical Forum for Nurse Anesthetists, 11*(4), 190–196.

Eslinger, M. R. (2000b). Foreword. *CRNA: The Clinical Forum for Nurse Anesthetists, 11*(4), 159.

Fairman, J. A., Rowe, J., Hassmiller, S., & Shalala, D. (2011). Broadening the scope of nursing practice. *New England Journal of Medicine, 364*(3), 193–196.

Fazzino, D.L, Quinn Griffin, M.T., McNulty, R., Sr., & Fitzpatrick, J. J. (2010). Energy healing and pain. *Holistic Nursing Practice, 24*(2), 79–88.

Fenton, M. V., & Morris, D. L. (2003). The integration of holistic nursing practices and complementary and alternative modalities into curricula of schools of nursing. *Alternative Therapies in Health and Medicine, 9*(4), 62–67.

Fitzgerald, M. A. (2007, December). Herbal facts, herbal fallacies. *American Nurse Today, 2.*

Hanley, M.A., Hines, M., Koithan, M., Sierpina, V., Krietzer, M. J., (2010, July). AHNA: Providing Transformative Innovations in Holistic Nursing Praxis. *The Journal of Science and Healing,* 6(4), 271–274.

Garner, B. (2007). Aromatherapy for you and your patient. *American Nurse Today, 2*(9), 53–54.

Good, M., Albert, J. M., Andersen, G. C., et al. (2010). Supplementing relaxation and music for pain after surgery. *Nursing Research, 59*(4), 250–269.

Hess, D. (2011). Defining holistic coaching. *Beginnings, 31,* 16–19.

Holistic nurse coaching. (2011). *Beginnings, 31.* Issue devoted to holistic nurse coaching.

Institute of Medicine. (2010). *The future of nursing: Leading change, advancing health.* Washington, DC. Retrieved July 5, 2011, from http://www.IOM.edu/Reports/2010/The-Future-of-Nursing-Leading-change-Advancing-health.aspx.

Janin, S. S., & Mills, P. (2010). Biofield therapies: Helpful or hype? A best evidence synthesis. *International Journal of Behavioral Medicine, 17,* 1–16.

Jonas, W. B. (1997). Alternative medicine: Editorial. *Journal of Family Practice, 45*(1), 34.

Jonas, W. (2009). *The wellness initiative for the nation, 2009.* Retrieved July 9, 2011, from http://www.samueliinstitute.org/news/news-home/WIN-Home/WIN-Updates.html.

Kaler, M. M., & Ravella, P. C. (2002). Staying on the ethical high ground with complementary and alternative medicine. *Nurse Practitioner, 27*(7), 38–42.

Kaptchuk, T. J., Friedlander, E., Kelley, J. M., et al. (2010). Placebos without deception: A randomized controlled trial in irritable bowel syndrome. *PLoS One, 5*(12), 1–7.

Kitko, J. (2007) Rhythmic breathing as a nursing intervention. *Holistic Nursing Practice, 21*(2), 85–88.

Kubsch, S., O'Shaughnessy, J., Carrick, J., Willihnganz, T., Henricks-Soderberg, L., & Sloan, S. A. (2007). Acceptance of change in the healthcare paradigm from reductionism to holism. *Holistic Nursing Practice, 21*(3), 140–151.

Macrae, F. (2011). The *genetic clue that may explain why women get more migraines.* Retrieved August 15, 2012, from http://www.dailymail.co.uk/health/article-2002789/The-genetic-clue-explain-women-migraines.html#ixzz247nGuPWw.

Mariano, C. (2007). Holistic nursing as a specialty: Holistic nursing—Scope and standards of practice. *Nursing Clinics of North America, 41*(2), 165–188.

McCaffery, R. (2007). The effect of healing gardens and art therapy on older adults with mild to moderate depression. *Holistic Nursing Practice, 21*(2), 79–84.

McCaffery, R., Hansen, C., &McCaffery, W. (2010). Garden walking for depression. *Holistic Nursing Practice, 24*(5), 252–259.

McCloskey, J. C., & Bulechek, G. M. (1992). *Nursing interventions classification.* St. Louis: Mosby.

McCloskey, J. C., & Bulechek, G. M. (2000). *Nursing interventions classification* (3rd ed.). St. Louis: Mosby.

Miles, P., & True, G. (2003). Reiki—A review of biofield therapy history, theory, practice and research. *Alternative Therapies, 3*(9), 62–71.

National Center for Complementary and Alternative Medicine. (2008). *2007 statistics on CAM use in the United States.* Retrieved December 15, 2008, from http://nccam.nih.gov/news/camstats.htm.

National Center for Complementary and Alternative Medicine. (2010). *What is complementary and alternative medicine?* Retrived July 2, 2011, from http://nccam.nih.gov/health/whatiscam/.

Nightingale, F. (1859/1969). *Notes on nursing.* New York: Dover Publishing.

North American Nursing Diagnosis Association. (2005) *NANDA: Nursing diagnoses: Definitions and classification, 2005–2006.* Philadelphia: Author.

Peters, R. M. (1999).The effectiveness of therapeutic touch: A meta-analytic review. *Nursing Science Quarterly, 12*(1), 52–61.

Purnell, M. J., & Lange, B. (2011). Creating a graduate holistic nursing program. *Holistic Nursing Practice, 25*(3), 140–146.

Quinn, J. F., Smith, M., Ritenbaugh, C., Swanson, K., & Watson, M. J. (2003). Research guidelines for assessing the impact of the healing relationship in clinical nursing. Definitions and standards in healing research: The first American Samueli symposium, Ed. Jonas, W., & Chez, R. A. A supplement to *Alternative Therapies in Health and Medicine, 9*(3), A65–A79.

Radzyminski, S. (2007). Legal parameters of alternative-complementary modalities in nursing practice. *Nursing Clinics of North America, 41*(2), 189–212.

Rakel, D. (2007). *Integrative medicine* (2nd ed.). Philadelphia: WB Saunders.

Reed, T. (2007). Imagery in the clinical setting. *Nursing Clinics of North America, 41*(2), 279–294.

Rew, L. (1996). *Awareness in healing.* Albany, NY: Delmar Publishers.

Rosenfeld, I. (2008, March 16). Do herbal remedies work? *Parade Magazine.* Retrieved May 5, 2012, from www.parade.com.

Ross, S. M. (2008). Osteoarthritis: A proprietary arnica gel is found to be as effective as Ibuprofen gel in osteoarthritis of the hands. *Holistic Nursing Practice, 22*(4), 237–239.

Ross, S. M. (2011). Research in review: The role of herbal medicine in women's health. *Holistic Nursing Practice, 25*(2), 105–110.

Sand-Jecklin, K., & Emerson, H. (2010). The impact of a live therapeutic music intervention on patients' experience of pain, anxiety, and muscle tension. *Holistic Nursing Practice, 24*(1), 7–15.

Schaub, B. G., & Dossey, B. M. (2009). Imagery: Awakening the inner healer. In B. M. Dossey & L. Keegan, (Eds.), *Holistic nursing: A handbook for practice* (5th ed., pp. 295–305). Sudbury, MA: Jones & Bartlett.

Shames, K. H. (1996). *Creativity in nursing.* Albany, NY: Delmar Publishers.

Smith, M. C., & Kyle, L. (2008). Holistic foundations of aromatherapy for nursing. *Holistic Nursing Practice, 22*(1), 3–9.

Snyder, M. (1985). *Independent nursing interventions.* New York: John Wiley & Sons.

Sok, S. R., Erlen, J. A., & Kim, K. B. (2004). Complementary and alternative therapies in nursing curricula: A new direction for nurse educators. *Journal of Nursing Education, 43*(9), 401–405.

Sparber, A. (2001). State boards of nursing and scope of practice of registered nurses performing complementary therapies. *Online Journal of Issues in Nursing, 6*(3), 1–10. Retrieved October 3, 2002, from www.nursingworld.org/ojin.

United States Department of Health and Human Services. (1998). *Healthy people 2010 objectives: Draft for public comment.* Washington, DC: Government Printing Office.

Vitale, A. (2009). Nurses' lived experience of Reiki for self care. *Holistic Nursing Practice, 23*(3), 167–179.

Vitale, A., & O'Connor, P. C. (2006). The effect of Reiki on pain and anxiety in women with abdominal hysterectomies. *Holistic Nursing Practice, 20*(6), 263–272.

Wardell, D. W., & Engebretson, J. (2001). Ethical principles applied to complementary healing. *Journal of Holistic Nursing, 19*(4), 318–334.

Wardell, D. W., & Weymouth, K. (2004). Review of studies of healing touch. *Journal of nursing scholarship, 36*(2), 147–154.

White House Commission on Complementary and Alternative Medicine Policy. (2002). *White House Commission on Complementary and Alternative Medicine Policy: Final report.* Retrieved July 19, 2002, from http://whccamp.hhs.gov/finalreport.html.

Winstead-Frye. P. Wijeck, J. (1999). An interpretative review and meta-analysis of therapeutic touch research. *Alternative Therapies in Health and Medicine*, 5(6), 58–67.

Zahourek, R. P. (1982a). Hypnosis in nursing practice—Emphasis on the problem patient who has pain. [Part 1.] *Journal of Psychosocial Nursing and Mental Health Services, 20*(3), 13–17.

Zahourek, R. P. (1982b). Hypnosis in nursing practice—Emphasis on the problem patient who has pain. [Part 2.] *Journal of Psychosocial Nursing and Mental Health Services, 20*(4), 21–24.

Zahourek, R. P. (1985) *Clinical hypnosis and therapeutic suggestion in nursing.* Orlando: Grune & Stratton, Inc.

Zahourek, R. P. (1988). *Relaxation and imagery: Tools for therapeutic communication and intervention.* Philadelphia: WB Saunders.

Zahourek, R. P. (2002). Imagery. In M. A. Bright, *Holistic health and healing.* Philadelphia: F.A. Davis.

Zahourek, R. P. (2009). Healing through the lens of intentionality. *International Journal of Healing and Caring, 9*(2). Retrieved July 10, 2012, from www.IJHC.org.

18

Basic Skills for Teaching and the Advanced Practice Nurse

Marilyn H. Oermann

In today's health-care environment, the advanced practice nurse (APN) serves a critical role in educating patients, students, staff, and other learners. The extensive knowledge base, clinical competencies, and communication skills of the APN prepare the nurse for carrying out this role across practice settings. Patient education is an important part of managing the patient's care to achieve optimal outcomes. Through this education, patients gain an understanding of their health problems and treatments, how to care for themselves at home, and health-promoting behaviors. By learning about their conditions and treatment options, patients can participate more fully in health-care decisions.

Teaching patients and their families, however, is only one role of the APN. In many settings the APN also teaches staff, assisting them in developing the knowledge and skills essential for providing care, keeping them up-to-date with advances in clinical practice, and mentoring nurses in the practice setting, ultimately improving the quality of patient care. For some APNs the educator role extends to nursing students, with the APN serving as a preceptor to nursing students and guiding their learning in the practice setting.

The purposes of this chapter are to describe the qualities of an effective teacher in nursing, the educational process from assessment through evaluation, strategies for teaching, and the role of the APN as educator. The chapter provides an overview of these topics as a way of preparing the APN for teaching patients, staff, students, and others.

FRAMEWORK FOR TEACHING

Every APN needs an understanding of the concepts of learning and teaching. These concepts provide a framework for the APN to use when making educational decisions.

Learning

Learning is a process of gaining new knowledge and skills as a result of experiences in which the learner engages. These experiences may be planned activities intended to guide the learner in acquiring this knowledge and these skills, or they may be unplanned experiences that lead to a new understanding. Learning may result in an overt and measurable change in behavior, such as patients' ability to perform a procedure after teaching by the APN, or the outcomes of learning may not be readily apparent, such as gaining a new perspective on a chronic illness or insight about one's own condition. Although learning has occurred, it may be more difficult to assess those outcomes.

Teaching

Teaching is a series of planned actions by the APN to facilitate learning. Teaching is not merely giving information, although that might be included in the process. Instead, teaching is identifying individual needs, setting goals in collaboration with the learner, planning experiences that guide the learner toward meeting those goals, and monitoring the learner's progression and determining where further learning is indicated (Gaberson & Oermann, 2010). Teaching is facilitating learning through experiences that actively involve the learner. Rather than telling a nurse what care to provide, the APN asks higher level questions about the patient to guide the nurse in thinking through possible options.

Supportive Environment for Learning

The relationship between teacher and learner is critical to the educational process. Learning is facilitated in a supportive environment in which there is mutual trust and respect (Gaberson & Oermann, 2010). Establishing this environment is particularly important when working with new graduates and students in the clinical setting. Clinical practice is stressful for new graduates (Beecroft, Santner, Lacy, Kunzman, & Dorey, 2006; Duchscher, 2008; Welding, 2011) and students (Galbraith & Brown, 2011; Hensel & Stoelting-Gettelfinger, 2011; Moscaritolo, 2009).

Although education is a shared experience between the APN and learners, the APN has the ultimate responsibility for establishing a supportive learning environment. When working with new graduates and students, the APN should remember that they are beginning practitioners and have varying clinical knowledge and competencies. The expectations set by the APN for these learners should be realistic considering their background and prior experiences.

Qualities of Effective Teachers in Nursing

Research conducted over the years has established the qualities of an effective teacher in nursing, particularly for teaching in the clinical setting. The findings of this research are significant because they guide the APN in developing skills that promote learning and avoiding behaviors that might impede learning. There are five predominant qualities of effective teaching: (a) expert knowledge, (b) clinical competence, (c) teaching skills, (d) positive relationships, and (e) personal characteristics. **Table 18-1** describes these qualities in more detail.

ASSESSMENT OF LEARNER

The teaching process begins with an assessment of learning needs and other determinants of learning and progresses through planning, implementation, and evaluation. The process, however, is not linear; teaching does not necessarily start with assessment and end with evaluation. For example, the APN may plan a program for staff education following a needs assessment, but he or she may realize at the start of the program that most of the nurses lack the knowledge base for understanding the new content. This in turn suggests that different content should be presented to assist staff in gaining the prerequisite knowledge.

Assessment of Learning Needs

Assessment is the first step in the teaching process because it determines the learner's present knowledge and skills, and examines other characteristics, such as readiness to learn and health status, which may influence achieving the objectives. The goal of assessment is to identify the knowledge

TABLE 18-1

The Five Predominant Qualities of Effective Teaching

Quality	Details
Expert knowledge	Has expertise in content area to be taught Is up to date with interventions and new developments in that area Is aware of and able to translate current research findings and evidence into clinical practice
Clinical competence	Knows how to care for patients Uses sound clinical judgments Has advanced clinical skills in area of practice and can guide learners in developing these skills
Teaching skills	Knows how to teach and has the ability to use those principles in teaching Assesses learning needs and plans instruction that meets those needs Explains ideas clearly at a level each learner can understand Asks thought-provoking questions that promote critical thinking and clinical judgment Effectively demonstrates procedures and technical skills Evaluates learners fairly, corrects mistakes without embarrassing them and decreasing their self-confidence, and gives immediate, specific, and instructional feedback
Positive relationships	Has strong interpersonal skills and an understanding of the importance of communication in the student–teacher relationship Provides support for students Communicates clearly
Personal characteristics	Includes enthusiasm for teaching, patience, a sense of humor, friendliness, and willingness to admit mistakes

and skills the learner has already acquired and the needs for learning. Assessment reveals gaps in learning to be met through education. Questions that guide assessment of learning needs are highlighted in **Box 18-1.**

Learners frequently have more needs than the time and resources available for teaching. As a result, the APN prioritizes the learning needs, focusing the instruction on the essential knowledge and skills for self-care if teaching patients and for safe, effective practice if teaching staff. For example, the mother of a toddler recently diagnosed with asthma needs to know warning signs of an asthma episode and how to manage it, her child's asthma medications, the correct use of inhalers, asthma triggers for her

BOX 18-1

Questions That Guide Assessment of Learning Needs

What does the learner already know about the content?

What competencies does the learner already have?

Is this knowledge and are those competencies sufficient to learn the new content?

Based on this information and the goals or objectives to be achieved, what should be taught?

child and how to prevent them, and when to seek treatment. These are immediate learning needs and should be the priorities for teaching by the APN. Although the mother may ask about the relationship between asthma and participating in organized sports, this information is not essential and is a low priority for teaching.

There also is limited time for educating staff, and the APN needs to focus the instruction on knowledge and skills essential for safe and competent practice. What are the most common practice problems new graduates and nursing staff are likely to encounter? What content must be learned to understand those problems and provide effective nursing care? What knowledge and competencies are required for safe care of patients? Once these essential learning needs are met, the APN can extend the instruction to other areas of learning.

Assessment of Readiness to Learn

A second area to assess is the learner's readiness to learn. Readiness is the point in time when the learner demonstrates an interest in learning and is able to participate in the teaching process (Bastable, 2008). The learner must be ready physically, psychologically, and cognitively to engage in learning, otherwise, learning will not occur regardless of the importance of the content and skills.

In assessing *physical readiness,* the APN focuses on whether the learner has the physical ability to learn the skill. For example, a patient must have a certain degree of strength to learn to transfer from bed to wheelchair. Health status also affects physical readiness because it often influences the energy the learner has to engage in learning and degree of comfort. A patient experiencing acute pain following a surgical procedure or who is fatigued because of a treatment may not have the energy to learn and may be too uncomfortable to participate. Teaching the family or planning instruction for the follow-up visit may be more appropriate.

Psychological readiness includes the degree of anxiety and stress experienced by the learner, motivation to learn, and developmental stage. The learner needs to be able to focus on learning and be actively involved in it. The stress associated with the diagnosis of a serious health problem, fear of losing one's job because of illness, and concern about not being successful in an educational program, to name a few, may influence readiness to learn. In assessing psychological readiness, it is important for the APN to get a sense of the learner's state of mind and determine whether the learner is emotionally ready to engage in learning.

Motivation is the desire of an individual to learn—the drive to gain new knowledge and skills or to change a behavior. Differences among staff and students in their motivation to learn are often apparent in the effort they give to learning, their desire to achieve at a high level of performance rather than meet minimal expectations, and their willingness to engage in remedial learning and practice. Motivation may change over time and with different learning situations. Strategies for motivating learners as part of the teaching process are presented in **Box 18-2.**

Readiness to learn also is determined by the learner's developmental stage. Pediatric nurses are well aware of differences in how children learn based on their ages and development. Knowledge of growth and development guides the APN in determining the complexity and outcomes of learning and the types of teaching strategies that are appropriate.

Cognitive readiness relates to the knowledge base of the learner—whether the learner has the prerequisite knowledge and skills for beginning the instruction. This is a critical area of assessment, particularly for content and skills that build on one another. When lacking the prerequisites, it is up to the APN to fill in these gaps and guide learners to resources and experiences they can complete on their own. Assessment of cognitive readiness also allows the APN to determine if the learner has already mastered the objectives and is ready to progress to a new area of learning.

BOX 18-2
Strategies for Motivating Learners as Part of Teaching

Teach *for* the learner based on the learner's needs, not the educator's needs.

Teach when ready to learn or develop alternate strategies, such as teaching family members and planning instruction for follow-up visits.

Set small and attainable goals so learners can meet them.

Focus the learner's attention on what needs to be learned.

Explain why this content and these skills are important.

Divide information to be learned into small segments, organize them logically, and teach only the amount learners can retain at a time.

Provide frequent and positive reinforcement (e.g., praise, for correct answers and accurate performance of skills).

Give immediate feedback at the time of learning, clarifying incorrect responses and errors in performance, and reteaching as needed.

Allow for practice so the learner develops skill and confidence in abilities.

Review essential content and skills over a period of time to improve retention.

Other Assessment Areas

Other areas to assess depend on the educational situation and type of learner. In teaching patients and families, the APN should be aware of their culture and how that might influence their education and methods selected for teaching. The patient's cultural values, health practices, and literacy are important to assess before teaching (Chang & Kelly, 2007; Gordon, Caicedo, Ladner, Reddy, & Abecassis, 2010; Michaels, McEwen, & McArthur, 2008; Wright, 2011).

Cultural differences also may exist when teaching staff and students, and should be assessed by the APN. The educational level of learners is often an important area for assessment, although the highest grade achieved in school does not necessarily indicate the learner's knowledge of a health problem or how that person will respond to the instruction.

Strategies for Assessment

Questioning Learners

One of the most effective strategies for assessment is questioning learners about their understanding of the content and what they believe are their educational needs. These questions can be planned in advance and asked in a structured interview, or they can be integrated in the interactions between the APN and learner, a more informal means of assessing needs. For patient education, it is valuable to develop a list of questions about the conditions and treatments commonly found in the APN's practice; a standardized list of questions facilitates assessment and enables the APN to document the learning needs, instruction provided to patients and family, and outcomes.

Questions for assessment need to be open ended and probing to be effective. Asking patients, "Do you have any questions about your asthma?" is of limited value in assessing their understanding of asthma and self-care. A more effective line of questioning is, "Tell me about the medications you are taking for your asthma and whether they are helping. What problems are you still having, and what are you doing about them?" Using open-ended and higher level questions is particularly important when assessing the learning needs of staff and students. Learners may be able to answer questions that ask for recall of facts and specific information but be unable to answer those that require application to new situations, analytical thinking, and clinical judgment. By asking different levels of questions, the APN can identify more clearly the actual learning needs.

Questionnaires

A second strategy for assessment is to develop a questionnaire that lists content areas and asks learners to identify where they need further instruction. One problem with questionnaires, however, is that learners rate their own instructional needs, which may not reflect an accurate assessment. A second problem when used for staff development is the length of time between conducting the assessment and planning and implementing the educational program. In that period, the learning needs of staff may change significantly.

Pretests

Written tests given before the instruction provide a reliable and valid means of assessing learning needs. By using pretest results, the APN can determine the content already mastered and identify gaps in learning that become the focus of the instruction. An advantage of using written tests is the opportunity to administer both a pretest and posttest as a means of evaluating the effectiveness of the instruction and educational programs offered by a facility. Although staff and students are conditioned to testing as a way of measuring learning, patients may be uncomfortable with written tests, and care should be used to write questions at a level patients can understand.

Observations

There is no better means of assessing psychomotor and technical skills than by observation of the learner performing them. Ideally, the APN should observe performance more than once.

Development of Objectives

Assessment reveals the knowledge and skills that the learner needs to acquire to meet the educational goals and the characteristics that might influence the learning process. From these needs the APN specifies the objectives to be met by the learner. These objectives reflect the outcomes of learning—the knowledge, psychomotor and technological skills, and values to be attained by the learner. The objectives also guide the selection of content and teaching strategies; assessment determines the extent to which learners have achieved the objectives and where further learning is indicated (Oermann & Gaberson, 2009). The planning phase of the teaching process includes the development of objectives and the selection of content, teaching methods, and learning activities.

Some educators prepare detailed objectives such as, "After reading an article on nursing management of patients in heart failure, the staff nurse identifies two nursing interventions with supporting evidence." Other educators prepare more general objectives that specify at minimum who the learners are and what they will know or be able to do at the end of the instruction. Using the previous example, a general objective would be: "The staff nurse identifies nursing interventions with supporting evidence for care of patients in heart failure." In most teaching situations, a general objective is sufficient.

Objectives should be clear, measurable, and attainable, considering the level of the learner and time frame allotted for the instruction. Behaviors such as list, identify, apply, and compare are measurable in contrast to terms such as know and understand. The time frame for teaching also dictates the number of objectives and their complexity.

Taxonomies of Objectives

There are three domains or areas of learning: cognitive, psychomotor, and affective. Objectives may be written in each of these domains and leveled using the taxonomies, which are classification systems for objectives.

Cognitive Domain Learning in the cognitive domain relates to the acquisition of knowledge and development of intellectual skills such as problem solving. In many teaching situations, the outcome of learning is memorizing facts and specific information; however, at other times, the goals are learning to apply concepts to new situations, analyze complex data about patients, arrive at decisions about patient problems and alternative possibilities that exist, and make decisions about the most appropriate course of action.

The taxonomy of the cognitive domain enables the teacher to organize the learning outcomes in a logical way from memorization to increasingly more complex cognitive skills. There are six levels in the cognitive taxonomy, beginning with recall of specific facts and information, the lowest, and progressing through comprehension, application, analysis, synthesis, and evaluation (Bloom, Englehart, Furst, Hill, & Krathwohl, 1956). A definition and sample objective for each of the six levels of the cognitive taxonomy are found in **Table 18-2.**

Anderson and Krathwohl (2001) updated the taxonomy, rewording the categories as verbs (e.g., remembering instead of knowledge), and reordering synthesis and evaluation. The highest level of learning in the adapted taxonomy is creating—synthesizing elements to form a new or different product.

Psychomotor Domain Psychomotor learning results in the development of motor skills, ability to perform technical procedures, and other competencies that involve physical coordination. In developing psychomotor skills, learners progress through different phases: cognitive (learning about the skill and how to perform it), associative (refining movements until they become more consistent), and autonomous (practicing the skill, until one can perform it automatically without thinking about each step) (Oermann, 2011; Schmidt & Lee, 2005). In teaching skills these phases are important to keep in mind. In the cognitive phase learners are attempting to understand the skill and how to accurately perform it. In this phase questions from the teacher about the rationale for the skill and its underlying principles are appropriate. However, in the other phases in which learners are developing and refining their performance

TABLE 18-2

Cognitive Taxonomy and Sample Objectives

Levels of Cognitive Taxonomy	Sample Objective
Knowledge: Ability to recall facts and specific information	The patient identifies side effects of medications.
Comprehension: Ability to understand and explain information	The nurse explains the underlying pathophysiology of the patient's condition.
Application: Ability to use knowledge in a new situation and apply concepts and theories to practice	The student plans interventions for critically ill patients that are based on current evidence.
Analysis: Ability to identify relevant parts and their relationships	The manager analyzes the outcomes of the new staffing pattern on patients and nursing staff.
Synthesis: Ability to develop a new product	The nurse designs a protocol for pain management.
Evaluation: Ability to arrive at judgments based on internal and external criteria	The student evaluates research studies on the use of relaxation for adults with chronic pain.

of the skill itself, the teacher should not ask questions about the "why" of the skill. When learning to drive a car, the instructor does not ask how the engine works. Similarly, as the patient is learning to draw up the insulin, or the student is setting up an infusion pump, the focus of the teacher and any questions asked should be on guiding performance, not on the underlying principles of the skill.

Progressing through these phases of learning and developing motor skills requires deliberate practice. Practicing a skill one time is generally not sufficient. Learners need an opportunity to practice a skill multiple times with specific feedback from the teacher on their performance and how to improve it (Ericsson, 2004; Ericsson, Whyte, & Ward, 2007; McGaghie, Issenberg, Petrusa, & Scalese, 2006, 2010). Feedback should focus on the motor components of the skill. Although objectives can be written for psychomotor learning, similar to the cognitive domain, in most situations skills are taught using a checklist of the steps of the procedure.

Affective Domain In some educational situations, the APN assists learners in developing values important in professional practice. Value development in this context builds on an understanding of the values and beliefs that are essential to practice as a professional, such as confidentiality and privacy. From this knowledge base, learners need to then accept these values and beliefs as their own and internalize them as a basis for their own professional practice (Oermann & Gaberson, 2009). In most teaching situations, the APN would not specify values to be taught to patients and other learners in the form of objectives but would be aware of these outcomes when planning the instruction.

DEVELOPMENT OF A TEACHING PLAN

The objectives represent the outcomes of learning based on the APN's assessment and form the basis for the teaching plan. The aim of the teaching plan is to guide learners in achieving the objectives, considering other characteristics of the learner also examined during the assessment. The APN plans and organizes content related to the objectives, selects teaching methods, and plans learning activities, all with the intent of assisting the learner in meeting the objectives or outcomes of learning.

In developing the teaching plan, the APN should consider the level of learning to be achieved as a result of the instruction. If the outcome of learning is to recall facts, the teaching methods could be lecture, discussion, and readings. When the objective is to *use* the knowledge gained from the instruction to decide on the most effective nursing interventions for a patient (application) or to determine the priority problem (analysis), the teaching strategies need to extend beyond lecture and discussion. For example, with those outcomes of learning, the APN might develop a short case in which the learner applies the concepts to a hypothetical patient scenario or have a discussion with staff about how to manage a patient's care, considering the evidence on interventions that might be used.

Although teaching often occurs without a written plan or by using or adapting a standardized plan, having a teaching plan is useful because it specifies the intended learning outcomes or competencies to be developed, content, teaching methods, time allotted for the instruction, and strategies for assessing if learning occurred. When offering an educational program for a group of learners, a written plan guides the teacher in the depth of content to present and types of teaching methods that can be used within the time frame. For programs that provide contact hours for continuing education, written plans are required, and the organization offering the contact hours specifies the form to be used.

There are many formats for developing written plans for teaching and educational programs. Generally, they include at least six components that relate to one another: (a) purpose of the education, (b) objectives or outcomes to be met, (c) outline of the content, (d) teaching methods for presenting the content and guiding learners in meeting the objectives, (e) time frame for the instruction, and (f) evaluation methods. **Figure 18-1** provides a sample teaching plan developed for a continuing education program; this can be used as a template for the development of teaching plans by the APN.

Continuing Education Offering: Documentation Form
Title of Offering: Clinical Teaching and Evaluation
Purpose: Examine a variety of clinical teaching and evaluation methods for use in nursing education.

Objectives	Content	Teaching Methods	Time Frame	Evaluation Methods
1. Examine varied clinical teaching methods and related evidence. 2. Describe clinical methods and principles for assessing clincal performance in nursing.	I. Lack of evidence base for clinical teaching II. Guidelines for good clinical teaching II. Clinical teaching methods A. Patient assessment B. Higher level questions and what research shows C. Case method D. Unfolding cases E. Short papers for clinical courses and why to use them F. Conferences G. Media clips H. Others	Lecture/discussion, PowerPoint, handouts, examples, small group work: develop each clinical teaching method and share with large group	1 hour	Questioning, review of clinical teaching methods
	I. Framework for evaluating clinical performance II. Methods for assessing clinical competencies A. Observation of performance and need for recording observations B. Problems with observations C. Rating forms 1. Types 2. Validity, reliability, and other standards D. Preparing teachers to rate performance: what can be done? E. Multiple assessment methods III. Summary and evaluation	Lecture/discussion, PowerPoint, handouts, role play (teacher observing student performance and giving feedback on it), video clips: observe performance and rate using forms	1 hour	Questioning, feedback during discussions of video clips, self assessment

FIGURE 18-1 Sample teaching plan.

The content is organized logically from simple to complex, with prerequisite content presented first. The extent of content to include depends on the objectives and the amount of time allotted for the instruction. If there is only a limited time available, the goal is to present the content that is critical to foster achievement of the outcomes. The content is usually listed on the teaching plan in outline format with sufficient detail for other educators to know what to teach and in what order. If only a brief outline is required in the setting, the APN can develop a more detailed one for personal use in delivering the instruction.

The next component of the plan is a list of the teaching methods, the strategies the APN will use to help learners achieve the outcomes and gain the knowledge and skills they need. Methods should be appropriate for the content to be presented and for achieving the objectives. The type of learner patients, students, new graduates, or experienced staff; size of the group; and time frame also influence the selection of teaching methods.

With patient education, discussion, handouts, visuals, and demonstration are effective because they lend themselves to individualized instruction and allow the APN to gear the teaching to the particular needs of the patient. With students and staff, there are many teaching methods from which to choose, but some, such as written assignments, are more appropriate for students than staff.

The group size is significant in that some methods are best used for individual instruction and with small groups such as discussion and demonstration, whereas others are useful for larger groups such as lecture. Along the same line, some strategies are more time consuming to implement. For example, games and role-play provide for experiential learning and actively involve learners, but they often are time consuming to set up and implement (Gaberson & Oermann, 2010). Discussion and small group activities add time to the instruction compared with presenting the content in a lecture format, but activities such as these might be critical considering the outcomes to be met and learner needs.

The next component of the teaching plan specifies the time frame for the instruction. The time allotted for teaching determines the depth and complexity of the content and also influences the selection of teaching strategies. The APN should carefully plan the content to avoid running out of time and to include essential information that the learner needs. It is less of a problem when the instruction is completed early because the APN can review the content, ask questions to ensure learner understanding, and provide additional practice for skill learning.

The last component of the teaching plan is the evaluation methods used to measure achievement of the outcomes. Evaluation may be formative, providing feedback to learners on their progress in meeting the objectives, or summative, measuring achievement of the outcomes of learning. Evaluation methods are described later in this chapter.

Teaching Methods

Many teaching methods are available for use by the APN in educating patients, students, and staff. This section presents a number of these methods. The goal is to choose methods that facilitate achievement of the objectives and are appropriate for the learner. The APN should be aware of different teaching methods that can be used and the evidence on their effectiveness (Oermann, 2009).

Lecture

Lecture is a structured means of presenting information to a group. In recent years with the focus on higher level thinking, there has been a shift from lecturing, in which students are usually passive participants, to more active learning methods. However, a lecture that synthesizes from multiple sources, is well organized, is delivered with skill, and allows for questions and open discussion is an effective method for presenting a large body of content in a short period (Oermann, 2007). Lectures can be efficient in that the teacher can emphasize key points to learn and can integrate different sources of information not available to the learners. To promote thinking and higher level learning, the teacher can include examples that apply content from the lecture to clinical situations and can ask questions about alternative perspectives and different possibilities (Oermann, 2007). By adapting the traditional lecture with minimal learner involvement to an interactive format with open-ended questions and discussion, lecture can be used for higher level learning.

A lecture begins with an introduction that presents the objectives to be met, an overview of the content, and why this information is important. The content presented during the lecture should reflect a synthesis from multiple sources of information rather than repeating what could be read in an article or a textbook. The intent of the lecture is to synthesize from resources not available to learners. Content should be clear and organized logically, beginning with simple concepts and progressing to more complex ones, consistent with the outline in the teaching plan. Questions and examples integrated throughout allow for higher level learning and actively involve the participants. Small group activities within the lecture or at the end serve a similar purpose, as well as encourage collaborative learning. Moellenberg and Aldridge (2010) recommended that teachers approach the lecture as a discussion or conversation, asking questions and incorporating other strategies such as film clips and examples from clinical practice. The lecture ends with a summary that reviews the main points, and for students and staff, their relevance to clinical practice.

The use of multimedia in the lecture provides for visualization of the content, allows the teacher to highlight key points as the lecture progresses, and adds variety to the presentation. Some important principles for developing media for presentations are shown in **Box 18-3.** In addition, there are many online tutorials that prepare teachers for developing quality media for their lectures and other types of presentations. Other guidelines for presenting an effective lecture or speech are also found in Box 18-3. Inexperienced teachers should practice their lectures in front of a mirror or have them video-recorded for self-assessment or critique by a colleague.

BOX 18-3
Guidelines for Presentations (Lectures, Speeches, and Other Types)

Identify Learners and Objectives

Know your learners and their background.

If presenting to learners about whom you have limited information, review materials that describe the educational program and ask program planners about learners.

Review objectives for presentation.

Plan Presentation

Plan content to meet objectives, considering learners and time allotted.

Do not develop content from one article or textbook; synthesize literature and resources not available to learners.

Develop list of topics and subtopics to be presented or use outline format.

Prepare introduction that includes objectives to be met, an overview of content, and why the information is important.

Do not write out presentations in sentence form to avoid reading to group; use short phrases.

Next to list of topics or outline, include sample questions to ask learners.

Continued

BOX 18-3

Guidelines for Presentations (Lectures, Speeches, and Other Types)—cont'd

Develop clinical scenarios and examples of how content applies to practice; integrate these throughout presentation, use for small group work, or save for end of presentation if presentation is finished early.

Underline or highlight with color key points to make during presentation so they are easy to see in notes.

List key points to include in summary.

Develop Media

Develop media, such as a PowerPoint presentation, that emphasize major points.

When using PowerPoint:

- Check that each slide presents one idea and begins with a clear title.
- Use key words and short phrases rather than sentences and keep to a minimum so slide is not too "busy."
- Make sure font is large enough, at least 24-point or larger, for everyone to read.
- Choose contrasting colors for text and background so text is easy to read.
- Avoid changing format, such as adding underlining, **bold**, *italics;* changing font size; or using different fonts on same slide.
- Combine uppercase and lowercase letters instead of all uppercase.
- Avoid varying transitions between slides to avoid distracting learner from content.
- Mark on list of topics or outline when to change slides or introduce new media.

Deliver Presentation

Practice in front of mirror or be video-recorded to assess style and gauge time.

Open with interesting anecdote, question, photo, humor, or another statement to get learners' attention.

During presentation, repeat and emphasize important points.

Include transitions between different content areas. Be enthusiastic.

Speak clearly, loud enough for everyone to hear, and at an appropriate speed.

Scan learners as you speak to gauge their attentiveness.

Never tell learners you "ran out of time"; if you finish early, move to your clinical scenarios and extra learning activities, then summarize the content.

Discussion

Discussion is an exchange of ideas between teacher and learner to meet an educational goal (Gaberson & Oermann, 2010). Although the teacher often plans the topic, the intent of the discussion is for learners to express their views, not to provide a forum for teachers to express their own. Both teacher and learner should actively participate.

Discussions are particularly valuable for students and staff to express their feelings and beliefs about a situation, examine values that influence patient care and their interactions with others, and explore ethical issues. Discussions also are effective for encouraging higher level thinking and development of clinical judgment because the teacher can ask the "right" questions—open-ended questions that ask learners to think beyond the obvious, consider alternative perspectives, and examine different options (Alfaro-LeFevre, 2008; Facione & Facione, 2008; Goodin & Stein, 2008; Oermann, 2008).

The cognitive taxonomy described previously in the chapter is a valuable tool to guide the level of questions asked in a discussion. The APN can begin with recall questions that assess the learners' knowledge of facts and can then progress toward higher level questions. **Table 18-3** illustrates questions at each level of the taxonomy. It is important to ask questions at higher levels because these encourage learners to think critically.

A discussion can occur on a one-to-one basis with a learner or in a small group. Gaberson and Oermann (2010) recommended limiting small group discussions to 10 people to provide an opportunity for everyone to talk. Learners need to know that their views and opinions in a discussion are accepted even if different from the teacher's. Some guidelines for conducting an effective discussion follow.

- Focus the discussion on the outcomes to be met.
- Encourage the participation of each learner, but do not force a learner to participate.
- Actively participate as a means of guiding the discussion toward the outcomes but do not dominate the discussion.
- Ask open-ended questions that cannot be answered with a "yes-no" response.
- Sequence questions from low to high level; the taxonomy is useful for this purpose.
- Do not accept the first answer to a question, even if correct; explore other possibilities and ask for a rationale.

TABLE 18-3

Levels of Questions for Discussion

Level	Sample Questions
Knowledge: Questions that ask for recall of facts and specific information	What is this type of breath sound called? Define peak expiratory flow rate.
Comprehension: Questions that explore understanding of content	What is the difference between emphysema and chronic bronchitis? Give an example of a short-acting bronchodilator.
Application: Questions that examine ability of learners to relate content to new or different situation	How do your patient's symptoms compare with what you read about chronic obstructive pulmonary disease? Why is it important to monitor these symptoms?
Analysis: Questions about analyzing data and relationships	What data support your diagnosis, and why are these data relevant? What are alternative interventions that might work in this situation and why?
Synthesis: Questions that ask for development of new ideas and plans	How would you modify this teaching plan to better meet your patient's needs? Tell me about two new interventions that would be effective in your patient's care, their evidence base, and how you would decide whether to use them.
Evaluation: Higher level questions that ask for judgments, critical thinking	Are your interventions effective, and how can you determine that? Your patient is still coughing. What changes can be made in the plan of care, and why would these be appropriate?

- Prevent side-tracking of ideas and help learners return to the topic.
- Summarize what was learned and how it relates to the objectives set for the discussion (Gaberson & Oermann, 2010).

Clinical Conference

Clinical conferences are specific types of discussions held with students and staff in the clinical setting. They can precede the clinical experience to ensure that learners have the prerequisite knowledge and skills to provide patient care and engage in other learning activities planned by the teacher. Often the APN can use these conferences to explain patient problems, interventions, and underlying rationales to learners if they lack the knowledge base to care for those particular patients.

Conferences held after the clinical experiences provide an opportunity to review patient care; discuss patient problems, interventions, and other possible approaches; apply concepts to clinical practice; and explore issues in practice. Conferences also provide a forum for learners to express feelings about patients and experiences in clinical practice (Stokes & Kost, 2009). In clinical conferences, similar to other types of discussions with staff and students, the APN should ask open-ended and probing questions that encourage learners to think about alternative ways of addressing clinical problems. The need for these questions and examples of them were described previously. The APN should be creative in planning conferences to provide variety and maintain learner interest, particularly at the end of a tiring clinical day.

Clinical Case

Clinical cases are actual or simulated scenarios for analysis. This method is effective for learning how to apply content to clinical practice and gaining skill in analyzing data, identifying problems, and deciding on possible solutions (Gaberson & Oermann, 2010). The value of cases for analysis is that they provide experience for learners in thinking through clinical decisions before they are faced with those decisions in actual practice.

With this strategy, the APN develops a case followed by open-ended and higher level questions about it. The cases should be short, a few sentences to a paragraph, and present only essential information. Questions can be directed toward assessment, focusing on missing data in the case and what additional information is needed for decision making. They also can be geared to identifying problems in the case, interventions for immediate action and for planning care, their evidence base, alternative decisions and consequences, and how concepts and theories can be used as a framework for understanding the case and answering the questions.

The questions focus on the objectives to be met by analyzing the case. For example, if the outcome is to select appropriate nursing interventions for a patient with delirium, the APN could ask learners about guidelines to use, early recognition, and how they would manage the patient's care. In analyzing a case, learners should describe the thought process they used and the rationale for their answers. Because the cases are short, they can be integrated easily within a lecture, used at the end of a class as small group work, discussed in clinical conferences, and explored on a one-to-one basis with the learner. Examples are provided in **Box 18-4.**

Case Study

A case study provides an in-depth description of a patient, family, or community, including background information. Case studies can be developed based on actual or simulated clinical situations, similar to shorter cases. With case studies questions can ask learners to differentiate significant from nonsignificant information in the case and examine the effect of the patient's background on current problems and situations. A sample case study is presented in Box 18-4.

BOX 18-4
Examples of Clinical Case and Case Study

Examples of Clinical Cases

Mrs. B, a 46-year-old, is brought to the clinic by her husband with complaints of weakness of the left arm and difficulty "getting her thoughts." The husband tells you that his wife was treated a few months ago for a cerebral aneurysm but has been fine since then. Mrs. B's blood pressure is 210/90. She slowly answers your questions with long pauses in between sentences.

1. What information would you collect from the husband as a priority? Provide a rationale why this information is critical to deciding on the diagnosis and actions to take.
2. What are possible problems that Mrs. B might be encountering? Describe why each of these is a possibility.

You are working in home health care and have a new patient with edema of both legs and extreme fatigue. The patient has no family in the area.

1. What additional data would you collect in your first home visit? Why is this important?
2. Summarize the information you might obtain in the home visit and identify a priority problem. What resources are needed for this patient's care?

You believe your patient may be experiencing side effects from her medication, but your preceptor does not agree and tells you to give the medication to the patient.

1. What are two possible approaches you could take in this situation?
2. What are the advantages and disadvantages of those options?
3. What would you do? Why?

Your patient who is increasingly restless pulls out her endotracheal tube. What should you do first? Include evidence to support this action.

You are working in the emergency department when a young man is admitted following a motor vehicle accident. His larynx appears to be fractured, and there are many facial cuts and bruises. You suction him only to find large amounts of blood; you determine that the only way to keep the airway clear is by suctioning.

1. What are your options for managing his airway?
2. What observations would you make and what other data would you collect that might affect your decision about how to manage his airway?
3. How would you manage this patient's airway? Provide a rationale.

Example of Case Study

Sally is a 6-year-old who has been complaining of pain in her abdomen off and on for the last week. Two weeks ago, she was seen by the pediatrician for a respiratory flu. Sally's current symptoms are two episodes of vomiting this morning, abdominal cramps, no appetite, and a rash on her back. Vital signs, blood pressure, height, and weight are normal. Sally is holding her abdomen and tells you it hurts. When you palpate her abdomen, you find diffuse tenderness without any rebound. There are no masses that you can detect. Sally's past medical history is unremarkable. She has never had any serious illnesses and has never been hospitalized. Her mother tells you that there are no changes in the family or home situation; they recently returned from a camping trip that Sally enjoyed.

1. What laboratory tests would you expect to be ordered? Explain each test and its relationship to this case.
2. What is the significance of "diffuse tenderness without any rebound"?
3. Name all possible problems Sally might have and why.
4. If Sally asks you what's wrong, how would you respond? Provide a rationale based on her age and development.

Unfolding Cases

Cases can be developed to represent a simulated clinical situation that changes over time, similar to patients whose conditions change. These are called unfolding cases (Azzarello & Wood, 2006; Ulrich & Glendon, 2005). A simulated or hypothetical case is presented first, followed by questions for learners. After they analyze the case, the teacher presents more information that modifies the clinical scenario, for example, by adding data or changing the patient's health status. Learners critique the new scenario and again answer questions about it. The teacher can continue to add data to the case to demonstrate changes in the patient's condition and related nursing care.

Grand Rounds

One other teaching method that also revolves around analysis of a case is grand rounds. In grand rounds the teacher presents an update on a clinical topic or care of a patient with a particular diagnosis or treatment. Observation and assessment of the patient, typical patient problems encountered, interventions, and evaluation of outcomes are often described. In some settings the grand rounds presentations are video-recorded and available on the Web for nurses and other health providers to view at a time and place convenient for them. For example, Cincinnati Children's Hospital (2011) presents their Nursing Grand Rounds via streaming media. Many of the programs are offered for continuing education contact hours. Nursing grand rounds also can be conducted in the clinical setting with observation of the patient and discussion about care.

Multimedia

Multimedia provide for multisensory learning. Depending on the type of media, they teach by using different sensory modes. In many teaching situations, it is easier to learn when more senses are involved in communicating the message. Learners can see a patient in a video clip or watch a DVD rather than imagining what the patient looks like or how the intervention should be implemented from the verbal description by the APN or from their readings. Multimedia are useful for demonstrating procedures and technological skills, from gathering the equipment through each step to follow. As learners practice their skills, they can record their performance and replay the video-recording when questions arise or they are unsure about their performance.

Multimedia also are valuable for exploring ethical issues and values. A short segment from a DVD or a YouTube video, for example, can be used to present clinical situations for learners to examine their values and beliefs, and consider how they would respond in those situations. Scenarios can be used to present ethical dilemmas for individuals and groups of students and staff to analyze; small group activities accompanying the media can teach valuable lessons in analyzing and resolving ethical issues.

The growth of the Internet and related technological innovations has resulted in new strategies for educating patients, students, and staff. It is beyond the scope of this chapter to examine the multiple types of technology available for teaching in nursing, but the APN should keep current with the development of these technologies and their use in nursing education.

Selecting Media for Teaching Considering the variety of multimedia available for teaching, the APN first needs to evaluate the quality of any multimedia program or Web-based method under consideration. Not every teaching situation needs the addition of multimedia. The goal is to use media when they clarify the content better than an explanation alone, such as by depicting a patient with the condition being discussed or demonstrating a procedure. Multimedia should not be used only for the sake of incorporating technology into teaching; instead, they should be selected based on the outcomes to be achieved and individual learner needs. In addition to evaluating the quality of the multimedia as a basis for their selection, the second area of concern is their appropriateness for the intended learners.

Questions the APN can use to guide this evaluation are the following:

1. Is the content presented in the multimedia accurate?
2. Is the content up to date?
3. Is the content organized effectively and presented clearly?
4. Are procedures, techniques, and equipment illustrated consistent with current practice in the setting or can they be adapted easily?
5. Are the multimedia of high technical quality (e.g., graphics, sound, interaction with learner, feedback mechanism, etc.)?
6. Are the multimedia appropriate for the outcomes to be met, and will they meet the learner's needs?
7. Are the multimedia appropriate for the learning situation (e.g., patient versus student education, setting for the education, time frame, etc.)?

Readability One additional consideration in evaluating print materials and Web sites for use in patient education is their readability. The reading level of patient education materials should be no higher than the sixth-grade level (Badarudeen & Sabharwal, 2008, 2010; Cotugna, Vickery, & Carpenter-Haefele, 2005; National Institutes of Health, 2011); however, most educational materials for patients are written above this level. This discrepancy inhibits many patients and families from understanding the information in written materials, including important documents such as consent forms, medication package inserts, educational pamphlets, handouts, and discharge instructions, among others.

Early research on readability focused on print materials, but patients accessing health information on the Internet also need to understand what they are reading on the Web. Studies have examined the readability of Web sites for patients, revealing that much of the health information on the Web is at too high a reading level for many consumers (Badarudeen & Sabharwal, 2008; Dornan & Oermann, 2006; Elliott & Shneker, 2009; Kaicker, Debono, Dang, Buckley, & Thabane, 2010; McInnes & Haglund, 2011; Oermann & McInerney, 2007; Washington, Fanciullo, Sorensen, & Baird, 2008).

There are different readability formulas for assessing patient education materials. These include the Flesch Reading Ease (FRE) score, which ranges from 0 (unreadable) to 100 (most readable) based on the average number of syllables per word and length of the sentences; the Flesch-Kincaid grade uses the score to determine a grade level. Another readability formula is the Fry Readability Graph. This formula assesses readability based on the average word length but requires only three 100-word samples from the document rather than the full text (Badarudeen & Sabharwal, 2010). Another readability formula is the Simple Measure of Gobbledygook (SMOG). This measure is determined based on the number of words with more than two syllables: a grade of 7 means the patient education materials could be understood by individuals with a seventh-grade reading ability. Developed specifically for assessing the readability of patient education materials, the New Dale-Chall Readability formula is based on sentence structure and the number of unfamiliar words in the text (Badarudeen & Sabharwal, 2010; Wang, Capo, & Orillaza, 2009). Badarudeen and Sabharwal reported that the New Dale-Chall Readability formula had the highest validity among these formulas (p. 2,574).

One easy way of estimating readability is by using the spelling and grammar function in Microsoft Word. The first step is to generate a Word file of the materials to be assessed; documents from Web sites can be copied and pasted as plain text (without the HTML tags), deleting information not relevant to the content such as the citations and copyright statement. In the Word file to be checked, the APN should omit the headings, tables, figures, and illustrations. To check readability, these steps can be followed:

1. Click the Microsoft Office button, then Word Options, and then Proofing.
2. In the section, "When correcting spelling and grammar in Word," select the check boxes "Check grammar with spelling" and "Show readability statistics," and click OK.
3. Perform a spelling and grammar check.
4. When completed, a pop-up screen will appear with the readability scores.

The APN has an important role in assessing the readability of patient education materials, discharge instructions, and documents given to patients. Before recommending health Web sites to patients, the quality of those sites including readability should be evaluated first. When teaching patients and families who lack the ability to read and understand the information, the APN should focus on key concepts to be learned, use easy-to-understand words, and use varied teaching strategies that rely on visuals. Murphy-Knoll (2007) recommended always speaking in "simple and nonmedical terms" and asking patients and families to repeat back the information in their own words (p. 207).

Self-Directed Instructional Methods

Self-directed instructional methods are completed by learners on their own to meet remedial needs, acquire prerequisite knowledge and skills, and fulfill personal interests. These methods include modules, independent study, multimedia programs, and a wide range of instructional technologies that learners complete independently. Self-directed methods are well suited for learners who are motivated, committed, and independent because they can be completed at a time and in a setting of the learner's choice. A major advantage from an educational point of view is the ability of learners to progress through the instruction at their own rates of learning. This affords learners the opportunity to repeat the instruction when unsure or until competent and to omit content areas already mastered.

Although self-directed methods may be planned for all students, the advantages they offer in terms of individualizing the instruction make them a better resource for meeting remedial needs and gaining prerequisite knowledge and skills. That way, learners who have already met the objectives and can demonstrate the competencies can progress to new areas of learning. Self-directed learning places the responsibility for achieving the competencies on the learner rather than the teacher. The teacher, however, might establish time frames for completion for certain activities and monitor learner progress by asking for a self-assessment or by periodic quizzing.

Demonstration

Demonstration is the presentation of how to perform a procedure or skill with the intent for learners to model that performance and implement the skill on their own. Before demonstrating the procedure, the APN should explain its purpose, equipment to gather, and steps to follow. Any explanation of the principles underlying the skill and discussion about its use in clinical practice should occur at this point in the instruction. As learners practice, feedback from the APN should focus on the performance itself. Because psychomotor learning is egocentric, learners need to focus on manipulating the equipment and refining their skill.

All learners must be able to see each step to be performed and hear any explanations. By observing the demonstration, learners develop an image of what the skill looks like and how to perform it, which then guides their practice of the skill. The return demonstration is when the learner performs the skill and the APN gives specific, instructional feedback to improve the performance. Once competent, learners can practice skills on their own. Practice is critical to refine performance, become more consistent, and develop the ability to carry out the skill in a reasonable period of time. Practice also is essential to retain the skill over time. With human patient simulators, students and nurses can practice and develop competency in the skill before performing it in the clinical setting.

Simulations

With simulations learners have an opportunity to practice and develop their skills, psychomotor, cognitive, communication, and others, in a safe environment. They can analyze scenarios, conduct assessments, make decisions and view the outcomes of those decisions, communicate with team members, and develop their ability to think critically and act quickly before caring for a real patient. With procedures and technologies that require costly equipment and supplies, learners need an opportunity to practice those procedures in a controlled environment before trying them with patients in the clinical setting. Jeffries (2006) indicated that simulations are useful as a competency check for new graduates and individuals being oriented to the clinical setting.

With simulations, learners should have an opportunity to review and reflect on their experiences and decisions; this occurs in the debriefing session after the simulation. In the debriefing, the discussion also may include how their personal values influenced their decisions. In developing values, learners need to experience situations to determine how they will respond to them; simulations provide this type of experience and help learners develop a sensitivity to how others may feel in a situation.

Evaluation of Learning

Evaluation is an integral part of any teaching situation and serves different roles. In working with patients, students, and staff, individually and in small groups, the APN continually assesses how well learners are acquiring an understanding of the content and developing ability to perform skills. Using this information, the APN modifies the teaching, perhaps explaining the content again and in a different way, adding media, suggesting remedial instruction, and allowing the individual more practice time for skills. This type of evaluation is diagnostic; it represents feedback to the learner about progress in meeting the objectives and provides the basis for developing a plan for improvement (Oermann & Gaberson, 2009). This is referred to as formative evaluation.

A second type of evaluation is summative. As the name suggests, this type of evaluation summarizes what has been learned rather than providing feedback to learners. Examples of summative evaluation are final examinations in a course and annual performance evaluations.

With both formative and summative evaluation, the objectives to be met or competencies to be developed serve as the framework for evaluation. The evaluation determines the progress of learners in meeting the objectives and developing clinical competencies or for summative evaluation if they have achieved them.

There are many methods for evaluating learning. The APN selects methods that provide information on the outcomes to be assessed and are appropriate for the learner. Evaluation methods include the following:

- *Questioning:* Questions are asked to assess the extent of learning.
- *Observation of performance:* Learners are observed while performing procedures, providing care, and carrying out interventions in clinical practice. Often a summary of the observations is recorded in a narrative note or on a checklist of performance.
- *Rating scale:* Performance of competencies is rated on a scale.
- *Checklist:* Steps in a procedure or skill are checked off as the learner performs them.

- *Test:* The learner is asked to answer a set of written questions about the content.
- *Written assignment:* Students complete papers of varying length.

ROLE OF ADVANCED PRACTICE NURSE AS EDUCATOR

Providing education to patients, students, and staff is an integral part of the APN role. The APN has a critical role in teaching patients about their illness and preventing further complications, treatments and medications, how to provide self-care, and the importance of follow-up care. In many settings it is up to the APN to prepare the patient for discharge and managing own care at home.

Teaching about the illness and self-care is only one of the areas of education provided by the APN. The APN also teaches patients and families about preventing illness and staying healthy. Without education by the APN, few patients would be informed about their health and how to maintain it. APNs are well suited to provide health-related patient education because they understand interventions for both health and illness.

In some settings, the APN also may be involved in teaching graduate and undergraduate nursing students. The APN may serve as a preceptor for students or guide student learning for individual clinical experiences. Because of their extensive clinical knowledge and skills, APNs may participate in classroom teaching and give lectures and speeches in their area of expertise.

Another component of the APN role is to educate nursing staff and health providers. This education may be informal, teaching in the clinical setting as the need arises, and through formal continuing education programs. As APNs become known for their particular areas of expertise, they are often asked to organize and present continuing education programs.

CONCLUSION

The APN has an important role in educating patients, students, and staff. The teaching process described in this chapter, assessing learner needs, planning instruction, selecting varied teaching methods, and evaluating learning, provides a framework for teaching any of these groups of learners. Nurses in advanced practice are well prepared for their role as educator with their extensive knowledge base, expert clinical skills, and strong communication skills. The knowledge and expertise of the APN combined with an understanding of the educational process prepare the APN to meet the learning needs of patients, families, students, and staff regardless of the setting in which the APN chooses to practice.

REFERENCES

Alfaro-LeFevre, R. (2008). *Critical thinking and clinical judgment: A practical approach to outcome-focused thinking* (3rd ed.). St. Louis: Saunders.

Anderson, L. W., & Krathwohl, D. R. (Eds.). (2001). *A taxonomy for learning, teaching, and assessing: A revision of Bloom's taxonomy of educational objectives.* New York: Longman.

Azzarello, J., & Wood, D. E. (2006). Assessing dynamic mental models: Unfolding case studies. *Nurse Educator, 31*(1), 10–14.

Badarudeen, S., & Sabharwal, S. (2008). Readability of patient education materials from the American Academy of Orthopaedic Surgeons and Pediatric Orthopaedic Society of North America Web sites. *Journal of Bone and Joint Surgery, American Volume, 90*(1), 199–204.

Badarudeen, S., & Sabharwal, S. (2010). Assessing readability of patient education materials: Current role in orthopaedics. *Clinical Orthopaedics and Related Research, 468*(10), 2572–2580.

Bastable, S. B. (2008). *Nurse as educator: Principles of teaching and learning for nursing practice* (3rd ed.). Sudbury, MA: Jones & Bartlett.

Beecroft, P. C., Santner, S., Lacy, M. L., Kunzman, L., & Dorey, F. (2006). New graduate nurses' perceptions of mentoring: Six-year programme evaluation. *Journal of Advanced Nursing, 55*(6), 736–747.

Bloom, B. S., Englehart, M. D., Furst, E. J., Hill, W. H., & Krathwohl, D. R. (1956). *Taxonomy of educational objectives: The classification of educational goals. Handbook I: Cognitive domain.* White Plains, NY: Longman.

Chang, M., & Kelly, A. E. (2007). Patient education: Addressing cultural diversity and health literacy issues. *Urologic Nursing, 27*(5), 411–417.

Cincinnati Children's Hospital. (2011). *Nursing grand rounds.* Retrieved April 1, 2011, from http://www.cincinnatichildrens.org/ed/cme/library/nursing.htm.

Cotugna, N., Vickery, C. E., & Carpenter-Haefele, K. M. (2005). Evaluation of literacy level of patient education pages in health-related journals. *Journal of Community Health, 30*(3), 213–219.

Dornan, B. A., & Oermann, M. H. (2006). Evaluation of breastfeeding Web sites for patient education. *MCN: Maternal and Child Nursing, 31*(1), 18–23.

Duchscher, J. B. (2008). A process of becoming: The stages of new nursing graduate professional role transition. *Journal of Continuing Education in Nursing, 39*(10), 441–450.

Elliott, J. O., & Shneker, B. F. (2009). A health literacy assessment of the epilepsy.com website. *Seizure, 18*(6), 434–439.

Ericsson, K. A. (2004). Deliberate practice and the acquisition and maintenance of expert performance in medicine and related domains. *Academic Medicine, 79*(10), S70–S81.

Ericsson, K. A., Whyte, J., IV, & Ward, P. (2007). Expert performance in nursing: Reviewing research on expertise in nursing within the framework of the expert-performance approach. *Advances in Nursing Science, 30*(1), E58–E71.

Facione, N. C., & Facione, P. A. (Eds.). (2008). *Critical thinking and clinical reasoning in the health sciences: An international multidisciplinary teaching anthology.* Millbrae, CA: California Academic Press.

Gaberson, K., & Oermann, M. H. (2010). *Clinical teaching strategies in nursing* (3rd ed.). New York: Springer.

Galbraith, N. D., & Brown, K. E. (2011). Assessing intervention effectiveness for reducing stress in student nurses: Quantitative systematic review. *Journal of Advanced Nursing, 67*(4), 709–721.

Goodin, H., & Stein, D. (2008). Deliberative discussion as an innovative teaching strategy. *Journal of Nursing Education, 47*(6), 272–274.

Gordon, E. J., Caicedo, J. C., Ladner, D. P., Reddy, E., & Abecassis, M. M. (2010). Transplant center provision of education and culturally and linguistically competent care: A national study. *American Journal of Transplantation, 10*(12), 2701–2707.

Hensel, D., & Stoelting-Gettelfinger, W. (2011, January 31). Changes in stress and nurse self-concept among baccalaureate nursing students. *Journal of Nursing Education,* pp. 1–4. DOI: 10.3928/01484834-20110131-09. [Epub ahead of print.]

Jeffries, P. R. (2006). Designing simulations for nursing education. In M. H. Oermann & K. T. Heinrich (Eds.), *Annual review of nursing education* (Vol. 4, pp. 161–177). New York: Springer.

Kaicker, J., Debono, V. B., Dang, W., Buckley, N., & Thabane, L. (2010, October 8). Assessment of the quality and variability of health information on chronic pain websites using the DISCERN instrument. *BMC Medicine, 8,* 59.

McGaghie, W. C., Issenberg, S. B., Petrusa, E. R., & Scalese, R. J. (2006). Effect of practice on standardised learning outcomes in simulation-based medical education. *Medical Education, 40*(8), 792–797.

McGaghie, W. C., Issenberg, S. B., Petrusa, E. R., & Scalese, R. J. (2010). A critical review of simulation-based medical education research: 2003–2009. *Medical Education, 44*(1), 50–63.

McInnes, N., & Haglund, B. J. (2011, February 18). Readability of online health information: Implications for health literacy. *Informatics for Health and Social Care.* [Epub ahead of print.]

Michaels, C., McEwen, M. M., & McArthur, D. B. (2008). Saying "no" to professional recommendations: Client values, beliefs, and evidence-based practice. *Journal of the American Academy of Nurse Practitioners, 20*(12), 585–589.

Moellenberg, K., & Aldridge, M. (2010). Sliding away from PowerPoint: The interactive lecture. *Nurse Educator, 35*(6), 268–272.

Moscaritolo, L. (2009). Interventional strategies to decrease nursing student anxiety in the clinical learning environment. *Journal of Nursing Education, 48*(1), 17–23.

Murphy-Knoll, L. (2007). Low health literacy puts patients at risk. *Journal of Nursing Care Quality, 22*(3), 205–209.

National Institutes of Health. (2011, January 4). *How to write easy to read health materials.* National Library of Medicine Web site. Retrieved April 2, 2011, from http://www.nlm.nih.gov/medlineplus/etr.html.

Oermann, M. H. (2007). Lectures for active learning in nursing education. In L. E. Young & B. Paterson (Eds.), *Teaching nursing: Developing a student centered environment* (pp. 279–294). Philadelphia: Lippincott Williams & Wilkins.

Oermann, M. H. (2008). Ideas for postclinical conferences. *Teaching and Learning in Nursing, 3,* 90–93.

Oermann, M. H. (2009). Evidence-based programs and teaching/evaluation methods: Needed to achieve excellence in nursing education. In M. Adams & T. Valiga (Eds.), *Achieving excellence in nursing education* (pp. 63–76). New York: National League for Nursing.

Oermann, M. H. (2011). Toward evidence-based nursing education: Deliberate practice and motor skill learning. *Journal of Nursing Education, 50*(2), 63–64.

Oermann, M. H., & Gaberson, K. (2009). *Evaluation and testing in nursing education* (3rd ed.). New York: Springer.

Oermann, M. H., & McInerney, S. M. (2007). An evaluation of sepsis Web sites for patient and family education. *Plastic Surgical Nursing, 27*(4), 192–196.

Schmidt, R. A., & Lee, T. D. (2005). *Motor control and learning: A behavioral emphasis* (4th ed.). Champaign, IL: Human Kinetics.

Stokes, L. G., & Kost, G. C. (2009). Teaching in the clinical setting. In D. M. Billings & J. A. Halstead (Eds.), *Teaching in nursing: A guide for faculty* (3rd ed., pp. 283–299). St. Louis: Saunders.

Ulrich, D. L., & Glendon, K. J. (2005). *Interactive group learning: Strategies for nurse educators* (2nd ed.). New York: Springer.

Wang, S. W., Capo, J. T., & Orillaza, N. (2009). Readability and comprehensibility of patient education material in hand-related Web sites. *Journal of Hand Surgery, 34*(7), 1308–1315.

Washington, T. A., Fanciullo, G. J., Sorensen, J. A., & Baird, J. C. (2008). Quality of chronic pain websites. *Pain Medicine, 9*(8), 994–1000.

Welding, N. M. (2011). Creating a nursing residency: Decrease turnover and increase clinical competence. *Medsurg Nursing, 20*(1), 37–40.

Wright, P. R. (2011). Care of culturally diverse patients undergoing ophthalmic surgery. *Insight, 36*(1), 7–10.

19

Culture as a Variable in Practice

Mary Masterson Germain

This chapter is an invitation to step into other worlds—worlds where experiences may be quite different from your own. You will be asked to reflect on the beliefs and values that make you who you are and to examine how they affect you as a healer and caregiver. Directly and indirectly, as an advanced practice nurse (APN) you play a pivotal role in shaping the quality of care that patients receive. You are privileged to share in some of your patients' most profound and intimate experiences. To fully enter into the patient's experience and to provide comprehensive care that is respectful of the patient's cultural beliefs and practices, nurses need to find ways to bridge the linguistic and cultural challenges that are inherent in caring for increasingly diverse populations. It is uncomfortable to stretch our ethnocentric boundaries; it is much easier to care for replicas of ourselves. However, if you are open to learning from your patients, the transient discomfort that you experience from having your time-honored interventions and teaching strategies tested and found wanting by patients with different cultural perspectives will be rewarded by gaining rich insights into cultural beliefs and practices that will inform your practice for years to come. Let us begin the journey.

SCOPE OF THE NEED

The challenge for APNs is to institute care in populations and practice settings that are increasingly diverse. Between 2000 and 2010, the Asian population in the United States grew faster than any other major racial group, increasing by 43%. In contrast, the White racial group had the lowest rate of growth, increasing only 5.7% during that same period (Humes, Nicholas, & Ramirez, 2010).

Every 10 years, the U.S. Department of Health and Human Services produces a comprehensive assessment of the health of Americans and sets goals and objectives for improving their health and well-being. See *Healthy People 2010* and *Healthy People 2020.* In 2000, when *Healthy People 2010* was published, the document established two overarching goals for improving the health of U.S. residents and communities in the first decade of the 21st century:

Goal 1: Increase quality and years of healthy life
Goal 2: Eliminate health disparities

These two goals, representing 28 focus areas and 467 measurable objectives, had a single, overarching purpose of promoting health and preventing illness, disability, and premature death, and a unifying vision: healthy people living in healthy communities (U.S. Department of Health and Human Services [USDHHS], 2000). Note that goal 2 does not say *reduce.* It says *eliminate;* a lofty goal. It is also critical to note that ethnicity and the social determinants of health care are inextricably linked in the discussion of the disparities in health status and access and use of health-care services presented in both *Healthy People 2010* and *Healthy People 2020 (AHRQ, 2007b).* This chapter will approach cultural competence in advanced practice nursing from a similar frame of reference and will examine how much progress has been made in achieving the objectives of *Healthy People 2010.*

Of the 309.3 million people living in the United States in 2010, 40 million persons (12.9% of the population) were foreign born, an increase of 1.4 million (0.4%) from 2009. The largest percentage, more than one-half (53.1%), were from Latin America, followed by Asians (28.2%) and Europeans (12.1%). The population of foreign-born residents from Latin America tended to be concentrated in four states: California (26%), Texas (14%), Florida (13%), and New York (10%) (U.S. Census Bureau, 2010a).

Because these data represent nationwide statistics, they do not capture the complexity of delivering culturally competent care, especially in urban settings that traditionally have large immigrant populations. The data on racial origin reported by the Bureau of the Census are associated with significant differences in health status and disease, condition-specific morbidity and mortality, and socioeconomic status:

- The infant mortality rate (2007) for non-Hispanic Black women was 2.4 times greater than that for non-Hispanic White women. Puerto Rican women also experienced significantly greater infant losses compared to non-Hispanic White women. The increased infant mortality for both racial groups was related to greater rates of preterm birth and preterm causes of death. Non-Hispanic Black women had a preterm delivery rate of 18.3%, 60% higher than that for non-Hispanic white women (MacDorman & Mathews, 2011).
- The Centers for Disease Control and Prevention (CDC) has documented increases in the age-adjusted percentage of persons diagnosed with diabetes from 1980 to 2009: Blacks (100%); Whites (123%); and Asians/Pacific Islanders (1997–2009: 51%) (CDC, 2011).

Clearly, racial origin alone does not account for these disparities in health and health outcomes. Health status is influenced by a multiplicity of factors, as reflected in **Figure 19-1.** Key determinants associated with poor health status and outcomes also tend to reflect economic status and household composition (DeNavas-Walt, Proctor, & Smith, 2010):

- The number of people in poverty in 2010 (46.2 million) is the largest number in the 52 years for which poverty estimates have been published (p. 14).

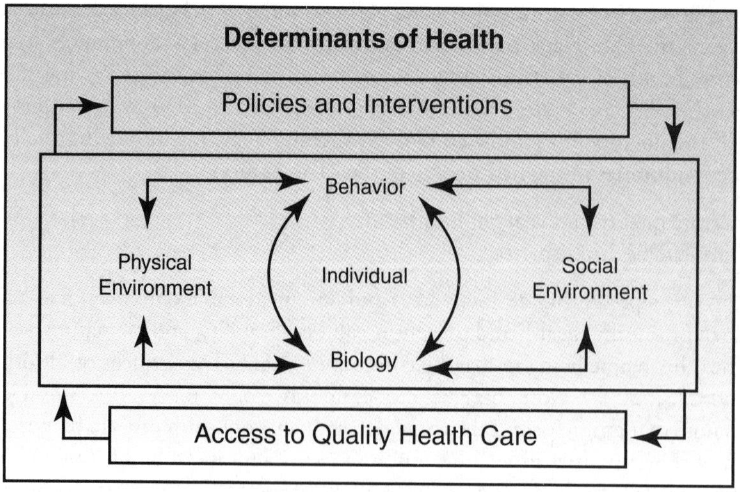

FIGURE 19-1 Healthy people in healthy communities. *(Source: USDHHS, 2000, p. 18.)*

- The uninsured rate was higher among people with lower incomes and lower among people with higher incomes. In 2010, 26.9% of people in households with annual incomes less than $25,000 had no health insurance coverage (p. 27).
- Children in poverty were more likely to be uninsured (15.4%) than all children (9.8%) (p. 28). Related children in households headed by a female were significantly more likely to be in poverty than related children in households headed by married couples—46.9% compared to 11.6% (pp. 17–18).

Level of education is a critical variable affecting economic status and health. There is a direct relationship between education and income. Analysis of American Community Survey (ACS) data from 2006 to 2008 demonstrates that a person's level of education affects work-life earnings five times more than other demographic characteristics, such as gender (Julian & Kominski, 2011, p. 10). The health status and survival of children of undereducated women differs significantly from that of their better-educated peers. One goal set by *Healthy People 2010* was to have a minimum of 90% of pregnant women accessing prenatal care during the first trimester. Only college-educated Asians/Pacific Islanders (90.0%) and non-Hispanic Whites (93.2%) achieved the *Healthy People 2010* target of 90% of women receiving prenatal care in the first trimester. The percentage was significantly lower for women with less than a high school education (72.8%) and high school graduates (82.0%) than for women with any college education (91.2%) (Agency for Healthcare Research and Quality [AHRQ], 2008, p. 231).

Another goal set by *Healthy People 2010* was for 100% of Americans to have health insurance. The 2010 *National Healthcare Disparities Report* (NHDR) cites the following (AHRQ, 2011b):

- In 2008, the percentage of people with health insurance was significantly lower for poor, near-poor, and middle-income people than for high-income people (71.0%, 69.4%, and 83.4%, respectively, compared with 93.8%) (p. 231).
- In 2008, the percentage of people with health insurance was about one-third lower for people with less than a high school education than for people with at least some college education (56.9% compared with 89.0%) (p. 231).
- From 2002 to 2007, the percentage of people who were uninsured all year was nearly three times higher for people who spoke another language at home as that for people who spoke English at home (in 2007, 33.7% compared with 12.2%) (p. 237).

In 1997, President Clinton appointed an Advisory Presidential Commission on Consumer Protection and Quality of Health Care in the Health Care Industry. On March 12, 1998, the Commission completed its final report to the President, "Quality First: Better Health Care for All Americans." The report called for the President to take a leadership role in developing a broad national consensus on the need to improve the quality of health care. The Commission recommended six national goals and the development of measureable objectives for each goal. It also recommended the development of core sets of quality measures that should be standardized and utilized across the entire health-care industry. The national goals and objectives were to be revised as improvement was documented and new areas of need arose.

The Agency for Healthcare Research and Quality (AHRQ) has played a pivotal role in implementing the recommendations of the Commission. Since 2003, the AHRQ has produced two annual comprehensive reports, the *National Healthcare Quality Report* (NHQR) and the *National Healthcare Disparities Report* (NHDR). After generating the fifth set of reports, the AHRQ asked the Institute of Medicine (IOM) to make recommendations as to how the reports could be improved. The IOM, founded in 1970 as the health arm of the National Academies of Science, is a nonprofit, independent organization of renowned scholar-clinicians in health care that advises the government on issues related to improving health. The IOM formed a Consensus Committee to study the reports, headed by Sheila Burke, RN, MPH, former chief of staff to Senator Robert Dole and currently Faculty Research Fellow at the Malcolm Weiner Center for Social Policy, John F. Kennedy School of Government, Harvard University. The Committee's report, titled *Future Directions for the National Healthcare Quality and Disparities Reports,* was released by the IOM in April 2010. The report acknowledged how essential it is to continuously assess quality and equity in health care on an ongoing basis, and commended the AHRQ for developing the annual set of reports. The Committee also made recommendations as to how the reports could be made more effective in promoting the reduction of disparities and improving the quality of health care. The report brief released by the IOM on April 14, 2010, summarized the recommendations of the IOM's authoring committee as follows: select measures that reflect health-care attributes or processes that are deemed to have the greatest impact on population health; affirm that achieving equity is an essential part of quality improvement; increase the reach and usefulness of AHRQ's family of report-related products; analyze and present data in ways that will inform policy and promote best-in-class achievement for all actors; and identify measure and data needs to set a research and data collection agenda (IOM, 2010).

The 2010 National Health Care Quality and Disparities Reports (NHQR and NHDR) reflect the recommendations made by the IOM. The 2010 NHDR identifies four priority populations: racial and ethnic minorities; low-income groups; residents in rural areas; and individuals with disabilities or special health-care needs. It is interesting to note that as of 2009, women were dropped as a priority population. Thus, critical data regarding access to, and utilization of, prenatal care is no longer presented in the report. The only data presented in either the NHQR or the NHDR relates to obstetric trauma. Children and older adults are also no longer considered to be priority populations. The data from both reports have been aggregated to present a unitary set of conclusions and to identify major areas of unmet needs. Health-care quality and access are suboptimal, especially for minority and low-income groups.

- Quality is improving; access and disparities are not improving.
- Urgent attention is warranted to ensure improvements in quality and progress on reducing disparities with respect to certain services, geographical areas, and populations, including cancer screening and management of diabetes, states in the central part of the country, residents of inner-city and rural areas, and disparities in preventive services and access to care.
- Progress is uneven with respect to eight national priority areas. Two are improving in quality: (1) palliative and end-of-life care and (2) patient and family engagement. Three are lagging: (3) population health, (4) safety, and (5) access. Three require more data to assess: (6) care coordination, (7) overuse, and (8) health system infrastructure.
- All eight priority areas showed disparities related to race, ethnicity, and socioeconomic status (AHRQ, 2011a; AHRQ, 2011b, p. 2).

We have a long way to go if we are to achieve the goals of equitable, high-quality health care for all of our people, as echoed in *Healthy People 2020.* Building on the goals set by *Healthy People 2010* and a vision of "a society in which all people live long, healthy lives," it establishes four goals encompassing almost 1,200 objectives spanning 42 important topic areas related to public health. Thirteen of the topical areas are new. They include adolescent health; global health, genomics; health-related quality of life and well-being; and transgender health. The four overarching goals are as follows:

- Attain high-quality, longer lives free of preventable disease, disability, injury, and premature death.
- Achieve health equity, eliminate disparities, and improve the health of all groups.

- Create social and physical environments that promote good health for all.
- Promote quality of life, healthy development, and healthy behaviors across all life stages (USDHHS, 2010).

Progress in meeting these goals will be assessed using four foundational measures: general health status, health-related quality of life and well-being, determinants of health, and disparities.

Some of the data that led to the NHDR's conclusions are given in **Box 19-1.** It is clear that there is no simplistic solution to the issue of disparities in health care. The causal factors are multiple and interactive. What is clear is that issues of access and quality will become even more pronounced as the health-care needs of an ever-growing elderly population compete for already limited resources. Designing and funding a system of care that will ensure equitable access to high-quality health-care services for all is a challenge that APNs must play a pivotal role in solving.

As is evident from the 2010 National Health Care Quality and Disparities Reports, the goals and objectives espoused in *Healthy People 2020* continue to present APNs with an unparalleled opportunity to lead; to practice; to develop high-quality, cost-effective health-care delivery systems that empower patients and promote self-care; and to conduct seminal research documenting the positive health outcomes associated with advanced practice nursing interventions. This is especially true in the context of the Patient Protection and Affordable Care Act (Public Law [PL] 111-148), commonly referred to as the Affordable Care Act (ACA), which was passed by the 111th Congress and signed into law by President Obama on March 23, 2010 (Kaiser Family Foundation, 2011). The provisions of the ACA

BOX 19-1
2010 National Healthcare Quality Report and National Healthcare Disparities Report Data

- Blacks and American Indians and Alaska Natives received worse care than Whites for about 40% of core measures (AHRQ, 2011b, p. 4).
- Hispanics received worse care than non-Hispanic Whites for about 60% of core measures (AHRQ, 2011b, p. 4).
- Poor people received worse care than high-income people for about 80% of the core measures (AHRQ, 2011b, p. 4).
- **Access is not improving.** Across the 22 measures of health care access tracked in the reports, about 70% did not show improvement and 40% were headed in the wrong direction (AHRQ, 2011c, p. 6).
- Fewer than 20% of disparities in quality of care faced by Blacks, American Indians and Alaska Natives, Hispanics, and poor people showed evidence of narrowing (AHRQ, 2011c, p. 7).
- **Effectively navigating and managing care:** Ethnicity, income, and education were associated with the need for language assistance when navigating the health-care system (AHRQ, 2011b, p. 22).
- **Selected process measures getting worse over time** (AHRQ, 2011c, p. 10):

Women age 40+ who received a mammogram in the last 2 years
Women age 18+ who received a Pap smear in the last 3 years
Adults age 50+ who received a fecal occult blood test in the last 2 years
Children ages 19–35 months who received 3 doses of *Haemophilus influenzae* type B vaccine
Adults age 40+ with diabetes who received a hemoglobin A_{1C} measurement in the calendar year
Adults age 40+ with diabetes who received a dilated eye examination in the calendar year

have the potential to bring more than 30 million additional persons into the health-care system. Meeting the goals of *Healthy People 2020* will demand a passionate commitment to professional activism, basic human rights, and a vision of high-quality health care for all peoples in the United States. Never before has the choice been so clear. We can lead, follow, or get out of the way. As Robert Frost wrote, "I took the road less traveled by, and that has made all the difference" (Frost, 1961, p. 84).

APNs frequently face a dual challenge: to provide high-quality, evidence-based care to culturally diverse populations and to do so in communities that are often socially and economically disadvantaged. Our profession's response to this challenge is found in the American Nurses Association's (ANA's) *Code of Ethics for Nurses,* particularly Provision 1 (ANA, 2001, p. 7):

> *The nurse, in all professional relationships, practices with compassion and respect for the inherent dignity, worth and uniqueness of every individual, unrestricted by considerations of social or economic status, personal attributes, or the nature of health problems.*

Central to the concept of ethical practice is the principle of justice: fair and equitable access to high-quality health-care services. That this access is not available for many Americans is indisputable, and it has served as the focal point for the debate over whether health care is a right or a privilege. In a quote attributed to the late Dr. Martin Luther King Jr., he addressed the inherent injustice in disparities in health care by saying, "Of all the forms of inequality, injustice in health is the most shocking and inhumane" (Changing the present, (2012). The racial, ethnic, and social factors creating existing disparities in health and access to health-care services create a moral imperative for APNs to integrate cultural competence into all their direct and indirect care roles. Cultural competence demands not only incorporation of our patient's cultural beliefs and practices into our caregiving, but also broader application of the principles of cultural competence in the management of clinical services and professional activities such as the formulation of health policy. It is inadequate for APNs to simply do no harm. APNs represent the majority of our profession's most highly educated nurses. It is their responsibility to do more than just render high-quality care on a one-to-one basis with their patients. They are also accountable for continually improving the systems within which that care occurs.

WALK A MILE IN SOMEONE ELSE'S SHOES

Imagine that you are an elderly U.S. tourist participating in an Elder Hostel tour abroad. This is the first time that you have ever been out of the United States. You have a history of hypertension and coronary artery disease, as well as myopia and moderate, bilateral hearing loss. While abroad, you experience recurrent chest pain. The tour guide tries unsuccessfully to locate an English-speaking physician, so you are brought to the local hospital where you are admitted for observation. Your glasses and clothing have been removed, and you are on bedrest and are receiving nitroglycerin intravenously and oxygen by nasal cannula. You are unable to reach the bedside table and you cannot see the other patients or the staff in the ward clearly. You are unable to speak or understand the language, so you have no idea of the severity of your condition or its treatment. The tour guide, who initially served as your interpreter, has had to return to the group that is departing for the next tour destination in the morning.

If this were you, how would you feel? Vulnerable? Frightened? At the mercy of a health-care system and care providers whose language, and perhaps beliefs and practices, are totally unfamiliar to you? Now imagine that you and your family recently immigrated to the United States. You may or may not speak and read English. The health-care beliefs and practices of your culture may differ significantly from those of Western medicine. You may be an undocumented alien, fearful of detection, and reticent to seek care. Superimposed on your ethnic and racial status may be the social implications of coming from the culture of poverty, or the drug culture.

In short, you would be a prototype for many of the patients cared for by APNs. How would you want to be treated if the roles were reversed and you were the patient?

THEORETICAL BASIS FOR CULTURAL COMPETENCE IN ADVANCED NURSING PRACTICE

Leininger's (2001) pioneering work in transcultural nursing and the development of her culture care theory provides a framework for the practice of APNs who care for culturally diverse populations. Care and caring, distinguishing characteristics of professional practice to which APNs lay particular claim, are central to her theory: "Care is the essence of nursing and the central, dominant and unifying focus of nursing" (p. 35). Leininger holds that for too long, caring has been the "covert, unknown, and almost invisible aspect of nursing and health services" (p. 32).

Leininger's commitment to the development of a theoretical framework that would assist nurses and other health-care providers to deliver culturally congruent care to patients from diverse populations evolved from a commitment to improve the health of clients, families, and cultural groups; to better help patients from diverse cultural groups to maintain or regain their health; or to experience death in a manner compatible with their cultural beliefs and practices. Leininger's theory of culture care acknowledges both universal and culture-specific care patterns. For instance, although beliefs and expressions associated with caring may vary widely from one cultural group to another, human care practices have been documented from the beginning of recorded history.

Formulated from an anthropological perspective, the theory questions nursing's traditional reliance on the concepts of person, health, and the environment. Leininger (2001) notes that, in many non-Western cultures, family and social institutions are primary and that the language may not even have a word for person. She also notes that although nurses and nursing exert significant influence over individual and societal health and the environment, these concepts are hardly unique to our profession or its practice. In place of these generic concepts, Leininger proposes that care and caring are the central core of nursing, stating, "Care is the nurse's way of being with and helping people" (p. 40).

Leininger's theory and the Sunrise Model in **Figure 19-2,** which depicts both the universality and diversity of cultural care, provide a framework for the APN to examine the dynamic interplay of the many forces that influence the delivery of care.

The culture care theory incorporates three major approaches to the delivery of culturally congruent nursing assessment, decision making, and interventions. Leininger defines these modalities as the following:

1. **Cultural care preservation and maintenance.** "Professional actions and decisions that help people of a particular culture to retain and/or preserve relevant care values so that they can maintain their well being, recover from illness, or face handicaps and/or death" (p. 48).
2. **Cultural care accommodation and negotiation.** "Creative professional actions and decisions that help people of a designated culture to adapt to, or to negotiate with others for a beneficial or satisfying health outcome with professional care providers" (p. 48).
3. **Cultural care repatterning or restructuring.** "Professional actions and decisions that help a client(s) reorder, change, or greatly modify their lifeways for new, different, and beneficial health care patterns while respecting the client(s) cultural values and beliefs and still providing a beneficial or healthier lifeway than before the changes were coestablished with the client(s)" (p. 49).

Inherent in each of these modalities are three of the core values that underlie all of advanced practice nursing: respect, advocacy, and partnership. The culturally competent APN is knowledgeable and

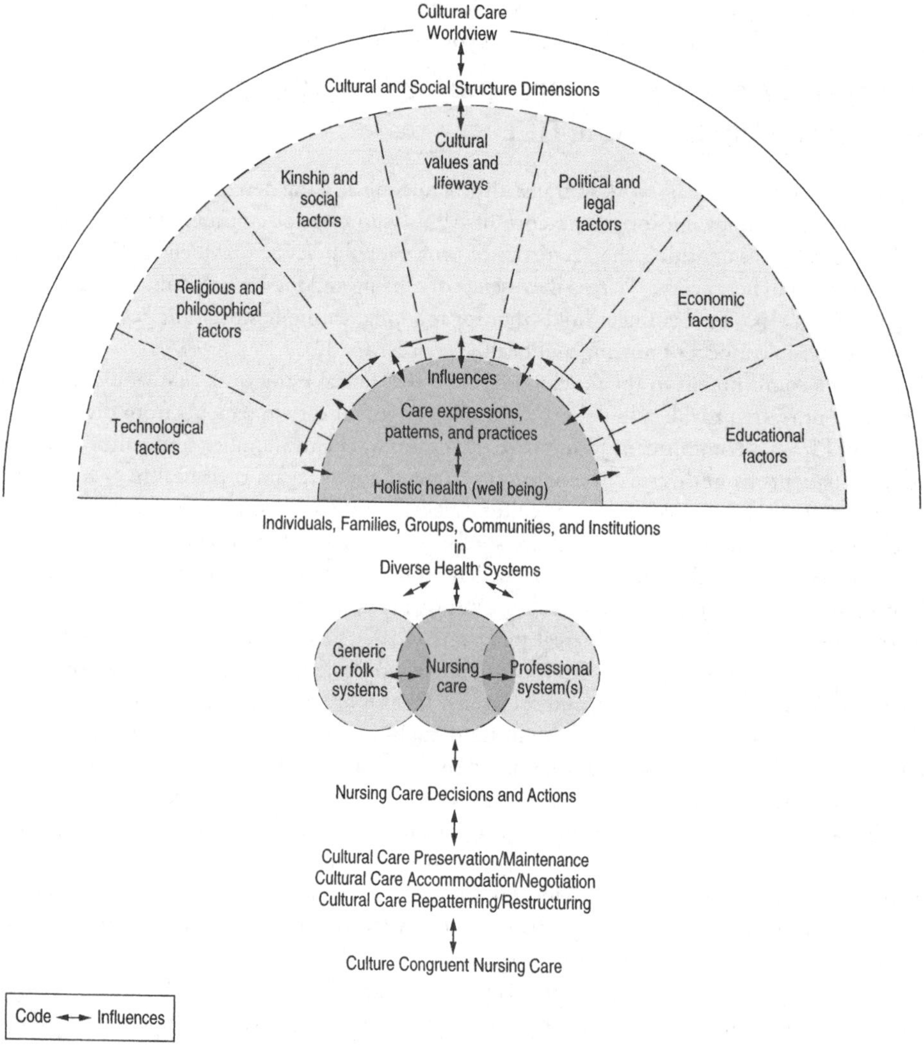

FIGURE 19-2 Leininger's sunrise model to depict the theory of cultural care diversity and universality. *(Source: Leininger, 1991, p. 43, with permission of the National League for Nursing.)*

respectful of diverse cultural beliefs and practices, partners with the patient to develop a care regimen that produces the desired health outcomes within the context of the patient's cultural values, and advocates for the development of culturally appropriate patient care services.

APNs who apply these modalities in their care of patients provide what Leininger (2001) terms *culturally congruent (nursing) care.* Leininger (2001, p. 49) states that this term

> *refers to those cognitively based assistive, supportive, facilitative, or enabling acts or decisions that are tailor made to fit with individual, group or institutional cultural values, beliefs, and lifeways in order to provide or support meaningful, beneficial, and satisfying health care, or well-being services.*

MOVING FROM THEORY INTO PRACTICE

There are multiple definitions of cultural competence. The pioneering work that established cultural competence as an essential component of quality health care was conducted by Cross and colleagues (1989). Adaptations of their definition of cultural competence are used throughout the USDHHS, including the AHRQ and the Office of Minority Health (OMH), as well as the National Center for Cultural Competence (NCCC). The OMH defines cultural competence as follows (adapted from Cross, 1989):

Cultural and linguistic competence is a set of congruent behaviors, attitudes, and policies that come together in a system, agency, or among professionals that enables effective work in cross-cultural situations. "Culture" refers to integrated patterns of human behavior that include the language, thoughts, communications, actions, customs, beliefs, values, and institutions of racial, ethnic, religious, or social groups. "Competence" implies having the capacity to function effectively as an individual and an organization within the context of the cultural beliefs, behaviors, and needs presented by consumers and their communities.

The NCCC expands on the OMH definition by identifying organizational requirements based on the five essential elements that Cross identifies as being necessary for culturally competent organizations. Cultural competence requires that organizations

- Have a defined set of values and principles, and demonstrate behaviors, attitudes, policies, and structures that enable them to work effectively cross-culturally.
- Have the capacity to (1) value diversity, (2) conduct self-assessment, (3) manage the dynamics of difference, (4) acquire and institutionalize cultural knowledge, and (5) adapt to diversity and the cultural contexts of the communities they serve.
- Incorporate the above in all aspects of policy making, administration, practice, and service delivery, and systematically involve consumers, key stakeholders, and communities.

Cultural competence is a developmental process that evolves over an extended period. Both individuals and organizations are at various levels of awareness, knowledge, and skills along the cultural competence continuum (NCCC, 2011; adapted from Cross et al., 1989).

Note that the NCCC definition highlights the developmental nature of cultural competency as applied to individual practitioners and organizations. The development of cultural competency occurs on a continuum, with the ultimate goal of cultural proficiency. The definitions speak to the requirements for achieving organizational, as well as individual, competence. In an environment in which health-care delivery systems are increasingly held accountable for continuous quality improvement and cost containment, APNs often straddle dual roles as clinicians and managers of clinical services. Thus, the APN must not only be skilled in the direct delivery of culturally competent care, but also in the implementation of policies and procedures that ensure cultural competence at the organizational level.

Cultural competence is inextricably linked to linguistic competence. The essence of advanced practice nursing is communication. Our ability to engage our patients as true partners in their care, to establish the trust relationship that is essential to building that partnership, requires that we exhibit linguistic competence. Every aspect of our practice, from initial assessment to teaching, counseling, and support, depends on our being linguistically competent. The NCCC (2009) defines *linguistic competence* as follows (Goode & Jones, 2009):

The capacity of an organization and its personnel to communicate effectively, and convey information in a manner that is easily understood by diverse groups including persons of limited English proficiency, those who have low literacy skills or are not literate, individuals with disabilities, and those who are deaf or hard of hearing. Linguistic competency requires organizational and provider capacity to respond effectively to the health and mental health literacy needs of populations served. The organization must have policy, structures, practices, procedures, and dedicated resources to support this capacity.

The definition is accompanied by a set of values and guiding principles that lay the foundation for demonstrating linguistic competence at both the individual and organizational levels. Services must be offered in the preferred language and/or mode of delivery comfortable to the population served; written materials are translated, adapted, and/or provided in alternative formats based on the needs and preferences of this population; interpretation and translation must comply with all relevant federal, state, and local mandates governing language access; and consumers are engaged in evaluation of language access and other communication services to ensure for quality and satisfaction (NCCC, 2009). APNs are responsible for taking leadership in reviewing not only their personal level of linguistic competence, but also for assessing the adequacy of the patient education materials and organizational services that support their practice.

In 2003, the American Hospital Association (AHA) replaced the Patients' Bill of Rights with *The Patient Care Partnership* (AHA, 2003). It is in the form of an easy-to-read brochure, which seeks to integrate patients' values and beliefs into their care, and describes what patients should expect during their hospitalization with respect to their rights and responsibilities. The brochure is available in eight languages (English, Arabic, traditional and simplified Chinese, Spanish, Russian, Vietnamese, and Tagalog) and may be downloaded from the AHA Web site (http://www.aha.org/advocacy-issues/communicatingpts/pt-care-partnership.shtml). The AHA has also produced two products for use by staff and an organization's leadership team, to enhance culturally competent care within in the United States:

- A Diversity and Cultural Proficiency Assessment Tool for Leaders: Does Your Hospital Reflect the Community it Serves? (April 2004), accessible at www.aha.org
- The Health Research and Educational Trust of the AHA (HRET) Disparities Toolkit, accessible at http://www.hretdisparities.org/

It is important to note that the diversity assessment tool, developed in collaboration with the National Center for Healthcare Leadership, the American College of Healthcare Executives, and the Institute for Diversity, moves the goal from competence to proficiency. The tool is comprehensive, containing not only an evidence-based diversity checklist, but also recommended action steps, case studies, and an extensive bibliography. The HRET Toolkit is designed for use in a wide variety of settings, ranging from hospitals to private health-care practices and community health centers, and specifically addresses best practices for obtaining accurate race, ethnicity, and primary language data from persons with limited English proficiency and/or visual/hearing deficits. Both resources are invaluable tools for promoting staff and organizational linguistic proficiency.

Health Literacy

Cultural competence must be operationalized in the context of health literacy. The definition of health literacy that was used in *Healthy People 2010* (USDHHS, 2000) was presented by the National Library of Medicine (Selden, Zorn, Ratzan, & Parker, 2000): the degree to which a person can obtain, process, and understand basic health information and services needed to make appropriate health decisions (Ratzan & Parker, 2000).

Multiple tools are available to clinicians to assess the literacy of their patients. As examination of **Table 19-1** reveals, these tools assess the literacy component of health literacy. Although reading comprehension and an understanding of commonly used medical terms are essential components of health literacy, such understanding does not necessarily translate into the ability to navigate the system to obtain the health-care services that promote improved health outcomes.

The last major study of adult literacy to be conducted in the United States was the National Assessment of Adult Literacy (NAAL). Citing data from the NAAL (Kutner, Greenberg, & Baer, 2003), the AHRQ reports that 9 out of 10 adults in the United States are not health literacy proficient, and as a

TABLE 19-1

Health Literacy Assessment Tools

Name of Tool	Format of the Tool	Test Administration	Approximate Completion Time(s)
Rapid Estimate of Adult Literacy in Medicine (REALM)	66-item word recognition test of commonly used medical terms. The REALM has a visually impaired version using a font size of 28.	The individual is asked to pronounce words in ascending order of difficulty.	2–6 minutes (Wallace, 2006)
Rapid Estimate of Adult Literacy in Medicine–Short Form, revised (REALM-SF)	7-item, rapid screening, word recognition test.	The individual is asked to pronounce words in ascending order of difficulty.	Under 2 minutes (AHRQ, 2009)
Rapid Estimate of Adolescent Literacy in Medicine: REALM-Teen	66-item word recognition test. Appropriate for adolescents in grades 6–12. Available only in English.	The individual is asked to pronounce words in ascending order of difficulty.	Under 3 minutes (Davis et al., 2006)
Test of Functional Health Literacy in Adults: original and short versions (TOFHLA and S-TOFHLA	The original TOFHLA is a 67-item, timed test of reading comprehension (50 items) and numerical ability (17 items). Available in both English and Spanish.	The individual replaces the missing words in paragraphs from four multiple-choice options for each missing word.	22 minutes (TOFHLA); about 7 minutes (S-TOFHLA) (Wallace, 2006)
Short Assessment of Health Literacy for Spanish Adults (SAHLSA-50)	50-item tool, based on the REALM, that measures the ability of Spanish-speaking adults to read and understand commonly used medical terms.	Each medical term is followed by two words, one of which is similar in meaning to the medical term; the other is a distracter. The person is asked to read the medical term aloud and to select the word that is similar in meaning.	Several minutes; time varies (AHRQ, 2009)

Continued

TABLE 19-1

Health Literacy Assessment Tools—cont'd

Name of Tool	Format of the Tool	Test Administration	Approximate Completion Time(s)
Newest Vital Sign (NVS)	6-question tool that tests the ability to read, comprehend, and apply the nutritional information on an ice cream label; tests both reading comprehension and numeracy skills. Available in both English and Spanish.	The person is given the NVS label to read and refer to as needed. The practitioner then asks the 6 questions.	3 minutes (Weiss et al., 2005)

result, may lack the skills to engage in successful health promotion, disease prevention, and management of acute and chronic diseases for themselves and their families (AHRQ, 2007a, p. 1). Health literacy is directly linked to English language proficiency. The American Community Survey reported that more than 20% of the population 5 years of age and older speak a language other than English at home. The majority, 12.8%, almost 37 million people, reported speaking Spanish or Spanish Creole at home (U.S. Census Bureau, 2010d). Over 40% of these respondents had not graduated from high school and 44.7% of them characterized themselves as speaking English "less than well" (U.S. Census Bureau, 2010c). Of the 26 million persons ages 16 to 64 who reported speaking Spanish at home, more than 8 million reported that they spoke English "not well" or "not at all" (U.S. Census Bureau, 2010b). These data paint a picture of millions of potential patients, many of whom are children, who are at high risk for limited access, inadequate care, and inability to acquire the self-care management knowledge and skills essential to maintain health and optimum function. Cultural beliefs and practices, low educational attainment, limited English proficiency, and poverty are all barriers to accessing and effectively using health-care resources. When they converge, the negative effects of each individual barrier are magnified.

In 2000, the IOM issued a report titled *America's Health Care Safety Net: Intact but Endangered* (Lewin & Altman, 2000). As if anticipating the demographic data previously cited and the AHRQ's definition of health literacy, the report states: "Compared with privately insured persons, Medicaid beneficiaries tend to be far more vulnerable, their needs more diverse, and their experience with and capacity for exercising choice more limited. In addition, non-medical services of special importance to vulnerable populations (e.g., enabling services such as translation services, transportation to clinic visits, and the provision of child care services, and outreach) may not be part of the managed care contract or amenable to managed care infrastructure" (Lewin & Altman, 2000, p. 7). Managed care has become the predominant model for Medicaid recipients.

In 2004, the IOM conducted a comprehensive study of health literacy and its impact on health outcomes: *Health Literacy: A Prescription to End Confusion*. Key findings can be found in **Box 19-2.** The report brings the impact of deficient health literacy dramatically to light in a case example (Parker, Ratzan, & Lurie, 2003, p. 150):

> *A two-year-old is diagnosed with an inner ear infection and prescribed an antibiotic. Her mother understands that her child has an ear infection and knows she should take the prescribed medication*

BOX 19-2
Institute of Medicine Key Findings

- Finding 3-3: "Adults with limited health literacy, as measured by reading and numeracy skills, have less knowledge of disease management and of health-promoting behaviors, report poorer health status, and are less likely to use preventive services" (Nielsen-Bohlman et al., 2004, p. 8).
- Finding 3-4: "Two recent studies demonstrate a higher rate of hospitalization and use of emergency services among patients with limited literacy. This higher utilization has been associated with higher health-care costs" (Nielsen-Bohlman et al., 2004, p. 9).
- Finding 4-1: "Culture gives meaning to health communication. Health literacy must be understood and addressed in the context of culture and language" (Nielsen-Bohlman et al., 2004, p. 10).
- Finding 6-2: "Health literacy is fundamental to quality care, and relates to three of the six aims of quality improvement described in the IOM Quality Chasm Report: safety, patient-centered care, and equitable treatment. Self-management and health literacy have been identified by IOM as cross-cutting priorities for health-care quality and disease prevention" (Nielsen-Bohlman et al., 2004, p. 12).

twice a day. After looking at the label on the bottle and deciding that it does not tell how to take the medicine, she fills a teaspoon and pours the antibiotic into her daughter's ear.

The IOM has held six major workshops on various aspects of health literacy since their groundbreaking report in 2004. Topics range from strategies to improve safe medication use and patient communication, including e-Health, to their most recent workshop, Health Literacy Implications for Health Care Reform. Free downloads of the Executive Summaries of these, and all of the IOM reports, are available at www.iom.edu.

For many of us, our practice environments have seen an exponential growth in patients from a wide variety of cultures; our knowledge of these cultures may be limited at best. For example, the University of Washington's Medical Center in Seattle reported 20,000 patient encounters requiring the use of interpreters. The five major non-English languages spoken by these patients were Russian, Spanish, Korean, Vietnamese, and Chinese. In contrast, the caregivers at the medical center were white (64%), African American (7%), Native American (1%), Hispanic (3%), and Asian (25%) (Abbott et al., 2002). The influx of culturally diverse patients, many with multiple health and social needs, may tax an organization's ability to provide translators. Similarly, patient education materials, essential to patient welfare and to meeting institutional accreditation standards set by The Joint Commission (TJC), are often not available in languages other than English and Spanish. These are but two of the challenges that confront the practitioner in a multicultural care environment.

Health literacy is not simply about English proficiency. Even if one is proficient in speaking, reading, and writing English, all of us process communication with our health providers in terms of interpersonal dynamics and through the lens of cultural beliefs and practices. Literal translation of patient education materials, discharge instructions, consent forms, and other written and multimedia patient materials often does not achieve their intended purpose because the content is not presented in a culturally congruent manner. We need to move from *translation* to *transcreation,* which is development of all forms of information within a cultural context.

A seminal study conducted in 2005 by Aguirre, Ebrahim, and Shea compared the performance of three groups of Medicaid and Medicare patients on the English and Spanish versions of the short form of the Test of Functional Health Literacy in Adults (S-TOFHLA). The 2,370 participants in the study attended eight clinics in Philadelphia, which serve predominantly African American and Hispanic populations. The English S-TOFHLA was completed by 1,304 participants (936 self-identified as non-Hispanic, 91% of whom were African American, and 368 as Hispanic) and 1,066 completed the Spanish version of the S-TOFHLA (self-identified as Hispanics, 93% of whom reported being Puerto Rican). Analysis of the findings revealed that 33% of the Hispanic, Spanish-version participants received scores indicating inadequate health literacy, compared to 19% of the non-Hispanic, English-version subjects and 8% of the Hispanic, English-version participants (p. 334). Hispanic participants who chose to complete the English version of the S-TOFHLA achieved the highest scores of all subgroups of participants. Hispanics who indicated a preference for speaking Spanish and who chose to complete the Spanish S-TOFHLA had the lowest scores (p. 338). Of particular interest in this study was the finding of significant differences in health literacy between men and women, a finding not seen in previous studies. Women performed better than men in this study on both the English and Spanish versions of the S-TOFHLA (p. 337).

In March 2011, the AHRQ released *Evidence Report/Technology Assessment 199: Health Literacy Interventions and Outcomes: An Updated Systematic Review.* The report used the definition of "health literacy" proposed by Ratzan and Parker (2000), which encompasses oral communication skills and numeracy, and which was used in *Healthy People 2010* and by the IOM in their 2004 report on health literacy. Review of research studies rated as being "fair" or "good" demonstrated that lower health literacy was associated with increased hospitalization, increased used of emergency care, lower use of influenza vaccine, and lower use of screening mammography (Berkman et al., 2011, p. ES-4). Two of the studies reviewed suggested that lower numeracy skills mediated the relationship between race and hemoglobin A_{1C} values, and between gender and self-care management of human immunodeficiency virus (HIV) medication regimens (Berkman et al., 2011, p. ES-6).

Asian Americans are the fastest growing population group in the United States, increasing by 43.3% from 2000–2010 to 14.7 million, 5% of the total U.S. population (Humes et al., 2010, pp. 3–4). This population is more at risk for developing type 2 diabetes than non-Hispanic whites, even though their body weight is lower. Chinese Americans, 50% of whom self-report being "linguistically isolated," constitute the greatest percentage of Asian Americans. The Joslin Clinic, a teaching affiliate of the Harvard Medical School, took the lead in developing culturally appropriate care sites and educational materials for Asian Americans with, or at risk for, diabetes. All of the educational materials, including the Joslin Clinic's clinical guidelines for the prevention, detection, and treatment of diabetes, are available in English, traditional Chinese, and simplified Chinese.

A driving force for the development of the transcreated educational materials and interactive Web site were findings from a pilot study of Chinese Americans between the ages of 18 and 70 who were diagnosed with diabetes for at least 1 year and who were taking either oral agents or insulin. The study, conducted by Hsu and colleagues (2006), consisted of 52 subjects, 91% of whom had type 2 diabetes. Twenty-two of the subjects indicated a preference for English, and 30 indicated Chinese as their preferred language. The Chinese American subjects who indicated a preference for Chinese demonstrated less knowledge about their disease process and had higher hemoglobin A_{1C} levels than did the subjects for whom English was the preferred language. These differences occurred even though the care to all subjects in the study was delivered in culturally competent sites with ready access to translation services. Another interesting finding of the study was that a significantly greater proportion of the English-language preference Chinese immigrant subjects (36.4%) reported diabetes educators as a source of information, compared to Chinese-language preference Chinese immigrant subjects (3.3%).

An increasing number of other health-care organizations are developing educational materials and programs that reflect transcreation; that are both linguistically and culturally appropriate for the target populations that they serve. Three of the more notable examples are as follows:

- Memorial Sloan-Kettering Cancer Center's (MSKCC's) Immigrant Health and Cancer Disparities Service (MSKCC, 2011): the newly formed Service, directed by Dr. Francesca M. Gany, incorporates many community outreach programs that were formerly under the auspices of New York University's (NYU's) Langone Medical Center and the NYU Cancer Institute, including the Center for Immigrant Health, the Cancer Awareness Network for Immigrant Minority Populations (CANIMP), and the Arab American Breast Cancer Education and Referral Program (AMBER). The new Service also houses MSKCC's South Asian Health Initiative (SAHI) and the Chinese American Cancer Access Program. The Service's Web site (http://www.mskcc.org/mskcc/html/103456.cfm) is currently being updated to provide users with a more comprehensive description of the resources available to consumers and health-care practitioners.
- National Cancer Institute's (NCI's) Office of Communications and Education at http://www.cancer.gov/. Services to consumers and clinicians include a publications locator, which is updated daily and from which publications may be viewed, printed as pdf documents, and ordered (https://cissecure.nci.nih.gov/ncipubs/detail.aspx?); personalized, confidential cancer information services by e-mail, telephone, or Chat through the LiveHelp link on NCI's Web site (www.cancer.gov); and tobacco cessation services, including NCI's Smoking Quitline (1-877-44U-QUIT, 1-877-448-7848), 8 a.m.–8 p.m. Eastern Standard Time (EST) in both English and Spanish. One of the NCI's transcreated booklets, *Facing Forward: Life After Cancer Treatment* (NCI, 2011) (Spanish version: *Siga Adelante: La Vida Después del Tratamiento del Cáncer*), designed for cancer survivors, is particularly useful in patient education. Other patient education materials have been translated into Spanish, Tagalog, Chinese, and Vietnamese, including *Do It for Yourself, Do it for Your Family,* about the importance of mammograms.
- Office of Minority Health (OMH) of the U.S. Department of Health and Human Services at http://minorityhealth.hhs.gov/. The OMH houses the Center for Linguistic and Cultural Competence in Health (CLCCH), which you can join by registering online (https://www.thinkculturalhealth.hhs.gov/) at no cost. Registration provides preferential access to a wide variety of resources, the quarterly *Think Cultural Newsletter,* and initiatives being undertaken by the OMH and/or the CLCCH. Both Web sites provide access to the National Standards on Culturally and Linguistically Appropriate Services (CLAS), online training, and continuing education.

Patient Navigator Programs

In addition to empowering patients through the development of transcreated educational materials, vulnerable populations are known to experience significant difficulty in "navigating" the health-care system. The interplay of barriers such as poverty, limited English proficiency, and dependence on overburdened, publicly funded health facilities that often lack evening and weekend services for nonurgent care leaves many patients feeling overwhelmed by the complexity of the system. Patients' failures to follow through on diagnostic tests and referrals, to obtain and take their medications as prescribed, and the like are usually ascribed to being "noncompliant." If you dig deeper, often noncompliance represents an inability to access the services necessary to facilitate adherence to their prescribed health-care regimen. In *Crossing the Quality Chasm,* the IOM, quoting the Picker Institute and the AHA, put it bluntly: "It is not surprising, then, that studies of patient experience document that the health system for some is a 'nightmare to navigate'" (IOM, 2001, p. 4).

The potential for wide-scale implementation of patient navigator programs to reduce disparities in health and access to high-quality health-care services garnered support in Congress. On April 25, 2005, Representative Robert Menendez introduced H.R. 1812: The Patient Navigator, Outreach and Chronic Disease Prevention Act of 2005 to amend the Public Health Service Act. The amendment authorized the Secretary of Health and Human Services (HHS), acting through the administrator of the HRSA, to award grants to health-care facilities to develop and implement patient navigator services to reduce barriers to care and to improve health outcomes. Facilities receiving the grants would be required to establish benchmarks and identify outcome criteria to measure the effectiveness of the program. Its companion bill in the Senate was S. 898, introduced by Senator Kay Bailey Hutchison. The proposed legislation had broad, bipartisan support and passed both houses of Congress. On June 29, 2005, President George W. Bush signed the Patient Navigator, Outreach and Chronic Disease Prevention Act (PL 109-18, Section 340A) into law (GovTrack, 2005). In fiscal year 2008, $2,948,000 was appropriated for competitive grants. HRSA awarded six grants, totaling almost 2.4 million dollars (USDHHS, 2008b).

Studies attest to the importance of patient navigators in minority populations. Researchers at the City University of New York, and Mount Sinai School of Medicine in New York City, conducted a cohort study of Hispanic patients referred for screening colonoscopies from their primary care clinics between November 2003 and May 2006. Of the 688 patients who were eligible to participate in the study, 532 had a female, bilingual, Hispanic patient navigator assigned to assist them with successfully completing the procedure. Of the navigated patients, 66% completed their screening colonoscopies. The vast majority—95%—had adequate bowel preparation; 16% were found to have adenomas. The "no-show" rate for urban minority patients dropped from a high of 40% before implementation of the navigator program, to a low of 9.8%. Most (98%) of the patients reported being satisfied with the navigator program, and 66% indicated that they probably, or definitely, would *not* have completed the procedure if the patient navigator program had not been in effect (Chen et al., 2008).

In 2009, citing the demonstrated effectiveness of patient navigation programs, especially in minority communities, HRSA chose to not allocate any additional funding for ongoing research in this area after 2008 (USDHHS, 2008a). This is a good object lesson about competing demands in an environment of increasingly scarce resources. It is incumbent on APNs to translate their patient advocacy role into political and legislative action. Public laws that are unfunded, such as the Patient Navigator, Outreach and Chronic Disease Prevention Act (PL 109-18, Section 340A), cannot deliver on the legislative intent for which they were enacted.

Even in the best of worlds, with full funding of PL 109-18, Section 340A, successful patient navigator programs present a real conflict to their parent health-care institutions or plans. Implementation of a successful program requires a substantial investment in personnel and training. A successful program will produce measureable improvements in patient outcomes, such as fewer patient visits to emergency departments for routine care, decreased incidence and severity of complications in patients with chronic disease processes, fewer hospital admissions, and so on. Although all these are highly desirable outcomes for patients, these outcomes translate into significantly less reimbursement to health-care facilities and providers. From a business perspective, it makes no sense to implement a program that will generate less revenue. A similar situation is seen in managed care programs weighing the pros and cons of implementing or expanding health promotional programs. If a few managed care plans take the lead in offering such expanded programs, they run the real risk that the long-term benefits that would accrue to the programs through a reduction in the care costs of their enrollees, will not be realized to the investing program if the enrollees subsequently switch to another managed care plan. The managed care plans that exhibited a commitment to health promotion could end up bearing all the costs for implementing these programs and realize none of the benefits. Indeed, the benefits could flow to other managed care plans that had not made such an investment in the health of their enrollees. Reimbursement needs to be redesigned to incentivize and reward delivery systems that produce positive health outcomes and lower overall health-care costs.

Assessment

The first step in providing culturally competent care is assessment—of ourselves, of our patients needs, and of our existing organizational resources. Each of us brings the influence of our own cultural heritage, experiences, biases, beliefs, and expectations about patient–provider relationships to the care that we give. Evaluation of the effect of these influences on our caregiving practices is the first step to achieving cultural competence as a practitioner. The National Center for Cultural Competence (NCCC) at the Georgetown University Center for Child and Human Development offers an exceptional array of tools for assessing cultural competence in individuals and organizations, as well as a wealth of instructional materials. Two of the self-assessment tools deserve particular mention. The Cultural Competence Health Practitioner Assessment (CCHPA) tool, developed at the request of the HRSA's Bureau of Primary Care, may be completed online in about 20 minutes. The tool contains six subscales: Values and Belief Systems; Cultural Aspects of Epidemiology; Clinical Decision-Making; Life Cycle Events; Cross-Cultural Communication; and Empowerment/Health Management. On completion of the tool, the practitioner receives immediate assessment of his or her performance on each of the subscales, as well as a list of recommended resources for addressing any identified deficiencies. Another excellent self-assessment tool is a 37-item checklist, Promoting Cultural and Linguistic Competency Self-Assessment Checklist for Personnel Providing Primary Health Care Services. Its content is applicable to all advanced practice nursing roles. The individual responds to specific examples about values, attitudes, communication styles, the practice environment, and patient materials and resources. For example, item 7 asks the practitioner to indicate the frequency with which he or she would do the following:

> *For individuals and families who speak languages or dialects other than English, I attempt to learn and use key words so that I am better able to communicate with them during assessment, treatment or other interventions.*

The tool may be downloaded by visiting the NCCC Web site at http://nccc.georgetown.edu and clicking on Self-Assessments.

Language gives voice to cultural expression. Many cultures have rich oral traditions that transmit the stories, traditions, and beliefs that define their cultural heritage from generation to generation. Language serves as the primary vehicle for most of our interpersonal communication, from patients' descriptions of their health-care needs to interprofessional collaboration. Linguistic competence is essential to the delivery of culturally competent health care. A fundamental tenet of advanced practice nursing is patient empowerment: patients as informed, full partners in decision making about their health care. Operationalizing this core belief clearly requires effective provider–patient communication, a condition that does not exist when linguistic barriers are present. At the very least, lack of linguistic competence makes patient assessment and intervention difficult; at worst, patient safety may be fundamentally compromised. See **Box 19-3.**

BOX 19-3
Buenos Días, Señora

Mrs. W, a 43-year-old married Hispanic woman with three children, came to the neighborhood health center complaining of tightness in her chest and difficulty in coughing up her secretions. Her usual bilingual care provider was unavailable, so she was seen by another practitioner who was not proficient in Spanish. Her records revealed that she had been diagnosed with mild intermittent asthma, for which she had been prescribed albuterol to be used as necessary. Mrs. W reported that she had not filled her last prescription because of the cost.

Mrs. W's physical examination was unremarkable except for a slight increase in respiratory rate and scattered expiratory wheezes. To save her the cost of prescription medication, the provider recommended that she purchase the over-the-counter product Robitussin and take it four times per day. She was advised to return to the clinic if her symptoms did not improve. No written follow-up instructions were available in Spanish.

Four days later, Mrs. W came to the clinic in acute distress. Because of her limited understanding of English, she had purchased Honey Cough by Robitussin. The provider had not thought to explain, or to give her written instructions, about the difference between guaifenesin (the active ingredient in plain Robitussin, which acts to liquefy pulmonary secretions and promote expectoration) and Honey Cough, which contains only dextromethorphan, a potent cough suppressant. Instead of relieving Mrs. W's symptoms, the provider's lack of linguistically appropriate intervention significantly worsened her condition by depressing the very mechanism that would have allowed her to expel her secretions.

The process of self-assessment must be approached with a willingness to confront and modify or discard those inaccurate and uninformed preconceived cultural beliefs and attitudes that detract from the care we provide. Many of our attitudes and beliefs are so ingrained that we may never scrutinize them in the course of our daily practice until, and if, we become aware of their negative effect on our care. Even then, long-held biases may limit our introspection. Ethnocentrism, or the belief in the relative superiority of one's own cultural group, is a common phenomenon. Often operating at an unconscious level, ethnocentrism can exert a powerful influence on our patient interactions and care practices.

The NCCC has produced another excellent tool that details the process for conducting an organizational self-assessment (Goode, Jones, & Mason, 2002). The process, which stresses community involvement and a nonpunitive approach with an emphasis on self-knowledge and growth, is also available at the NCCC Web site listed previously. Knowledge of our individual and institutional strengths and weaknesses in the area of cultural competence is a prerequisite to corrective action.

Culturally competent patient assessment is indispensable to appropriate diagnosis and treatment, and promotes patient participation in decision making about health and treatment regimens. Although an understanding of the beliefs and practices of a patient's cultural group facilitates such assessment, respectful questioning wherein the patient becomes the teacher about his or her culture produces data to support your clinical judgments and helps build trust between patient and provider. See **Box 19-4.** A particularly valuable resource for drawing out a patient's beliefs about health and illness is a work by an early pioneer in culturally competent care, "Understanding, Eliciting and Negotiating Clients' Multicultural Health Beliefs" (Jackson, 1993).

Note that all of the questions in Box 19-4 are framed from the perspective of the patient. They acknowledge the patient's ownership of his or her unique illness experience. Framing the questions in this way allows the APN to enter into the patient's lived experience. By exploring the patient's

BOX 19-4
Questions to Elicit Beliefs and Treatment Expectations from Patients Seeking Illness Care

- What do you think caused your problem?
- Why do you think it started when it did?
- What do you think your sickness does to you?
- How does it work?
- How severe is your sickness?
- Will it have a short or long course?
- What kind of treatment should you receive?
- What are the results you hope to receive from this treatment?
- What are the problems your sickness has caused you?
- What do you fear most about your sickness?

Adapted from Jackson, 1993, p. 30.

perceptions and expectations, the provider is better able to propose a treatment plan that is compatible with the patient's cultural beliefs and practices.

Culturally competent assessment also requires that the clinician apply ethnically appropriate parameters when interpreting physical findings. Body mass index (BMI) is widely used as a tool to assess patients' risk for diabetes and cardiovascular disease. There is a growing body of evidence to suggest that the current, European-derived, "one size fits all" BMI classifications for overweight (25.0 kg/m^2 or greater, but less than 30.0 kg/m^2) and obese (equal to or greater than 30 kg/m^2) may not be appropriate across all ethnic groups. A seminal study (Razak et al., 2007) reported in *Circulation* sought to determine if the current cut point for determining obesity that is used in clinical practice is appropriate for use in non-European populations. A random sample of 1,078 subjects was recruited from participants in the Study of Health Assessment and Risk in Ethnic Groups (SHARE) and Risk Evaluation in Aboriginal Peoples (SHARE-AP). The subjects, from four ethnic groups: South Asians (n = 5,289), Chinese (n = 5,281), Aboriginals (n = 5,207), and Europeans (n = 5,301) were evaluated for 14 variables: 2 clinical (systolic and diastolic blood pressure) and 12 biochemical (fasting and 2-hour glucose; fasting and 2-hour insulin; HbA_{1C}, Homeostasis Model Assessment–insulin resistance [HOMA-IR]; high-density and low-density lipids and triglycerides [HDL and LDL, respectively]; fasting and 2-hour free fatty acids) cardiometabolic markers. Factor analysis revealed three latent factors that accounted for 56% of the variation in the subjects' cardiometabolic markers and blood pressure. The main effect of ethnicity was highly significant for each factor (P) 0.001). Compared to European subjects for a given BMI, South Asian, Chinese, and Aboriginal subjects had elevated glucose and lipid metabolism-related factors. The South Asian subjects had the worst glucose and lipid profiles, the highest 2-hour oral glucose tolerance tests levels, the highest LDL levels, and the lowest HDL levels (Razak et al. 2007, p. 2113). Elevated blood-pressure–related factor was found in Chinese subjects at a BMI of 25.3 kg/m^2 compared to a BMI of 30.0 kg/m^2 in Europeans (p. 2,114). In discussing their findings, the authors conclude the following (Razak et al., 2007, p. 2,114):

> *Use of BMI cut points derived among Europeans understates the cardiometabolic risk associated with weight gain in other ethnic groups. The pathway linking obesity to clinical events is mediated*

partially through its strong association with the development of diabetes, hypertension, and dyslipidemia. This suggests that to minimize the development of cardiometabolic risk factors, lower BMI targets should be used by healthcare professionals in some non-European populations.

Major sources of best practices, such as the Joslin Clinic, have already incorporated ethno-specific and gender-specific BMI recommendations in their clinical guidelines. The Joslin Diabetes Center and Joslin Clinic Clinical Nutrition Guideline for Overweight and Obese Adults with Type 2 Diabetes, Those with Prediabetes, or Those at High Risk for Developing Type 2 Diabetes uses BMI or waistline measurements to identify target populations. Persons from Asian populations (South Asian Indians, East Asians and Malays) with a BMI greater than 23 kg/m^2 and a waistline greater than 35 inches (90 cm) in men, or greater than 31 inches (80 cm) in women, are considered to be target individuals. This is in contrast to the guideline's generic criteria of BMI greater than 25 kg/m^2 and/or a waistline greater than 40 inches (102 cm) (men) and 35 inches (88 cm) (women) (Joslin Diabetes Center & Joslin Clinic, 2011).

Treatment regimens should always strive to incorporate the cultural practices and preferences that are most valued by the patient. For example, Muslim patients observe strict dietary laws that include a prohibition against eating any pork products. Practicing Muslims also pray five times a day and may be reluctant to eat or to take medications during daylight hours at certain periods of the year. For example, tradition dictates that Muslims fast while the sun is up during the observance of Ramadan. The scheduling of diagnostic testing and use of treatment plans that are congruent with patients' valued cultural beliefs and practices are more likely to generate positive outcomes. Outcomes data are key determinants of reimbursement, provider recognition by third-party payers, and institutional accreditation. Culturally and linguistically competent patient assessment is the foundation of successful outcomes.

Knowledge

As an APN, you are well aware of the value of knowledge. Evidence- and research-based practice is the standard to which you are held. Many of the national guidelines for clinical assessment of wellness and major health conditions affecting large segments of the U.S. population reflect a cultural congruence not seen in previous guidelines, as in the Centers for Disease Control and Prevention (CDC) growth charts released in 2000. Before the release of the revised guidelines, clinicians had to rely on growth charts developed in 1977 by the National Center for Health Statistics (NCHS), which were derived from data drawn primarily from 10,000 White, middle-class infants and children living in Ohio between 1929 and 1975. In contrast, the current CDC guidelines are based on survey data of children from diverse ethnic and racial groups, and incorporate data on breastfed children in proportion to the rate of breastfeeding in the general population. Fourteen percent of the data from which the current guidelines were developed represent information collected in surveys of African American children. This figure reflects the proportion of African American children living in the United States from 1971 to 1994 ("New Growth Charts a Welcome Improvement," 2002).

Just as you are expected to incorporate the latest clinical guidelines for the management of conditions such as diabetes and lipid disorders into your practice, so, too, must you inform yourself about the beliefs and practices of the cultural groups in your patient population. This can seem like a daunting task, especially if your patient population is quite diverse. The task becomes even more complex if you have a rapid influx of immigrants from a cultural group new to the setting. Many sources of help are available to assist the individual practitioner and organization to care effectively for diverse populations. Every cultural group has its community leaders. Often they are religious leaders and professionals who are more than willing to assist local health and social agencies in meeting the needs of their community. Many culturally affiliated church and social organizations have developed literature and other materials to help noncommunity members better understand their cultural beliefs and practices.

All APNs are partners with their patients in providing culturally competent care. Recognizing that individual patients may or may not adhere to cultural norms, key questions to explore about any cultural group for whom you care are in **Box 19-5.** Here is a phrase that may help you to remember these key questions and be a better partner:

Partners in delivering culturally competent research-based care for diverse populations.

The Internet is an extremely valuable resource for gathering information on various cultural groups. The culture-specific materials developed by the University of Washington Medical Center are invaluable to APNs practicing in culturally diverse settings. Culture Clues are brief, provider-friendly overviews of the dominant beliefs and practices of the major cultural groups cared for by the medical center staff. Examples of the types of information included in the clues are essential information about the cultural group's perception of illness, how medical decisions are made, how prognostic information should be handled, and cultural norms about touch and modesty, among others. Culture Clues have been developed for the care of Albanian, Chinese, Korean, Latino, Russian, Somali, and Vietnamese patients, as well as deaf and hard-of-hearing patients. End of Life Culture Clues for the Latino,

BOX 19-5
Key Questions Used to Explore Cultural Groups: PIDCCRCFDP

Partners In Delivering Culturally Competent, Research-based Care for Diverse Populations

- **P**erceptions: How are health and illness defined?
- **I**nterpersonal behavior: Does the cultural group have particular norms for interpersonal behavior regarding beliefs about touch, eye contact, personal space, modesty, sexuality ...?
- **D**ecision making: Who makes health-care decisions?
- **C**ommunication needs: Be particularly sensitive to how the patients wish to be addressed and how and by whom health-care information is communicated **Box 19-6.**
- **C**omplementary medicine: What are the group's folk medicine beliefs and practices to maintain wellness and to treat illness or injury? Explore their use of complementary and alternative medicine.
- **R**eligion/spirituality: To what extent does spirituality or religious belief affect health-care beliefs and practices (e.g., specific dietary practices, prayer rituals, and such)?
- **C**are: What are the patient's expectations for the outcomes of health and illness care? What cultural preferences and practices does the patient wish to have incorporated into his or her plan of care (e.g., the diet of some Chinese patients may include the use of selected foods or herbs to maintain a balance between complementary forces [yin and yang] of hot and cold, light and dark)? Is this the patient's first formal experience with receiving care in a structured health-care setting; the first experience of being cared for by an APN?
- **F**amily: What is the primary social unit—the individual, the family, or the community? What are the family and kinship structures and roles in health care?
- **D**eath and dying: Explore the meaning of and rituals associated with death and dying.
- **P**sychiatric/mental health: How are mental health issues perceived by the group?

BOX 19-6

My Name is Mr. Roberts

Mr. John Roberts, a widower, was a 68-year-old Black man of African American descent. Retired for 10 years, he lived independently in his private home. His civilian and military pensions allowed him to live comfortably and to meet his health-care costs. He was active in several church and community groups and expressed a high degree of satisfaction with his life. A heavy smoker for many years, he had recently agreed to enroll in a smoking cessation program in an effort to better control his hypertension. A chest x-ray examination performed during a comprehensive physical examination revealed a large, previously undetected mass in his right lung. Further testing determined that the mass was malignant and that metastases had occurred. Mr. Roberts declined any treatment, saying that he wanted to live out his remaining life as fully as possible.

When his condition deteriorated to the point at which his comfort and safety were at risk, he agreed to enter a hospice home-care program. The APN coordinating Mr. Robert's care collaborated with him and his son in ensuring that all aspects of his physical and psychosocial needs were respected and met. Late in the terminal phase of his illness, Mr. Roberts fell and fractured his right hip, necessitating hospitalization. In the hospital, he was frequently addressed by his first name, especially by younger staff members. Despite his repeated admonishment that his name was Mr. Roberts, many of the staff persisted in calling him John.

The small, community hospital to which Mr. Roberts was admitted did not have pain management specialists. The attending hospitalist physician and the nursing staff caring for Mr. Roberts were predominantly Caucasian and found him to be very resistant to switching from the oral analgesic medications that he had taken for pain while at home, to intramuscular and/or intravenous administration of his analgesics. His primary nurse consulted with the clinical nurse specialist for the unit and a meeting was set up with Mr. Roberts's son. His son revealed that Mr. Roberts had always been fearful of being hospitalized, or taking anything other than oral medications, after he read about the Tuskegee Study of Untreated Syphilis, begun in 1932 and continuing until 1972. The 600 study participants were all Black males, 299 of whom had syphilis, none of whom gave informed consent. The men with syphilis were followed for the next 40 years to determine the natural course of untreated syphilis. None of the men received penicillin, even after it became known as the drug of choice for treatment in 1947. Mr. Roberts's son also shared that his father had preferentially sought out an African American as his primary care physician. The hospitalist asked Mr. Roberts's son for help in allaying Mr. Roberts's fears so that his analgesics could be administered by injection. His son helped to bridge the cultural gap and his father experienced significantly better pain relief.

Mr. Roberts died while hospitalized. He had been brought up in a traditional home in which older persons were addressed by their last name by all except family members and close friends. Younger individuals never presumed to call an older person by their first name. To do so would have been considered disrespectful and rude.

An accident denied the fulfillment of Mr. Roberts's wish to die at home. However, the indignities that he experienced while hospitalized were totally preventable, had his caregivers been more respectful of his communication needs and knowledgeable about the potential for patients to mistrust medical recommendations based on their own personal experiences of racism or knowledge of unethical medical practices in the past. A useful article is Benkert, Hollie, Nordstrom, Wickson, and Bins-Emerick (2009).

Russian, and Vietnamese cultures have also been developed. They are available at http://depts.washington.edu/pfes/CultureClues.htm.

Each of the Culture Clues provides the reader with additional resources about the cultural group and health care. The University of Washington also maintains a Web site called EthnoMed at www.ethnomed.org that is a treasure trove of information. The culture-specific materials include comprehensive discussion of the barriers to health care. The Web site provides access to an extensive compendium of clinician support resources in the following areas:

- Cultures—cultural profiles on multiple cultural groups, including Soviet Jewish and Arab cultures.
- Clinical topics (including clinical pearls and case studies). The topics range from commonly encountered disease conditions such as asthma and diabetes, to modesty, sexuality, and breast-feeding in specific cultures, domestic violence, genetics, and end-of-life care.
- Patient education, including low literacy patient education materials in 18 languages.

Diversity Rx (www.diversityrx.org) and the National Multicultural Institute (http://www.nmci.org) are additional useful sites.

The AHA is a rich source of cultural information that improves patient care. Two products designed to improve cultural competence in individual caregivers and health-care facilities are:

- Strategies for Leadership: Does your hospital reflect the community it serves? A Diversity and Cultural Proficiency Assessment Tool for Leaders. Access the resource at http://www.aha.org/content/00-10/DiversityTool.pdf.
- A toolkit for collecting race, ethnicity, and primary language information from patients, the HRET Disparities Toolkit, is accessible at http://www.hretdisparities.org.

The AHA was also instrumental in the development of the Institute for Diversity in Health Management, founded in 1994, which is a nonprofit organization that works with educational institutions and health-care organizations to expand leadership opportunities for ethnic minorities in management of health care. Its Web site is www.DiversityConnection.org. The AHA also has a particular focus on end-of-life care. A national center to improve the palliative care of patients has been established at the Mount Sinai School of Medicine in New York City—the Center to Advance Palliative Care (CAPC; http://www.capc.org). The CAPC is a valuable resource for palliative care tools and for your own professional development. E-learning is available through the CAPC's Campus Online. The Center also sponsors a Web site for patients and families seeking palliative care: www.getpalliativecare.org (CAPC, 2011).

Finally, honesty is the best policy. If you are unsure whether your approach to a patient is culturally appropriate, acknowledge your unfamiliarity with the patient's cultural norms and ask for guidance in how to best deliver care. Most patients perceive this as being a thoughtful response to their right to respect and will be happy to help inform you. They may become your best teachers. It will enhance their trust in you and allow you to provide care until you research additional information on the patient's cultural group.

COMMUNICATION

Communication is a critical element in the self- and institutional-assessment process. It encompasses provider–patient communication in all its forms, from assessment to patient education, counseling, and documentation. How do you assess a patient or community whose primary language is other than English? What technologies (e.g., Language Line Services) or interpreters are at your disposal to facilitate assessment, intervention, and teaching? What is your own level of proficiency in languages other than English? Linguistic competence is essential to quality patient care. With our multicultural patient populations, most of us are, or soon will be, linguistically challenged. This becomes a practice issue only if we ignore the need and make no attempt to modify our practice environment to meet the comprehensive needs of our patient base. Multiple texts and e-learning programs exist to develop basic foreign language skills.

Patient teaching raises major ethical issues regarding equality of treatment. Whether the patient is an individual, family, or community, many patient education materials are available primarily in English. A substantial number have also been translated into Spanish; fewer into other languages. For most other languages, the practitioner depends on interpreters or English-speaking family members to assist in the education process. The availability of these supports may be limited, and as we know, patients need supplemental materials to reinforce direct teaching, especially if the patient is anxious or the encounter is hurried. Cost-containment efforts focus on increased staff productivity, which translates into more patients in less time. This, coupled with a linguistic barrier to teaching, is a recipe for a poor outcome. Collaborative decision making with your patients, a defining characteristic of advanced nursing practice, mandates the ability to communicate effectively. Advocacy begins in your own practice environment, with your own patients. You have an ethical and legal obligation to work toward ensuring equality in the treatment of all patients.

Federal agencies have multiple online resources that you can use to develop more culturally and linguistically appropriate patient education materials. Download *Simply Put: A Guide for Creating Easy-to-Understand Materials* and *Toolkit for Making Written Materials Clear and Effective* from the HRSA Web site (http://www.hrsa.gov/culturalcompetence/index.html), and AHRQ's *Health Literacy Universal Precautions Toolkit* (DeWalt et al., 2010), at http://www.ahrq.gov/qual/literacy/healthliteracytoolkit.pdf.

The National Institute of Diabetes and Digestive and Kidney Diseases (NIDDK) Web site, at www.niddk.nih.gov/health/spanish.htm, provides a fairly extensive listing of patient education materials that are available in Spanish, as well as English, for urologic diseases, kidney diseases, diabetes, digestive diseases, and weight control and physical activity. Many of the materials may be downloaded and reproduced. Another helpful resource is the Babel Fish Translation Service (http://babelfish.yahoo.com/). The latter resource allows you to input up to 150 words per entry, which can then be translated into multiple languages ranging from Spanish to Japanese and Korean. A word of caution, however: the "translation" may only be a rough approximation of the English content that you entered. It is helpful if you want to translate basic assessment questions or simple instructions such as "Where is your pain?" or "Do not eat for 8 hours before your blood tests."

In most cases, a translator who is proficient in the language should review the patient instructions or educational materials translated from this source before you give them to patients. As the provider, you are ultimately responsible for the accuracy of the patient education materials that you use.

Many additional organizations and concerned individuals are actively engaged in addressing health literacy. Two of the most innovative resources now available to APNs are the Asian American Diabetes Initiative (AADI) sponsored by the Joslin Diabetes Center and "The Debilitator." The ADDI, co-directed by Dr. William C. Hsu, author of "Identification of Linguistic Barriers to Diabetes Knowledge and Glycemic Control in Chinese Americans with Diabetes," previously discussed in the health literacy section of this chapter, has developed a wide range of teaching-learning tools for use by patients and health-care professionals. The tools range from clinical guidelines and video clips to the interactive Wok, which teaches the patients and their families how to calculate the caloric value, fat, and sodium content of Asian recipes and commonly used foods. Materials developed by the AADI may be found on the Internet at www.aadi.joslin.harvard.edu; click on "Joslinville" to access the Wok. "The Debilitator," developed by African American independent filmmaker Maurice Madden, is a 30-minute DVD designed to increase awareness of the devastating effects of diabetes in the black community. "The Debilitator" won a 2006 "Life Making a Difference in Diabetes Award" and is available through the National Diabetes Education Program (NDEP) at http://www.millenniumfilmworksinc.com./store/form2.htm (Chwedyk, 2007). Two facilitator's guides for leading group discussions on the themes portrayed in "The Debilitator" are available from the National Diabetes Education Program at ndep.nih.gov/media/. Enter the titles "Power to Prevent" and "New Beginnings, a Discussion Guide" in the search box on the Web site.

Another thought for consideration is your indirect role as a nurse researcher. Do you, or the institutions with which you are affiliated, conduct evaluation research to determine whether you are accomplishing desired patient outcomes in your area of specialty practice? Would it be interesting to collect and analyze outcomes data and not only compare the relative efficacy of the different types of practitioners, but also to examine outcomes as a function of patient cultural groupings, primary languages spoken and read, and other factors? Outcomes data from evaluation research are often the catalyst for bringing about organizational change.

Professional Accreditation and Legal Considerations

Commitment to the provision of culturally competent care is an integral component of advanced practice nursing, as reflected in *Nursing: Scope and Standards of Practice,* second edition (ANA, 2010). The document reemphasizes the client's right to self-determination, privacy, confidentiality, full and truthful disclosure, and care that is respectful and inclusive of the client's cultural beliefs and practices. The client advocacy role of the nurse is stressed, as is the importance of empowering the patient for effective clinical decision making and self-care.

In addition to the professional imperative, three other major external forces mandate that APNs be culturally competent. Of most immediate importance are the legal implications of failing to practice in a culturally appropriate manner. The care that is documented in a patient's clinical record is a direct reflection of your practice. If cultural and linguistic barriers exist between you and your patients and you have not instituted action to address these in your history taking, clinical decision making, and patient education, treatment failure and adverse outcomes may well occur. From a legal perspective, what is not documented has not been done. In our increasingly litigious society, failure to document culturally appropriate care may well serve as an ethical and legal indictment of your practice with very real professional repercussions.

Individual and organizational and system vulnerability to legal action may also result from failure to comply with the provisions of Section 601 of Title VI of the Civil Rights Act of 1964, as amended, 42 U.S.C. §2000d et seq., which states the following (U.S. Department of Justice [USDOJ], Civil Rights Division, 1998):

> *No person in the United States shall, on the ground of race, color, or national origin, be excluded from participation in, be denied the benefits of, or be subjected to discrimination under any program or activity receiving Federal financial assistance.*

Previous court decisions involving Title VI have employed the Fourteenth Amendment's standard of proof of intentional discrimination, as well as Title VI's requirement for demonstration of "disparate impact." Health-care institutions receiving federal assistance whose programs or policies discriminate against particular cultural groups are liable to be held accountable under the provisions of Title VI.

For example, the Supreme Court has held that undocumented aliens fulfill the definition of "persons" in the context of the Fifth and Fourteenth Amendments to the U.S. Constitution. As such, they are, by extension, included under the protections afforded by Title VI. Keep in mind that federal assistance has been broadly defined as encompassing not only direct financial assistance, but also forms of indirect aid such as subsidies, loans, and federal training (USDOJ, Civil Rights Division, 1998).

On August 11, 2000, Executive Order 13166 was issued: *Improving Access to Services for Persons with Limited English Proficiency.* The Executive Order required all federal agencies that funded non-federal program(s) to publish guidance to recipients of such funding as to how they could comply with the provisions of Title VI. To minimize confusion and maximize compliance across all federal agencies, adoption of the uniform criteria established by the USDOJ was encouraged. The current regulatory guidelines of the USDHHS went into effect in October 2004. Limited English proficiency (LEP) persons are defined as follows (USDHHS, 2004, p. 7):

> *Individuals who do not speak English as their primary language and who have a limited ability to read, write, speak, or understand English may be limited English proficient, or "LEP," and may be eligible to receive language assistance with respect to a particular type of service, benefit, or encounter.*

The regulations forbid "restrict[ing] an individual in any way in the enjoyment of any advantage or privilege enjoyed by others receiving any service, financial aid, or other benefit under the program" or from "utiliz[ing] criteria or methods of administration which have the effect of subjecting individuals to discrimination because of their race, color, or national origin, or have the effect of defeating or substantially impairing accomplishment of the objectives of the program as respects individuals of a particular race, color, or national origin" (USDHHS, 2004, pp. 2–3).

The guidelines identify the types of USDHHS recipients who must comply with the provisions of Title VI, including hospitals and nursing homes, state Medicaid programs, Head Start programs, managed care organizations, and state, county, and local health agencies. They also identify the four criteria that programs and institutions can use to determine the level of resources that must be invested to ensure compliance: (a) the number or proportion of LEP persons eligible to be served or likely to be encountered by the program or grantee; (b) the frequency with which LEP individuals come in contact with the program; (c) the nature and importance of the program, activity, or service provided by the program to people's lives; and (d) the resources available to the grantee/recipient and costs (USDHHS, 2004, p. 7).

The Patient Protection and Affordable Care Act of 2010, PL 111-148, contains provisions that will facilitate the development of health policy that more accurately reflects the health-related needs of Americans. Title XXXI, Data Collection, Analysis, and Quality, Sec. 3101, mandates that within 2 years of enactment of PL 111-148, the Secretary of the Department of Health and Human Services will ensure that any health-care or public health program conducted or supported by the federal government, and any data collection mechanism that provides essential data for such programs, such as the American Community Survey conducted by the Bureau of the Census, will collect cultural and linguistic data on the populations served or surveyed.

The Joint Commission (TJC) is increasingly incorporating culturally and linguistically appropriate care as a key element in the accreditation standards that are used in its institutional evaluation process. New accreditation standards for Patient-Centered Communication, approved in December 2009, were released to the field in January 2010 and are incorporated in the 2011 *Comprehensive Accreditation Manual for Hospitals* (CAMH), the *Official Handbook.* TJC surveyors began assessing compliance to the new standards in an implementation pilot project that started on January 1, 2011. The findings from the pilot project will be used to assess and respond to questions and issues of compliance raised by the sites being surveyed, and do not affect accreditation decisions. Full implementation of the new standards as a factor in accreditation decisions will occur no earlier than January 2012. To assist institutions to prepare to meet the new standards, TJC (2010) has developed a monograph titled *Advancing Effective Communication, Cultural Competence, and Patient- and Family-Centered Care: A Roadmap for Hospitals.* To access a free copy, go to http://www.jointcommission.org/assets/1/6/ARoadmapforHospitalsfinalversion727.pdf.

Another useful resource from TJC focuses on assessing the spiritual needs of patients (TJC, 2008). TJC recommends that the minimum data set for assessment of a patient's spirituality include the patient's denomination (if any), beliefs, and important spiritual practices. The standards require that the organization define the elements and breadth of its spiritual assessment of patients, as well as the qualifications of the practitioners conducting the assessment. In an effort to assess the potential impact of patients' spiritual beliefs on care requirements and service delivery, TJC provides examples of elements that can facilitate assessing the spiritual needs of patients: http://www.jointcommission.org/standards_information/jcfaqdetails.aspx?StandardsFaqId=290&ProgramId=1.

NEXT STEPS

I submit that the defining characteristic that has led to widespread use of APNs across multiple care settings and earned them unparalleled patient acceptance is their ability to truly partner with their patients to provide care that the patient perceives as being respectful and inclusive of his or her uniqueness as a human being. A major component of that uniqueness is associated with culture, its values, beliefs, and attitudes toward caring.

The delivery of culturally congruent care is not optional, but mandated by the ethical standards of our profession, as well as by legal and accreditation requirements. The challenge is for us as individual APNs, and collectively as practitioners within a variety of health-care institutions, to consistently practice in a manner that is personally sensitive to our own biases and culturally astute.

REFERENCES

Abbott, P. D., Short, D., Dodson, S., Garcia, C., Perkins, J., & Wyatt, S. (2002). Inproving your cultural awareness with culture cues. *Nurse Practitioner*, 27(2), 44-47, 55.

Agency for Healthcare Research and Quality. (2007a). *Health literacy program brief.* Rockville, MD: U.S. Department of Health and Human Services, Agency for Healthcare Research and Quality. Retrieved August 21, 2011, from www.ahrq.gov.

Agency for Healthcare Research and Quality. (2007b). *2007 National healthcare disparities report* (AHRQ Pub. No. 08-0041). Rockville, MD: U.S. Department of Health and Human Services, Agency for Healthcare Research and Quality. Agency for Healthcare Research and Quality. (2008) *National healthcare disparities report* (AHRQ Pub. No. 09-0002). Rockville, MD: U.S. Department of Health and Human Services, Agency for Healthcare Research and Quality. Retrieved September 22, 2011, from www.ahrq.gov/qual/qrdr08.htm.

Agency for Healthcare Research and Quality. (2009). *Health literacy measurement tools.* Rockville, MD: U.S. Department of Health and Human Services, Agency for Healthcare Research and Quality. Retrieved September 18, 2011, from http://www.ahrq.gov/populations/sahlsatool.htm.

Agency for Healthcare Research and Quality. (2011a). *Highlights from the National healthcare quality and disparities reports.* Rockville, MD: U.S. Department of Health and Human Services, Agency for Healthcare Research and Quality. Retrieved August 22, 2010, from http://www.ahrq.gov/qual/nhdr10/Key.htm.

Agency for Healthcare Research and Quality. (2011b). *2010 National healthcare disparities report* (AHRQ Pub. No. 11-0005). Rockville, MD: U.S. Department of Health and Human Services, Agency for Healthcare Research and Quality. Retrieved August 18, 2011, from http://www.ahrq.gov/qual/nhdr10/nhdr10.pdf.

Agency for Healthcare Research and Quality. (2011c). *2010 National healthcare quality report* (AHRQ Pub. No. 11-004). Rockville, MD: U.S. Department of Health and Human Services, Agency for Healthcare Research and Quality. Retrieved August 18, 2011, from http://www.ahrq.gov/qual/nhqr10/nhqr10.pdf.

Aguirre, A. C., Ebrahim, N., & Shea, J. A. (2005). Performance of the English and Spanish S-TOFHLA among publicly insured Medicaid and Medicare patients. *Patient Education and Counseling, 56*(3), 332–339.

American Hospital Association. (2003). *The patient care partnership.* Retrieved September 17, 2011, from http://www.aha.org/advocacy-issues/communicatingpts/pt-care-partnership.shtml.

American Nurses Association. (2001). *Code of ethics for nurses with interpretive statements* (Publication No. CEN21). Silver Spring, MD: American Nurses Publishing.

American Nurses Association. (2010). *Nursing: Scope and standards of practice* (Pub No. PUB# 978155810282803SSNP). Silver Spring, MD: Nursesbooks.

Benkert, R., Hollie, B., Nordstrom, C.K., Wickson, B., & Bins-Emerick, L. (2009). Trust, mistrust, racial identify and patient satisfaction in urban African American primary care patients of nurse practitioners. *Journal of Nursing Scholarship, 41*(2), 211–219.

Berkman, N. D., Sheridan, S. L., Donahue, K. E., Halpern, D. J., Viera, A., Crotty, K., et al. (2011). *Health literacy interventions and outcomes: An updated systematic review. Evidence report/technology assessment No. 199.* (Prepared by RTI International–University of North Carolina Evidence-based Practice Center under contract No. 290-2007-10056-I. AHRQ Publication No. 11-E006.) Rockville, MD: Agency for Healthcare Research and Quality. Retrieved September 24, 2011, from http:www.ahrq.gov/downloads/pub/evidence/pdf/literacy/literacyup.pdf.

Center to Advance Palliative Care. (2011). *About CAPC.* Retrieved September 8, 2011, from http://www.capc.org.

Centers for Disease Control and Prevention (2011). *Age-adjusted percentage of civilian, noninstitutionalized population with diagnosed diabetes, by race, United States, 1980–2009.* Page reviewed and last modified April 5, 2011. Retrieved August 8, 2011, from http://www.cdc.gov/diabetes/statistics/prev/national/figbyrace.htm.

Changing the present. (2012). *Health.* Retrieved August 20, 2012, from http://changingthepresent.org/global_health/quotes.

Chen, L. A., Santos, S., Jandorf, L., Christie, J., Castillo, A., Winkel, G., et al. (2008). A program to enhance completion of screening colonoscopy among urban minorities. *Clinical Gastroenterology and Hepatology, 6*(4), 443–450.

Chwedyk, P. (2007). Targeted tools: Resources for creating culturally competent diabetes interventions. *Minority Nurse, 16*(1), 34.

Cross, T. L., Bazron, B. J., Dennis, K. W., Isaac, M. R., and Campinha-Bacote, J. (1989). *Towards a cultural competent system of care: A monograph on effective services to minority children who are severely emotionally disturbed.* Washington, DC: Georgetown University Child Development Center, CASSP Technical Assistance Center.

Davis, T. C., Wolf, M. S., Arnold, C. L., Byrd, R. S., Long, S. W., Springer, T., et al. (2006). Development and validation of the rapid estimate of adolescent literacy in medicine (REALM-Teen): A tool to screen adolescents for below-grade reading in health care settings. *Pediatrics, 118*(6), 1707–1714.

DeNavas-Walt, C., Proctor, B. D., & Smith, J. C. (2011). *U.S. Census Bureau, Current Population Reports, P60-239: Income, poverty, and health insurance coverage in the United States: 2010.* Washington, DC: U.S. Government Printing Office. Retrieved September 28, 2011, from http://www.census.gov/prod/2011pubs/p60-239.pdf.

DeWalt, D. A., Callahan, L. F., Hawk, V. H., Broucksou, K. A., Hink, A., Rudd, R., et al. (2010). *Health literacy universal precautions toolkit* (AHRQ Pub. No. 10-0046-EF). Rockville, MD: U.S. Department of Health and Human Services, Agency for Healthcare Research and Quality. Retrieved October 8, 2011, from http://www.ahrq.gov/qual/literacy/healthliteracytoolkit.pdf.

Fact sheet: Creating jobs and increasing the number of primary care providers. (2011). Retrieved October 3, 2011, from http://www.healthreform.gov/newsroom/primarycareworkforce.html.

Frost, R. (1961). *You come too.* New York: Holt, Rinehart & Winston.

Goode, T., Jones, W., & Mason, J. (2002). *A guide to planning and implementing cultural competence organization self-assessment.* Washington, DC: National Center for Cultural Competence, Georgetown University Child Development Center.

GovTrack. (2005). U.S. H.R. 1812-109th Congress. *Patient navigator outreach and chronic disease prevention act of 2005.* Retrieved March 10, 2008, from http://www.govtrack.us.

Guerra, C. E., Krumholz, M., & Shea, J. A. (2005). Literacy and knowledge, attitudes and behavior about mammography in Latinas. *Journal of Health Care for the Poor and Underserved, 16*(2), 152–156.

Hsu, W. C., Cheung, S., Ong, E., Wong, K., Lin, S., Leon, K., et al. (2006). Identification of linguistic barriers to diabetes knowledge and glycemic control in Chinese Americans with diabetes. *Diabetes Care, 29*(2), 415–416.

Humes, K. R., Jones, N. A., & Ramirez, R. R. (2010). *C201BR-02: 2010 Census Briefs: Overview of race and Hispanic origin: 2010.* Retrieved August 18, 2011, from http://www.census.gov/prod/cen2010/briefs/c2010br-02.pdf.

Institute of Medicine. (2001). *Crossing the quality chasm: A new health system for the 21st century.* Retrieved August 20, 2011, from www.nap.edu/catalog/10027.html.

Institute of Medicine. (2010). *Report Brief: Future directions for the national healthcare quality and disparities reports.* Retrieved September 15, 2011, from http://iom.edu/Reports/2010/Future-Directions-for-the-National-Healthcare-Quality-and-Disparities-Reports/Report-Brief-Future-Directions-for-the-National-Healthcare-Quality-and-Disparities-Reports.aspx.

Jackson, L. E. (1993). Understanding, eliciting and negotiating clients' multicultural health beliefs. *Nurse Practitioner, 18*(4), 30–32, 37–38, 41–43.

Joslin Diabetes Center & Joslin Clinic. (2011). *Clinical nutrition guideline for overweight and obese adults with type 2 diabetes, prediabetes or those at high risk for developing type 2 diabetes: 8-07-2011.* Retrieved October 5, 2011, from http://www.joslin.org/bin_from_cms/Nutrition_Guidelines-8.22.11(1).pdf.

Julian, T., & Kominski, R. (2011). *Education and synthetic work-life earnings estimates.* U.S. Census Bureau, American Community Survey Reports (ACS-14), September 2011 (p. 10). Retrieved September 23, 2011, from http://www.census.gov/prod/2011pubs/acs-14.pdf.

Kaiser Family Foundation. (2011). Summary of new health reform law (Publication # 8061). Retrieved October 2, 2011, from http://www.kff.org/healthreform/upload/8061.pdf. Kutner, M., Greenberg, E., & Baer, J. (2003). *2003 National assessment of adult literacy.* Washington, DC: U.S. Department of Education, Institute of Education Sciences, National Center for Education Statistics.

Leininger, M. M. (1991). *Ethnonursing: A research method with enablers to study the theory of culture care.* New York: National League for Nursing.

Leininger, M. M. (2001). *Culture care diversity and universality—A theory of nursing.* Boston: Jones & Bartlett.

Lewin, M. E., Altman, S. (Eds.). (2000). *America's health care safety net: Intact but endangered.* Washington, DC: Institute of Medicine of the National Academies.

MacDorman, M. F., & Mathews, T. J. (2011). *Understanding racial and ethnic disparities in U.S. infant mortality rates.* National Center for Health Statistics (NCHS) data brief, No. 74. Hyattsville, MD: National Center for Health Statistics.

Memorial Sloan-Kettering Cancer Center. (2011). *Immigrant Health and Cancer Disparities Service (2011).* Retrieved October 6, 2011, from http://www.mskcc.org/mskcc/html/103456.cfm.

National Cancer Institute of the National Institutes of Health, USDHHS. (2011). *Facing forward: Life after cancer treatment.* Retrieved October 5, 2011, from http://www.cancer.gov/cancertopics/coping/life-after-treatment.pdf.

National Center for Cultural Competence, Georgetown University, Center for Child and Human Development. (2009). *Linguistic competence: Definition.* Retrieved September 4, 2011, from http://nccc.georgetown.edu/foundations/frameworks.html.

National Center for Cultural Competence, Georgetown University, Center for Child and Human Development. (2011). *Cultural competence: Definition and conceptual framework.* Retrieved August 28, 2011, from http://nccc.georgetown.edu/foundations/frameworks.html.

New growth charts a welcome improvement. (2002). *Clinician Reviews, 12*(7), 5.

Nielsen-Bohlman, L., Panzer, A. M., & Kindig, D. A. (Eds.). (2004). *Health literacy: A prescription to end confusion.* Washington, DC: Institute of Medicine of the National Academies.

Parker, R. M., Ratzan, S. C., & Lurie, N. (2003). Health literacy: A policy challenge for advancing high-quality health care. *Health Affairs, 22*(4), 147–153.

President's Advisory Commission on Consumer Protection and Quality in the Health Care Industry. (1998). *Quality first: Better health care for all Americans: Summary of recommendations.* Retrieved August 24, 2011, from http://www.hcqualitycommission.gov/final/.

Public Law 111-148, Patient Protection and Affordable Care Act. 42 USC 18001 (2010, March 23). Retrieved on October 6, 2011, from http://www.gpo.gov/fdsys/pkg/PLAW-111publ148/pdf/PLAW-111publ148.pdf.

Ratzan, S. C., & Parker, R. M. (2000). Introduction. In C. R. Selden, M. Zorn, S. C. Ratzan, & R. M. Parker (Eds.), *National Library of Medicine current bibliographies in medicine: Health literacy* (p. 5) (NLM Pub. No. CBM 2000-1). Bethesda, MD: National Institutes of Health, U.S. Department of Health and Human Services.

Razak, F., Anand, S. S., Shannon, H., Vuksan, V., Davis, B., Jacobs, R., et al. (2007). Defining obesity cut points in a multiethnic population. *Circulation: Journal of the American Heart Association, 115,* 2111–2118.

Selden, C. R., Zorn, M., Ratzan, S. C., & Parker, R. M. (2000). *National Library of Medicine current bibliographies in medicine: health literacy* (NLM Pub. No. CBM 2000-1). Bethesda, MD: National Institutes of Health, U.S. Department of Health and Human Services.

The Joint Commission. (2008). *Frequently asked questions: Spiritual assessment (Revised 11-24-2008).* Retrieved July 13, 2011, from http://www.jointcommission.org/standards_information/jcfaqdetails.aspx?StandardsFaqId=290&ProgramId=1.

The Joint Commission. (2010). *Advancing effective communication, cultural competence, and patient- and family-centered care: A roadmap for hospitals.* Retrieved October 4, 2011, from http://www.jointcommission.org/assets/1/6/ARoadmapforHospitalsfinalversion727.pdf.

U.S. Census Bureau. (2010a). *2010 American Community Survey highlights.* Retrieved August 15, 2011, from http://www.census.gov/newsroom/releases/pdf/acs_2010_highlights.pdf.

U.S. Census Bureau. (2010b). *B16004: Age by language spoken at home by ability to speak English for the population 5 years and over. Universe: Population 5 years and over, 2010 American Community Survey 1-year estimates.* Retrieved September 30, 2011, from http://factfinder2.census.gov/faces/tableservices/jsf/pages/productview.xhtml?pid=ACS_10_1YR_B16004&prodType=table.

U.S. Census Bureau. (2010c). *S1603: Characteristics of people by language spoken at home. Data Set: 2010 American Community Survey 1-year estimates.* Retrieved September 30, 2011, from http://factfinder2.census.gov/faces/tableservices/jsf/pages/productview.xhtml?pid=ACS_10_1YR_S1603&prodType=table.

U.S. Census Bureau. (2010d). *S1601: Language spoken at home. Data Set: 2010 American Community Survey 1-year estimates.* Retrieved September 30, 2011, from http://factfinder2.census.gov/faces/tableservices/jsf/pages/productview.xhtml?pid=ACS_10_1YR_S1601&prodType=table.

U.S. Department of Health and Human Services. (2000). *Healthy people 2010: Understanding and improving health* (Volume I, Conference edition). Washington, DC: Author.

U.S. Department of Health and Human Services, Office of Civil Rights. (2004). *Guidance to federal financial assistance recipients regarding Title VI prohibition against national origin discrimination affecting limited English proficient persons (revised).* Retrieved October 8, 2011, from http://www.hhs.gov/ocr/civilrights/resources/specialtopics/lep/HHSLEPguidancepdf.pdf.

U.S. Department of Health and Human Services. (2008a). *Health Resources and Services Administration justification of estimates for appropriations committees for fiscal year 2009.* Washington, DC: Health Resources and Services Administration, U.S. Department of Health and Human Services. Retrieved September 8, 2011, from www.hrsa.gov/about/budgetjustification09.

U.S. Department of Health and Human Services. (2008b). *Press release dated October 2, 2008: HRSA awards $2.4 million for patient navigator demonstration.* Washington, DC: Health Resources and Services Administration, U.S. Department of Health and Human Services. Retrieved October 3, 2011, from http://archive.hrsa.gov/newsroom/releases/2008/patientnavigatoroct.htm.

U.S. Department of Health and Human Services. (2010). *Healthy people 2020: About healthy people.* Retrieved August 15, 2011, from http://www.healthypeople.gov/2020/about/default.aspx.

U.S. Department of Justice, Civil Rights Division. (1998). *Title VI legal manual.* Retrieved October 6, 2011, from www.usdoj.gov/crt/grants_statutes/legalman.html.

Wallace, L. (2006). Patients' health literacy skills: The missing demographic variable in primary care research. *Annals of Family Medicine, 4*(1), 85–86.

20

Conflict Resolution: An Essential Competency in Advanced Practice

Phyllis Beck Kritek
Lucille A. Joel

Conflict happens. Few nurses find this startling news, and most nurses can, with little effort, describe in detail several conflicts currently swirling about them in their daily practice. As scope of practice expands, so also do the conflicts nurses face. This chapter explores that reality and its implications for the nurse facing the challenges of advanced practice. It also posits that expanding conflict resolution competency is an opportunity to improve our work environments, and a choice worth making.

Conflict resolution, also called alternative dispute resolution (ADR), is a relatively young but burgeoning academic discipline, developing a sophisticated body of literature, including formal research, best practices commentary, compelling case histories, and evocative emerging theories. As such, it provides a rich array of insights for persons confronted with conflict in their work situations. Interestingly, the discipline has only minimally explored the utility of ADR in health care. Were it to do so, it would find a gold mine.

Because the ADR community has had limited involvement within health-care environments, most health-care professionals also have limited information about ADR. In addition, early efforts to address health-care conflicts tended to focus on malpractice, union disputes, and other structural conflicts that may have seemed remote to the practicing nurse. Yet even a casual assessment of health-care environments reveals the central role conflict plays in the daily life of the practicing nurse. Recent studies about the dissatisfactions of nurses clearly support the centrality of such conflict. Some examples may help.

The June 2002 issue of the *American Journal of Nursing* reported on a survey about nurse–physician relationships in Voluntary Hospitals of America (VHA) on the West Coast, part of a national network of community-owned hospitals and health-care systems (Rosenstein, 2002). Reporting on the analysis of the first 1,200 responses to the survey, Rosenstein, himself a physician, reports that "although all respondents saw a direct link between disruptive physician behavior and nurse satisfaction and retention," the three respondent groups of administrators, physicians, and nurses differed in their beliefs about the outcomes of these conflictual situations (Rosenstein, 2002, p. 26). Nurses scored the administrative support they received in nurses' conflicts with physicians significantly lower than either administrators or physicians. Their lowest rating in the study, also statistically significant, was their reported perception of physician support in nurse–physician conflict. Nurses do not feel supported in such conflicts, either by their bosses or by physicians. They also fear retribution and do not believe that physician counseling processes are adequate. Research has shown that patient outcomes are adversely affected by team conflict. Coworker interactions are among the most essential to high-quality of care. Effective teamwork becomes even more critical as care becomes more complex (Baker at al., 2005).

These findings substantiate some significant job dissatisfiers for nurses, reasons they may leave practice and never return. They are more compelling when juxtaposed with the growing body of literature focusing on the importance of registered nurses to high-quality patient care and their impact on outcomes. By way of example, concurrent with Rosenstein's study, the *New England Journal of Medicine* published two related articles. Needleman, Buerhaus, Mattke, Stewart, and Zelevinsky (2002) reported on a nurse-staffing levels and quality-of-care study that concluded that "a higher proportion of hours of nursing care provided by registered nurses and a greater number of hours of care provided by registered nurses per day are associated with better care for hospitalized patients" (p. 1,716). Steinbrook (2002), a physician, provided his analysis of the current nursing shortage. He noted that many of the tensions currently shaping the health-care environment "will be difficult, if not impossible, to resolve" (p. 64). He then offered an example of a path to better care as one linked to nurses with advanced education. Steinbrook stated, "Such a workforce, however, would expect more responsibility and greater independence and would be more expensive to hire and retain" (p. 64). This statement sets the stage for advanced practice nurses and development of skills in conflict resolution as part of the required course of studies.

Knickle and McNaughton (2008) find that we are statistically more active and effective in resolving conflict with clients and students than we are with peers. These researchers have incorporated simulations and components of role playing and role reversal in learning conflict resolution skills, allowing the participants to move from adversarialism to an effective dialogue with their simulated colleague. The results have been positive, but require more investigation of the retention of these skills and long-term application in the real world. This represents one piece of research that is contributing to a body of knowledge comparing classroom-based techniques with simulations in teaching conflict resolution strategies.

Another variable in conflict resolution is the issue of culture, which is operative with clients, with peers, and interprofessionally. We are a multicultural society and guaranteed to become more so with time. The mosaic versus the melting-pot analogy is appropriate here. Whereas earlier immigrants were assimilated into the U.S. culture, today's global environment promotes accommodation of a new standard, but not necessarily adoption of all of its ways. Significant differences have been noted among ethnic groups as they deal with conflict, and this deserves to be researched (Gunia et al., 2011).

These examples point toward some of the inherent glitches in health-care environments today and strategies that offer hope. Conflict is a reality and guaranteed to be an escalating and intensifying phenomena. Avoiding conflict is simply not an option, so we had best learn how to understand and deal with it.

CONFLICT MANAGEMENT STRATEGIES OF NURSES

The issue of conflict avoidance is critical. Valentine (2001) reported a synthesis of research findings about nurses' conflict management strategies as identified by use of the Thomas-Kilmann Index (TKI). The TKI is a conflict mode index that identifies preferred conflict management strategies from a set of five options: avoiding, compromising, collaborating, competing, and accommodating. Eight studies were analyzed.

Two conflict strategies were used predominantly by all categories of nurses: avoiding and compromising. The third strongest preference was for accommodation. These findings are sobering because avoiding and accommodating lead to outcomes where one disadvantages oneself. Compromising runs a weak second because in this strategy all parties are equally disadvantaged. The remaining two strategies least often used by nurses, collaborating and competing, are the only strategies that ensure some type of gains for oneself. Richard Shell (1999), the director of the Wharton Executive Negotiation Workshop, observes, "Among the professional groups I have taught, hospital nurses are characteristically accommodating. Sometimes this works well for them. But they can also get squeezed between the demands of angry patients and impatient, authoritative physicians" (p. 12). A similar observation is made by Kelly (2006), who sees conflict within the nursing profession as traditionally generating negative feelings.

Taback and Orit (2007) studied the effect that different ways of resolving conflicts have on those involved. They examined the tactics nurses adopt to resolve conflicts with doctors and how these tactics affect their level of stress and job satisfaction. What they have called the integrating (collaborating) and dominance (competing) approaches to conflict resolution are associated with low occupational stress levels, whereas the obliging (compromising/accommodating) and avoidance approaches are linked to higher stress. In this study, there was evidence that the seniority and status of nurses drive both their choice of tactics and the associated stress/satisfaction level. Similar outcomes were found in a study that focused on the occurrence of conflict in an assisted living facility and nursing home, and how staff as compared to residents of each handled the situation. Results indicate that staff in each care context showed a preference for a solution-oriented approach, whereas residents reported an equal use of nonconfrontational and solution-oriented approaches. The authors propose that the conflict resolution style may vary most as a function of the role of the communicator (Small & Montoro-Rodriguez, 2006). Do not residents often see themselves as being at the mercy of staff, powerless and unsupported in their interpersonal disputes?

In a study by Siu, Spence Laschinger, and Finnegan (2008), investigators identified a link between the nurses' perception of the quality of their practice environment and their self-evaluation to success in conflict resolution. A positive professional practice environment and a high self-evaluation explained over 46% of the variability in nurses' constructive conflict management and effectiveness of the solutions. Put simply, if you see yourself as a skilled particpant in a high-quality work environment, you have a good chance of resolving disputes in an effective manner.

Hence, we find that although the levels of conflict in health-care environments, and specifically those faced by nurses, are indeed escalating, the strategies nurses are using are often those most likely to ensure an undesirable outcome. As the shortages deepen, and as nurses seek advanced practice responsibilities, this troublesome state of affairs will worsen. Increasing one's scope of competence, expertise, and authority is actually a sufficient catalyst to increasing one's exposure to conflicts.

It would seem nursing is at something of a crossroads in relationship to conflict and the possibilities of ADR. Reframing our options and learning new strategies appears to be in our best interest, and probably, therefore, also in the best interest of those for whom we care. Becoming a skillful manager of conflict is a goal that would wisely replace our naïve embrace of conflict avoidance and delimiting compromise.

A simple literature review indicates that there is a growing consciousness about this concern. Five years ago, the *Cumulative Index to Nursing and Allied Health Literature* identified few sources connected with the terms *conflict* and *conflict resolution.* Today, the listings number more than 3,000. Most of these manuscripts advocate for ADR and encourage nurses to master this area. However, we do not yet have comprehensive research in this area, and the options for learning about ADR are too often incongruous with nursing's realities. There is work to be done here.

CHANGING PARADIGMS OF ADR

Initial development in ADR was heavily influenced by the work done by a network of innovators at Harvard University, perhaps best exemplified by the best-selling primer on ADR, *Getting to Yes: Negotiating Agreement Without Giving In* by Roger Fisher, Bill Ury, and Bruce Patton (1991). This classic in ADR sets forth the basic tenets of interest-based negotiation, an approach that encourages disputing parties to find common interests that could serve as the basis for a settlement of the conflict. Because both Fisher and Ury were part of my earliest training in ADR, it is a perspective that shaped my original understanding of the field, and also evoked some degree of resistance. I have since learned that this is a resistance shared by many nurses.

Happily, the field of ADR is expanding its horizons and supplementing this initial theoretical posture with several that probably will be experienced as more congruent with professional nursing's values and traditions. Nurses often find themselves negotiating on behalf of patients and their families. Hence, although they may be able to identify the interests of a given disputant with whom they are in conflict, trying to present their interests as "representing the patient's interests" can be viewed as offensive and presumptuous, and can simply escalate the conflict. Alternatives are needed.

Bush and Folger (1994) broke new ground by positing an approach to ADR they called *transformative practice,* in which the goal shifted from interest-based settlement to empowerment and recognition of the disputing parties, a model more deliberately focused on the relational and social interaction dimensions of conflict. Others have followed. Mayer (2000), with more than 25 years of ADR experience, looks back reflectively on what he has learned and posits that communication and attitudes toward conflict are more compelling than settlement. He views ADR as a process that can help people solve their problems in ways that are not only collaborative but also just and powerful.

Winslade and Monk (2000) have recast the initial model of ADR to one congruent with postmodernity, creating a process they call *narrative mediation,* building relationships that start with story. They too focus on collaboration as a central dimension of hearing and understanding the stories of disputants. Cloke and Goldsmith (2000) also use stories as a central component of their approach to ADR. They posit a model of mediation that focuses on transformation and forgiveness, once more focusing on relationships.

Shell (1999) makes a case for switching from interest-based to information-based negotiation. He places emphasis on the uniqueness of each conflict and actively discourages the illusion of thinking a single approach or set of guidelines can ensure mastery of ADR. He also posits that the essential attributes of an effective negotiator are "a willingness to prepare, high expectations, the patience to listen, and a commitment to personal integrity" (p. 15). His description stands in sharp contrast to many interest-based descriptions of ADR in which manipulation and cunning are covertly posited as indicators of skill.

Each of these ADR experts is providing leadership in moving away from perceiving conflicts as situations in which the personal interests of two or more parties are dissonant and require intervention and settlement. They are ushering in an alternative viewpoint, one with an emphasis on relationship building, collaboration, authenticity, and self-management. These models augur well for nurses interested in ADR.

THE WORD FROM THE TRENCHES

My personal interest in ADR emerged from a growing frustration with the effect of conflict in our practice settings and a personal hunger for "something better." This led me to 3 years of intensive ADR training during a Kellogg Leadership Fellowship (1986–1989), my involvement in a variety of negotiation and mediation program initiatives, the writing of a book on the subject (Kritek, 2002), and an ever-expanding investment in training nurses in ADR. If we are going to have to manage a good deal of conflict anyway, I believed that it made sense to learn how to do it well. Hence, the lion's share of my energy in ADR has focused on training nurses throughout the United States to become more knowledgeable and competent in their management of conflict.

The training work with nurses has taught me a good deal about conflict in our times. I have done workshops all over the United States (and a few elsewhere), and I have developed some insights, and some convictions, along the way. Sharing some of each makes up the central message in this chapter. All emerge from repetitious experiences during training sessions with nurses and hence lack formal empirical grounding. Nonetheless, their very repetitiousness is instructive. Although this results in something of a "grocery list" of the following observations, it is hoped that these ideas can be catalytic in propelling advanced practice nurses (APNs) toward exploration and mastery of ADR and its potential for good.

- Many nurses are extremely conflict avoidant. Some, trying to overcome this tendency, become attacking and aggressive. Neither posture appears to meet the ADR needs of nurses and those with whom they work.
- Many nurses want an "easy" answer to learning ADR, a set of rules or guidelines that can be applied much like one applies the step-by-step process of learning how to use a new piece of equipment. Conflict is about relationship. The very values that have made nursing a powerful health-care force—the respect for humans, the compassion, the commitment—are the very factors that also shape the ADR enterprise. There are no short cuts.
- Many nurses make snap judgments about a conflict rather than conducting a conflict analysis. They create a quick story in their minds that explains the conflict, preferably one that casts "the other" as at fault or "in the wrong." This pattern of snap judgments short-circuits the process of ADR before it can get started. All conflicts are complex, and it takes time to really understand them.
- Many nurses believe they should prevail in conflicts because they know that they have good motives and feel comfortable questioning the motives of others. Others sometimes contribute to this tendency by indeed having questionable motives. Resolving conflict, however, is not about differentiating the good guys from the bad guys. Judgment and blaming rarely further the effort or assist in meeting the goal. The search is for common ground, points of agreement and collaboration, not the creation of moral hierarchies.
- Many nurses hope to resolve conflicts they confront while remaining personally unchanged by the process. All effective conflict resolution changes the parties involved, for good or ill. It is the intent of ADR to make the outcome for the "good." Conflict unveils the dark and edgy side of all of us, and running from it can seem quite reasonable. Working hard to avoid authenticity and self-insight keeps conflicts going. Wanting to resolve them does require change, even transformation, of both oneself and one's relationships.
- Many nurses make declarative sentences to insist on their viewpoint during a conflict when they might more constructively ask questions that evoke from the other disputants needed information and understanding of the issues. Declarative sentences tend to lock positions; questions open avenues of thought.
- Many nurses confuse accommodation and collaboration. They smooth over a conflict without resolving it, only to find it will return the next day or the next week . . . with a vengeance. Part of conflict resolution is truth telling, and this means neither verbal assault nor coy innuendo,

but simple candor without judgment and blaming. One has to slog through the messy part of conflict to get to a real resolution.

- Many nurses deny or avoid recognition of the overt structured inequity designed into healthcare systems in the United States. They ignore this when it involves patients, and they deny it when it involves nurses. Many believe that to honestly face these facts will be disempowering, an admission of disadvantage. However, although persons can treat me as a victim, it does not mean I must become one or act as one. To deny the efforts of others to diminish or victimize me usually leads to my collusion in this process. This may be difficult to accept.
- Many nurses rush to settlement too quickly, eager to end the discomfort of conflict. Hence, they fail to look at the range of choices they have available to resolve the conflict and the consequences of each. Rather than seeing ADR as a creative process, they are eager to make it a quick process. This diminishes the outcomes and their potential for good.
- Many nurses give away their personal power as a solution to keeping conflict at bay. They keep silent, or go along, or compromise their integrity. Somewhere, their authentic selves know that they have done this. This can enrage or depress them, and make them cling even more tenaciously to their conflicts. This is a sad thing, and not seeing it in oneself is often tragic.

This list is not exhaustive, but does capture the challenges before nurses, and the options they have to change their current conflict styles. In addition, it highlights some of the serious losses nurses are taking by their unwillingness to become conflict experts. Few disciplines are as well equipped as nursing to actually become ADR-proficient. Perhaps the time has come to lay claim to this unique possibility.

RESPONDING TO THE CHALLENGE: EXERCISES IN ADR

Nurses who take on expanded practice roles often experience a sense of personal satisfaction about this achievement. They tend to have worked hard to get where they are and know the path before them will evoke new professional experiences that will enhance their sense of personal satisfaction. Conflict can sometimes seem like the "spoiler," the irritating situation that deflects from the task at hand.

One option is obvious: One can elect to become more proficient at conflict management. Having previously provided a list that essentially serves as a self-assessment inventory, the following list of opportunities that address the inventory outcomes may prove useful. These exercises are available for APNs to improve their participation in ADR activities. This list, again, is not exhaustive, but does provide a reality map of options for the path unfolding before all of us.

- Read about ADR. The reference list at the end of this chapter can be a starting point. The books that have been identified as more recent may offer paradigms of conflict management more attractive to nurses.
- Participate in an ADR training program. There are a variety of options out there. Watch for opportunities, and sign on. Make it part of your planned continuing education.
- Look in your phone book for available mediation programs and services available in your area. Call to find out what opportunities might be available for you.
- Go to the Internet and search for options that might fit your needs, including additional books, programs, training options, and online courses.
- Find an ADR mentor. Any of the resources listed previously might reveal one and give you a chance to start working with an expert. The idea of coaching for conflict resolution is one that shows merit (Brinkert, 2011).

- Start deliberately practicing what you are learning. Take a small, easy conflict and try your new skills.
- Systematically study your own conflict behaviors. Find out what ways you tend to engage in conflict. Keep a journal of this, if possible, to increase your self-honesty and your awareness. Determine whether your current practices are enough and what added skills you would like to acquire.
- Ask peers or colleagues to critique your conflict behaviors. Ask them to tell you how they see you responding to conflict. After you ask, listen carefully. Many people do not like to answer this question for fear of starting a conflict, so assure your informant of your openness before you ask.
- Do environmental scans of your workplace. Train yourself to conduct comprehensive and objective conflict analyses, and observe the ways that your understanding of conflict shifts as you expand your understanding of a given conflict. Systematically teach yourself new modes of thought about conflict, and reinforce them through practice.
- Form a coalition with other colleagues interested in improving their conflict management skills; share learning experiences, assessments, and analyses of conflict situations. Learn from one another and normalize dealing with conflict as a group expectation.

This is a starter set of ideas. Any or all of them can be helpful in moving toward enhancing your conflict management skills and in accessing the many skills you currently have that can be helpful in conflict situations. You elected to prepare yourself for an APN role because you wanted to give care, not slog through conflicts. The efficient and skillful management of conflict as it emerges can ensure that you spend as much time as possible focused on your primary goal of patient care and as little time as possible on the sometimes onerous, yet often transformative task of resolving conflict.

Surprisingly, your patients are watching. They may find your new skills and competencies worthy of modeling and assuredly worthy of their trust. It is nice to know that the person taking care of you knows what to do with conflict. It increases one's sense of safety, a belief that the care provider is an advocate with the necessary ability to advocate well, even in the face of conflict.

CONCLUSION

Nurses who elect to expand their practice roles will find that along with the increased ability to deliver care, they will also confront a larger and more complex array of conflicts in their work settings. To date, nurses have not invested in increasing their ability to improve their conflict management skills. This has a deleterious effect not only on nurses, but also on other providers, and more poignantly, on patients and their families. Hence, improved mastery of ADR abilities is an idea whose time has come.

The field of ADR has minimally invested in health-care environments to date. More recent theoretical developments in the field have yielded models of ADR that show high congruence with the values and traditions of nursing. Nurses who wish to enhance their ADR competencies would be wise to first conduct an honest self-assessment of current skill levels, both acknowledging existing strengths and identifying learning needs. Having done this, they have a wide range of options available that can be accessed as resources for further building conflict management skills. The decision to do such building benefits not only the nurse, but also all persons who come in contact with the nurse, particularly patients and their families. ADR is indeed an idea whose time has come for the nursing profession.

REFERENCES

Baker, D. P., Gustafson, S., Beaubien, J. M., Salas, E., & Barach, P. (2005). Medical team training programs in health care. In *Advances in patient safety: From research to implementation. Volume 4: Programs, tools and products.* AHRQ Publication No. 05-0021-4. Rockville, MD: Agency for Healthcare Research and Quality (AHRQ) and the Department of Defense (DoD)–Health Affairs.

Brinkert, R. (2011). Conflict coaching training for nurse managers: A case study of a two-hospital health system. *Journal of Nursing Management, 19* (1), 80–91.

Bush, B. R. A., & Folger, J. P. (1994). *The promise of mediation: Responding to conflict through empowerment and recognition.* San Francisco: Jossey-Bass.

Cloke, K., & Goldsmith, J. (2000). *Resolving personal and organizational conflict.* San Francisco: Jossey-Bass.

Fisher, R., Ury, W. & Patton, B. (1991). Getting to Yes: Negotiating Agreement Without Giving In, New York: Penguin Books.

Gunia, B. C., Brett, J. M., Nandkeolyar, A. K., & Kamdar, D. (2011). Paying a price: Culture, trust, and negotiation consequences. *Journal of Applied Psychology, 96*(4), 774–789.

Kelly, J. (2006). An overview of conflict. *Dimensions of Critical Care Nursing, 25*(1), 22–28.

Knickle, K., & McNaughton, N. (2008). Collegial conflict: Experiencing attribution theory through simulation. *Medical Education, 42*(5), 541–542.

Kritek, P. B. (2002). *Negotiating at an uneven table: Developing moral courage in resolving our conflicts* (2nd ed.). San Francisco: Jossey-Bass.

Mayer, B. (2000). *The dynamics of conflict resolution: A practitioner's guide.* San Francisco: Jossey-Bass.

Needleman, J., Buerhaus, P., Mattke, S., Stewart, M., & Zelevinsky, K. (2002). Nurse-staffing levels and the quality of care in hospitals. *New England Journal of Medicine, 346,* 1715–1722.

Rosenstein, A. H. (2002). Nurse–physician relationships: Impact on nurse satisfaction and retention. *American Journal of Nursing, 102,* 26–34.

Shell, G. R. (1999). *Bargaining for advantage: Negotiation strategies for reasonable people.* New York: Penguin Books.

Siu, H., Spence Laschinger, H. K., & Finegan, J. (2008). Nursing professional practice environments: Setting the stage for constructive conflict resolution and work effectiveness. *Journal of Nursing Administration, 38*(5), 250–257.

Small, J. A., & Montoro-Rodriguez, J. (2006). Conflict resolution styles: A comparison of assisted living and nursing home facilities. *Journal of Gerontological Nursing, 32*(6), 39–45.

Steinbrook, R. (2002). Nursing in the crossfire. *New England Journal of Medicine, 346,* 1757–1766.

Tabak, N., & Orit K. (2007). Relationship between how nurses resolve their conflicts with doctors, their stress and job satisfaction. *Journal of Nursing Management, 15*(3), 321–331.

Valentine, P. E. B. (2001). A gender perspective on conflict management strategies of nurses. *Journal of Nursing Scholarship, 33,* 69–74.

Winslade, J., & Monk, G. (2000). *Narrative mediation: A new approach to conflict resolution.* San Francisco: Jossey-Bass.

21

Leadership for APNs: If Not Now, When?

Edna Cadmus

Over the last 10 years an infrastructure for radical change of the health-care system in the United States has been created. Both of the Institute of Medicine (IOM) reports, *To Err Is Human* (IOM, 2000) and the recent *The Future of Nursing: Leading Change, Advancing Health* (IOM, 2011), were prominent in prompting these changes. The latest IOM report has provided nurses, more specifically APNs, with a blueprint to be part of that change. It addresses adjusting their role and functions to ensure access, quality, and value at a reduced cost. The blueprint is further advanced through the Campaign for Action sponsored by the Robert Wood Johnson Foundation in collaboration with the Association for the Advancement of Retired Persons (AARP). Their campaign vision is to ensure that "all Americans have access to high-quality, patient-centered care in a health-care system where nurses contribute as essential partners in achieving success (Center to Champion Nursing in America, 2011). Currently, Campaign for Action is providing support to Action Coalitions at the state level in 15 states with the goal of all states by 2012. These Action Coalitions are charged with implementing the recommendations described in the IOM *Future of Nursing* report. To learn more about these initiatives, visit http://thefutureofnursing.org.

Legislation, including the American Recovery and Reinvestment Act of 2009 (ARRA) and the Patient Protection and Affordable Care Act of 2010 (PPACA), have also contributed to an uncertain health-care environment, but one that holds promise for APNs. These legislative actions provide the technological and financial framework for resource allocation in an evolving health-care delivery system. ARRA defines meaningful use regulations for informational technology. It requires hospitals and physicians' offices to create an electronic health-care record with an incentive to those who comply by 2014 and reduced reimbursement for those who do not. The focus of the meaningful use standards are to track a patient's clinical conditions for better coordination across settings and to provide clinical decision support for providers. The anticipated outcomes are to improve quality and safety by providing information in a more efficient and effective manner (Burchill, 2010). The PPACA has established the Center for Medicare and Medicaid Innovations to ensure coordinated care across the health-care continuum through delivery models that predict improved outcomes for patients. These new care delivery models span the spectrum from preventive to end-of-life care opportunities. In 2007 the Health Workforce Solutions Program was commissioned by the Robert Wood Johnson Foundation to identify criteria and an evaluation process to review 24 innovative delivery models across the spectrum of care needs. A list of these innovative models and opportunities for further exploration can be found in **Table 21-1.**

This is a unique occasion for APNs to develop and implement evidence-based models of care and to reframe traditional definitions of health and health care. Yet opinion leaders in general do not see nurses as having a great deal of influence in health-care reform. A survey was conducted by Gallup for the Robert Wood Johnson Foundation (2010), *Nursing Leadership from Bedside to Boardroom:*

TABLE 21-1

Care Delivery Models Across the Continuum

Acute Care	Bridge Continuum	Comprehensive Care
12-Bed Hospital	11th Street Family Health Services	Comprehensive Rural Care Collaborative
Med/Surg Unit Team Nursing Model RN Line	Care Transitions Intervention	Evercare Care Model
	Chronic Care Coordination	Living Independently for Elders
Nurse Caring Delivery Model	Collaborative Patient Care Management	Values-Driven System
Patient-Centered Care	Heart Failure Resource Center	
Planetree Patient-Centered Care	Home Healthcare	
	Telemedicine	
Primary Care Coordinator	Nursing Model for Anticoagulation Management	
Self-Organized Agile Teams	The Little Clinic	
Unit-Based Care Manager	Transitional Care Model	

Adapted with permission from Health Work Force Solutions, LLC & The Robert Wood Johnson Foundation. (2008). Innovative care models. Retrieved June 8, 2011, from http://innovativecaremodels.com.

Opinion Leaders' Perceptions. Telephone interviews with 1,504 opinion leaders throughout the country were conducted from August 19 to October 30, 2009. This study sought to determine the role of nursing in the future and barriers to nurses assuming leadership roles in health care. The key barriers identified were that nurses are not seen as significant decision makers or revenue generators. Several strategies were offered for nurses to overcome barriers and become more influential, including the following: (1) nurses need to make their voices heard through a unified focus on key issues in health policy; (2) nurses need to demonstrate an interest in health policy; and (3) society and nurses need to have higher expectations for what they can achieve and be held accountable not only for providing high-quality care but also for health-care leadership.

So what does leadership mean for the APN? APNs have a responsibility to lead health-care reform that improves access, quality, and value-based care. Leadership frameworks and theories that have evolved over time will be described and then applied to the APN role. Further, the environments in which APNs practice are described as complex and uncertain; therefore, APNs have a responsibility to make the changes needed for Americans as they traverse this complex health-care system.

EVOLUTION OF LEADERSHIP FRAMEWORKS AND THEORIES

The ongoing changes in the health-care landscape are most influenced by globalization, economic and technological factors, and the aging of the population. The complexity of the health-care environment requires us to examine the leadership theories that are applicable for today and the future. Leadership is often oversimplified into one theory or framework, but the reality is that each situation and how the leader interprets the environment determines the leadership framework that is needed and the process to be employed. To better understand these theories and how they apply to the APN, it is important to appreciate how they have evolved over time.

There have been many definitions of leadership. Leadership has been described as a person or group, a process or an outcome, depending on the theory utilized. Leadership has moved from leader-centered or focusing on an individual to an orientation of mutual power and influence that results in collaboration and innovation. In the industrial age, leadership was more about control and structure, and people were treated as things. It was defined as mechanistic and leadership was considered reductionist. Leadership in the postindustrial age requires a different skill set for both the designated leader and leadership qualities within every follower. Today's leaders must embrace new ways of being and interacting for success.

In the knowledge worker age, Covey (2007) describes the "whole person paradigm," in which the leader taps into each person and maximizes an individual's contributions to create results. In the whole person paradigm people are engaged in a four-dimensional way, tapping into their mind, body, spirit, and heart. Covey (2007) further describes the four imperatives of great leaders: (1) inspiring trust, (2) clarifying purpose, (3) unleashing talent, and (4) aligning systems. In many situations a lack of any one of these imperatives will not allow the organization to move forward with the speed and efficiency to remain competitive. These imperatives can be applied by the APN in working with patients and other professionals as well. As the frameworks and theories are described, you will see an emphasis on many of these imperatives.

Situational or Contingency Leadership

Situational leadership has been evolving since 1967, starting with the works of Vroom and Yetton (1973), Fielder (2012), and most recently Hersey and Blanchard (2007).

Contingency or situational theories are based on the premise that different styles of leadership are needed in different circumstances. In all these models the most effective style is contingent on the maturity and competence of the subordinates and the situation that is presented to the leader. For example, Hersey and Blanchard's model identifies four combinations that can occur in leadership style based on the situation/level of employee or group that the leader is interacting with. Maturity in this model is focused on competence, which is signified by the knowledge, skills, and commitment of the participants (Blanchard, 2008). The activities of leadership can include (1) "telling" when there is very low maturity, (2) "selling" to those with moderate maturity, (3) "participating" for those with moderately high maturity, and (4) "delegation" for those with very high maturity (Thompson & Vecchio, 2009). Leadership style depends on the difficulty of the task and the maturity of the persons responsible for carrying out the task.

Servant Leadership

In the early 1970s Robert Greenleaf defined servant-leadership as a leader who wants to serve first versus being the leader first (Greenleaf Center for Servant Leadership, 2010). Servant-leaders focus on meeting the needs of others and accomplishing the work. In this model anyone can be a servant-leader by meeting the needs of others. McCrimmon (2010) describes it as meeting the needs of followers so that they can perform optimally. Spears (2004) defined the characteristics of servant-leadership to include active listening, empathy, healing, awareness, persuasion, stewardship, commitment to the development of others, foresight, and building community. Sipe and Frick (2009) further developed the work of Greenleaf by defining the seven pillars on which servant-leadership will grow and flourish: (1) personal character, (2) an ethic of people first, (3) skilled communicator, (4) compassionate collaborator, (5) possessing foresight, (6) systems thinker, and (7) a leader with moral authority (Sipe & Frick, 2009). These seven pillars translate into specific competencies that define servant-leadership: being visionary, being a good listener, recognizing that there is a higher purpose other than oneself, respecting others, and holding oneself and others accountable for actions that affect the organization as a whole. Although all these competencies are not expected to be fully met by the leader, a large proportion must be part of the persona of the servant-leader.

Some of the advantages of this model are that it introduces the concept of caring and creates a nurturing environment for the followers and ultimately the patient/client. Some of the disadvantages are that it is often confused with transformational leadership, and is also seen as a weak form of leadership due to the connotation of the word "servant." Servant symbolizes the historical religious heritage of nursing where the nurse was called to serve and therefore today seems outmoded. Many of the pillars described in servant-leadership are important characteristics that should be incorporated into a leader's competencies regardless of the model.

Transformational and Transactional Leadership

Transformational leadership has received considerable attention. Burns (1978) defined transactional leadership and transformational leadership. He connected leadership with the need for purpose. Transactional leaders work with their followers to gain some type of exchange for services that are contracted by the leader. Transformational leaders look for the motives of their followers and engage the full person in reaching a mutual purpose. Burns (1978) identified a strong link with morality and ethics in the transformational model, placing emphasis on the wants and needs of the followers as opposed to the leader or the situation at hand. Bass (1985) further defined and challenged transformational leadership, defining the art of transformational leaders as being able to elevate the interests of their followers and their ability to look beyond their own self-interest to that of the group. This type of leadership is most effective in turbulent markets. He further defined transactional leadership as working on the promise of reward or the fear of penalties by the followers. This type of leadership is more effective in a stable marketplace. Bass differs from Burns in that he saw transformational leadership as elevating the performance of followers, yet holding significant cost for them were they to fail. Burns saw transformational and transactional leadership as opposites. Therefore, leaders were either transformational or transactional, but not both. Bass on the other hand stated that leaders use both transformational and transactional behaviors based on the situation, and even within the same situation. Transformational leaders are described as being charismatic and are able to bring out the best in their followers. They tend to exude competence and confidence. They are inspirational, individualize the consideration of their followers, and are intellectually stimulating (Bass, 1985; Bass and Riggio, 2008).

Using transformational leadership as a springboard, Kouzes and Posner (2007) developed 5 practices and 10 commitments of leadership behaviors. They defined leadership not by title, power, or authority but by relationships, credibility, and what we do. The relationship is between the person who aspires to lead and those who choose to follow. Credibility includes being honest, competent, and inspiring, and is the foundation of leadership. Credibility is established by doing what you say you will do. Kouzes and Posner's work is different from that of Bass because they put an emphasis on behaviors. Their five principles of leadership are (1) modeling the way, (2) inspiring a shared vision, (3) challenging the process, (4) enabling others to act, and (5) encouraging the heart (Kouzes & Posner, 2007). In each of these principles, there are valuable lessons that the APN can apply in practice.

In practice one, "modeling the way," you need to find your voice and articulate your values. Based on these values, common principles and ideals can be generated with others. Set an example by using actions to speak louder than words. In practice two, "inspiring a shared vision," it is the vision that creates the future state and the enthusiasm helps in getting others engaged. Engaging others through shared dreams is key to successful change. In practice three, "challenging the process," leaders are willing to challenge the status quo and take risks by experimenting with new ways of doing things. Leaders learn from their successes and their failures, and continue to adapt to new ways of operating. In practice four, "enabling others to act," the leader recognizes the importance of the team. Building trust and collaboration with others make them successful. They are considered authentic leaders. In the fifth practice, "encouraging the heart," leaders provide support and encouragement through the change process and recognize the contributions of their team. They celebrate their successes regularly (Kouzes and Posner, 2007).

Relational Leadership

Uhl-Bien (2006) and Rost (1995) describe relational leadership theory as occurring in any direction and reflecting a mutual agenda between follower and leader. It requires an inclusiveness of others and their viewpoints, and the ability to persuade others to your way of thinking. This model of leadership focuses on the team as a process, and the team works collectively for the common good of the organization. This is not a single role. In this model teams also evolve their own culture. In the relational leadership model, each individual brings his or her leadership skill set to the table and the collective learning and abilities enable an adaptation to complexity. An example of this type of leadership can be found in the virtual team leadership, in which the primary work is conducted using electronic media modalities. This model can be used by APNs as they frequently work in interprofessional teams where they may need to use their expertise in dealing with patient care needs or practice changes.

Clinical Leadership/Congruent Leadership

Theories described in the management literature may not completely translate for those in clinical practice. Congruent leadership may be a more appropriate theory for the clinician. Stanley (2008) defines congruent leadership theory as "matching the clinical leaders' action and their values and beliefs about care and nursing and is the theoretical foundation on which clinical nurses can build their capacity to be clinical leaders" (p. 519). The concepts that are embedded in transformational leadership—namely, vision and creativity—may not be appropriate to explain clinical leadership; however, the other characteristics remain (Stanley, 2008). Hamric, Spross, and Hanson (2009) further describe clinical leadership as focusing on the patient first and on building working relationships to problem solve as part of an interprofessional team. Stanley (2006) further identifies the key characteristics of clinical leaders as being approachable and open; having strong values and beliefs that are displayed in their practice; being effective communicators, role models, and decision makers; and being visible and clinically competent. They do not exhibit the creativity and vision described in transformational leadership (Stanley, 2006). Clinical leaders are not commonly in management positions. This framework may fit more appropriately for the APN.

REFRAMING LEADERSHIP THROUGH MENTAL MODELS

Bolman and Deal (2008) use the concept of framing as a mental model and reframing based on the situation. These frames are filters for problem solving and getting things done in organizations. There are four frames: (1) structural, (2) human resource, (3) political, and (4) symbolic. Leaders of today and the future need to be able to use all four frames, based on the situation with which they are presented.

The structural frame focuses on the organization's circumstances, goals, rules, technology, and environment. It addresses how the organizational chart is structured and how work is distributed in the organization. It is the old adage, does form follow function or does function follow form? In times of certainty, relationships are usually hierarchical. Organizations focus on structure in times of uncertainty, looking to reestablish stability (Bolman & Deal, 2008). For example, with health-care reform impending, redesign of the system needs to focus on the needs of the population in the community, building from bottom up, from the smallest to the largest unit of service. Organizations such as hospitals will shrink over time and other models of care and mental models will substitute, creating newfound relationships.

Structure also applies to teams and requires changes based on the situation. Katzenbach and Smith (1993) identified six characteristics of high-functioning teams: (1) the team shapes purpose in response to a demand or opportunity identified by the leaders in the organization; (2) the team translates purpose into measurable goals; (3) the team itself is a manageable size; (4) the team has the right expertise; (5) the team has a common commitment to the work; and (6) the team members hold themselves collectively accountable. These characteristics should be adapted by APNs as they work in team environments. In comparison, Senge (1994) calls "team" an antiquated concept and claims it takes more effort to maintain the team than to do the team's work. This opinion may be outdated or contingent on the sophistication of team members.

The human resource frame focuses on the alignment between human and organizational needs. The decision that leaders need to make is to either invest in their people or to be lean and mean. Organizations that engage employees and can connect to meaningful work are the organizations that are most successful. How engagement is demonstrated varies based on the organization and the situations. Relationships are key to being flexible and nimble, and are the key to organizational effectiveness (Bolman & Deal, 2008).

The political frame redefines organizations as coalitions in which individuals and groups are competing for scarce resources. Exercising the use of power and influence to negotiate resources as needed is a key skill set for individuals and groups. Being effective politically requires leaders to set an agenda, scan the environment, develop networking skills, and negotiate with those who support their agenda, as well as create relationships with those who do not (Bolman & Deal, 2008).

The symbolic frame focuses on how meaning is perceived by the individual or group. Symbols create that perception and include rituals, values, stories, and myths that are evidenced in our culture. Symbols are created in times of uncertainty and ambiguity to try to make sense of reality and to create a more rational world. Organizations are frequently measured by appearance as well as outcomes (Bolman & Deal, 2008).

Application of Leadership Theories for APNs

APNs are leaders both formally and informally in the practice setting. As clinical leaders they serve as the leader or the follower, depending on the situation. There are many common characteristics of leadership regardless of the theory one identifies with. The key characteristics include strong values, clear purpose, bringing out the best in others on the team, strong interprofessional relationships, mutual power and influence, and clinical competence.

The APN uses evidence to support practice, ensures that quality indicators are met, works with the team (having strong collaboration skills), and focuses on the patient and the family. The APN can be the leader as in the primary care model in which he or she manages a practice of patients, or be a member of a team, depending on the environment in which he or she works. In either situation, the APN focuses on the patient and family to ensure that their needs are met and will advocate for them as required to achieve high-quality outcomes. APNs need to be innovators in creating new models of care delivery for the future. Current models under review include accountable care organizations, medical homes, and transitional care delivery models. With the current gap in primary care, APNs need to fill the gap and create new models that are valued by the consumer at a lower cost.

OTHER ASPECTS OF LEADERSHIP

Emotional and Social Intelligence

Goleman, Boyatzis, and McKee (2002) define *emotional intelligence* as "how leaders handle themselves and their relationships" (p. 6). They describe learned abilities that include 4 domains and 18 competencies. The domains and competencies are listed in **Table 21-2.** The competencies are categorized as either *personal,* how we manage ourselves, or *social intelligence,* how we manage our relationships. All four domains are interwoven and connected to the neural anatomy of the brain. Leaders do not need to meet all of the competencies, but must meet a substantive proportion of them to be considered emotionally intelligent leaders.

The four domains are self-awareness, self-management, social awareness, and relationship management. The personal competencies focus on self and include self-awareness and self-management. Self-awareness requires the leader to be honest with himself or herself and with others about the leader's strengths and weaknesses. The leader is considered reflective and clear on values and goals, and acts with authenticity. Self-management requires us to control our emotions. Leaders who demonstrate self-management are seen as optimistic, enthusiastic, transparent, and adaptable. They are perceived as positive leaders (Goleman et al., 2002).

TABLE 21-2

Domains and Competencies of Emotional Intelligence

Emotional Intelligence Domains	Competencies *Personal*
Self-awareness	Emotional self-awareness Self-assessment Self-confidence
Self-management	Emotional self-control Transparency Adaptability Achievement Initiative Optimism
	Social
Social awareness	Empathy Organizational awareness Service
Relationship management	Inspirational Influence Developing others Change catalyst Conflict management Teamwork and collaboration

Adapted with permission from Goleman et al. (2002). *Primal leadership.* Boston: Harvard Business School Press (p. 39).

The social competencies are focused on how we manage relationships and include social awareness and relationship management. Social awareness requires the leader to be empathetic, a good listener, and attuned to the needs of others. In relationship management it requires the leader to have a tool set that includes conflict management and collaboration skills. The leader is able to find a common ground in various situations. He or she is considered inspirational, with an ability to influence and develop others on the team. The emotionally intelligent leader is seen as a change catalyst and has the ability to create effective teams (Goleman et al., 2002).

Goleman and Boyatzis (2008) have further developed emotional intelligence based on the breakthroughs in brain science that focus on the emotional centers of the brain. Social intelligence is "a set of interpersonal competencies built on specific neural circuits in the brain and (endocrine system) that inspire others to be effective" (p. 76). They include mirror neurons, which mimic other behaviors; spindle cells, which provide a gut reaction to a situation or person; and oscillators, which coordinate our physical movements with those of others (Goleman & Boyatzis, 2008; Veronesi, 2009). Socially intelligent leaders are tuned in to others so that they can communicate effectively and be effective leaders. The brain can be reprogrammed to learn how to become more socially intelligent through strategies that change behaviors. This requires the individual to be motivated to make the change in behaviors, obtain feedback from others on one's strengths and weakness using tools such as a 360-degree assessment, and setting a learning agreement between oneself and a mentor. This calls for intense work on the part of the leader and a socially intelligent mentor. If a leader is mentored by someone who is strong and socially intelligent, who is able to provide immediate feedback on a consistent basis, the neural circuits can be changed (Veronesi, 2009).

Power, Authority, and Influence

Power can occur through persuasion/influence or control. Bolman and Deal (2008) compare and contrast power from the perspective of structural and human resource theorists. Through the structural theorists lens power is focused around authority. The leader makes a decision and then monitors if the followers carry out the directive. In addition, power is given because of the leader's control of resources. This is an old-world view of power. The human resource theorist changes the concept of power to empowerment. Empowerment fits more appropriately in today's world.

Power is often considered in a negative light. Power can be both negative and positive, depending on how it is used. In the new age, power is needed by leaders in building relationships and getting results. There are various sources of power. These sources can come from one's position, persona, reputation, or expertise, or can come from being coercive or controlling of information or others. Leadership and authority do not necessarily go together. Both are considered voluntary. Leaders cannot lead without legitimacy from their followers. Legitimate authority is a product of influence and acceptance by a group of people. More important than hierarchical authority is the ability to influence others through motivation, persuasion, and negotiation (Jooste, 2004).

Leaders motivate or influence others to follow by creating a shared vision and purpose, and providing the environment where change can happen. Alignment of values and purpose is essential to success. This is not an optional step in the leadership sequence; leaders need followers, and vice versa. Both the leader and the follower depend on each other for success, yet each has different talents and skills. Although much has been discussed about leadership, it is just as important to describe key components of being a "good follower." These components include (1) clear role comprehension, (2) service attributes for self and others, (3) integrity, and (4) support for the leader. It is key that the follower be engaged in the organization. The leader needs to create an environment where there is both trust and respect so that the follower can flourish.

ENVIRONMENT

Complexity Science and Chaos Theory

Complexity science and chaos theory create the platform for looking at leadership and organizations collectively in the 21st century. Looking through this lens focuses on leadership as a process and not as an individual. To help explore this basic understanding of complexity science, complex adaptive systems and chaos theory are needed.

Complexity science looks at relationships between and among all things, and defines the nature of the relationship by its actions and impact (Malloch & Porter-O'Grady, 2005). Plsek (2003) defines health care systems as complex adaptive systems. A complex adaptive system (CAS) is defined as "a collection of individual agents who have the freedom to act in ways that are not always predictable, and whose actions are interconnected such that one agent's actions change the context for other agents" (p. 2). A CAS has the ability to adapt to change. Plsek (2003) defines the following properties of a CAS: (1) relationships as central to understanding the system (i.e., the way in which the system behaves comes from the interactions of the individuals); (2) structures, processes, and patterns; (3) actions based on internalized simple rules and mental models (i.e., the individual's mental model contributes to the patterns in the environment); (4) attractor patterns (i.e., those that help facilitate a change are close to the individual's values); (5) constant adaptation; (6) experimentation and pruning (i.e., support for new ways of doing things and eliminating those that no longer work); (7) inherent nonlinearity (i.e., there is no predictable cause and effect; the shortest distance between two points is not always a straight line); and (8) systems are embedded within other systems and co-evolve (i.e., formal and informal leadership can advance simultaneously and often in different directions). A CAS defines a healthy system as one that is always ready to change because if it is not it cannot survive (Lindberg et al., 2008). Chaos is a key component of change and, in fact, a necessary catalyst for change. Change is constant in the new age, and therefore we need to create spaces for new interactions, structures, and patterns that will be formed (Lindberg et al., 2008).

Wheatley and Frieze (2010) urge us to let go of the traditional paradigm of leadership, which preaches that leaders have the answers and know what to do; people do what they're told and just have to be given good plans and instructions; and high risk requires high control, and as situations grow more complex and challenging, power needs to shift to the top (with the leaders, who know what to do). If we want these complex systems to work better, we need to abandon our reliance on the leader-as-hero and invite in the leader-as-host. We need to support those leaders who know that problems are complex, who know that to understand the full complexity of any issue, all parts of the system need to be invited in to participate and contribute. We, as followers, need to give our leaders time, patience, and forgiveness, and we need to be willing to step up and contribute. These leaders-as-hosts are candid enough to admit that they don't know what to do; they realize that it's foolish to rely only on them for answers. But they also know they can trust in other people's creativity and commitment to get the work done. They know that other people, no matter where they are in the organizational hierarchy, can be as motivated, diligent, and creative as the leader, given the right invitation.

Wheatley (2007) brings together chaos and complexity theories with leadership. She believes that leaders were traditionally focused on transactional functions and that in the new age it is about decentralizing, differentiation of tasks, spanning boundaries, collaboration, flexibility, adaptability of structures and processes, participation, and autonomy. The journey for the leader is from hero to host. Leaders-as-hosts don't just benevolently let go and trust that people will do good work. As hosts, leaders have a great many things to attend to, but these are quite different from the work of heroes. Hosting leaders must do the following (Wheatley & Frieze, 2010):

- Provide conditions and good group processes for people to work together
- Provide resources of time, the scarcest commodity of all
- Insist that people and the system learn from experience
- Offer unequivocal support—people know the leader is there for them
- Keep the bureaucracy at bay, creating oases (or bunkers) where people are less encumbered by senseless administrative trivia
- Play defense with other leaders who want to take back control, who are critical that people have been given too much freedom
- Reflect back to people on a regular basis how they're doing, what they're accomplishing, how far they've journeyed
- Work with people to develop relevant measures of progress to make their achievements visible
- Value conviviality and *esprit de corps*—not false rah-rah activities, but the spirit that arises in any group that accomplishes difficult work together

The Wheatley model is based on four core principles, which drive change for the host-leader (Wheatley, 2007): (1) Participation is not a choice; in other words, "people only support what they create" (p. 89). (2) Life always reacts to directives; it never obeys them, therefore "people accept partners not bosses" (p. 90). (3) We do not see reality; we each create our own interpretation of what reality is. (4) To create better health in a living system, connect it to more of itself; therefore, leaders need to increase the number and variety of connections. An underpinning of Wheatley's principles is therefore engagement. The leader needs to encourage engagement and create an environment where there is conversation that fleshes out different perspectives and increases the connections by changing or expanding those needing to be involved.

Change in a Complex World

Understanding complexity science and chaos theory can help create the linkage to change. Porter-O'Grady and Malloch (2011) describe change as a dynamic journey that is everywhere and cannot be avoided but needs to be embraced by leaders. The leaders' responsibility is to help translate the change for their followers and role model a comfort level with the ambiguity generated from uncertainty. The leader is the change agent or catalyst for change in an organization and is under constant observation by followers to determine how he or she adapts to the change. If the leader does not adapt to change, the followers will not adapt.

Creating a vision for the change and why it is needed is key to success. The leader needs to work with all of the stakeholders in the organization to bring about change. In any change process there are resisters. Resistance occurs if there is a perceived change in vision or values, or if the proposed actions cause the stakeholders to be disenfranchised (Raza & Standing, 2011; Trader-Leigh, 2001). Change is not often resisted because of the change itself but because of the role the person or group plays or does not play in the change process. Conflict occurs as an output of resistance. In dealing with conflict the leader needs to create an environment that is supportive so that the conflict can be discussed and ultimately resolved. It is the leader who needs to bring the resisters on board with the change through engagement and facilitated dialogue.

Tools are needed to lead change. One approach to change is to use the traditional approach, which is problem solving. Hammond (1998) describes the basic assumption in this approach as "an organization IS a problem to be solved" (p. 24; emphasis in original). In today's organizations that are viewed as organic and whole systems, appreciative inquiry (AI) has been found to be more successful. Hammond (1998) describes the assumption of appreciative inquiry as "an organization is a mystery to be embraced" (p. 24). In conducting an appreciative inquiry approach, we look at what is working and through asking guided questions explore where an organization wants to base and create new energy and positivism. The appreciative inquiry model consists of the "four *D's*"—Discovery, Dream, Design, and Destiny. In the Discovery phase stories are told about when the qualities of the organization were at their best. The Dream phase explores what it could and should look like. In the Design phase the new norms, values, structures, patterns of relationships, and systems emerge. In the Destiny phase transformation occurs through innovation (Ludema et al., 2003). Using the AI process facilitates engagement, strengthens relationships, and produces results.

Learning Organizations

Senge (1990) defined the five disciplines of a learning organization: personal mastery (members of the organization develop themselves based on goals and purpose), mental models (how we shape actions and decisions), shared vision (building mutually agreeable images of the future), team learning (the sum of individual talents), and systems thinking (interrelationships that shape the system—the whole is greater than the sum of its parts) (Senge, 1990). Creating a learning organization is important in today's environment. The impact of implementing a successful learning organization is that it helps in improving quality, creating a competitive environment, gaining commitment of the workforce, managing change, being proactive, and generating collective thinking opportunities to improve organizational performance.

Many of the five disciplines have been described in the various leadership frameworks and in the complexity theory of previous sections. For the APN it is important to align yourself with an environment where you can practice in a learning organization. This is an organization where your talents will best be utilized and where positive outcomes will be achieved.

Disruptive and Catalytic Innovation

Christensen, Baumann, Ruggles, and Sadtler (2006) created the disruptive innovation model, which challenges leaders to offer simpler, more convenient, and less expensive alternatives to underserved customers. There are many examples in industry, such as Southwest Airlines, which offered inexpensive no-frills flights that served an unserved market and had a major impact on the travel industry. Frequently leaders are either resistant to or cannot see the innovation because of their mental model or patterns of thinking. Christensen and colleagues (2006) developed a subset of disruptive innovation called catalytic innovation with a focus on social change at a national level. They described the five qualities of catalytic innovators: (1) creating systemic social change through scaling and replication; (2) meeting the needs of the overserved (people who receive too many services that are not needed) or underserved; (3) offering services that are simpler and less costly, but perceived as appropriate for what is needed; (4) generating resources that are considered unattractive by competitors; and (5) tolerating being disparaged by their competitors, who see their market as unprofitable or unattractive (Christensen et al., 2006). Being a disruptive innovator requires creativity at all levels within the organization or as an individual.

At a national level, the changes predicted to characterize health-care reform could lead to catalytic innovation. Realigning the health-care system to ensure access, improve quality, and add value while slowing the rate of inflation offers attractive opportunities for innovation. Those who are creative and can adapt their mental models will be successful in future health-care delivery. Transforming the system requires several changes, including (1) matching clinician skills to the level of the problem, (2) investing in technology that simplifies complex problems, (3) creating new care delivery systems, and (4) changing regulations that impede progress toward this end (Christensen, Bohmer, & Kenagy, 2000). These changes require collaboration across the spectrum of health care.

One prime example of disruptive innovation is the role of the APN. The APN offers services that meet the needs of both the overserved and the underserved. APNs provide services in communities that physicians may view as unprofitable or unattractive for their practice. The services provided are frequently simpler and less costly, and meet the needs of the consumers in different ways from those physicians provide.

Blue Ocean Strategy

Kim and Mauborgne (2005) describe the differences between blue ocean and red ocean strategies in their book *Blue Ocean Strategy*. Blue ocean is a strategy used to "grow demand and break away from the competition" (p. x), whereas red ocean is a strategy used when there is bloody competition for the same market space. The differences in approach surface from how organizations approach the marketplace, competition, demand, value, cost, and differentiation.

The key to blue ocean success is that it is focused on differentiation of services and providers and low cost. It is not an either/or proposition. In providing a framework to create the new value curve, the authors identify four areas where questions should be asked: raise, reduce, create, and eliminate. For example, in looking at an opportunity for an APN in the new health-care reform environment he or she might ask, What factors should be *created* in the new health-care industry that have never been offered before? Similarly, one might ask, What factors should be *eliminated* in the new health-care industry that have previously been taken for granted? Blue ocean strategy is defined through a "reconstructionist" lens. In the reconstructionist view there are no boundaries and there is demand that is untapped. The focus is on creation of value innovation similar to disruptive innovation described earlier.

If we look at the current health-care system and the role of the APN, blue ocean strategy is a perfect framework to change health care and to lead change. Instead of competing in the current market, APNs need to think about creating new models across the system rather than competing from within the system.

An example of blue ocean strategy is the transitional care model defined by Mary Naylor. Naylor and her colleagues (2004) conducted a randomized controlled trial to examine the effectiveness of a transitional care intervention delivered by APNs to elders hospitalized with heart failure. The sample included 239 patients age 65 and older hospitalized with heart failure. A 3-month, APN-directed discharge planning program and home follow-up protocol was implemented. Results demonstrated that there was an increase in the length of time between hospital discharge and readmission or death, and reduced health-care costs. If we look at this model in terms of blue ocean strategy, the APNs were not competing with other services, but rather served as a liaison between hospital and home care services. They recognized no boundaries and offered a service that was in demand. They differentiated themselves from other markets at a lower cost and improved outcomes.

NETWORKING

Networking is defined by Merriam-Webster's dictionary as "the exchange of information or services, among individuals, groups, or institutions; specifically, the cultivation of productive relationships for employment or business." Professional networks are important for job opportunities, professional identity, or obtaining available resources for the patients being served. Rojas-Guyler, Murnan, & Coltrell (2007) described some of the key ways to develop a network: (1) identifying contacts from current or past experiences; (2) getting involved in voluntary agencies outside of your work; (3) attending professional association meetings; (4) accepting leadership roles within those voluntary agencies or professional associations; (5) publishing your findings in your area of practice; (6) presenting at national, state, or community groups or associations; and (7) simply providing your business card to others.

For new and experienced APNs the professional organizations at both a state and national level provide a formal structure for networking. Frequently, there are specific forums that both address professional development opportunities and bring APNs together to deal with political or legislative issues related to practice. As the health-care landscape changes, it is critical that APNs network to determine opportunities for new areas of practice.

Looking for forums that are interprofessional is also important to gaining perspective from outside of the profession. This can be through participation in committees or consortia that are formed at a community, state, or national level.

MENTORING

Dorsey and Baker (2004) describe mentoring as a planned relationship between an experienced person and one with less experience for the purpose of achieving identified outcomes. Joel (1997) describes mentorship as a "patron relationship/system" with varying levels of power, influence, and engagement on a continuum. The continuum goes from the mentor level, which is the most intense, to the level of "peer pals" (peers helping peers), which is the least intense. Mentors may have been role models or preceptors, but the opposite may not be true. Mentoring is helping the protégé develop professionally. Mentoring can be either formal or informal in design. Formal mentoring is where a mentor is assigned in an organization. The question of being assigned a mentor is controversial. Mentor–protégé relationships cannot be forced but must be considered mutually acceptable by both parties. Informal mentoring is where the two parties find each other. Barker (2006) identifies key aspects of the mentor–protégé relationship that should be considered from the beginning. They include the following:

1. Select a mentor who communicates with, and does not talk at, the protégé.
2. It is best if there is no line authority between the mentor and protégé where job security is at issue.
3. The mentor and protégé should have a "good fit" (similar styles, communication patterns, availability, and focus on goal attainment).
4. Mentors who derive energy from oppressive relationships should be avoided.
5. The mentor and protégé should both recognize that relationships will change over time.

When considering a mentor, it is not essential that the mentor be within one's own field but that he or she can meet the professional growth need identified.

The Fellows of the American Academy of Nurse Practitioners (AANP, 2006) conducted a 1-day think tank with new and experienced NPs. They separated their findings based on years of experience in the field. The areas where they found that new NPs needed mentoring included time management and productivity, managing caseloads of patients, developing clinical skills, overcoming fear and anxiety, dealing with isolation, business practices, and work-life balance issues (AANP, 2006). This list could help set goals for new APNs in their mentor–protégé relationships (Harrington, 2011).

Mentoring for experienced NPs took on different areas of need. Their needs included networks for communication; dealing with burnout; development in education, research, and publishing; need for a change; keeping up skills; and the ability to be a mentor themselves (AANP, 2006). Mentors that could be helpful for this group of NPs included peers, educators, researchers, and leaders both inside and outside the profession (AANP, 2006).

Mentorship is even more critical when there are times of uncertainty. As previously discussed, anticipated health-care reform creates both uncertainty and opportunities for APNs. A mentor can help the APN identify new opportunities and provide advice and support for career development, which is vital. Joel (1997) describes how we can help build strength in the nursing ranks by mentoring others. It is the responsibility of those who have the experience and expertise to become mentors to new APNs. It is also the responsibility of the protégé to ensure that his or her objectives and needs are made evident to the mentor and that there is follow-through with the protégé's career plan.

CONCLUSION

This chapter has provided an overview of the various leadership theories and frameworks, and applied them to the role of the APN. There is no more critical time than now for APNs to take the lead in changing the health-care system. This requires engagement by the individual APN, as well as courage to lead in this complex world. Failure to take on a leadership role is not an option. APNs need to be disruptive innovators and seek out the "blue ocean" opportunities to make a difference in U.S. health care. Networking through professional organizations and utilizing mentors can help provide the support needed to move ahead of the curve.

REFERENCES

American Academy of Nurse Practitioners. (2006). *Mentoring assessment.* Retrieved July 14, 2011, from http://www.annp.org.

Barker, E. (2006). Mentoring—A complex relationship. *Journal of the American Academy of Nurse Practitioners, 18,* 56–61.

Bass, B. (1985). *Leadership and performance beyond expectations.* New York: The Free Press.

Bass, B.M., and Riggio, R.E. (2008). *Transformational Leadership, 2nd Ed. Mahwah, NJ: Erlbaum Associates.*

Blanchard, K. (2008, May). Situational leadership. *Leadership Excellence,* 19.

Bolman, L., & Deal, T. (2008). *Reframing organizations.* San Francisco: Jossey-Bass.

Burchill, K. (2010). ARRA and meaningful use: Is your organization ready? *Journal of Healthcare Management, 55*(4), 232–235.

Burns, J. (1978). *Leadership.* New York: Harper & Row.

Center to Champion Nursing in America. (2011, March 1). Retrieved August 15, 2012, from http://championnursing.org/news/regional-action-coalitions.

Christensen, C., Baumann, H., Ruggles, R., & Sadtler, T. (2006). Disruptive innovations for social change. *Harvard Business Review, 12,* 94–101.

Christensen, C., Bohmer, R., & Kenagy, J. (2000). Will disruptive innovations cure health care? *Harvard Business Review, 9,* 102–112.

Covey, S. (2007). *Leadership in the 21st century.* Everest DVD. Franklin Covey.

Dorsey, L., & Baker, C. (2004). Mentoring undergraduate nursing students. *Nurse Educator, 29,* 260–265.

Fielder, F. (2012). *Fielder's Contingency Model.* Retrieved August 15, 2012, from http://www.coachingcosmos.com/38.html

Gallup & The Robert Wood Johnson Foundation. (2010). *Nursing leadership from bedside to boardroom: Opinion leaders' perceptions.* Retrieved June 11, 2011, from http://www.rwjf.org/files/research/nursinggalluppolltopline.pdf.

Goleman, D., & Boyatzis, R. (2008). Social intelligence and the biology of leadership. *Harvard Business Review, 86,* 74–81.

Goleman, D., Boyatzis, R., & McKee, A. (2002). *Primal leadership.* Boston: Harvard Business School Press.

Greenleaf Center for Servant Leadership. (2010). *What is servant leadership?* Retrieved June 20, 2011, from http://www.greenleaf.org.

Hammond, S. (1998). *The thin book of appreciative inquiry* (2nd ed.). Bend, OR: Thin Book Publishing Company.

Hamric, A., Spross, J., & Hanson, C. (2009). *Advanced practice nursing: An integrative approach* (4th ed). St. Louis: Saunders, Elsevier.

Harrington, S. (2011). Mentoring new nurse practitioners to accelerate their development as primary care providers: A literature review. *Journal of the American Academy of Nurse Practitioners, 23,* 168–174.

Health Work Force Solutions, LLC & The Robert Wood Johnson Foundation. (2008). Innovative care models. Retrieved June 8, 2011, from http://innovativecaremodels.com.

Hersey, P., Blanchard, K.H. and Johnson, D.E. (2007). 9th Ed., *Management of organizational behavior: Leading human resources.* Englewood Cliffs, NJ:Prentice Hall.

Institute of Medicine. (2000). *To err is human: Building a safer health system.* Washington, DC: National Academy Press.

Institute of Medicine. (2011). *The future of nursing: Leading change, advancing health.* Washington, DC: National Academies Press.

Joel, L. (1997). Charged to mentor. *American Journal of Nursing, 97*(2), 7.

Jooste, K. (2004). Leadership: A new perspective. *Journal of Nursing Management, 12,* 217–223.

Katzenbach, J., & Smith, D. (1993). *The wisdom of teams: Creating the high performance organizations.* Boston: Harvard Business School Press.

Kim, C., & Mauborgne, R. (2005). *Blue ocean strategy.* Boston: Harvard Business School Publishing.

Kouzes, J., & Posner, B. (2007). *The leadership challenge* (4th ed.). San Francisco: John Wiley & Sons.

Lindberg, C., Nash, S., & Lindberg, C. (2008). *On the edge: Nursing in the age of complexity.* Bordentown, NJ: Plexus Press.

Ludema, J., Whitney, D., Mohr, B., & Griffin, T. (2003). *The appreciative inquiry summit.* San Francisco: Berrett-Koehler Publishers.

Malloch, K., & Porter-O'Grady, T. (2005). *Quantum leader.* Sudbury, MA: Jones & Bartlett.

McCrimmon, M. (2010). *Servant leadership.* Retrieved June 20, 2011, from http://www.leadersdirectlcom/servant-leadership.

Naylor, M., Brooten, D., Campbell, R., Maislin, G., Mc Cauley, K., & Schwartz, J. (2004). Transitional care of older adults hospitalized with heart failure: A randomized controlled trial. *Journal of the American Geriatric Society, 52,* 675–684.

Plsek, P. (2003, January 27 & 28). *Complexity and the adoption of innovation in health care.* Convened by the National Institute for Health Care Management Foundation and the National Committee for Quality Health Care. Washington, DC.

Porter-O'Grady, T., & Malloch, K. (2011). *Quantum leadership* (3rd ed.). Sudbury, MA: Jones & Bartlett Learning.

Raza, S., & Standing, C. (2011). A systemic model for managing and evaluating conflicts in organizational change. *Systems Practice Action Research, 24,* 187–210.

Rojas-Guyler, L., Murnan, J., & Coltrell, R. (2007). Networking for career-long success: A powerful strategy for health education professionals. *Health Promotion Practice, 8*(3), 229–233.

Rost, J. (1995). Leadership: A discussion about ethics. *Business Ethics Quarterly, 5*(1), 129–142.

Senge, P. (1990). *The fifth discipline.* New York: Doubleday.

Sipe, J., & Frick, D. (2009). *Seven pillars of servant leadership: Practicing the wisdom of leading by serving.* Mahwah, NJ: Paulist Press.

Spears, L. (2004). *Practicing servant leadership.* Retrieved June, 20, 2011, from http://www.sullivanadvisorygroup.com.

Stanley, D. (2006). In command of care: Clinical nurse leadership explored. *Journal of Research in Nursing, 11*(1), 20–39.

Stanley, D. (2006). In command of care: Toward the theory of clinical leadership. *Journal of Nursing Research, 2*(2), 132,144.

Stanley, D. (2008, July). Congruent leadership: Values in action. *Journal of Nursing Management, 16(5),* 519–524.

Thompson, G., & Vecchio, R. (2009). Situational leadership theory: A test of three versions. *Leadership Quarterly, 20,* 837–848.

Trader-Leigh, K. (2001). Case study: Identifying resistance in managing change. *Journal of Organizational Change Management Decisions, 36*(8), 543–548.

Uhl-Bien, M. (2006). Relational leadership theory: Exploring the social processes of leadership and organizing. *Leadership Quarterly, 17,* 654–676.

Veronesi, J. (2009). Breaking news on social intelligence. *Journal of Nursing Administration, 39*(2), 57–59.

Vroom, V., & Jago, A. (2007). The role of situation in leadership. *American Psychologist, 62*(1), 17–24.

Vroom, V. H., and Yetton, P. W. (1973). *Leadership and decision-making.* Pittsburg: University of Pittsburg Press.

Wheatley, M. (2006). *Leadership and the new science* (3rd ed.). San Francisco: Berrett-Koehler Publishers.

Wheatley, M. (2007). *Finding our way: Leadership for an uncertain time.* San Francisco: Berrett-Koehler Publishers.

Wheatley, M., & Frieze, D. (2010). Leadership in the age of complexity: From hero to host. Retrieved September 1, 2011, from http://www.margaretwheatley.com/articles/Leadership-in-Age-of-Complexity.pdf.

UNIT 4

Ethical, Legal, and Business Acumen

22

Measuring Advanced Practice Nurse Performance: Outcome Indicators, Models of Evaluation, and the Issue of Value

Shirley Girouard

INTRODUCTION

Although all nurses are critical to improving quality and safety outcomes, advanced practice nurses (APNs) must provide leadership to meet professional and societal obligations throughout the health-care system. Recently, several major national-level initiatives have "pushed the envelope" for the profession and the health-care system. Passage of the Patient Protection and Affordable Care Act (Public Law [PL] 111-148) and the Health Care and Education Reconciliation Act (PL 111-152), modifying some elements of the Affordable Care Act, will continue to foster significant changes in the organization, delivery, and financing of health care and thus have implications for APNs. Also influencing the current climate and expectations for health and health care are the Institute of Medicine (IOM) reports on the future of the nursing profession (IOM, 2011) and on continuing education in the health professions (IOM, 2010).

The purpose of the health-care system is to continuously reduce the impact and burden of illness, injury, and disability and to improve the health and functioning of the people of the United States. Although providing direct care and influencing the direct care provided by others are necessary work and contribute to meeting this goal, they are not sufficient to meet growing professional and societal quality and accountability demands. The current health-care quality climate demands that APNs demonstrate their contributions; continuously improve their performance; and be accountable to the profession, employers, and the public for all components of their role.

As the nurse moves from novice to expert, responsibility for and accountability to self and others for the structures, processes, and outcomes of health care increase proportionally. Achieving the status of APN is not a terminal event, and the role assumes ongoing and increasing professional and societal obligations. Responsibility for health-care quality means that the APN must serve the profession and society as a primary agent for ensuring the quality of health care. In addition, the professional and societal trust afforded to the APN obliges meaningful contributions—beyond individual patient care—to meet the purpose of the health-care system. APNs must not only do good, they must demonstrate their value to society through performance assessment and its documentation and dissemination.

The Case for Accountability

Why should APNs be concerned about these issues? A Web search of the terms *health care AND accountability* resulted in more than 130 million hits. This reflects the importance of this issue in our society. The search revealed that accountability for the quality and costs of health care—its value—are of interest to consumers, purchasers/payers, employers, insurers, the government, and professional provider organizations. Although the demand for accountability for the value of health care is not new, growing complexity and changes in the health-care system raise the issue to a level that cannot be denied or minimized. This demand requires the APN to measure and disseminate information on the value of the role. Nurses in advanced practice, like other providers and health-care system components, need knowledge and skills to assess and measure quality and determine the costs of their services if they are to demonstrate value. It is not enough to "do good"; the APN must demonstrate how "doing good" translates into outcomes and costs.

As Buerhaus and Norman (2001) suggest, the improvement of health-care quality is an "authentic commitment" (p. 68) for all stakeholders and will shape how health-care services are delivered in the future. Given the definition of advanced practice and its role components, APNs must contribute to and lead broad efforts to improve quality. Their actions in defining, measuring, and reporting on their performance will determine their future and that of the health-care system. The advanced practice framework includes patients, health care, nursing, and individual outcomes. Thus, the APN is accountable for performance in all of these domains.

These concepts and obligations are further reflected for the graduate-level student (American Association of Colleges of Nursing [AACN], 2011) because, prepared at this level, the nurse is expected to have advanced role skills, possess refined analytical skills, operate from a broad-based perspective, have the ability to articulate views and positions, and connect theory and practice. The master's-prepared nurse is expected to engage in quality and safety initiatives and collaborate interprofessionally to improve patient and population health outcomes.

The Quality Context

If the health-care system is to reduce the effect and burden of illnesses, injuries, and disabilities and improve outcomes and functioning, all involved in the system must be responsible for identifying and improving the structures and processes for achieving positive outcomes. Research has shown that consumers and society are not getting what they want or need from the health-care system. The IOM (1999, 2001) identified problems with the quality of care and safety concerns. In a study of consumer satisfaction with the health-care system, the Commonwealth Fund (Davis et al., 2002) found that patients were not satisfied with the quality of care they were receiving. Managed care, cost concerns, and the growing consumer movement in health care increased the demand for information about the value (quality in relation to cost) of health-care services and the performance of health-care providers in delivering quality, cost-effective services across all components of the health-care system.

Led by advocacy organizations, consumers are demanding greater accountability from health-care providers and the health-care system. They want quality, cost-effective services delivered from a patient-centered perspective. Federal and state government agencies and other purchasers want to know if the services they pay for are achieving the best possible outcomes at the best price. Organizations that accredit health-care organizations are increasingly seeking evidence that the structures and processes of care produce positive health outcomes.

All these demands to demonstrate and be accountable for value- and cost-effective high-quality care require individuals and groups of providers to measure performance and share their assessments with stakeholders. Organizations such as the National Committee for Quality Assurance (NCQA), the National Quality Forum (NQF), The Joint Commission (TJC), and several agencies of the federal government lead efforts to measure and report on the quality of care provided by various health-care system components. Federal and state agencies, independently and in collaboration with private sector organizations, are collecting and disseminating information about the quality of services provided by the health-care system's various providers. Health-care "report cards" are mechanisms widely employed to address the concerns of consumers, payers, employers, and others about the quality of health care being provided. Report cards are done for hospitals, health plans, and provider groups with the intent of informing consumers and improving quality.

Public reports of health-care quality are done by state and federal governments and private sector organizations. Implementation of the Patient Protection and Affordable Healthcare Act will result in greater reporting at the state and federal levels. Although the impact of these types of reports is not well known (Rand Corporation, 2010), they are likely to proliferate and be increasingly tied to reimbursement as reflected in the Centers for Medicare and Medicaid efforts to tie reimbursement to outcomes of care.

The APN's role includes accountability for patient and systems outcomes. Thus, the APN must measure performance in relation to the outcomes and effect improvements. Assessing performance includes examining the structures and processes of care provided by the APN. In addition, involvement to more broadly influence the health-care system is an essential accountability component.

Values and Value in Health Care

To contribute effectively to fulfilling the purpose of the health-care system, the APN needs a clear vision derived from personal and professional values. The APN needs to embrace society's mandate for health-care value and clarify how the quality and cost issues relate to personal and professional goals. Explicit incorporation of quality and cost values and critical thinking about these issues will result in actions and activities consistent with social demand. Therefore, the APN role can be justified and the needs of society will be better served. APNs will be well positioned to provide leadership in affecting quality and costs, the "bottom line," of health-care system performance.

To be effective leaders and advocates for value issues associated with patients and the role, the APN must know and appreciate what other stakeholders want. Thus, it will be easier to understand their behavior and thinking about health and health care and to develop and implement strategies to address value conflicts, thereby resulting in better health-care outcomes. For example, the APN's employer may value reducing costs to ensure organizational survival, whereas the APN's highest value is meeting the diverse needs of patients served by the organization. Negotiation, compromise, and collaboration are necessary to incorporate both values into strategic planning efforts. Awareness of the importance of values, understanding the value equation, and possessing the skills to address value conflicts are critical for APN survival and health-care system improvement.

The purposes of this chapter are to introduce APN students to quality frameworks, performance measurement, and accountability and to suggest approaches to address current issues and respond to trends. For the graduate APN, this chapter can enhance knowledge and skills that will promote the APN's quality activities, better demonstrate accountability, and foster actions to justify the role of the APN in meeting societal demands for quality, cost-effective health care. The complexity of the quality movement and the value equation are discussed. As the health-care system becomes increasingly complex, as stakeholders' values and visions clash, and as there is growing dissatisfaction with the health-care system, APN leadership is critical. The challenge to establish value and be accountable at all levels may appear daunting, but it is exciting and potentially rewarding for the APN, the profession, and our society.

THE QUALITY ENVIRONMENT

Nursing, beginning with Florence Nightingale, has always given attention to quality issues. Despite our historical roots as leaders in this area, the profession has drifted to a more internal, narrow perspective. Until recently, this mirrored the attention our society gave to the quality of health care. In the United States especially, the values of individualism and self-determination, science and technology, a disease and medical focus, the free-market economy, and nongovernmental interference shaped both the structures and processes of the health-care system, and thus influenced its outcomes. Access and cost issues have, until recently, received more attention than quality, particularly at the societal level. As cost concerns increased and new delivery systems—such as managed care—were implemented, greater attention focused on quality and value. In addition, industry and quality theories and practices in business suggested that lessons learned in these arenas could be applied to the health-care sector.

Definitions and Frameworks

With greater attention being given to quality, long-standing terms and processes were dusted off and a new vocabulary evolved. As shown in **Table 22-1,** there are a plethora of terms used to describe quality concepts. The APN, to operate effectively in the new health-care quality climate, must be fluent in the new language.

One of the earliest conceptual frameworks to describe quality was developed by Donabedian (1966). It is widely used by the nursing community and others in the health-care system as a way to identify the structural and process factors that affect outcomes. Hamric (1983, 1989) provides a model for APN patient care evaluation using Donabedian's framework. Girouard (2000) identifies structural elements that include the APN's education, the time the APN spends in role components, reimbursement levels, and organizational characteristics. Process elements include APN behaviors, referral patterns, prescriptive practice behavior, collaboration, and APN satisfaction. The outcomes related to APN structures and processes include mortality, morbidity, patient knowledge, patient satisfaction, service use, and health status.

Quality of care can also be viewed from a micro or macro perspective. At the micro level, quality is conceptualized and assessed for the patient, the provider, or the institution. Clinical and technical care, satisfaction with care, and quality of life represent components of a micro view (Shi & Singh, 2005). Although always an important component of any quality approach, increasing attention is being given to the macro level—looking at outcomes and cost-effectiveness for populations and society. Examples include the efforts of private sector organizations such as TJC, NQF, NCQA, and the work supported by private foundations. State and federal legislatures and the agencies implementing public policy decisions are also involved in macro-level quality approaches.

CAHMI, in collaboration with consumers, developed an experience of care framework and measures for children and adults. This framework and the measures developed to date are widely used by such organizations as the NCQA, the NQF, the IOM, and the Robert Wood Johnson Foundation for measuring the quality of care provided to large population groups. In addition, federal government agencies such as the Agency for Healthcare Research and Quality (AHRQ) and the Centers for

TABLE 22-1

The Vocabulary of Quality

Access	Ability to obtain care or health and related services (also defined as use or insurance coverage)
Accountability	The demonstration of value (e.g., quality care, patient satisfaction, resource efficiency, and ethical practice); liability for actions
Cost	To the individual paying for services; to the provider to produce services; for society
Outcome	The end result of structures and processes of care; the goal or objective of health and health care
Performance	Assessment of how individual providers behave; measurement assessment of processes of care; may be compared against standards or benchmarks
Process	Method in which health care is provided; provider behaviors; includes technical and interpersonal elements
Quality	How well services increase chance for desired outcomes; knowledge based and evidenced based
Quality assessment	Process of defining and measuring quality Quality assurance Process of measurement and quality improvement; may also be defined as the minimum standards approaches
Quality indicator	Trait or characteristic linked with evidence to desirable health outcomes; may serve as proxy for outcome
Report cards	Collection and reporting of performance and other quality-related data to the public or other targeted groups
Structure	Tools and resources for care (e.g., facilities, licensing and regulation, staffing, equipment)
Total quality	Includes an environment for quality, involves continuous measurement and improvement activities (often called total quality management or continuous quality improvement)

Medicare and Medicaid Services (CMS) and state government agencies have adopted the framework and adapted the measures for a macro approach to quality.

Access, Cost, and Quality

The growing demand for quality requires that attention also be given to access because improved health status and other outcomes of care depend on the individual's ability to receive needed services across the continuum of care. Although often discussed as an issue of access to insurance, for the uninsured and the underinsured, a payment mechanism is not sufficient to improve outcomes. What providers, services, and goods individuals and groups have access to are major factors in achieving desired outcomes and cost efficiencies. Thus, payment levels, what is paid for, and who gets paid are important access considerations in the quality equation. Well-known deficiencies currently exist in mental health-care services, oral health-care services, and nursing services (e.g., the cyclical nursing shortage). The APN should pay particular attention to and justify the needs and benefits resulting from advanced practice nursing services in all health-care settings and for all levels of care.

Cost issues are the third component (along with access and quality) of the health-care system triangle and are essential to establish the value of health care. Cost can be considered from the perspective of the society at large—the total costs of health care, the percentage of national dollars for health-care expenditures. Global expenditures include provider services, insurance, goods and supplies, pharmaceuticals, research, education, core public health services, and institutional costs for delivering health-care services. Consumers and employers are concerned about the direct costs of care. For employers, their insurance costs, loss of productive work time, and health-care program administration costs are considered as a percentage of expenditures needed to conduct their business. Individual consumers, although most often focused on their out-of-pocket costs, are also concerned about the costs of insurance, the price of services and goods needed, and pharmaceutical costs. A third approach when considering health-care costs is the perspective of the health-care professional or health-care organization in which the focus is on expenditures, such as costs for personnel, administration, physical plants, and supplies and equipment, to produce services for groups of patients.

To adequately assess quality at the individual, societal, or organizational level, the APN must be cognizant of access and cost issues and the role they play in determining outcomes. Access and cost issues reflect structural and process elements, the factors that influence health-care outcomes. In addition, this approach holds opportunities for representing the APN as a solution to access and cost concerns. Thus, the APN can make a strong case for the role's value in the health-care system.

Recent Quality Initiatives

A growing number of national quality initiatives reflect the importance of this issue and support the assertion that quality efforts will remain a significant factor in shaping the future of the health-care system. The identification of standards and expected outcomes for access, costs, and quality; their measurement; and public dissemination and discourse are ongoing and expanding. To ensure quality and cost-effective care, quality must be defined; performance expectations specified; and performance and outcomes measured. These are the bases for the quality efforts of national health-care organizations.

Quality measurement is needed to understand the effects of services on individuals and populations and to make improvements in the organization, delivery, and financing of health care. According to the IOM's National Health Care Quality Roundtable (Donaldson, 1999), health-care quality measurement objectives include the following:

- Gathering and analyzing data to inform quality improvement efforts
- Assessing facilities and individual performance in relation to established standards
- Comparing providers to inform purchaser and consumer choice of providers
- Informing all stakeholders about decisions and choices
- Identifying, rewarding, and sharing best practices
- Monitoring and reporting on quality over time
- Addressing the health-care needs of communities

In response to the demand for quality, performance measurement, and accountability, federal and state governments and the private sector have taken action. Government agencies, with congressional policy direction and as major purchasers of health-care services, need information about the quality of health care to guide policy and program decision making. Two government agencies, the AHRQ and the CMS, are worthy of particular attention because quality is a major focus of their activities. The AHRQ, through its internal and external research programs and educational initiatives, is charged to improve the outcomes and quality of health care. In addition, the AHRQ's goals include addressing patient safety and errors, increasing access to effective services, and reducing costs. As a major purchaser (Medicare and Medicaid), the CMS must ensure that its program beneficiaries receive quality, cost-effective care. In addition, through its regulatory functions it sets quality standards for the health-care industry.

An example of a recent AHRQ initiative is a synthesis of completed research to answer questions about which prescriptive drugs reduce costs and improve outcomes. The AHRQ is also evaluating pilot projects that reward providers for delivering high-quality health-care services. They have disseminated a synthesis of studies so clinicians can make better decisions about treating patients with community-acquired pneumonia. Clinicians will also find the AHRQ's "Child Health Tool Box" and other collections of guidelines and measures useful in establishing their own performance measurement and quality programs. An exciting new initiative led by the AHRQ is the development of a national health-care quality report.

Because Medicare and Medicaid beneficiaries use a wide array of health-care services, CMS's quality efforts are far reaching. Among its initiatives are programs to assess quality and performance in hospitals, home care, and long-term care. The quality improvement system for managed care sets regulatory standards and guidelines for quality assessment and improvement and health services management in managed care organizations (MCOs). To address quality in nursing homes, the CMS is assessing and disseminating information about quality in Medicare- and Medicaid-certified long-term care facilities. Through the collection and analysis of uniform patient level data (outcome and assessment information set [OASIS]), CMS is fostering outcome-based quality improvement in home health care.

The initiatives described previously reflect only a few of the federal government's quality-related activities. Other Health and Human Services departments, such as the Centers for Disease Control and Prevention (CDC) and the Maternal and Child Health Bureau (MCHB), are actively engaged in similar activities. State governments are also involved in quality measurement and reporting. For example, New York, Florida, and Washington are measuring provider performance in children's health care.

Private sector organizations representing foundations, purchasers, employers, and professional organizations also measure and report on quality. Accrediting organizations, such as The Joint Commission (TJC, formerly the Joint Commission on Accreditation of Healthcare Organizations), are moving from assessing only structures and processes of care to outcome evaluation. For example, TJC-accredited organizations, through the ORYX initiative, are required to measure specific patient outcomes and provider performance standards. ORYX is TJC's performance measurement and improvement initiative, first implemented in 1997. Safety, medical errors, and infection rates are also being used by TJC as performance indicators. Through an annual report on health-care quality in 271 MCOs, NCQA looks at plan performance related to quality, access, and consumer satisfaction. NCQA's health plan report cards are shared with employers and purchasing groups and are made available for consumer use in choosing health-care plans.

Three national organizations exemplify the private sector's role and collaboration with government agencies to address quality: the Child and Adolescent Health Measurement Initiative (CAHMI), the American Health Quality Association (AHQA), and the NQF. The Foundation for Accountability (FACCT) was dedicated to help consumers make better decisions and choices by informing them about what to expect from the health-care system and by fostering their involvement in holding the health-care system accountable. The CAHMI evaluates health system performance for children covered by Medicaid and private insurance and reports on gaps in care to consumers.

The AHQA represents professionals involved in quality and CMS's quality improvement organization (formerly the peer review organizations) by implementing best practices and fostering quality improvement. By supplying providers and the public with regular updates on quality-of-care research, standards, and other related issues, they educate a wide audience of health-care system stakeholders. The NQF, created in response to the President's Commission on Quality in Health Care, states that its role is to develop and implement a national strategy for quality measurement and reporting. It uses its members and other experts to assess research and performance reports and provide guidance for improving health-care quality. For example, it issued a report that identified disparities in health care for minority populations and suggested priority activities to address these disparities.

Employers are also involved in health-care quality through their demand for information about quality and performance. Accountability is achieved through the measurement and reporting of performance measures and though incentives for providers. For example, large employers in Massachusetts are offering bonuses to providers who improve the care of patients with diabetes and who use an electronic database to follow chronically ill patients.

As these initiatives suggest, the APN's performance is already being measured—directly as a primary care provider and indirectly as a contributor to the health-care team's performance. Thus, the APN must be aware of national issues, trends, and approaches in quality measurement and improvement to guide practice and other professional activities. As is discussed later in this chapter, there are additional actions to be taken to participate more fully in the quality movement.

ADVANCED PRACTICE NURSE PERFORMANCE EXPECTATIONS

Because the core of advanced practice nursing is the clinical role, the APN is positioned to address quality issues and to be held accountable for quality provided. According to the American Association of Colleges of Nursing (AACN, 1996), advanced practice nursing education prepares the graduate to "assume responsibility and accountability for the health promotion, assessment, diagnosis and management of patient problems within a specialty area of clinical practice" (p. 12). As described by Brown (2000), the following are five characteristics of the clinical role:

- Use of a holistic perspective
- Formation of patient–APN partnerships
- Expert clinical thinking and skillful practice
- Research-based practice
- Diverse approaches to health and illness management

These characteristics parallel consumer and other stakeholder expectations for the health-care system and are expectations for which the APN can be held accountable. Each reflects quality concerns driving the value equation in health care.

Patient partnerships with providers are key to ensuring quality. Consumers want and need information about their care and their providers to be true partners. The APN's holistic perspective in caring for patients, when translated into practice behaviors, will meet consumer expectations. By partnering with patients, APNs guide patient decision making within the current health-care context. Because consumers desire these partnerships with providers, these aspects of quality are recognized as important determinants of quality. For example, questions about consumer experiences with these dimensions of health-care quality are contained in the Consumer Assessment of Health Plan Survey (CAHPS) tools. These tools are widely used by government and private agencies to assess health-care system quality.

The health-care system's providers are also expected to provide expert clinical thinking and skillful performance based on the best evidence. Quality health care is characterized by the use of evidence to identify the interventions and services that enhance outcomes. Patients want, need, and often seek (from a variety of sources) knowledge about all aspects of their health-care problem and its treatment, expected outcomes, health promotion, and disease prevention. APNs, with expertise in a specialized aspect of patient care, should have the knowledge to inform patients and make good clinical decisions in partnership with their patients or groups of patients.

Finally, the expectation that the APN uses diverse approaches to health and illness management suggests the need to identify best practices likely to improve outcomes for individual patients or groups of patients. Tailoring care decisions to patient needs and values within the current context requires APNs to understand both the patient and the context. Knowledge about what works in what situations and with what types of patients is essential, and along with skills to apply the knowledge, is an additional expectation of the APN.

Brown's (2000) characteristics are reflected in the U.S. Department of Health and Human Services (USDHHS) Health Resources and Services Administration, Bureau of Health Professions, Division of Nursing (2002) six domains and competencies for APNs. Four of the domains relate specifically to direct clinical practice: (1) management of patient health and illness status, (2) the nurse–patient relationship, (3) the teaching-coaching function, and (4) professional role. The remaining two domains are more global in scope: (5) managing and negotiating health-care delivery systems and (6) monitoring and ensuring quality of health-care practice. The APN is expected to perform competently in all six domains. Thus, the APN is accountable for the competencies within each domain. Domains one to four are patient care structures, processes, and outcomes amenable to evaluation by patients and other health-care system stakeholders. Domains five and six provide a framework for assessing the more global aspects of the APN's role, affecting patients less directly. Competencies associated with domain five, managing and negotiating health-care delivery systems, are directly applicable to the APN's role in quality. Competencies include the following:

Managing:

- Demonstrates knowledge about the role of the nurse practitioner in case management
- Provides care for individuals, families, and communities within integrated health-care services
- Considers access, cost, efficacy, and quality when making care decisions
- Maintains current knowledge of the organization and financing of the health-care system as it affects delivery of care
- Participates in organizational decision making, interprets variations in outcomes, and uses data from information systems to improve practice
- Manages organizational functions and resources within the scope of responsibilities as defined in a position description
- Uses business and management strategies for the provision of quality care and efficient use of resources
- Demonstrates knowledge of business principles that affect long-term financial viability of a practice, the efficient use of resources, and quality of care
- Demonstrates knowledge of relevant legal regulations for nurse practitioner practice, including reimbursement of services

Negotiating:

- Collaboratively assesses, plans, implements, and evaluates primary care with other health-care professionals, using approaches that recognize each one's expertise to meet the comprehensive needs of patients
- Participates as a key member of an interdisciplinary team through the development of collaborative and innovative practices
- Participates in the planning, development, and implementation of public and community health programs

- Participates in legislative and policy-making activities that influence health services and practice
- Advocates for policies that reduce environmental health risks
- Advocates for policies that are culturally sensitive
- Advocates for increasing access to health care for all

Monitoring and ensuring the quality of health-care practice, domain six, is specific to the APN's role in quality and performance measurement. In addition, the competencies speak specifically to APN accountability. The competencies are the following:

Ensuring quality:

- Interprets own professional strengths, role, and scope of ability to peers, patients, and colleagues
- Incorporates professional and legal standards into practice
- Acts ethically to meet the needs of patients
- Assumes accountability for practice and strives to attain the highest standards of practice
- Engages in self-evaluation concerning practice and uses evaluative information, including peer review, to improve care and practice
- Collaborates or consults with members of the health-care team about variations in health outcomes
- Uses an evidence-based approach to patient management that critically evaluates and applies research findings pertinent to patient care management and outcomes
- Evaluates the patient's response to the health care provided and the effectiveness of the care
- Uses the outcomes of care to revise care delivery strategies and improve the quality of care
- Accepts personal responsibility for professional development and the maintenance of professional competence and credentials
- Considers ethical implications of scientific advances and practices accordingly

Monitoring quality:

- Monitors quality of own practice and participates in continuous quality improvement based on professional practice standards and relevant statutes and regulation
- Evaluates patient follow-up and outcomes including consultation and referral
- Monitors research to improve quality care

Clearly, professional expectations, such as those discussed previously, embody quality and accountability expectations for the APN in direct clinical care and within the health-care system. The APN is expected to do good for patients, measure performance in relationship to best practices, and be held accountable for practice. But that is not enough; APN expectations include quality-related issues that extend beyond direct clinical care to the health-care system and its quality and accountability issues.

MEASURING QUALITY AND PERFORMANCE

During the past several years, there have been significant efforts to define and measure quality and performance as reflected in the literature. The APN will find the literature helpful to begin the development of a professionally and personally relevant framework to measure quality, evaluate performance, and identify meaningful indicators to justify the role and fulfill the expectations of the role. The structures, processes, and outcomes associated with APN practice can be evaluated at the individual's practice level, for groups of providers and organizations, for care systems (such as MCOs), and at the societal level. The APN should be knowledgeable about all of these approaches and involved at all levels. The intensity of involvement at a given level varies with the position held, employer expectations, level of knowledge, skill in evaluation, and other demands.

Individual Level

APNs can assess their ability to meet the expectations for advanced practice nursing by using core competencies promulgated by the National Organization of Nurse Practitioner Faculties (NONPF). The competencies are acquired through mentored patient care experiences with emphasis on independent and interprofessional practice; analytic skills for evaluating and providing evidence-based, patient-centered care across settings; and advanced knowledge of the health-care delivery system. Earlier versions of the core competencies authored in 2002 and 2006 were applicable for master's preparation, and for the doctor of nursing practice (DNP) graduate as additive to the core competencies for the master's graduate. As of 2011, there was one set of core competencies for entry into practice on graduation, regardless of whether preparation was in a master's or DNP program (NONPF, 2011).

Most APNs are probably already involved with directly measuring their individual performance. For example, annual performance reviews are a part of most employer–employee relationships. Generally, this type of evaluation focuses on the processes of care, productivity, and position description expectations. When outcomes, such as effectiveness of care, costs, or patient satisfaction with care, are measured by APNs, they generally apply to the individual's work or program-specific goals. Recent quality and performance measurement approaches suggest opportunities for the APN to evaluate performance more broadly and in other domains. For example, some state Medicaid programs are assessing their beneficiaries' experiences with care and providing feedback to individual providers. APNs can use such information to compare their care with other providers and state norms, thus identifying areas for improvement. Although these data are infrequently shared with consumers, it is likely to be made more widely available in the future.

Group Level

Evaluation of the structures, processes, and outcomes for groups of providers are a growing component of national initiatives to assess quality and performance. APNs may evaluate their practice as a group of APNs or in groups of diverse health-care providers. For example, nurse-midwives can join together to assess the costs, patient satisfaction, and birth outcomes associated with their practice. APNs in a family practice group that includes physicians can determine how their performance compares with that of other group practices. NCQA's performance health plan measurement data can be abstracted to the provider group level and thus can be compared to national or state norms. The hospital-based APN can participate in evaluating patient outcomes for specific populations of patients and in determining performance in relation to issues such as infection rates, antibiotic use, patient safety, and medication errors.

With the advent of setting- and group-specific data collection, analysis, and reporting, opportunities exist for the APN to use findings from these reviews to develop and implement quality improvement in the practice setting. For example, a geriatric nurse practitioner (NP) working with a long-term care facility can use the nursing home–specific reports generated by CMS to design programs to improve structures and processes of care related to specific outcomes. Findings of TJC can guide the hospital-based APN to identify goals for patient care, developing processes for improvement, and assessing the effect of changes made.

Systems Level

Health-care plans, MCOs, and Medicaid programs are being evaluated and held accountable to consumers and purchasers of care for the quality they provide. As panel or staff members in these health-care delivery systems, APN care is also being assessed. It is assumed that purchasers of care and consumers will use the information increasingly being made available to make purchasing decisions.

The Consumer Assessment of Healthcare Providers and Systems (CAHPS) Clinician and Group Surveys (CG-CAHPS) ask patients about their recent experiences with clinicians and their staff. These surveys, used by state Medicaid agencies, Medicare, NCQA, and others, ask consumers to report on their care in a number of domains. Survey questions ask about timeliness of care, provider communication, and satisfaction with the provider. NCQA uses these tools and the Healthplan Employer Data and Information Set (HEDIS) to evaluate the quality of care in more than 90% of the nation's health plans. HEDIS data are obtained from administrative data sources and chart audits to assess effectiveness of care using indicators derived from research and expert opinion (AHRQ, 2012).

State Medicaid programs use both CAHPS and HEDIS to assess the performance of care provided to beneficiaries. In addition, a number of states are assessing the quality of children's health-care services using tools such as those developed and tested by CAHMI. For example, one parent survey asks about providers' ability to meet expectations related to promoting healthy development (PHD) in young children.

CAHPS, HEDIS, and PHD measures, as well as other tools used to assess quality at the systems or health-plan level, are evidence based, psychometrically tested, and widely endorsed by providers, consumers, and other stakeholders. Given the current demand for quality information, these efforts are likely to grow in the future. APNs, as practitioners in most of these settings, should be familiar with the performance assessment measures used in their workplace and regularly review reports to continuously improve quality and meet national performance standards.

Societal Level

At the societal level, there are a number of existing and evolving approaches to assess the quality of the nation's health-care system and its outcomes. *Healthy People* (USDHHS, 2012) sets health outcome goals, identifies indicators to measure progress in achieving these goals, and lists structures and processes needed to meet the goals. The nation's health quality is also being assessed by a number of private sector organizations such as advocacy and consumer groups and foundations. For example, the Commonwealth Fund, using national databases, has issued a report card with information about the appropriateness and effectiveness of treatment and prevention in chronic disease, medical mistakes, costs, patient-centered care, and disparities in care (Commonwealth Fund, 2011).

Congress mandated that AHRQ produce an annual report to the nation on health-care quality. Also, the AHRQ produces a national report on disparities in health care. The National Healthcare Quality Report (AHRQ, 2008a) includes measures of effectiveness of care, safety, and patient-centered care. Disparities in quality, access, use, and costs for low-income groups, minority groups, women, children, older adults, and people with special health-care needs are reported in the National Health-care Disparities Report (AHRQ, 2008b).

The quality and performance measurement approaches discussed previously represent a sample of the increasing number of activities in this area. The models section of this chapter includes more detailed descriptions of these efforts, and the recommendations section contains specific actions for the APN's greater involvement at all levels. All are important to the APN to justify the role and to be accountable for meeting the expectations of society for the advanced practice role. All have strengths and weaknesses when considered from the perspective of the APN.

Individual-level performance, especially when evaluated using nonstandardized methodologies, provides information of value to only the APN and the employer. Without comparative data, the APN's performance cannot be assessed in relation to other providers; thus, it is more difficult to justify the role and identify APN contributions to outcomes. Individual-level performance evaluation may be necessary, but it is not sufficient to justify the role or its contributions to quality health care. When performance is assessed at the group, system, or societal level, especially when using standard, tested approaches, the APN is better positioned to justify the role and demonstrate contributions to health-care outcomes. In addition, quality improvement goals derived from these measurement efforts are those that are of greatest social value. However, doing only group-, system-, or societal-level evaluation means that APN-dependent performance may be more difficult to articulate.

APPROACHES AND MODELS FOR PERFORMANCE EVALUATION

As the APN begins or enhances strategies to evaluate performance, quality, and value, a framework is needed to guide decision making and plan for effective and meaningful assessments of the role and its contributions. There are many approaches and models for the APN to consider. The APN should assess the approaches and models in relation to their relevance and adaptability to meet the APN's specific needs, justify the role, and measure APN contributions to health and health care in choosing an approach to evaluation. The goals of APN quality measurement are the following:

- Develop new and adopt existing data collection methods relevant to the APN role
- Establish APN competency and practice standards aligned with facility, systems, and societal quality standards
- Compare APN practice with other providers and groups of providers
- Improve performance based on evidence
- Monitor and report quality over time to all stakeholders
- Address community and societal health-care needs

Donabedian (1966) provides a basic framework for quality measurement at all levels. Although structures, processes, and outcomes of care can all be examined and used as quality indicators, it is important to provide evidence that measures of specific structures and processes are related to outcomes. In addition, outcomes chosen should be those of importance to health-care stakeholders. Selecting indicators that are of interest only to the APN does not serve to establish the role's value or its contributions to meeting the purpose of health care and the health-care system. Studies of the relationship of nurse staffing (a structural measure) to patient outcomes demonstrate how this can be done (Aiken, Clarke, Sloane, Sochalski, & Silber, 2001, 2002; Needleman, Buerhaus, Mattke, Stewart, & Zelevinsky, 2002). The researchers provide evidence for selection of the structural variables (nurse staffing) and for the relationship between nurse staffing and patient outcomes. The importance of their work to a variety of stakeholders, such as TJC (Joint Commission on the Accreditation of Healthcare Organizations, 2002) and the American Hospital Association (AHA, 2002), is reflected in the media attention given to these studies.

Structure, Process, and Outcome Measures

Structural measures related to quality and specific to the APN role include characteristics of the APN (education, experience, legal aspects, and role expectations), the practice or organizational setting (group resources, organizational structure, and provider relationships), and access to services (referral mechanisms, collaboration, and geographical location). Process measures focus on the nature of the APN's interventions and interactions with patients. In current quality terminology, process and performance measures are synonymous. Process measures include the APN's competence in diagnosis and management of health-care problems, prevention, teaching, and counseling, interpersonal aspects of care, and technical care (e.g., errors and medication misuse). Outcomes reflect the results of structures and processes for individual patients, groups of patients, or society. Traditional quality outcome measures are mortality and morbidity. With increasing attention to assessing the quality of health care, patient experience or satisfaction with care, costs, and access are often considered as outcome measures. The framework and evaluation models selected for use by the APN and the purpose and goals of the quality assessment process determine how the APN views patient satisfaction, costs, and access as indicators of quality.

A common model for measuring APN effectiveness encompasses structures, processes, and outcomes. Structural variables include legal issues and funding, organization of care delivery, and use of the APN. Process and performance measures reflect the direct and indirect patient care activities of the APN. The model includes both short- and long-term outcomes. Short-term outcomes include accessibility, satisfaction, patient knowledge and health behaviors, and complications of care. Optimal health status, morbidity, mortality, and costs of care are long-term indicators of quality.

Individual Level

Because APNs are involved in evaluating their performance as a component of their organizational responsibilities, approaches to this level of evaluation are important. In addition, individual-level performance processes can be designed to address evaluation needs at the group and organizational, system, or societal levels. The purpose of the individual evaluation is to assess APN achievement of competencies and to measure performance in meeting position or job description expectations. The APN works with peers, physician collaborators, and supervisors to determine the specific factors to be assessed and to identify or design an evaluation methodology. Approaches to individual-level evaluation may include structures, processes, and outcomes. Mason and colleagues (1999) examined the structural issue of MCO credentialing and found that more than half of NPs had never sought MCO credentialing. Other studies focusing on structure have looked at patient characteristics within APN practices, providing valuable information about the types of patients served (Hamric, Worley, Lindeback, & Jaubert, 1999; Paine, et al., 1999). Other APN-related structural variables studied include uses of technology (Borchers & Kee, 1999), identification of activities (Knaus, Felten, Burton, Fobes, & Davis, 1997), and use of hospital data systems (Bozzo, Carlson, & Diers, 1998).

Satisfaction with APN care is a traditional part of APN evaluation. Oermann, Lambert, and Templin (2000) found that having access to nurse-midwives was an important quality of care element for parents. Larrabee, Ferri, and Hartig (1997) found high levels of satisfaction with most aspects of NP care and used those areas with lower ratings to guide quality improvement efforts. Numerous other studies have demonstrated that patients and other providers are satisfied with the care delivered by APNs (Aquilino, Damiano, Willard, Momony, & Levy, 1999; Garvisan, Grimsey, Littlejohns, Lownes, & Stacks, 1998; McMullen, 1999). Instruments have been developed, and their psychometric properties tested, that can be useful to the APN in determining patient satisfaction with NP care (Cole, Mackay, & Lindenberg, 1999).

Assessing the processes of APN care focuses on the nature of the APN's activities and interventions for direct patient care and their indirect patient care activities such as staff teaching and planning. Examples of instruments developed for this purpose include those of Ingersoll (1988); Tierney, Grant, and Mazique (1990); Kearnes (1992); Houston and Luquire (1991); and Girouard and Spross (1983).

Oermann (1999) studied consumer descriptions of quality of care and found that consumers believed quality nursing care meant having nurses who were competent and skilled, communicated effectively, conducted patient teaching, and demonstrated caring behaviors. These elements of quality are consistent with other reports of consumer expectations and thus should be included in the APN's measurement as indicators of care quality. Evaluation of these processes is important for role justification and the identification of nursing processes that affect quality outcomes. A number of studies have demonstrated APN contributions to process indicators of quality (Bozzo et al., 1998; Diers & Bozzo, 1997; Diers, Bozzo, Blatt, & Roussel, 1998; East & Colditz, 1996; Jacavone, Daniels, & Tyner, 1999; Pelletier-Hibbert, 1998).

APNs play a major role in the development, implementation, and evaluation of practice guidelines, clinical protocols, and clinical pathways that guide the processes of care. NPs, for example, develop protocols for their collaborative practices with physicians. APNs in hospitals, home care, long-term care, and other settings have leadership opportunities in this area as well. Examples in the literature include the work of Musclow, Sawhney, and Watt-Watson (2002); Morin and colleagues (1999); Sagehorn, Russell, and Ganong (1999); McDaniel (1999); Jacavone and colleagues (1999); Kee and Borchers (1998); and Card and colleagues (1998). APNs have also described and measured processes of care for a variety of patients (Barnason & Rasmussen, 2002; Beal & Philips, 1999; Brooten & Naylor, 1995; Coward, 1998; Strohschein, Schaffer, & Lia-Hoagberg, 1999).

Outcomes, as the result of the APN's clinical activities, given their importance in quality improvement and accountability, are the most meaningful components of the APN's evaluation process. The reference list at the end of this chapter includes a number of studies that illustrate how APNs evaluated the effectiveness of their practice and outcomes. Additional studies described the costs and demonstrated the cost-effectiveness of APN practice (Burl, Bonner, Rao, & Kahn, 1998; Dahle, Smith, Ingersoll, & Wilson, 1998; Lombness, 1994; Walker, Baker, & Chiverton, 1998). Studies linking structures, processes, and outcomes of APN care are particularly important to document APN effectiveness and to determine best practices for the organization and delivery of patient care services. For example, Rudy and colleagues (1998) examined relationships between staff type, activities of care giving, and patient outcomes. Other examples of this type of evidence include the work of Mundinger and Kane (2000) comparing NP and physician outcomes in primary care. (Additional examples, including the work of Aiken, Brooten, and others, are included in the reference list.)

Little information is available to describe the APN's contributions to achieving broad community- or societal-level health-care goals such as those in *Healthy People* (USDHHS, 2012). Although the effect of an individual APN or even a group of APNs may be difficult to measure on such outcomes as health promotion and disease prevention, given the number of contributing factors, APNs should begin to identify how to address these most important societal outcomes. As national assessments of quality and outcomes are developed, the APN has an opportunity to begin to examine practice in relation to these evolving indicators. The models for assessing health-care quality described in the following can be used to shape the APN's quality and performance assessment goals, especially at the systems and societal levels.

Group, System, and Societal Levels

During the past several years, there have been a number of organized efforts to evaluate the quality of health care in the United States. Some are well established as evaluation models, although they are constantly being refined and updated. Other efforts are in earlier stages of development. There is significant consistency and collaboration among all stakeholders to develop approaches and models that will better determine quality, measure performance, demonstrate value, and allow for health-care providers and systems to be held accountable. Nurses, including the APN, and organizations of nurses are increasingly involved in all phases of these activities. Some of the most promising and widely accepted approaches are described to provide the APN with a broad view of current approaches and models.

Although the individual's performance and the APN's care-related outcomes are important, they take on greater meaning when they can be compared. The APN is encouraged to participate in the development, testing, and use of standardized instruments to measure structures, processes, outcomes, and satisfaction with care to allow for comparisons. In the discussion of group, system, and societal measures that follows, it is clear that group- and system-level assessments will, in the near future, allow for individual provider tracking in relation to performance and outcomes of care. The APN can use these data for individual performance assessments.

One of the most widely used frameworks for quality and performance measurement reflects the way consumers think about their care (FACCT, 1999). The categories of the framework are the following:

- The basics: satisfaction with the delivery of care by providers, access to care, and receipt of information and services
- Staying healthy: avoiding illness, health promotion through preventive care, reduction of health risks, early detection of illness, and health education
- Getting better: appropriateness of treatment and follow-up care to help recover from illness or injury
- Living with illness: self-care guidance, symptom control, avoidance of complications, and maintaining daily activities for people with chronic illness
- Changing needs: comprehensiveness of services, caregiver support, and hospice care that helps individuals and families when needs change dramatically because of a severe disability or terminal illness

Evidence-based measures are identified or new measures are developed and field tested for each of the categories and are used as standards for accountability. FACCT's framework is widely used by national accrediting organizations, such as NCQA and TJC, federal and state agencies, and others, to measure quality and organize quality reporting. For example, the Commonwealth Fund's score card on health care quality (2011) uses the FACCT framework to organize the information contained in the report.

Another framework commonly used for quality and performance measurement is that put forward by the IOM (2001). Experts and a wide variety of health-care system stakeholders, including consumers, developed the framework. It includes six dimensions of quality: safety, effectiveness, equity, patient centeredness, efficacy, and timeliness. It, too, is the conceptual framework that guides other organizations and individuals in quality measurement, improvement, reporting, and research.

The Consumer Assessment of Health Plans (AHRQ, 2008a) is a national quality measurement initiative conducted by AHRQ through a number of research organizations. It uses elements of the FACCT framework to organize survey questions designed to assess consumer experience with care. There are general surveys and surveys specific to special populations such as children and people with chronic conditions. CAHPS is used by NCQA and others as a standardized approach to provider and health plan quality and performance measurement. The Obama administration established *Partnerships for Patients: Better Care, Lower Cost.* This public–private partnership focuses on safety and reducing unnecessary hospital admissions (USDHHS, 2011).

The NCQA assesses and reports on the performance and quality of MCOs and health plans, including those that serve Medicare and Medicaid beneficiaries in managed-care plans. Both the FACCT and IOM conceptual frameworks are used by NCQA. Data are collected on individual providers and aggregated to the health organization (plan) level. HEDIS and CAHPS serve as the measure sets for assessing quality and performance. HEDIS includes more than 60 evidence-based consensus measures of effectiveness of care. Measures such as immunization levels, breast and cervical cancer screening, chlamydia screening, antidepressant medication management, postcoronary beta-blocker medication use and cholesterol management, comprehensive diabetes care, hypertension control, follow-up after hospitalization for mental illness, prenatal and postnatal care, and appropriate medication treatment for people with asthma are included in the data set (NCQA, 2011). The HEDIS and CAHPS data are analyzed and reported publicly.

Another private sector initiative addressing quality and performance in the health-care system is the NQF (National Forum for Healthcare Quality Measurement and Reporting, 2002). NQF is a membership organization representing a diverse group of public and private sector stakeholders, and its mission is to standardize quality of care performance measurement and reporting mechanisms. NQF has endorsed a list of procedures to promote patient safety; developed a framework for achieving their mission; and identified strategies to reduce health-care disparities. Future plans include developing sets of performance measures for hospitals, nursing homes, cancer care, and diabetes care. The hospital performance measures are created using the IOM's six domains of quality: safety, effectiveness, equity, patient centeredness, efficacy, and timeliness.

Purchasers of care and the business community are adopting existing quality and performance measurement models and assessment methodologies to meet their needs to determine the value of the health care they purchase. For example, a Minnesota coalition of large purchasers, the Buyers Health Care Action Group, assesses quality to increase value, choice, and health-care accountability. The National Business Coalition has strategies to improve patient safety and reduce medical errors by fostering consumer awareness; promoting the use of standardized measurement and reporting; rewarding quality; and supporting and using contract standards for safety. Many business coalitions, employers, and purchasers use data from national organizations such as the NCQA to improve their and their employees' ability to make better health plan choices and to hold health plans accountable.

As the major accrediting organization for hospitals, TJC has a long history of assessing structures and processes of care. During the past several years, and with the introduction of ORYX (a performance and outcome measurement program), TJC has moved toward outcomes assessment. Patient safety, including medication errors and infection rates, are receiving greater attention as quality indicators. Nurses involved in the development and testing of models to improve access quality are also an important consideration. For example, patient satisfaction with hospital care was addressed by Dozier, Kitzman, Ingersoll, Holmberg, and Schultz (2001). They developed and tested a tool, Patient Perception of Hospital Experience with Nursing, to assess whether or not patients' needs were met by nurses. These tools, and others developed by nurses to assess other nurse-dependent outcomes, are an important alternative to traditional patient care satisfaction tools that focus on amenities of care rather than competencies of nursing practice and to evaluate nurse-dependent outcomes.

The federal government's Medicare, Medicaid, and State Child Health Insurance Program both use and drive quality efforts through the evaluation of care to their beneficiaries in health maintenance organizations and MCOs, long-term care, and home care. HEDIS and CAHPS are used to assess plan quality. As a purchaser of care, CMS is able to demand quality and accountability and does so through contracts that specify quality measures and the identification of specific performance improvement goals. For example, CMS and states are involved in a voluntary performance measurement project using HEDIS measures. CMS's OASIS uses patient-level home-health agency data to assess and improve quality in Medicare-certified home-health agencies (Shaughnessy, Crisler, Hittle, & Schenkler, 2002).

In November 2002, CMS released the Nursing Home Quality Report for 17,000 nursing homes across the country (CMS, 2002). The report includes information about quality, inspection results, and nurse staffing levels that can be compared to state and national norms. The quality measures include ability to perform activities of daily living, pressure sores, use of physical restraints, infection rates, delirium incidence, pain management, and ambulation. Mullan and Harrington (2001) used these data to confirm deficiencies in nursing homes.

Other federal agencies such as the Bureau of Primacy Health Care (BPHC) and the MCHB are implementing quality assessment and quality improvements initiatives. For example, BPHC's quality center coordinates quality initiatives and conducts strategic planning to enhance the quality of primary health care, especially for the community health centers it supports. MCHB, in part using CAHMI measures, has sponsored national surveys of children with special health-care needs to determine their health status and the quality of care they are receiving.

The federal government's Quality Interagency Coordination Task Force represents another model of collaboration in the quality arena. The task force is to coordinate efforts across all federal agencies involved in health and health-care quality and its improvement. Task force participants are the Departments of Health and Human Services, Labor, Defense, Veterans Administration, and Commerce; the Office of Management and Budget; the Coast Guard; the Federal Bureau of Prisons; the National Highway Traffic Safety Administration; the Federal Trade Commission; and the AHRQ. They are to improve safety, improve patient and consumer information on quality, develop the health-care workforce, and improve information systems. The AHRQ's National Healthcare Quality and National Healthcare Disparities Reports use a framework that includes the IOM's dimensions of care and FACCT's patient need frameworks.

State governments, advocacy organizations, professional organizations, provider organizations, foundations, and others are undertaking other efforts and using the conceptual frameworks offered by the IOM and FACCT to guide the development of measures or the use of existing measures in their quality strategies. For example, the states of Vermont and California are using the CAHMI performance measurement tools to assess quality of health care for children who are Medicaid beneficiaries. Children NOW, a California advocacy organization, issues report cards on child health status using the CAHMI measures. School-based clinics are using HEDIS-like measures to assess and improve the quality of care in these settings. FACCT, using its adult and child health quality measures, had consumer-centered tools for use by individuals, employers, and purchasers of care. For example, "Compare Your Care" was a computer-based program that helped consumers compare their care experience to national and regional benchmarks derived from evidence-based practice guidelines. One module provides a formulary to help inform consumers about 10 health conditions and what prescription medications are best for them.

As the preceding discussion suggests, there is consistency and collaboration across the health-care system in relation to the conceptual frameworks used for measuring health-care quality. The FACCT and IOM frameworks guide most of the assessment, research, and reporting related to quality. Similarly, there is a fast-growing consensus for the use of HEDIS, CAHPS, CAHMI, and similar measures to assess quality in the domains suggested by the conceptual frameworks. Another trend is the significant collaboration and cooperation among a wide variety of stakeholders at all levels. The current climate also strongly suggests that health-care quality models and approaches must include the assessment of care in relation to what consumers want from the system, must be evidence based, and must use standardized and tested measurement approaches. The APN will be well positioned to justify the role and operationalize the APN contribution to health and health care if these and related theoretical frameworks are used. In addition, collaboration, the use of evidence in measure development, rigorous measure testing (or the use of tested measures), and linking structural and process factors to outcomes or quality indicators are vital for APNs to achieve the purposes of their quality and performance assessment activities.

RECOMMENDATION FOR ACTION

To meet the expectations of advanced practice nursing, the APN must transform expert knowledge and skill into actions that contribute to meeting societal health-care goals. One of the most important opportunities for influence is to affect changes that improve outcomes for individual patients, groups of patients, health-care organizations, systems, and society. The APN can and should exert influence to make this change a reality. To improve quality, it must be defined from an evidence base, have outcome standards identified against which to measure quality and performance, have identified best structures and processes linked to outcomes, be tested and articulated, be assessed at all levels, and be shared with all stakeholders.

The sixth domain of advanced practices (USDHHS, 2002) is monitoring and ensuring the quality of health-care practice. Competency in this domain is demonstrated when the APN engages in quality monitoring and quality assurance activities. Knowledge and skill for these competencies begin with graduate education, building on the student's undergraduate education, and professional experience, and are continuously enhanced through education and practice experiences. In addition, nursing research and other health-care literature should be regularly scanned and the media closely followed to assess trends and keep knowledge up to date. Many of the quality-focused and professional organizations (such as the American Nurses Association, nursing specialty organizations, and nursing research societies) provide electronic and paper newsletters that can help the APN stay informed.

The skills needed to effect change in the quality arena are the core competencies of advanced practice, direct clinical practice, research skills, clinical and professional leadership, ethical decision-making skills, collaboration, consultation, and expert coaching and guidance. Applying these skills beyond the individual patient practice level increases the APN's ability to influence quality. Skills grow over time as the APN gets more involved in addressing quality concerns. As others become aware of the APN's expertise in patient care and quality, and as the APN seeks new opportunities, the sphere of influence will grow.

There are actions the APN can take at all levels and in relation to the practice, education, research, administration, and advocacy roles of advanced practice nursing. Each role component is discussed and examples of actions are provided. Although challenging, active engagement in the quality movement ensures recognition of the value of the APN role and better outcomes that will improve the health and reduce the burden of illness for U.S. citizens.

Practice

In direct clinical care, the APN should practice from an evidence base; deliver patient-centered care; be accessible to the patient; be responsive to patient needs, preferences, and concerns; and avoid missed opportunities to deliver preventive and health promotion services. The APN's role modeling and expertise in delivery system operations can guide others to provide quality patient care and engage in quality improvement activities. Operationalizing Brown's (2000) characteristics of the clinical role will also result in quality care and quality improvement. Noll and Girard (1993) provide a typology for quality activities related to APN competencies.

At the practice level, the APN can contribute to the quality movement by collecting accurate and timely data for research and quality assessment purposes. The APN should participate in group practice, organizational, and professional organization quality activities aimed at assessing quality, performance, access, and costs. Partnering with consumers on quality issues is also expected and desirable. For example, quality advisory committees that include consumers can be formed at the practice level to identify patients' quality concerns and approaches to quality improvement.

APNs must also participate in formal quality improvement programs and activities at the practice level. Participation and leadership in accrediting and quality reviews by regulators, including TJC, is another action the APN can take to engage in quality measurement and improvement.

Another practice-level set of activities that can be used for quality purposes is use of the position description and annual performance reviews. Position descriptions can be rewritten to reflect the elements of the IOM and FACCT models. Clear articulation of the goals and objectives of the review, and the use of standardized measures derived from these models, will foster more meaningful and relevant APN evaluation. Performance standards should reflect the purposes, goals, and objectives of the practice setting and meet external quality demands. For example, the APN in primary care can use an immunization benchmark from HEDIS to assess preventive care objectives and CAHPS questions about patient centeredness to determine patient experiences with the APN's care. Because standardized measures are used, the APN can compare performance to others or to national benchmarks.

The collection of data and information to justify the APN role, measure performance, demonstrate contributions to quality, and guide quality improvement efforts is critical. Suggested strategies include the regular collection and analysis of data on outcomes expected from the APN's practice; the collection of preintervention and postintervention data to track results over time; and assessment of patient experience and satisfaction with care. Possible data sources include administrative data (the data provided to regulators, accreditors, and insurers), chart audits, and client surveys. HEDIS, CAHPS, and other standardized measure use is encouraged to enhance the ability to compare data across individuals, groups, and settings. Data should be analyzed for trends over time: variations among groups of patients (e.g., age, gender, race, and ethnicity); variance from expected outcomes; differences among providers; and variations when compared with regional, state, or national norms. Performance data should be summarized and shared with consumers, other providers, and organizational leaders and used for accountability purposes.

Education

The APN has responsibility for his or her own, consumers', and other providers' education about quality issues and approaches. Consumers need information to be partners in their care, and other members of the health-care team need to better understand the value of APN practice. Sharing clinical expertise and participating in collaborative efforts to measure and improve quality best accomplish this. Offering information about best, evidence-based practices is one example of this type of activity.

Advanced practice and basic education should include content about and experience with all aspects of the quality process. Buerhaus and Norman (2001) give four reasons for including such information in formal educational programs: (a) given the current economic climate surrounding health-care delivery, competition will increase and providers will be competing on the basis of quality, using quality indicators to distinguish themselves to purchasers and consumers; (b) the nursing shortage will result in greater use of unlicensed personnel and foreign-educated nurses, but nurses will still be accountable for nursing care and will need to ensure quality and quality improvement; (c) nursing is responsible for quality and quality improvement to meet health system goals; and (d) nurses can capitalize on emerging evidence about the relationship of staffing to outcomes to advocate for structures and processes that will improve outcomes.

The APN may be involved in formal classroom or clinical teaching of undergraduate and graduate nursing students and should incorporate quality information and experiences in teaching strategies. The APN is also encouraged to include quality-related content during in-service and continuing education offerings. For example, the pediatric NP giving an in-service on assessing early childhood development should discuss how outcomes will be assessed using the CAHMI PHD measures.

Research

APN research-related competencies include critically evaluating and applying research to practice, monitoring and evaluating practice, and participating in research. Research knowledge and skills are directly applicable to quality measurement and the interpretation of data. APNs can contribute by building an evidence base for their practice through collaborative research efforts. Using data collected and analyzed to assess performance, the APN can use research knowledge and skills to promote and improve quality. APNs have contributed to building a knowledge base and the methodologies needed to assess quality. Duffy (2002) described the clinical leadership role of the APN in identifying nurse-sensitive and multidisciplinary-quality indicator sets. The author advocates for using a phased, organization-wide process for incorporating these indicators into data collection efforts. Dunbar-Jacob and Schron (2002) suggest using ancillary studies to clinical trails to study questions relevant to nursing practice. Both of these suggestions provide examples of actions the APN can adopt at the practice level.

Administration

APNs in leadership positions can create a climate that fosters and supports quality and quality improvement. They can also propose structures and processes needed for quality and quality improvement such as available information systems for patient-level data collection. Even if the APN does not have administrative functions, efforts can be made to promote the climate and the structures needed. Cubanski and Kline (2002) suggest a number of system challenges the APN can help address:

- Redesign care to better serve patient needs
- Improve the use of information technology for practice and make it available to clinicians
- Develop systems to coordinate care across conditions, services, and settings
- Promote team effectiveness
- Incorporate process and outcome measures into the delivery of health care

Another administrative opportunity is providing incentives and awards for quality performance or quality improvement. Praise, recognition, promotion, raises, or other monetary contributions can provide incentive to staff. Awards, public acknowledgment, and offering special educational opportunities are other possible actions to foster continuous attention to quality and its improvement. The APN may do these things directly or by promoting their use by leaders in the setting. Rewards and recognition can also be provided through professional nursing organizations.

Advocacy

As another core competency of APN practice, advocacy can be applied to advancing quality measurement performance and improvement. Clearly, patient advocacy has always been a hallmark of professional nursing practice. The APN can further develop this competency by providing consumers with quality-related information, including what they should expect from health care and the health-care system. Advocacy and the development of partnerships with patients can be enhanced when patients have their personal health record and information about their condition and treatment options (Davis et al., 2002). Armed with this information, patients can make better informed decisions and participate in all aspects of their care planning. The APN can also advocate for the practice, education, research, and administrative actions described previously.

APNs, especially those in direct practice roles, are not often involved with advocacy at the system or policy level. This is a loss to both the APN and society. With their expertise in practice, who better than the APN knows what is needed for quality care to become a reality?

Advocacy is needed at the systems and societal levels to promote more resources for quality measurement and research, improve access for all people, develop better measurement and reporting of quality, support financing of appropriate services, and support government quality efforts. Advocacy with government and private sector organizations means getting involved with the political and policy processes, lobbying, educating consumers and policy makers, and using the media to deliver quality and APN value messages. The APN's expert knowledge and skills should be used to influence legislators, regulators, insurers, and private sector organizations involved (or who should be involved). For example, the APN using the influence of a professional nursing organization should use public comment periods to influence new HEDIS measures, TJC standards, and state Medicaid performance measurement approaches.

The APN should become an insider in the quality movement by participating in local, state, and national committees that are addressing quality concerns. For example, the author serves on the advisory and executive committees of FACCT's CAHMI, thus having influence in the development and adoption of child health performance measures. Nurses are also staff at such organizations as TJC and the AHRQ and review quality-related grants for foundations and government agencies. The APN can also become a leader and advocate for quality in the community, in the state, or in the nursing organization. For example, the APN might chair the town health committee or advisory board and develop community health outcome measures for a report card or promote an annual quality conference by the state nurses association.

CONCLUSION

As the IOM report on the future of the profession (IOM, 2011) recommends, the transformation of the health-care system requires that nurses practice to the full extent of their legal scope and lead change to advance health. The Patient Protection and Affordable Health Care Act signals that our society is ready for change in health care. More attention will be directed to primary care, prevention, chronic care, coordination, and other services traditionally provided by nurses. It is also likely that initiatives to link outcomes to payment will continue. In addition, the demands created by an aging population will present opportunities and challenges to ensure the quality and quantity of health-care services.

APNs cannot escape the responsibility they have for clearly articulating their value to the health-care system. Because value equals quality and cost, without evidence of quality the case cannot be made for value. Advanced practice nursing cannot be supported and the purposes of the health-care system are not as well met as when the APN is a major player in the quality movement. Although efforts to define, assess, and improve quality have grown significantly in recent years, APN involvement in this arena has been less obvious. To move the health-care system toward quality, the APN, the health-care team, care organizations, and society must all participate and change. As this chapter has made clear, there are plenty of activities for engagement.

This chapter has made the case that the APN must be involved at all levels and in all aspects of the quality movement. The profession and the health-care system are ready for greater nursing and APN leadership. Recent and ongoing quality initiatives offer clear direction for the APN in evaluating performance, measuring quality, and articulating value to a variety of stakeholders. The competencies expected of the APN are explicit to the quality domain. If the profession's clinical leaders do not get involved, who will fill the gap? The challenges are many, but the potential outcomes for the APN and society are great.

REFERENCES

Agency for Healthcare Research and Quality. (2008a). *Key themes and highlights from the National Healthcare Quality Report.* Retrieved July 22, 2008, from www.ahrq.gov/qual/nhqr07/key.htm/.

Agency for Healthcare Research and Quality. (2008b). *Key themes and highlights from the National Healthcare Disparities Report.* Retrieved July 22, 2008, from www.ahrq.gov/qual/nhdr07/key.htm/.

Agency for Healthcare Research and Quality. (2012). *Surveys and tools to advance patient-centered care.* Retrieved February 20, 2012, from https://www.cahps.ahrq.gov/Surveys-Guidance/CG.aspx.

Aiken, L. H., Clarke, S. P., Sloane, D. M., Sochalski, J., & Silber, J. H. (2001). Nurses report on hospital care in five countries. *Health Affairs, 20*(3), 43–53.

Aiken, L. H., Clarke, S. P., Sloane, D. M., Sochalski, J., & Silber, J. H. (2002). Hospital nurse staffing and patient mortality, burnout and job dissatisfaction. *Journal of the American Medical Association, 288*(16), 1987–1993.

American Association of Colleges of Nursing. (2011). *Essentials of master's education in nursing.* Washington, DC: Author.

American Hospital Association. (2002). *In our hands: How hospital leaders can build a thriving workforce.* Chicago: American Hospital Association.

Aquilino, M. L., Damiano, P. C., Willard, J. C., Momony, E. T., & Levy, B. T. (1999). Primary care physician perceptions of the nurse practitioner in the 1990s. *Archives of Family Medicine, 8*(3), 224–227.

Barnason, S., & Rasmussen, D. (2002). Patient outcomes beyond hospitalization: Carotid endarterectomy surgical patient outcomes after a rapid recovery program. *Clinical Nurse Specialist, 16*(2), 100–105.

Beal, J. A., & Philips, M. (1999). *The nurse practitioner role in the NICU: A study of role turnover.* Presentation at the Eastern Nursing Research Society, New York.

Borchers, L., & Kee, C. C. (1999). An experience in telenursing. *Clinical Nurse Specialist, 13*(3), 115–118.

Bozzo, J., Carlson, B., & Diers, D. (1998). Using hospital data systems to find target populations: New tools for clinical nurse specialists. *Clinical Nurse Specialist, 12*(2), 86–91.

Brooten, D., & Naylor, M. D. (1995). Nurses' effect on changing patient outcomes. *Image: The Journal of Nursing Scholarship, 27*(2), 95–99.

Brown, S. J. (2000). Direct clinical practice. In A. B. Hamric, J. A. Spross, & C. M. Hanson (Eds.), *Advanced practice nursing: An integrative approach* (2nd ed., pp. 137–182). Philadelphia: W. B. Saunders.

Buerhaus, P. I., & Norman, L. (2001). It's time to require theory and methods of quality improvement in basic and graduate nursing education. *Nursing Outlook, 49*(2), 67–69.

Burl, J. B., Bonner, A., Rao, M., & Khan, A. (1998). Geriatric nurse practitioners in long-term care: Demonstration of effectiveness in managed care. *Journal of the American Geriatric Society, 46*(4), 506–510.

Card, S. J., Herrling, P. J., Matthews, J. L., Rossi, M. L., Spencer, E. S., & Lagoe, R. (1998). Impact of clinical pathways for total hip replacement: A community-based analysis. *Journal of Nursing Care Quality, 13*(2), 67–76.

Centers for Medicare and Medicaid Services. (2002). *Nursing home compare.* Retrieved June 1, 2003, from www.medicare.gov/nhcompare/home.asp.

Cole, F. L., Mackey, T., & Lindenberg, J. (1999). Search and research. Quality improvement: Psychometric evaluation of patient satisfaction with nurse practitioner care instrument. *Journal of the American Academy of Nurse Practitioners, 11*(11), 471–475.

Commonwealth Fund. (2011). *New national scorecard on U.S. health system performance.* Retrieved February 20, 2012, from http://www.commonwealthfund.org/Topics/Health-System-Performance-and-Costs.aspx/.

Coward, D. D. (1998). Facilitation of self-transcendence in a breast cancer support group. *Oncology Nursing Forum, 25*(1), 75–84.

Cubanski, J., & Kline, J. (2002). *Improving health care quality: Can federal efforts lead the way?* (Issue Brief #539). New York: The Commonwealth Fund.

Dahle, K., Smith, T., Ingersoll, R., & Wilson, J. (1998). Impact of a nurse practitioner on the costs of managing inpatients with heart failure. *American Journal of Cardiology, 82*(5), 686–688.

Davis, K., Schoenbaum, S. C., Collins, K. S., Tenny, K., Hughes, D., & Audet, A. J. (2002). *Room for improvement: Patients report on the quality of their health care.* New York: The Commonwealth Fund.

Diers, D., & Bozzo, J. (1997). Nursing resource definition in DRGs: RIMS/nursing acuity project. *Nursing Economics, 15*(3), 124–137.

Diers, D., Bozzo, J., Blatt, L., & Roussel, M. (1998). Understanding nursing resources in intensive care: A case study. *American Journal of Critical Care, 7*(2), 143–148.

Donabedian, A. (1966). Evaluating the quality of medical care. *Milbank Memorial Fund Quarterly, 44*(3 suppl), 166–206.

Donaldson, M. S. (Ed.). (1999). *Measuring the quality of health care.* Washington, DC: National Roundtable on Health Care Quality, Institute of Medicine.

Dozier, A. M., Kitzman, H. J., Ingersoll, G. L., Holmberg, S., & Schultz, A. W. (2001). Development of an instrument to measure patient perception of the quality of nursing care. *Research in Nursing and Health, 24*(6), 506–517.

Duffy, J. R. (2002). The clinical leadership role of the CNS in the identification of nursing-sensitive and multi-disciplinary quality indicator sets. *Clinical Nurse Specialist, 16*(2), 70–76.

Dunbar-Jacob, J., & Schron, E. (2002). Ancillary studies in clinical trials. *Nursing Research, 51*(5), 336–338.

East, C. E., & Colditz, P. B. (1996). Women's evaluations of their experiences with fetal intrapartum oxygen saturation monitoring and participation in a research project. *Midwifery, 12*(2), 93–97.

Foundation for Accountability. (1999). *The FACCT consumer information framework.* Retrieved June 1, 2003, from www.facct.org/FACC/doclibfiles/documentfile_203.doc.

Garvisan, L., Grimsey, E., Littlejohns, P., Lownes, S., & Sacks, N. (1998). Satisfaction with clinical nurse specialists in a breast care clinic: Questionnaire survey. *British Medical Journal, 316*(7136), 976–977.

Girouard, S. A. (2000). New directions for the advanced practice nurse in health care quality. In A. B. Hamric, J. A. Spross, & C. M. Hanson (Eds.), *Advanced practice nursing: An integrative approach* (2nd ed., pp. 755–795). Philadelphia: W. B. Saunders.

Girouard, S. A., & Spross, J. A. (1983). Evaluation of the CNS: Using an evaluation tool. In A. B. Hamric & J. A. Spross (Eds.), *The clinical nurse specialist in theory and practice* (pp. 207–218). New York: Grune & Stratton.

Hamric, A. B. (1983). A model for developing evaluation strategies. In A. B. Hamric & J. A. Spross (Eds.), *The clinical nurse specialist in theory and practice* (pp. 187–206). New York: Grune & Stratton.

Hamric, A. B. (1989). A model for CNS evaluation. In A. B. Hamric & J. A. Spross (Eds.), *The clinical nurse specialist in theory and practice* (2nd ed., pp. 83–104). New York: Grune & Stratton.

Hamric, A. B., Worley, D., Lindeback, S., & Jaubert, S. (1999). Outcomes associated with advanced nursing practice prescriptive authority. *Journal of the American Academy of Nurse Practitioners, 10*(3), 113–118.

Houston, S., & Luquire, R. (1991). Measuring success: CNS performance appraisal. *Clinical Nurse Specialist, 5*(4), 204–209.

Ingersoll, G. L. (1988). Evaluating the impact of the clinical nurse specialist. *Clinical Nurse Specialist, 2*(3), 150–155.

Institute of Medicine. (1999). *To err is human: Building a safer health system.* Washington, DC: National Academy Press.

Institute of Medicine. (2001). *Crossing the quality chasm.* Washington, DC: National Academy Press.

Institute of Medicine. (2010). *Redesigning continuing education in the health professions.* Washington, DC: National Academy Press.

Institute of Medicine. (2011). *The future of nursing: Leading change, advancing health.* Washington, DC: National Academy Press.

Jacavone, J. B., Daniels, R. D., & Tyner, I. (1999). CNS facilitation of a cardiac surgery clinical pathway program. *Clinical Nurse Specialist, 13*(3), 126–132.

Joint Commission on the Accreditation of Healthcare Organizations. (2002). *Health care at the crossroads: Strategies for addressing the evolving nursing crisis.* Chicago: Author.

Kearnes, D. R. (1992). A productivity tool to evaluate NP practice: Monitoring clinical time spent in reimbursable, patient-related activities. *Nurse Practitioner, 17*(4), 50–52, 55.

Kee, C. C., & Borchers, L. (1998). Reducing readmission rates through discharge interventions. *Clinical Nurse Specialist, 12*(5), 206–209.

Knaus, V. L., Felten, S., Burton, S., Fobes, P., & Davis, K. (1997). The use of nurse practitioners in the acute care setting. *Journal of Nursing Administration, 27*(2), 20–27.

Larrabee, J. H., Ferri, J. A., & Hartig, M. T. (1997). Patient satisfaction with nurse practitioner care in primary care. *Journal of Nursing Care Quality, 11*(5), 9–14.

Lombness, P. (1994). Differences in length of stay with care managed by a clinical nurse specialist or physicians assistants. *Clinical Nurse Specialist, 8*(5), 253–260.

Mason, D. J., Alexander, J. M., Huffaker, J., Reilly, P. A., Sigmund, E. C., & Cohen, S. S. (1999). Nurse practitioners' experiences with managed care organizations in New York and Connecticut. *Nursing Outlook, 47*(5), 201–208.

McDaniel, A. M. (1999). Assessing the feasibility of a clinical practice guideline for inpatient smoking cessation intervention. *Clinical Nurse Specialist, 13*(5), 228–235.

McMullen, M. (1999). *Satisfaction of patients, physicians and staff nurses with the care provided by nurse practitioners/attending collaborative service.* Presented at the 11th Annual Scientific Sessions Eastern Nursing Research Society Meeting, New York.

Morin, K. H., Bucher, L., Plowfield, L., Hayes, E., Mahoney, P., & Armiger, L. (1999). Using research to establish protocols for practice: A statewide study of acute care agencies. *Clinical Nurse Specialist, 13*(2), 77–84.

Mullan, J. T., & Harrington, C. (2001). Nursing home deficiencies in the United States. *Research on Aging, 23*(5), 503–531.

Mundinger, M. O., & Kane, R. L. (2000). Health outcomes among patients treated by nurse practitioners or physicians. *Journal of the American Medical Association, 283*(19), 2521–2524.

Musclow, S. L., Sawhney, M., & Watt-Watson, J. (2002). The emerging role of advanced practice nursing in acute pain management throughout Canada. *Clinical Nurse Specialist, 12*(2), 63–68.

National Committee for Quality Assurance. (2011). *HEDIS and quality measurement.* Retrieved February 15, 2012, from http://www.ncqa.org/tabid/59/Default.aspx/.

National Forum for Healthcare Quality Measurement and Reporting. (2002). *About the National Quality Forum.* Retrieved July 7, 2003, from www.qualityforum.org/about/home.htm.

National Organization of Nurse Practitioner Faculties. (2011). *Nurse practitioner core competencies.* Washington, DC: Author.

Needleman, J., Buerhaus, P. I., Mattke, S., Stewart, M., & Zelevinsky, K. (2002). Nurse-staffing levels and the quality of care in hospitals. *New England Journal of Medicine, 346*(22), 1715–1722.

Noll, M. L., & Girard, N. (1993). Preparing the CNS for participation in quality assurance activities. *Clinical Nurse Specialist, 7*(2), 81–84.

Oermann, M. H. (1999). Consumer's descriptions of health care quality. *Journal of Nursing Care Quality, 14*(1), 47–55.

Oermann, M. H., Lambert, J., & Templin, T. (2000). Patients' perceptions of quality health care. *MCN, American Journal of Maternal Child Nursing, 25*(5), 242–247.

Paine, L. L., Lang, J. M., Strobino, D. M., Johnson, T. R., DeJoseph, J. F., Declercq, E. R., et al. (1999). Characteristics of nurse-midwife patients and visits. *American Journal of Public Health, 89*(6), 906–909.

Pelletier-Hibbert, M. (1998). Coping strategies used by nurses to deal with the care of organ donors and their families. *Heart and Lung, 27*(4), 230–237.

Rand Corporation. (2010). *Report cards for health care: Is anyone checking them?* Retrieved February 15, 2012, from http://www.rand.org/pubs/research_briefs/RB4544-2/index1.html/.

Rudy, E. B., Davidson, L. J., Daly, B., Clochesy, J. M., Sereida, S., Baldisseri, M., et al. (1998). Care activities and outcomes of patients cared for by acute care nurse practitioners, physician assistants and resident physicians: A comparison. *American Journal of Critical Care, 7*(4), 267–281.

Sagehorn, K. K., Russell, C. L., & Ganong, L. H. (1999). Implementation of a patient-family pathway: Effects on patients and families. *Clinical Nurse Specialist, 13*(3), 119–122.

Shaughnessy, P. W., Crisler, K. S., Hittle, D. F., & Schenkler, R. E. (2002). *Summary of the report on OASIS and outcome-based quality improvement in home care.* Denver: Center for Health Services Research, University of Colorado Health Sciences Center.

Shi, L., & Singh, D. A. (2005). *Essentials of the U.S. health care delivery system.* Boston: Jones & Bartlett.

Strohschein, S., Schaffer, M. A., & Lia-Hoagberg, B. (1999). Evidenced-based guidelines for public health nursing practice. *Nursing Outlook, 47*(2), 84–90.

Tierney, M. J., Grant, L. M., & Mazique, S. I. (1990). Cost accountability and clinical nurse specialist evaluation. *Nursing Management, 21*(5), 26–28, 30–31.

U.S. Department of Health and Human Services. (2011). *Partnership for patients: Better care, lower costs.* Retrieved February 20, 2012, from http://www.healthcare.gov/compare/partnership-for-patients/index.html.

U.S. Department of Health and Human Services. (2012). *Healthy people.* Retrieved February 15, 2012, from http://www.cdc.gov/nchs/healthy_people.htm/.

U.S. Department of Health and Human Services, Health Resources and Services Administration, Bureau of Health Professions, Division of Nursing. (2002). *Nurse practitioner primary care competencies in specialty areas.* Washington, DC: U.S. Government Printing Office.

Walker, P. H., Baker, J. J., & Chivertons, P. (1998). Costs of interdisciplinary practice in a school-based health center. *Outcomes Management for Nursing Practice, 2*(1), 37–44.

23

Advanced Practice Registered Nurses: Accomplishments, Trends, and Future Development

Jane M. Flanagan
Dorothy A. Jones
Allyssa Harris

INTRODUCTION

The major roles within the framework of the advanced practice registered nurse (APRN) are the clinical nurse specialist (CNS), certified nurse-midwife (CNM), certified registered nurse anesthetist (CRNA), and nurse practitioner (NP) (APRN Consensus Work Group & National Council of State Board of Nurses Advisory Committee, 2008). Historically, the APRN roles developed out of an identified need for improved continuity of care and increased access to health services. Many APRNs work with diverse populations in a variety of settings, often where access to health care is limited.

According to the International Council of Nurses (ICN, 2002) key components of the APRN role include the integration of research, education, practice, and management; role autonomy; managing a direct patient case load; acquisition of advanced health assessment decision-making and diagnostic reasoning skills; advanced clinical role/skill competencies; independent consultation with patients and other providers; the aptitude to plan, implement, and evaluate care outcomes; and being designated a "first point of contact" to initiate patient care. The ICN also recognizes that individual countries and states within countries have regulations restricting practice and the full potential of patient care delivered by APRNs including the right to diagnose, prescribe, consult, and admit to a hospital.

Over the years, patients, administrators, family, and physicians have all acknowledged the contributions made by APRNs to enhance patient care (Horrocks, Anderson, & Salisbury, 2002; Ingersoll, McIntosh, & Williams, 2000; Institute of Medicine [IOM], 2010; McGee & Kaplan, 2007). The value and efforts of APRNs have extended well beyond the United States and are gaining increased attention worldwide. The demand for APRNs is even more pronounced in areas where there is pandemic disease and concerns about safe childbirth (Schober, 2006; World Health Organization, 2006). Despite this acknowledgement of APRN's contributions to health care, there are continued challenges that affect role implementation and utilization.

As APRNs continue to grow in number and their impact on health care is more widely acknowledged, new challenges have arisen about efficacy and practice impact of APRNs. The movement toward the preparation APRNs more aligned with the medical model of cure rather than the advanced practice nursing model of caring and healing stimulates further debate. Some have suggested that this expansion into medical practice is a "natural evolution" of the APRN role, whereas others have argued that the recent changes foster professional abandonment and the blurring or omission of a nursing-informed model of care. Unaddressed, this challenge could result in a diminished voice for nursing, decreased collaboration, a loss of professional autonomy, and reduced public legitimacy (Bryant-Lukosius, Dicenso, Browne, & Pinelli, 2004; Fawcett, Newman, & McAllister, 2004; Flanagan, 2008; Grace, 2008; Jones, 2006; Newman, Smith, Pharris, & Jones, 2008).

This chapter explores the current realities of APRN roles and the recent trends affecting APRN education and practice. APRNs are discussed within the context of nursing science and a changing clinical practice environment.

THE APRN: ROLES, PRACTICE SETTINGS, AND OUTCOMES

APRNs practice in the expanded role with increasingly diverse populations in a variety of settings including large medical centers, physicians' offices, community health centers, ambulatory care clinics, and emergency rooms, as well as the traditional community and rural hospitals and clinics. Nursing and other disciplinary knowledge, along with information about populations and settings, further inform and define each of the APRN roles.

The national consensus model for advanced practice nurses regulation (APRN Consensus Work Group & National Council of State Board of Nurses Advisory Committee, 2008) recognizes four roles—CNM, CRNA, CNS, and NP—working with six population foci: adult-gerontology, family, women's, pediatric, neonatal, and psychiatric. APRNs may choose to specialize in areas such as oncology or palliative care, but they cannot be solely licensed as an APRN within a specialty area. The scope of practice for APRNs is not setting specific, but varies according to the needs of the patient or population.

In a changing health-care environment driven by economics and physician residency education, some APRNs (NPs and CNMs) have been used as physician substitutes in disease-based specialty care (Steven, 2004) within the hospital setting. This phenomenon has resulted in shifts in practice settings for NPs and CNMs who formerly were more home and community based, but now are more acute and hospital based.

Certified Nurse-Midwives

The Health Resources and Services Administration (HRSA, 2010) reports that there are 18,492 CNMs. More than 30% of CNMs report having a diploma or associate's degree in nursing as the highest academic degree. This reflects the fact that early CNM programs did not require a baccalaureate preparation, nor did they award a master's degree at the completion of the program. Many CNMs (56%) complete programs of specialized education between 13 and 36 months beyond nursing school. Approximately 55% of CNMs are prepared at the master's level or greater. CNMs provide gynecological care to healthy women and low-risk obstetrical care. CNMs care for women in the home and the hospital setting.

Study findings support that CNMs have increased patient satisfaction with care, lower incidences of cesarean births, decreased use of forceps delivery, less medication use, decreased length of hospitalization, and, overall, fewer complications with the delivery (Davidson, 2002; Declercq, 2002;

De Koninck, Blais, Joubert, & Gagnon, 2001). Other studies have demonstrated that mothers cared for by CNMs have a greater tendency to breastfeed their babies, improving both infant immunity and rates of infant mortality (De Koninck et al., 2001; Raisler, 2000). Hellings and Howe (2000) found that CNMs and NPs had a better understanding of problems associated with breastfeeding, and provided the strategies needed to promote effective breastfeeding.

Collectively these studies suggest that CNMs provide effective prenatal, labor, and delivery care, and postbirth assistance. The evidence indicates that CNMs provide obstetrical care that is accessible, safe, and low cost with lower rates of neonatal mortality and cesarean births and higher rates of breastfeeding. CNMs have reinforced the fact that pregnancy is a normal health transition for many women, easily managed by the CNM.

Certified Registered Nurse Anesthetists

In 2008, a reported 34,821 CRNAs were practicing in the United States (HRSA, 2010). CRNAs are registered nurses who have completed 2 to 3 years of higher education beyond a bachelor's degree (typically a master's degree) and hold national certification to practice in this role. Most CRNAs have had previous experience in critical care, a criterion often used as part of the admission requirements to a graduate program.

CRNAs work in hospital settings and administer more than 65% of the anesthetics given annually to patients. From its inception, the role of the CRNA has focused on providing safe, effective anesthesia care to patients in the hospital setting. No particular groups of patients have been identified (i.e., healthier, more stable, poor, ethnically diverse, rural, or inner city) as a specific focus of CRNA care. In response to a critical shortage of anesthesia providers in the 1980s, the American Association of Nurse Anesthetists (AANA) established the National Commission on Nurse Anesthesia Education (NCNAE) to oversee all aspects of CRNA preparation and develop strategies that would enable nurses to respond to this crisis (Mastropietro, Horton, Ouellette, & Faut-Callahan, 2001).

Outcome studies associated with anesthesia administration by CRNAs suggest that when specialists provide anesthesia—whether it be a physician or CRNA—the outcomes are better than when care is provided by a nonspecialist (AANA, 2002). A comprehensive study reported that the care provided by CRNAs is comparable to care provided by anesthesiologists (Simonson, Ahern, & Hendryx, 2007). Despite these findings, physician anesthetists continue to regulate CRNA practice and limit their work as independent providers of anesthesia care; however, the CRNA role has prevailed, especially in underserved and rural settings (AANA, 2002; Simonson et al., 2007).

Nurse Practitioners

NPs have traditionally focused on primary care for underserved populations within the inner city, rural areas, and other nonhospital settings. NPs continue to deliver patient care in settings in which traditional physician providers are unavailable. More recently, and in growing numbers, NPs provide care in the hospital setting. Keough and colleagues (2011) found that among the American Nurses Credentialing Center (ANCC) certified NPs they surveyed, a large number (42%) of acute care nurse practitioners were practicing in nontraditional settings and of that 90% were practicing in primary care. Other findings of this study suggest that less than 10% of primary care nurse adult–gerontology and family nurse practitioners were practicing in acute care settings. Research conducted by Pulcini and colleagues (2005) suggested that NPs deliver direct patient care that includes prescription writing as well as the ordering of treatments and procedures. Some may also have hospital admitting privileges, conduct patient rounds, and participate in urgent care visits (Pulcini, Vampola, & Levine, 2005).

In 2008 there were an estimated 158,348 NPs in the United States, and the majority of NPs practiced in ambulatory care or hospital-based settings (HRSA, 2010). More than 88% of these NPs had a master's degree and 3.9% held a doctorate (HRSA, 2010). The majority of NPs practice in urban primary care settings providing care to elderly, poor, and ethnically diverse populations with otherwise limited, or no, access to health care (Pulcini et al., 2005).

Studies focusing on the care provided by NPs when compared to that provided by physicians for a variety of primary care–related conditions have demonstrated that NPs provide care that is as safe as and as effective as physicians. Additionally, patients often report higher levels of satisfaction with NP practice, particularly related to increased time spent with the patient for information gathering and teaching (Hayes, 2007; Hoffman, Tasota, Zullo, Scharfenberg, & Donaue, 2005; Mundinger et al., 2000). Another study comparing NPs with medical doctors indicated that NPs had significantly more patient "return visits," but overall there was no significant difference in prescribing practices or patient care costs between the two providers (Venning, Durie, Roland, Roberts, & Leese, 2000). These results are consistent with the findings of Horrocks and colleagues (2002) who reported that although NPs may order more tests, they focus heavily on teaching, health promotion, and self-care. These may be important behaviors contributing to a decrease in overall health-care costs.

NPs practicing within a nursing framework come to know the patient in a holistic way, including exploring meaning associated with sociocultural, financial, and other life situations as they relate to their health. This knowledge may significantly affect the NP's ability to provide care that is responsive to cost, quality, and effectiveness for both the organization and the patient. NP practice settings have expanded to include NPs in urgent care, emergency room, and acute care. Outcome studies are needed to understand and evaluate the effectiveness of the NP role in these care settings.

Clinical Nurse Specialists

There are 59,242 CNSs who are registered nurses with advanced degrees at either the master's level (92.8%) or doctorate level (7.2%). This number represents an 18.4% decline in the CNS (HRSA, 2010). The CNS role developed as a result of fragmented health-care services and a lack of expert nursing care at the bedside and limited continuity in care across settings, and, with changes that have emerged in health care and cost containment, the CNS role has been affected. More than any other group of APRNs, CNSs report not "functioning in the role" (18.8%). Some CNSs who are dually certified as NPs work in that role (15.8%). Other roles of the CNS include management (17.8%), instruction (21.1%,) and staff nurses (16%) (HRSA, 2010).

The CNS is an autonomous nurse clinician who provides specialized care in the community or hospital setting, usually through referral from other providers such as physicians and other nurses (Oermann & Floyd, 2002). The CNS is recognized as a clinical expert in a specialized area of patient care such as wounds, pain, or diabetes (Lyons, 2005). Most CNSs work directly with patients and staff and in conjunction and collaboration with multiple members of the health-care team. With the exception of the psychiatric/mental health CNS, most CNSs do not have prescriptive authority.

Although past research has provided supportive evidence to link the contributions of the CNS to (a) reduced length of hospital stay, (b) reduced use of emergency rooms for care, (c) decreased hospitalization admissions and recidivism after discharge, and (d) diminished cost and increased satisfaction with care received (Brooten, 1995; Brooten et al., 1995; Newhouse et al., 2011; Oermann & Floyd, 2002), the CNS has been challenged in many institutions by budget cuts. It is essential that CNSs conduct outcomes evaluation research that clearly links cost savings, patient care effectiveness, and improved satisfaction to their role (Oermann & Floyd, 2002).

APRN REIMBURSEMENT

The mean salary for the APRN varies by region within the United States and is also influenced by years of experience, practice setting, specialty area, and education. According to the 2010 National Salary of Nurse Practitioners, the average salary for an APRN is $90,770 (Perron Pronsati & Gerchufsky, 2011; Rollet, 2010). As in the general public, gender plays a significant role in APRN salaries, with women earning 12.8% less than men—$89,186 compared with $102,271 (Perron Pronsati & Gerchufsky, 2011). Salaries of CRNAs remain the highest of all APRNs, at an average salary of $154,221 per year. The average annual salary is $72,856 for CNSs, $85,025 for NPs, and $82,111 for CNMs (HRSA, 2010).

Rollet (2010) suggests that practice settings are the greatest determinate of salaries, with $30,000 separating the most profitable from the least profitable. Educational level and experience influence compensation. APRNs with approximately 11 to 15 years of experience earn the most. As more APRNs with a doctorate of nursing practice (DNP) enter practice settings, it is expected that APRN salaries will be increased to reflect this educational change. According to the 2009 National Salary and Workplace Survey of Nurse Practitioners, DNPs earn $7,688 more than their colleagues with a master's degree (Rollet, 2010). APRNs typically have additional benefits such as health insurance, paid vacation and sick time, malpractice insurance, and continuing education support.

The reimbursement rules detailed in the *Federal Register* (1998) that revised Medicare reimbursement for physicians also included other health-care providers. Currently, Medicare payment has allowed CNSs, NPs, and physician assistant services to be reimbursed in selected situations. The Balanced Budget Act of 1997 facilitated direct Medicare reimbursement for the NP (Richmond, Thompson, & Sullivan-Marx, 2000). Expanded Medicare reimbursement for acute-care NPs continues to be reviewed. The American Nurses Association (ANA) is working with a variety of federal agencies to improve direct reimbursement for APRNs, regardless of specialty and geographical location. Challenges associated with reimbursement in today's health-care environment are often linked to care outcomes and reimbursement policy established by insurers, mostly controlled at the state level. It is critical for APRNs to document their contributions to care and patient outcomes. Data that link the work of the APRN to improved patient outcomes, reduction in costs, enhanced patient and family satisfaction, and increased efficiency can be used to examine care and provide compensation recognizing the contributions of APRNs.

FUTURE TRENDS: THE IMPACT OF ADVANCED PRACTICE NURSES

Findings from many individual, as well as systematic, reviews of research comparing the effectiveness of APRN practice suggest that APRNs provide care that is comparable to and in some cases better than care provided by medical doctors (Newhouse et al., 2011). Key components of the APRN role include direct, comprehensive patient care; support and advocacy within the health-care system; monitoring and ensuring quality of service; and education, research, publication, and leadership (Cumbie, Conley, & Burman, 2004).

In 2000, the ANA identified nurse-sensitive indicators attributable to APRN practice in both the acute-care and community-based settings. They include care outcomes related to activities around pain management, patient satisfaction, cardiovascular disease prevention, pressure ulcer prevention and treatment, identification and prevention of risk for patient falls, nosocomial infection rate, and nurse satisfaction. Ingersoll and colleagues (2000) suggested nine nurse-sensitive indicators: satisfaction with care delivery; symptom resolution or reduction; perception of being well cared for; complication or adherence with treatment plan; knowledge of patients and families; trust in care provider; collaboration among care providers; frequency and type of procedures ordered; and quality of life. Kring (2008, p. 179) isolated five domains to promote CNS practice: discovery, summary, translation, integration, and evaluation. The author linked these competencies with CNS practice in the areas of expert practice, research, consultation, education, and leadership. Such indicators offer all APRNs a focus, as well as an opportunity to research and disseminate findings about practice outcomes.

The ANA's National Database of Nursing Quality Indicators (NDNQI, 2008) and the ANCC Magnet Designation initiatives have greatly affected the role of the CNS. Magnet Status, a designation developed and rewarded by ANCC, recognizes excellence and innovation in nursing practice as it relates to quality outcomes (ANCC, 2008). NDNQI outlines nurse-sensitive indicators such as falls, skin ulcerations, and hospital-acquired infections (including ventilator-associated pneumonia and catheter-associated urinary tract infections) as conditions responsive to nursing care. These quality indicators are now linked to Medicare reimbursement through the Centers for Medicare and Medicaid Services' (CMS's) program. These agendas have spurred studies that aim to link the work of the CNS to improved patient care outcomes. In one study, CNS initiatives resulted in an 86% reduction in the incidence of catheter-associated bloodstream infections, a 47% reduction in catheter-associated urinary tract infections, and a 39% reduction in hospital-acquired pressure ulcer prevalence (Muller, Hujcs, Dubendorf, & Harrington, 2010). This type of compelling evidence provides support for the CNS role and decreases their vulnerability. Other trends such as enhanced safety/risk reduction and the goal of achieving Magnet Status have the potential to revive the CNS role. Although these nurse-sensitive quality indicators do much to support the CNS role, more specific nurse-sensitive indicators are needed to distinguish the contributions of other APRNs such as the CNM, NP, and CRNA.

CHANGES AND CHALLENGES IN HEALTH CARE

The past decade has presented many challenges to health-care organizations and the delivery of safe, quality, timely, cost-effective patient care (IOM, 1999, 2001). Currently, reforms include an overhaul of the current health-care system, with increased emphasis on (a) the need for continued cost reduction, (b) the identification of potential risks to existing and new services, and (c) vigilance and monitoring over rare, serious, and reportable medical events termed *never events* by the National Quality Forum.

From a national health policy perspective, implementation of the Affordable Healthcare Act of 2009 will result in an increased demand for all APRNs and nurse practitioners in particular. Millions of previously uninsured people will be able to obtain health insurance, resulting in an increased demand for APRNs in primary, long-term, and community-based settings. Care groups made up of physicians and APRNs will be organized to provide care to patients with high-risk problems, such as diabetes and heart disease, and other high-risk chronically ill or dying patients. These care groups will bring both specialists and primary care providers together to provide the best, most cost-effective, high-quality care.

The Institute of Medicine (IOM) 2010 report calls for initiatives that focus on changes that will enhance the potential of nurses to have a positive impact on the future of health care. They include the following:

1. Nurses should practice to the full extent of their education and training.
2. Nurses should achieve higher levels of education and training through an improved education system that promotes seamless academic progression.

3. Nurses should be full partners, with physicians and other health-care professionals, in redesigning health care in the United States.
4. Effective workforce planning and policy making require better data collection and information infrastructure.

Collectively, these agendas will affect care delivery, outcomes, and reimbursements. Additional changes in the health-care landscape have affected and will continue to affect APRNs. Since 1980, emphasis has been given to preparing medical primary care providers.

Despite this emphasis, 75% of physicians chose specialty practice over primary care, and in the years between 1999 and 2006, the trend toward specialization continued despite federal government cuts in funding for residency programs in areas of specialization (Steven, 2004). In addition, federal regulations, which limit the resident work week to 80 hours, have added a new burden to health-care delivery, creating a void in medical management within the acute-care setting. This trend presents added challenges to NPs, requiring them to fill this gap in care. The added skills and competencies needed in such roles often focus more on medical specialty knowledge rather than on advanced nursing knowledge, such as being with, listening to, and coming to know the patient as a whole, complex person.

As the number of APRNs increases, competition for reimbursement and questions about the delivery of safe, effective, high-quality care and evidenced-based patient/family practice continue to present challenges. Limited time during patients' visits coupled with reduced follow-up visits due to cost constraints may compromise the full impact of APRNs on patient care immediately and over time.

FUTURE DIRECTIONS AND FUTURE CONSIDERATIONS

Emerging changes within professional nursing have affected and will continue to affect APRN practice. The Consensus Model (2008) introduced standards for the licensure, accreditation, certification, and education (LACE) of APRNs. This model seeks to provide consistency and clarity around population-based health and areas of specialization. Further, this model will affect blended education programs that have attempted to merge rather than distinguish roles such as the CNS and NP.

Concurrently, the American Association of Colleges of Nursing (AACN) suggests that by 2015 the doctorate in nursing practice (DNP) be the minimum degree for APRNs to enter practice and as an alternative to a research-focused doctorate (AACN, 2011). As a result, a growing number of APRNs are being prepared with a clinical doctorate. There has been a 51.2% increase in the number of nurses pursuing this degree since 2010. Although there has been tremendous growth in DNP programs, it is not yet clear what roles and responsibilities the DNP nurse will assume. The research-focused doctorate (doctorate of philosophy [PhD], doctor of education [EdD], or doctorate of nursing science [DNSc]) continues to be the highest academic degree for nurses, and currently all but seven states have research-focused doctorate programs. Recent statistics suggest that over 28,369 nurses have a research-focused doctorate in nursing (HRSA, 2010).

Skills Versus Knowledge

APRN preparation includes knowledge, skills, and the resultant competencies for a particular role and populations plus advanced knowledge in the discipline of nursing itself. The graduate curriculum includes content on role preparation, research, and health policy, as well as knowledge that reflects disciplinary theory and concepts (e.g., holism and healing). In addition, specialty content related to populations, diagnoses, procedures and treatments, and disease management enhances an APRN's ability to care for patients.

The ability to blend components of both medicine and nursing makes the APRN unique, but too often the work of nursing becomes invisible as APRNs assume more of the medical role while underutilizing the domains unique to advanced practice nursing (Bryant-Lukosius et al., 2004). This lack of nursing identity plagues the NP, while the CNS is devalued and job opportunities are diminished (Mick & Ackerman, 2002, p. 397).

Advancing the Discipline

The literature supports the need for APRNs to work together, increase their focus on cost-effective, outcomes-based practice, and demonstrate patient satisfaction (Mick & Ackerman, 2002; Oermann & Floyd, 2002; Prevost, 2002). Several troublesome issues emerge in APRN practice: (a) roles are consistently developed and morphed in a response to fill gaps in medicine, (b) there is a lack of distinction regarding the uniqueness of the role—either in comparison to medicine or to each other, and (c) there is a lack of evidence to support the contribution of APRNs to individuals' well-being and to the delivery system.

Despite the need for evidence-based practice, research supporting the APRN role is not a priority in clinical settings. When it does exist, the primary focus is to describe how APRNs are similar to rather than unique and distinct from their physician counterparts. The growth of the APRN role appears to be a response to shortages of physicians, rather than a complement or alternative in care, with clear distinctions about why a consumer would prefer one to the other. It is this lack of evidence that has negatively affected the CNS in the past decade. Some of the NP roles in acute care have been created in response to cuts in the hours worked by medical residents, and anecdotal evidence suggests NPs are "as good as" or a welcome complement to physician care teams, yet there is limited research to support these conclusions. Limited use of standardized nursing language that communicates NP care beyond medical concerns is needed to provide evidence linked to outcomes. It is suggested that these NPs do not distinguish their practice and knowledge, as compared to other providers (Hoffman et al., 2005; Steven, 2004). The care provided by NPs in acute and chronic care settings is comprehensive specialty care that is sought by patients with complex medical and psychosocial problems. This NP role mirrors CNS practice and has led to a blurring of the two roles.

Research, practice, and education are central to the APRN role. Without research that is sensitive to the breadth and depth of APRN practice, the role of the APRN will lack the needed evidence to advance professional nursing practice. Nursing studies that link nurse-sensitive quality indicators to patient care outcomes are essential to advancing the discipline. Doctorally prepared APRNs in clinical settings are critical to achieving this goal.

Often the most critical element in any health-care setting is the nurse–patient relationship. Within this context there is the potential to discover meaning, affect individual choices, and promote health and personal transformation (Flanagan, 2008; Grace, 2008; Jones, 2006; Newman et al., 2008). APRNs attending to this mandate may promote new behaviors that influence health-care outcomes in a cost-effective, efficient, timely, and safe manner.

CONCLUSION

This chapter focused on the role of APRNs and the contributions they have made to improve health care for all. Care provided by APRNs is safe, cost effective, and satisfying to patients and families. Trends in care suggest that both the practice settings and roles of APRNs have changed greatly since their inception. It is important for nurses practicing in these roles to continue to document and research practice outcomes, so that when evidence is needed to support a role, it can easily be made available.

As health care evolves, it is important that APRNs reflect a clear image of professional nursing, as opposed to changing in response to the call of medicine. Loss of disciplinary focus creates nurses who may be technically skilled and competent but unable to discuss their unique contributions. It is essential that an evaluation of the impact of the APRN take into account accomplishments that are often silent in a medically driven health-care system. These events may require the transition from "fix it" models of care delivery to frameworks guided by nursing knowledge to achieve personal changes and improved life for the patient.

REFERENCES

American Association of Colleges of Nursing. (2011). *The doctor of nursing practice.* Retrieved November 16, 2011, from http://www.aacn.nche.edu/dnp.

American Association of Nurse Anesthetists. (2002). *Patients: Quality of care in anesthesia—section two.* Retrieved September 20, 2011, from http://www.aha.org.

American Nurses Association. (2000). *Certified nurses report fewer adverse effects: Survey links certification with improved health care.* Retrieved September 20, 2011, from http://www.needlestick.org.

American Nurses Credentialing Center (2008). *A new model for ANCC's Magnet Recognition Program®.* Retrieved September 20, 2011, from http://www.nursecredentialing.org/MagnetModel.aspx.

APRN Consensus Work Group & National Council of State Board of Nurses Advisory Committee. (2008). *Consensus model for APRN regulation: Licensure, accreditation, certification and education.* Retrieved September 20, 2011, from https://www.ncsbn.org/1623.htm.

Brooten, D. (1995). Perinatal care across the continuum: Early discharge and nursing home follow-up. *Journal of Perinatal and Neonatal Nursing, 9*(1), 38–44.

Brooten, D., Naylor, M., York, R., Brown, L., Roncoli, M., Hollingsworth, A., et al. (1995). Effects of nurse specialist transitional care on patient outcomes and costs: Results of five randomized trials. *American Journal of Managed Care, 1*(1), 35–41.

Bryant-Lukosius, D., Dicenso, A., Browne, G., & Pinelli, J. (2004). Advanced practice nursing roles: Development, implementation and evaluation. *Journal of Advanced Nursing, 48*(5), 519–529.

Cumbie, S., Conley, V., & Burman, M. (2004). Advanced practice nursing model for comprehensive care with chronic illness: Model for promoting process engagement. *Advances in Nursing Science, 27*(1), 70–80.

Davidson, M. (2002). Outcomes of high-risk women cared for by certified nurse-midwifes. *Journal of Midwifery and Women's Health, 47*(1), 46–49.

Declercq, E. (2002). CNM birth attendance in the United States, 1999. *Journal of Midwifery and Women's Health, 47*(1), 44–45.

De Koninck, M., Blais, R., Joubert, P., Gadnon, C. (2001, March-April). Comparing womenril). C. n, C., C. alth,s, 1999. tates, 1999., 1999. d nurs. *Journal of Midwifery and Women's Health,* 46(2), 60-67.

Fawcett, J., Newman, D., & McAllister, M. (2004). Advanced practice nursing and conceptual models of nursing. *Nursing Science Quarterly, 17*(2), 135–138.

Federal Register. (1998, January). Medicare & Medicaid. Retrieved August 19, 2012, from http://www.netreach.net/~wmanning/mmov.htm

Flanagan, J. (2008). Ethical issues for advanced practice nurses caring for the adult health population. In P. Grace (Ed.), *Nursing ethics and professional responsibility in advanced practice.* Boston: Jones & Bartlett.

Grace, P. (2008). Nursing ethics. In P. Grace (Ed.), *Nursing ethics and professional responsibility in advanced practice.* Boston: Jones & Bartlett.

Hayes, E. (2007). Nurse practitioners and managed care: Patient satisfaction and intention to adhere to nurse practitioner plan of care. *Journal of the American Academy of Nurse Practitioners, 19*(8), 418–426.

Health Resources and Services Administration. (2010). *The registered nurse population: Findings from the 2008 national sample survey of registered nurses.* Washington, DC: U.S. Department of Health and Human Services.

Hellings, P., & Howe, C. (2000). Assessment of breastfeeding knowledge of nurse practitioners and nurse midwives. *Journal of Midwifery and Women's Health, 4*(3), 264–270.

Hoffman, L., Tasota, F., Zullo, T., Scharfenberg, C., & Donaue, M. (2005). Outcomes of care managed by an acute care nurse practitioner/attending physician team in a subacute medical intensive care unit. *American Journal of Critical Care, 14*(2), 121–130.

Horrocks, S., Anderson, E., & Salisbury, C. (2002). Systematic review of whether nurse practitioners working in primary care can provide equivalent care to doctors. *British Medical Journal, 324*(7341), 819–823.

Ingersoll, E., McIntosh, M., & Williams, M. (2000). Nurse-sensitive outcomes of advanced practice. *Journal of Advanced Nursing, 32*(5), 1272–1281.

Institute of Medicine. (1999). *To err is human: Building a safer health care system.* Washington, DC: National Academy Press.

Institute of Medicine. (2001). *Crossing the quality chasm.* Washington, DC: National Academy Press.

Institute of Medicine. (2010). *The future of nursing: Leading change, advancing health.* Washington, DC: National Academies Press.

International Council of Nurses. (2002). *Definition and characteristics of the (APRN)role.* Retrieved August 21, 2012 from www.icn-APRNetwork.org.

Jones, D. (2006). Are we abandoning nursing as a discipline? *Clinical Nurse Specialist: The Journal for Advanced Nursing Practice, 19*(6), 275–277.

Keough, V. A., Stevenson, A., Martinovich, Z., Young, R., & Tanabe, P. (2011). Nurse practitioner certification and practice settings: Implications for education and practice. *Journal of Nursing Scholarship, 43*(2), 195–202.

Kring, D. L. (2008). Clinical nurse specialist practice domains and evidenced-based practice competencies. *Clinical Nurse Specialist: The Journal for Advanced Nursing Practice, 22*(4), 179–183.

Lyons, B. (2005). Getting back to autonomous practice. *Clinical Nurse Specialist: The Journal for Advanced Nursing Practice, 19*(1), 25–27.

Mastropietro, C. A., Horton, B. J. Ouellette, S. M., & Faut-Callahan, M. (2001). The National Commission on nurse anesthesia education 10 years later—Part I: The commission years (1989–1994). *AANA Journal, 69*(5), 379–385.

McGee, L. A., & Kaplan, L. (2007). Factors influencing the decision to use nurse practitioners in the emergency department. *Journal of Emergency Nursing, 33*(5), 441–446.

Mick, D., & Ackerman, M. H. (2002). Deconstructing the myth of the advanced practice blended role: Support for role divergence. *Heart and Lung, 31*(8), 393–398.

Muller, A., Hujcs, M., Dubendorf, P., & Harrington, P., (2010). Sustaining excellence: Clinical nurse specialist practice and magnet designation. *Clinical Nurse Specialist, 24*(5), 252–259.

Mundinger, M., Kane, R., Lenz, E., Totten, A., Wei-Yann, T., Cleary, P., et al. (2000). Primary care outcomes in patients treated by nurse practitioners or physicians: A randomized trial. *Journal of the American Medical Association, 283*(1), 59–68.

National Database of Nursing Quality Indicators. (2008). Retrieved September 20, 2011, from https://www.nursingquality.org/.

Newhouse, R., Stanik-Hutt, J., White, K., Johantgen, M., Bass, E., Zangaro, G., et al. (2011). Advanced practice nurse outcomes 1990–2008: A systematic review. *Nursing Economics, 29*(5), 1–22.

Newman, M., Smith, M., Pharris, M., & Jones, D. (2008). The focus of the discipline revisited. *Advances in Nursing Science, 31*(1), 16–27.

Oermann, M., & Floyd, J. (2002). Outcomes research: An essential component of the advanced practice nurse role. *Clinical Nurse Specialist, 16*(3), 140–144.

Prevost, S. (2002). Clinical nurse specialist outcomes: Vision, voice and value. *Clinical Nurse Specialist, 16*(3), 119–124.

Pronsati, M.P., Gerchufsky, M., (2011, February 1). National Salary Report. *Advance for NPs & PAs,* Retrieved August 21, 2012 from http://nurse-practitioners-and-physician-assistants.advanceweb.com/features/articles/national-salary-report-2010.aspx

Pulcini, J., Vampola, D., & Levine, J. (2005). Nurse practitioner practice characteristics, salary, and benefits survey, 2003. *Clinical Excellence for Nurse Practitioners, 9*(1), 49–58.

Raisler, J. (2000). Midwives helping mothers to breastfeed: Food for thought and action. *Journal of Midwifery and Women's Health, 45*(3), 202–204.

Richmond, T. S., Thompson, H. J., & Sullivan-Marx, E. M. (2000). Reimbursement for acute care nurse practitioner services. *American Journal of Critical Care, 9*(1), 52–61.

Rollet, J. (2010). 2009 National salary and workplace survey. *Advance for Nurse Practitioners.* Retrieved September 20, 2011, from http://nurse-practitioners-and-physician-assistants.advanceweb.com/features/top-story/2009-national-salary-and-workplace-survey-results.aspx.

Schober, M. (2006). Advanced nursing practice: An emerging global phenomenon. *Journal of Advanced Nursing, 55*(3), 275–276.

Simonson, D. C., Ahern, M. C., & Hendryx, M. S. (2007). Anesthesia staffing and anesthetic complications during cesarean delivery: A retrospective analysis. *Nursing Research, 56*(1), 9–17.

Steven, K. (2004). APRN hospitalist: Just a resident replacement? *Journal of Pediatric Health Care, 18*(4), 208–210.

Venning, P., Durie, A., Roland, M., Roberts, C., & Leese, B. (2000). Randomised controlled trial comparing cost effectiveness of general practitioners and nurse practitioners in primary care. *British Medical Journal, 320*(7241), 1048–1053.

World Health Organization. (2006). *Strengthening nursing and midwifery care.* Retrieved September 20, 2011, from http://www.who.int/hrh/nursing_midwifery/resolutions/en/index.html.

24

Starting a Practice and Practice Management

Judith Barberio

Advanced practice nurses (APNs) increasingly strive for greater autonomy in their practice. This desire to have control over their work environment has led to the emergence of independent nurse-managed health-care practices. However, is an entrepreneurial spirit, a fine-tuned knowledge base and clinical skills, and the desire to provide quality health care enough? Over the past 20 years, individuals, as well as schools of nursing, have increasingly opened nurse-managed health centers, only to see their viability threatened because of a lack of financial self-sufficiency (Brown, 2007; King, 2008; Vincent et al., 1999). New areas of concern revolve around the doctor of nursing practice degree (DNP) and how it affects master's-prepared APNs and their ability to continue to practice, as well as the impact on health-care policy issues such as reimbursement and independent practice without joint protocols.

With the passage of the Affordable Care Act and its guarantee of health-care access for all Americans, there will be an increased need for more primary care providers and more cost-effective services. Nurse-managed practices are positioned to play an important role in access to cost-effective health care; however, for these practices to survive and grow, APNs must acquaint themselves with the emerging realities of the new health-care policy agenda and nursing education in addition to the business acumen and financial know-how that is essential to creating practices that are efficient and fiscally viable.

ADVANTAGES TO INDEPENDENT PRACTICE

Independent nursing practice continues to garner support and become a reality. The ability to maximize the care of the client and the time to provide the educational base is necessary to enable the client to become a true partner in the health-care regimen. An independent practice can provide the APN with many opportunities, such as those listed in **Box 24-1.**

The Affordable Care Act provides the opportunity for a major change in the U.S. health system. Millions of uninsured Americans will have access to health care, which presents a need for change in our current health-care systems. The Affordable Care Act, along with the American Recovery and Reinvestment Act, has the potential to remove many of the barriers to independent APN practice (Kocher, Emanuel, & DeParle, 2010). The time to embrace an entrepreneurial spirit may be *now.*

BARRIERS TO INDEPENDENT PRACTICE

With all the advantages to independent practice, why do so few APNs consider this alternative? APNs have long been lauded in the literature with respect to their high quality of patient care and cost-effectiveness (Carzoli et al., 1994; Newhouse et al., 2011); Office of Technology Assessment, 1986; Spitzer et al., 1974). Their practice has been compared to physicians in primary care practices,

BOX 24-1
Opportunities That Can Come With Independent Practice

1. The freedom to focus the practice and your energy on your interests, such as alternative therapy or acupuncture, or specialty populations such as women's health or geriatrics.
2. Time management becomes flexible. You have the ability to structure your workload and allow time to examine, counsel, and educate clients.
3. The quality of your practice becomes your responsibility and is under your control. You are able to include the preventive health care and education needed at each client encounter.
4. Multiple sources for reimbursement can be identified and pursued. Besides third-party reimbursement, contracts for service can be sought out in industry and community groups. Income can be tied to workload.
5. New opportunities and requests for service provide a challenge to expanding services and promoting the growth of the practice.
6. Staffing becomes your responsibility and provides the opportunity to work with people you respect and who share your philosophy of health care.
7. Enhanced problem-solving skills and self-esteem are positive by-products of independent practice for the entrepreneurial APN. Learning to constructively deal with change, resolve conflicts, and successfully implement strategies creates a profitable practice and enhances self-confidence and self-esteem.

and findings suggest that APNs provide comparable high-quality care with similar positive health outcomes (Mundinger et al., 2000; Newhouse et al., 2011). What barriers to practice are so prevalent that they dissuade this competent, highly educated, and cost-effective group of health-care providers from establishing independent practices?

Pearson (2007) identifies the four major roadblocks to independent APN practice:

1. The need for direct reimbursement from third-party payers
2. Statutory limitations to the APN's scope of practice
3. Inconsistent and restrictive prescriptive authority
4. The inability to obtain hospital privileges

Many factors contribute to the roadblocks that stand in the way of independent APN practice. Throughout the 20th century physicians have controlled health-care practice and health information, partially because they were the first health-care providers to be granted legislative autonomy. This legislative autonomy and recognition enhanced the public's confidence that the actions of physicians were always directed for the good of the public and not for personal gain. Financial security, legislative strength, and a unified medical community also played a role in organized medicine's control of hospital policy and third-party reimbursement (Brassard & Smolenski, 2011; Mirvis, 1999).

Over the past decade, the clinical doctorate with a focus on administrative leadership, clinical practice, and clinical education has evolved. Supporters of this terminal clinical degree cite the need for nursing to attain parity with other health-care disciplines. They argue that increased knowledge is needed to provide leadership in health-care system effectiveness and optimal patient outcomes. Advocates maintain that educational credentials are needed to be included in high-level health-care management and policy decisions (Cronenwett et al., 2011; Fain, Asselin, & McCurry, 2008). Some master's-prepared APNs fear being marginalized to second-class status as the DNP becomes the preferred educational degree for APNs. The potential for devaluation of MS-prepared APNs exists, as does the possibility of being replaced by APN providers with a clinical doctorate (Meleis & Dracup, 2005). This fear of becoming obsolete may discourage an entrepreneurial spirit.

In addition to persuasive national barriers, common problems applicable to most new start-up businesses contribute to the demise of independent APN practices. Major obstacles to overcome with the start of most new businesses include the following:

1. Start-up costs for the practice
2. Cash-flow and financing an ongoing practice
3. Accounting practices, billing, and collection of receipts
4. Day-to-day management of the practice
5. Compliance with city, state, and federal regulations
6. General and malpractice insurance for the practice and individual providers
7. Hiring, training, and retaining competent, enthusiastic personnel

The obstacles inherent in starting a business coupled with the unique barriers confronting the independent APN practice have provided a challenge to many individuals. This chapter acknowledges their struggles, learns from their mistakes, and provides guidance to the entrepreneurial APN who is about to embark on this journey.

FIRST THINGS FIRST

The decision has been made: you want to be your own boss and deliver health care *your* way. No more time clocks, overbooking clients, or cutting short the patient visit due to time constraints. But where do you go from here? Key considerations and decisions must be made to get your business up and running. The items listed in **Box 24-2** will focus your operation and provide the organizing details that determine start-up efficiency in the world of managed care.

BOX 24-2
Key Business Decisions

- Develop a clear-cut strategy
- Determine the area's need for the service
- Develop a timeline for business start-up
- Determine licensing, tax, and insurance requirements
- Select your consultants
- Decide on the appropriate business structure
- Create the business name and image
- Select a practice location
- Develop a business plan
- Determine financing options
- Develop fees, reimbursement, and billing procedures
- Purchase equipment and select suppliers
- Hire and manage personnel
- Develop an organized documentation and quality assurance process
- Develop policies and procedures
- Develop marketing strategies

KEY QUESTIONS

As you embark on the key start-up decisions to be made, pay attention to the questions that may arise. A major question to consider is the scope of independent APN practice in the state in which you practice. Thirty-five states currently have statutory or regulatory requirements for physician collaboration, direction, or supervision. Only 15 states and the District of Columbia have independent prescriptive authority that does not require physician involvement or delegation (Pearson, 2011). If your practice is not located in one of these enlightened states, carefully read and clarify the policies regarding collaboration or supervision of your practice and the regulation of your prescriptive authority. Developing a collaborative agreement with a physician and creating appropriate protocols, including protocols for controlled dangerous substances (CDSs), are other areas to investigate if this is a state requirement for APN practice.

Reimbursement is another major question to consider. Where will it come from and will it be enough to cover your expenses? Investigate how pervasive managed care is in your practice location and determine if APNs are admitted to managed care panels and are listed as primary care providers (PCPs). If APNs are accepted in your state as PCPs and practice independently, how do you deal with the patient whose condition exacerbates and needs hospitalization? Investigate the area hospitals to determine if APNs are given hospital privileges. Even if APNs are admitted to hospital panels in your area, you will need a collaborative arrangement or referral agreement with various physicians in the area for management of your patients when they are acutely ill.

These and other questions will arise as you carry out the myriad tasks needed to launch a new business. Pay attention to detail and carefully consider each question and decision you make. These decisions will structure your practice operations and ultimately enable you to attain your personal and professional goals.

DEVELOP A CLEAR-CUT STRATEGY

Strategy distinguishes your business. It tells the consumer what differentiates your practice from the competition. It is the foundation of your business plan and dictates the day-to-day operations of your practice. How does one develop a strategy? Look around you and consider the market, consumer needs, the competition, your practice's strengths and weaknesses, and your philosophy of health care and personal goals.

Focus the nature of your practice and do not try to be all things to all patients. Competitive personal service businesses, such as a health-care practice, will commonly use the strategy of specialization. Specialization reduces competition and drives reimbursement. Initially, you may want to see any patient who elects to seek your help. As you begin to develop your practice, simultaneously begin to advertise, write articles for the local newspaper, and hold seminars on topics that focus on your expertise. This exposure will promote the area in which you wish to specialize and will allow you to phase out other aspects of your practice.

Specialize by developing a niche market, one that you know extremely well. A niche market is one with a unique service or product that services a particular clientele. You may decide that you want the focus of your practice to be on wellness. You can then tailor your practice to offer individual health risk assessments, counseling on behavior change, work site wellness programs, smoking cessation and weight loss programs, and countless other health promotion activities that may be needed in your location. One word of advice: know your service. Do not begin a practice marketing alternative therapy without an exhaustive knowledge of these services or competent, knowledgeable staff. Remember that your competition is already established and knows the business aspects of the practice better than you do. You want to present yourself as an expert in the field.

DETERMINE THE AREA'S NEED FOR THE SERVICE

Determine who the potential clients are and then attempt to ascertain their needs. If you decide that your practice will serve the health-care needs of inner-city, low-income residents, you must investigate the most prevalent reasons for health-care use and follow-up care. This information can be gathered from various sources. The state nurses association, state division of health, and county and local health departments may be helpful in providing important data. Topics you may want to explore include health provider demographics for an area, medically underserved areas, and health-care delivery systems in an area such as ambulatory care centers, urgent care centers, and family planning clinics. Local businesses, such as pharmacies and medical device companies, may also provide information about the health-care needs of the local population, as well as advertising and articles in the local newspaper.

DEVELOP A TIMELINE FOR BUSINESS START-UP

Organization is the key ingredient to developing a business plan and moving your practice from the planning stage into action. A minimum of 9 months should be allowed to complete this project. Designate yourself as the project leader and determine other individuals who may assist you with start-up tasks. The key undertaking of business start-up is persistence and attention to detail. A sample timeline for completing major tasks is presented in **Box 24-3.**

BOX 24-3
Practice Start-up Timeline

Nine Months Before Practice Start-up

1. Select a geographical location.
2. Obtain contracts from third-party payers and hospitals you wish to join.
3. Determine start-up costs of a practice and your net worth.
4. Develop a business plan.
5. Investigate sources of capital investment in your practice.
6. Obtain loan applications, speak to various loan officers, and submit applications.
7. Determine when telephone books are printed and list your practice.
8. Open a business checking account.
9. Obtain state nursing license, advanced practice license, and federal Drug Enforcement Administration (DEA) number.
10. Investigate potential physician collaborators if needed in your state.

Six Months Before Practice Start-up

1. Investigate practice locations for rent or purchase.
2. Inquire about zoning laws regarding your type of practice and signage requirements.
3. Determine utility requirements for your practice, sources, and cost.
4. Determine office layout, design, and necessary structural improvements.
5. Determine needed office and medical equipment and determine cost of lease versus buy.
6. Explore and select business consultants, specifically a lawyer, accountant, banker, insurance broker, and medical biller.

Continued

BOX 24-3
Practice Start-up Timeline—cont'd

7. Determine form of the practice, such as solo practice, partnership, or corporation, and have your attorney draw up all legal documents for your signature.
8. Evaluate all contracts with your attorney before signing.
9. Investigate medical practice systems that contain scheduling, billing, and records.
10. Make application for federal Medicare, Medicaid, and national provider identifier (NPI) numbers and obtain fee schedules.
11. Obtain current procedural terminology book (CPT-4) and International Classification of Diseases, Ninth Revision, Clinical Manual (ICD-9-CM) and the HCFA 1500 insurance claim forms.
12. Formalize a collaborative agreement with an area physician if required by law.
13. Apply for an office laboratory license or a Clinical Laboratory Improvement Amendments (CLIA) waiver.
14. Apply for provider status to managed care provider panels.
15. Apply for hospital privileges to local health-care institutions.

Three Months Before Practice Start-up

1. Arrange for professional malpractice insurance for providers and liability insurance for the practice and equipment.
2. Arrange for health and disability insurance for yourself and employees.
3. Arrange for telephone service installation and an answering service for the practice, beeper service, and call forwarding service.
4. Order signage for the practice.
5. Investigate and arrange for the acceptance of credit cards as a payment option.
6. Design and order announcements for the opening of your practice.
7. Apply for your federal and state employer identification number (EIN) through your local Internal Revenue Service (IRS) office and state labor department.
8. Review federal and state tax requirements with your accountant and obtain booklets describing federal, state, and city tax withholding requirements.
9. Develop a policy and procedure manual for the practice.
10. Develop job descriptions for all employees.
11. Begin advertising and interviewing for office personnel.
12. Arrange for needed services such as biomedical waste management, specimen pickup, janitorial services, laundry services, and ground maintenance and snow removal.
13. Order clinical supplies and set up an inventory control system.
14. Order business supplies such as state prescription pads (if mandated), appointment cards, business cards, letterhead stationery and envelopes, stationery supplies, deposit stamp for checks, petty cash vouchers, purchase order forms, telephone message pads, and patient referral forms and disposition forms.
15. Order office equipment and arrange for delivery.
16. Determine office hours.
17. Determine fee schedule.

BOX 24-3
Practice Start-up Timeline—cont'd

18. Develop advertising information such as a patient booklet of services, press release, and introduction letters to local health-care providers, pharmacy and medical equipment suppliers, and pharmaceutical representatives in your area.
19. Develop your practice Web site and professional Facebook page, and explore Twitter and YouTube for their advertising potential for your practice.

One Month Before Practice Start-up

1. Set up your office.
2. Arrange for utility start-up, including telephone, gas, electric, and water.
3. Hire a medical biller and obtain your Medicare, Medicaid, NPI, and managed care organization provider numbers.
4. Hire office personnel and train them with respect to office policies, telephone procedures, appointment scheduling and collection of fees, and use of the medical office system.
5. Establish the office cash flow procedures and a petty cash fund.
6. Install your office sign.
7. Accept patient appointments.
8. Place announcements, advertisements, and press releases in local newspapers and send to local community groups and area professionals.

Opening Day

Congratulations, you have started an independent APN practice!

DETERMINE LICENSING, TAX, AND INSURANCE REQUIREMENTS

To open an independent APN practice, a number of licenses must be obtained. After choosing a location for your practice, the process of applying for all state and federal licenses should be your next priority. Besides state licensure for nursing and advanced practice nursing, you must also obtain state and federal identification numbers and a federal Drug Enforcement Administration (DEA) number, as well as others to open your door and do business. The most commonly required licenses and tax identification numbers have been listed.

State Nursing License and Advanced Practice License or Certification

The state board of nursing will be able to provide information and a list of documents you need to apply for these licenses. Be aware that in some states the board of nursing and the board of medicine oversee the advanced practice nursing license or certification.

State Narcotics License

Check with your state concerning the requirement for a state narcotics license. This is not a requirement of all states, but if it is, it must be obtained before application for a federal narcotics license.

Your state's board of nursing will be able to inform you if this license is necessary and the procedure to obtain this license.

Federal Narcotics License

APNs do not have legal authority in all states to dispense narcotics. You will be able to obtain the necessary information from the board of nursing in the state. DEA numbers are assigned for your lifetime; they will not be reassigned if you move to another location. If you move to another state, you are required to notify the DEA authorities of your new address. If you do not have a DEA number and can legally prescribe narcotics in your state, you can obtain this license from the Department of Justice at:

Registration Unit
Drug Enforcement Administration
PO Box 28083 Central Station
Washington, DC 20005
Drug Enforcement Administration (DEA), Office of Diversion Control, Registration Unit, toll-free number, 24 hours a day: 1-800-882-9539

The DEA also has forms online for registration of APNs. The application form can be found on the Web at the Diversion Control Program Web site at www.DEAdiversion.usdoj.gov.

Medicaid Provider Number

Medicaid is a jointly funded, federal-state health insurance program for certain low-income people. The people covered include children, the aged, blind, disabled, and people who are eligible to receive federally assisted income maintenance payments.

You can apply for this provider number through the state Medicaid agency. Obtain a provider application for APNs from the provider relations department of your state health department. The state Medicaid agency is billed using the Centers for Medicare and Medicaid Services (CMS) 1500 form unless the client is enrolled in Medicaid managed care.

The number you receive from your state Medicaid agency will remain with you while you practice in the state. If you move within the state, you only need to notify the carrier of your new address. If you move out of state, you will need to obtain a new number in the new state.

Medicaid Managed Care

Some patients who have health insurance through the state Medicaid program will be covered under a managed care organization (MCO). To obtain a provider number for Medicaid MCOs, you must contact the provider relations for each MCO and apply for admission to the panel of providers. APNs are not admitted to provider panels in all MCOs. In some states, MCOs cannot discriminate among providers on the basis of type of license held. In other states, an MCO can accept or reject any provider. Check your state law concerning managed care and provider panels. If you are initially rejected, request a meeting to present your case. Pursue the MCO to reevaluate your application and go up the chain of command with your request.

Medicare

Medicare is a federal health insurance program for certain groups of people including the elderly over age 65 and the permanently disabled. This program covers hospitalization (Part A); provider services, home care, and outpatient health care (Part B); and medication (Part D).

If you will be providing health-care services to this population, you need to apply for a Medicare number. This number will be valid only in the state in which you currently practice. If you move out of state, you will be assigned a new Medicare number for that state.

An insurer in each state that has contracted with the CMS manages the administration and payment services for Medicare. You can find the Medicare carrier for your state by going to the CMS Web site at www.cms.hhs.gov/ or Medicare at www.medicare.gov/. Once you are aware of the carrier for your state, you can obtain an application and apply for a provider number. Medicare is billed on a form called the CMS 1500. The preferred method of billing for Medicare is electronic funds transfer (EFT), and this can be elected when enrolling in Medicare for the first time or when making a change to your existing enrollment information. If a patient is enrolled in Medicare managed care, reimbursement is handled by an MCO, and the provider must be admitted to the MCO provider panel.

National Provider Identifier

The national provider identifier (NPI) is a unique identification number given to each health-care provider and used in standard transactions, such as claims for reimbursement for health-care services. This number may be used to identify health-care providers on a number of documents including prescriptions, patient medical records, and coordination of benefits between health plans. Once assigned, the NPI is expected to remain the same regardless of change of name, change of address, or change of other information provided on the original application. The compliance date for all entities to use the NPI number on transactions was May 23, 2008. The NPI is the only health-care provider identifier that can be used for identification purposes in standard transactions including electronic billing.

Health-care providers may apply for an NPI number through the national plan and provider enumeration system (NPPES) available at https://nppes.cms.hhs.gov. Providers may also apply for the NPI number on a paper application by requesting form CMS-10114 through the NPI enumerator or by downloading the paper application. The phone number for the NPI Enumerator is 1-800-465-3203, and the paper application can be downloaded from www.cms.hhs.gov/NationalProviderStand/ and mailed to the address on the form. There is no fee associated with obtaining an NPI.

If health-care providers do not have a Medicare or Medicaid provider number, they are encouraged to apply for the NPI before enrolling in these programs. Health-care providers who already have enrolled in these programs are encouraged to include their Medicare identification number, Medicaid identification number and state, and any other provider numbers issued by health plans in which they are enrolled when applying for the NPI.

Clinical Laboratory License

CMS regulates all laboratory testing performed on humans in the United States through the Clinical Laboratory Improvement Amendments (CLIA). The objective of the CLIA program is to ensure quality laboratory testing. These amendments require that all health provider office laboratories must be licensed according to the types of tests they perform. Office laboratories are subject to federal and state inspection and approval. The more complex the testing, the more stringent the state and federal laboratory requirements. However, any laboratory testing done on site will require the facility to have a CLIA number.

Laboratory tests are divided into categories, and there are a number of waived tests that can be performed in the office setting. A practice that only performs waived tests can apply for an exemption from inspection and the requirement of a medical director to oversee the laboratory. Federal CLIA regulations can be found on the Internet at www.cms.hhs.gov/clia/, and state CLIA regulations can be obtained from the state health department. The state will provide forms for the federal and state application for a CLIA number. Pay particular attention to the state regulations because many times the state regulations are more restrictive than the federal guidelines.

Employer Identification Number

The employer identification number (EIN) is a tax identification number and is needed for all communication with the Internal Revenue Service (IRS). Contact your local IRS office or Social Security office and request Form SS-4 to apply for an EIN. This number can also be applied for by phone with the local IRS Service Center. Once an EIN is obtained, the IRS will send a booklet of payment coupons (Form 8109) for depositing your withholding taxes. The EIN will also be used to report compensation from third-party payers such as private insurance companies, Medicare, or Medicaid.

State Tax Identification Number

Contact your state to confirm whether there is an additional need to apply for a state tax identification number. The local phone number can be found in the white pages listed under United States or the name of your state. Your accountant will be able to inform you of all identifying numbers needed to satisfy federal and state regulations.

Professional Liability Insurance

Many carriers cover APNs, including traditional insurance companies, self-insured companies, and group purchasing programs. Not all companies conduct business in every state. Choose a company that has experienced claim adjusters and a formidable legal network. Inquire about the company's service orientation and its capacity to offer risk management and loss prevention assistance and advice. Consider a company that has been in business for at least 10 years and has a good financial standing. Litigation can take many years to come to fruition, and you want a company with the capability to remain in business to defend you.

Some points to consider when evaluating insurance policies:

1. How comprehensive is the policy? Make sure you read the policy thoroughly and note the inclusions, as well as the exclusions. Question anything you do not understand; it may save you a great deal of stress and money if litigation ensues.
2. What type of insurance should you purchase: "claims made" or "occurrence"? A claims made policy will cover the APN only when the insurance policy is active, no matter when the incident occurred. If you were to retire and cancel your insurance policy, you would no longer be covered for any prior incident if litigation ensues at a later date. An occurrence policy will cover the APN for any incident that occurred while the insurance policy was in place.
3. Are the limits of coverage adequate? Many APNs purchase insurance based on the minimal coverage of $1,000,000 per occurrence and $3,000,000 cumulative. We reside in a litigious society, and this amount of coverage can easily be exhausted. Consider purchasing cumulative insurance that is at least double to triple the occurrence amount.
4. Should you purchase "tail coverage"? Frequently, APNs may join a group practice that already has a group policy for professional liability coverage. If you currently have malpractice insurance that you plan on canceling, consider purchasing tail coverage. This policy will cover any prospective legal action from events before joining the group practice.

5. Do you own the practice? If so, you may want to name the practice on your insurance policy. If litigation ensues, usually the practice, as well as an individual, is named.
6. Is business malpractice insurance necessary? Absolutely. Cover the practice. Inquire with the insurance company about the rates for covering an independent APN practice. This coverage will be in addition to your individual plan and can prove quite cost effective in the event of litigation.

Conventional Commercial Insurance Policies

Besides professional and business malpractice insurance, consider purchasing insurance protection for your office, the employees, and the equipment you have purchased. Some types of insurance to consider:

1. *Equipment insurance:* The expenditure for medical and office equipment is costly. A reasonably priced property insurance policy will cover the cost to replace the tangible assets of the practice. This policy should cover all medical equipment and supplies, office equipment and supplies, textbooks, and journals. Insurance premiums typically decrease as deductibles rise.
2. *Equipment malfunction insurance:* Many companies sell product warranties to cover equipment malfunction, repair, and replacement. Investigate commercial insurance companies for a blanket policy that covers all major equipment purchases. Many policies will also cover lost revenue for the time period that the equipment is unproductive.
3. *General liability coverage:* This is comprehensive insurance coverage that protects your practice in the event of litigation by a third party. It does not cover the policyholder or other parties specifically excluded. This policy typically includes lawsuits for personal injury, equipment failure, contractual liability, and advertising liability.
4. *Office disability insurance:* If your office becomes inaccessible as a result of property loss, your practice could go out of business in a short period of time. This policy should include reimbursement for lost revenue and profit; continuous expenses such as the lease on the copy machine; funding to temporarily relocate your office, purchase supplies, and advertise your new location; and finally the cost to return to your office after it has been restored.
5. *Workers' compensation insurance:* Most states require this insurance for any business that has employees. The owner of the business is usually not covered by this insurance unless the business is a corporation. This policy can be purchased from a commercial insurance company, but the state will regulate the benefits and cost of the policy. Therefore, most policies are comparable.

SELECT YOUR CONSULTANTS

Starting a health-care practice requires knowledge of state and federal laws, as well as general legal and accounting procedures. It is highly advisable to consult with these professionals as you set up your practice. Seek recommendations from other APNs, colleagues, business associates, the state nursing organization, and the board of nursing.

Attorney services will focus on setting up the legal structure of your practice and provide legal advice, contract development, and review. When you interview attorneys, pay particular attention to their health-care law experience, especially with respect to independent APN practice.

An *accountant* is another professional whose expertise can be cost effective for the short term, as well as the long term. Initially, consult with this professional to develop an accounting system, initiate internal controls, and establish an operating budget. As the practice develops, the accountant may suggest operating procedures that will provide the best tax advantage and provide tax-planning consultation.

A *medical biller* is an essential component of any health-care practice that intends to receive reimbursement from third-party payers. Medical billers will be involved in all aspects of billing and collecting accounts receivable. They may set up and track a charge account with a major credit card company for patients who are self-pay and send billing statements to patients who have been extended credit by the health-care practice. Medical billers frequently make application to insurer provider panels for the health-care providers in the practice. Additionally, they will make applications to NPI, Medicare, and Medicaid for provider numbers for the practice and all professional staff. Once avenues of reimbursement are established, the medical biller will ensure that the patient and medical information requested by the payer is completed and will submit the bill for payment. Tracking accounts receivable and questioning and resubmitting denial of payments is another aspect of the services provided by a medical biller. The scope of services from a medical biller will depend on the expertise and experience of this consultant. Many practices find it more cost effective to hire a full-time medical biller, whereas smaller practices may hire an off-site independent service to handle the billing aspect of the practice. Judiciously assess the qualifications and reputation of the employee or service you are contemplating.

A *practice manager* might be just the person or service you need if you are taking over an established practice or have a large patient following. An experienced practice manager may provide accounting and bookkeeping services, as well as total practice management. Services offered can vary greatly by consultant, and fees will increase as services provided increase. Practice managers may perform such services as hiring employees, maintaining bank accounts, paying practice bills, billing and account receivables for services rendered, staffing, payroll, tracking and ordering supplies, and contracting for laboratory, biomedical waste, and janitorial services. Many practice management consultants will develop employee job descriptions, policy and procedure manuals, and fee schedules that are consistent with the local market. Always ask for local references, preferably from other health-care providers, especially other APN practices. Remember to always check references and qualifications to get an idea of the types of services provided by this consultant, his or her experience and expertise, and his or her ability to competently complete the project in a timely manner.

DECIDE ON THE APPROPRIATE BUSINESS STRUCTURE

There are basically four types of business structures for a practice: sole proprietorship, partnership, corporation, or a limited liability corporation. The legal differences between these forms of business are contained in three issues: liability, the number of owners, and tax ramifications.

Sole Proprietorship

This is the simplest form of business, where the owner of the business and the business are one and the same. All of the assets and liabilities of the business are also the personal assets and liabilities of the owner. The owner of an independent APN practice is personally liable for any debt or legal infractions of the practice. There are no explicit prerequisites to establishing a sole proprietorship. A sole proprietorship can have only one owner of the business and is established when you go into business by yourself. This gives the APN the advantage of "running her own show" and establishing a practice according to specific beliefs and preferences. A sole proprietorship is not taxed *per se*. Because the business and the owner are one and the same, the owner completes an individual tax return along with a Schedule C. A Schedule C is a "profit and loss from business" form, which is used to file the practice earnings and expenses. Year-end profits and losses from the practice will be added to or subtracted from the owner's personal income.

Benefits from this type of business structure include autonomy, flexibility, and the ability to make practice decisions based on your individual philosophy. Any losses suffered by the practice, which is common in the start-up phase of a business, can be deducted from your personal income. Control of the profits is another benefit of this business structure along with a simplified tax return. A major disadvantage of a sole proprietorship is the total liability for all start-up and maintenance costs of the practice, as well as the negligence of any employees.

Partnership

A *partnership* is defined as the association of two or more people to carry on as co-owners of a business to make a profit. Although a partnership agreement is not required by law, most parties will spell out the relationship in a legal agreement. In a partnership there is a differentiation between the partnership and the partners. Partnerships cannot sue or be sued. However, all partners are personally liable for losses, wrongful acts, and omissions or commissions assumed by the partnership. Partners share in the profits, administration, decision making, and workload of the practice as defined in the partnership agreement. In this type of practice, earnings or losses pass through to the individual partners and appear on each partner's personal tax return.

A major benefit of this type of business structure is the shared financial and professional risks and responsibilities. Decision making remains fairly flexible, and it is generally easier to attract venture capital for financing the practice. The disadvantages of a partnership include the unlimited personal liability of each partner and the responsibility of each partner to pay taxes on business income.

Corporation

A corporation is an individual legal entity without ties to the individual business owner and is generally formed as a C corporation. It has the legal status to buy and sell assets and enter into contracts. It has its own tax identification number, as well as tax return. A professional corporation enjoys limited liability in that only the corporate assets can be used to satisfy judgments and thereby reduces the personal and financial risk of the APN owner and shareholder. In a professional practice, the APN is paid a salary, and as an owner or shareholder receives the profits of the corporation as dividends throughout the year. The downside of this arrangement is that the corporation is taxed on its profits and then the individual is taxed on the dividends. The owner of a small corporation can elect to be an S corporation that offers special tax advantages. All profits of an S corporation are taxable only as they are distributed as dividends to shareholders. Because of the intricacies of the law and the ever-changing tax laws, it is essential that the APN consult a tax professional.

Advantages of a corporate structure is the limited liability of the shareholders, centralized management, tax advantages for pension and profit-sharing plans, and a larger talent pool for decision making. Disadvantages of a corporation include the costs involved to establish and operate the corporation. There are also time-consuming federal, state, and local government requirements and filings to deal with, as well as the possibility of double taxation on corporate profits and shareholder dividends.

Limited Liability Corporation

A limited liability corporation (LLC) is another form of corporate structure that provides the best aspects of a partnership and a corporation. Income and losses pass through to the shareholders or owners as in a partnership, and there is no limit on the number of owners or shareholders. Legal liability is also limited, and members are not liable for the overall obligations of the LLC, although an individual would still be liable for professional malpractice. This type of corporate structure is also easier to set up and is subject to less government regulation. Be aware that LLCs are not recognized in all states, so be sure to check with your accountant or attorney.

Benefits of this type of corporate structure include limited liability and taxation only on the member's share of the LLC's income. An unlimited number of shareholders are allowed, and the shareholders or an appointed manager can manage the LLC. Disadvantages include limited recognition of this corporation by individual states and limited legal precedent addressing this form of corporate structure.

CREATE THE BUSINESS NAME AND IMAGE

Image plays an important role in how your practice is perceived in the marketplace. Your image is reflected in the office environment, advertising materials, your personal presentation and that of your staff, and written communication. Determine what image you want to present to your patients and convey this in your business name and practice style.

Ascertain what image would generate a positive response from prospective patients. Would a warm, homey atmosphere or a high-tech, professional office create more appeal for your target population? Are you trying to convey the notion of alternative therapy or new concepts in health-care delivery? Investigate what the potential consumer expects in his or her health-care provider. Above all, project high quality in every aspect of your practice, from the service you provide to the image you present.

Carefully evaluate the image you project in every patient encounter. Pay attention to every detail of the practice even if you delegate responsibilities to staff or consultants. Make sure the staff conveys their commitment to patient care and service during each interaction with patients. Consider the advantages of consulting with experts for certain aspects of the practice. A graphic artist may be better able to create a logo or brochure for the practice. Perhaps a marketing expert can develop a more effective advertising strategy. Keep in mind that image considerations play a part in all your practice decisions and should be used as a guide for future decision making.

A business name should convey the image you want to present to the public and will basically take one of two forms: your name or a name you have created for the practice. By selecting your name as the legal name of the practice, you are conveying a professional image and making the patient aware of the health-care provider in this practice. If you have been part of another practice in the area or are well known in this location, your name recognition may draw in a number of patients. The addition of "and Associates" to your name will convey the appearance of a larger practice with additional resources.

Professional practices do not always convey the names of the health-care providers. Many APNs prefer to project the name of what they do to reflect their business focus. Lois Brenneman of NPCEU (www.NPCEU.com) decided to market her product versus her name. NPCEU offers continuing education programs to APNs nationally. An individual was purposely not identified with this practice to project the image of large numbers of programs with a variety of speakers. *Elder Choices* is a health-care counseling practice that was developed by a group of APNs with expertise in gerontology and counseling. The name of this practice conveys the target population and the focus of the practice. Ultimately the choice is yours. Consider the image you want to project and use this as a guide in choosing a name.

SELECT A PRACTICE LOCATION

Location, location, location. This will be one of your most important business decisions. Think about your ideal geographical location, knowledge of the marketplace, professional relationships, and professional climate. Remember, health care is local, not global. The highs and lows of the local economy will have an effect on the success of your practice. Several factors will play into your ultimate choice of practice location.

Geographical Location

When you consider your practice location, think about convenience for your patients and the niche market you want to attract. A pediatric practice located in a downtown business location will not be as appealing as a practice location in a growing suburb. Ascertain parking availability in your practice location and determine if it is adequate to meet the needs of your clients. If on-site parking is limited or unavailable, investigate the proximity of public transportation to your practice location. If you hope to attract walk-in patients, determine if your practice is located in a heavily used pedestrian area. Remember that your services must not only be high quality, be cost effective, and have public appeal, but they must also be convenient.

Economics

The demographic makeup of your location will provide a snapshot of your market. The U.S. Census Bureau, local, county, and state governments, and private demographic services can provide the data necessary to evaluate a location. Pay particular attention to a few key factors.

1. *Male versus female population in a given area.* Women are the primary purchasers of health care and typically direct the health care of their families.
2. *The age distribution of the local population.* Age dictates the type of services chosen. New-age therapies might not be as eagerly accepted by a rural aging clientele as they would by upwardly mobile city dwellers. Age also influences the types of care used. Pediatric and midwifery services are sought after in a childbearing, child-rearing population, whereas wellness programs, health education, and chronic illness management may have a higher use among an older population.
3. *The income distribution in the local population.* Income influences the probability of and type of health insurance coverage, as well as disposable dollars for noncovered therapies and preventive programs. A stable or growing population is frequently associated with higher incomes and employment security.
4. *Cultural and language influences on the local population.* Cultural background, values, and practices of particular groups of people will influence their use of health care and wellness programs. Language barriers can be a significant factor in patient use of your services. Consider hiring personnel from the neighborhood who are familiar with the culture and speak the language of the local population.

Professional Relationships

Do not discount the professional relationships you have made along your professional career path. Prior employment, educational training, preceptorships, and professional associates are all sources of reference and referrals for your practice. These people already know you, your competence, and your skill. They can provide references or testimonials to your practice, as well as opportunities to expand the services provided by your practice.

Professional Climate

Consider the professional climate in the area you are considering opening an independent APN practice. What are the legal restrictions to practice in your state? How will the local medical and nursing community respond to your practice? Will collaborative protocols with an area physician and hospital privileges be difficult to obtain? Will physician consultation and referrals pose a problem? Do not abandon a location because of these obstacles, but know if they exist. When you are aware of potential barriers, you can address them and seek solutions.

DEVELOP A BUSINESS PLAN

A business plan is a written document that encapsulates the practice strategy for the future direction of the business and an action plan to achieve the practice objectives. Formulating a business plan is an effective way to plan for the practice and anticipate business decisions. Business plans may be developed for several reasons, such as a new business start-up, business expansion, financing of the business, or as an ongoing plan to manage the business. An effective business plan will describe the elements needed to run the business. Items should include a summary, business concept, market analysis, competition, competitive analysis, marketing plan, management team and personnel, operations, financial plan, and repayment projections. A business plan should give a clear picture of what is really required to start the business.

Summary

This should be a short and concise explanation of the major features of the practice. In one to two pages you should describe your practice strategy, practice development, financial objectives, and business organization. It is important to describe your service, and why it has promise. Describe the status of the practice with respect to a start-up timeline and marketing research. Include information about the business structure and the location of the practice, as well as financial projections, financing needs, and the projected return on investment. Be sure to focus on the key elements of the plan. Give the reader an overview of the practice, not a reiteration of the business plan.

Business Concept

This section should contain a clear explanation of the practice strategy. What sets your practice apart from other health-care practices in the area? Focus on the individuality of the practice and how this compares to the competition. Include areas that might have a significant impact on your strategy such as unique services, marketing ploys, or management team.

Market Analysis

This is where you document the need for your practice in a specific location. Has your location been designated as a health professional shortage area (HPSA)? If so, you must include citations of the documentation that supports this statement. Describe the marketplace and your potential competition. Discuss the size of the potential market and where patients are currently obtaining health care. Assess your competitors with respect to the size of their health-care practice, the clientele, the types of insurance accepted, and their fee structure. Determine if the population of the area is generally growing or shrinking and if there is a segment of the population that is medically underserved. Learn all you can about the population of your targeted location and consider this information when developing your marketing plan.

Where do you obtain this information? Seek out reports from various area trade associations and the chamber of commerce, as well as city, county, and state government reports. Research published material distributed by your competitors and reports published by area nursing organizations, hospitals, medical associations, and health departments. Conduct focus groups of area residents to determine what residents identify as a priority and the extent of these types of services in the specific location.

Competition

Know your competition and exactly what threat they are to your practice. Do they have a better location or a more convenient public transportation network than your practice? How do the services they offer and the quality of care compare to those of your practice? What are their practice fees and insurance reimbursement arrangements? Explore the reputation and image of your competition and the appearance they present to the public. Research the stability of the other health-care practices in your area, paying particular attention to staff turnover, reorganizations, and the announcements and cancellations of new initiatives. Pay attention to the advertising and marketing efforts of your competition and new health-care practices that may open in your area within the near future.

Competitive Analysis

This section of the business plan deals with an analysis of the strengths and risks associated with your practice. Be sure to include in your business plan a strategy to address these risks. An example of a business risk might be two established family medical practices within a 10-mile radius of your practice, thereby contributing to the risk of an inadequate patient caseload to financially sustain your practice. You can address this risk by renting highly visible space in a heavily trafficked area and target your services to a segment of the health-care market. A suburban storefront operation with convenient hours and walk-in appointments located in a strip mall next to the grocery store and cleaners may appeal to a large segment of the busy, well-woman population.

Marketing Plan

Develop and describe your overall promotional plan. What strategies will you use to reach your target population? Explain the reasoning behind your choice of advertising media, use of publicity, and other promotional plans and how they will enable you to get your message across to the target audience. Be realistic in your determination of a marketing budget and advertising timeline. Remember that effective marketing relies on repetition of your message. If your marketing budget is limited, concentrate your efforts on a smaller geographical area and the target population.

Management Team and Personnel

Focus your attention on key personnel. Describe the skills and competencies your staff and consultants bring to the practice. This is the section to highlight the relevant experience of your consultants, management team, and personnel. Stress the training and experience of your team and correlate their abilities to their role in your practice. Résumés of each team member should be included in the appendices. Include an organizational chart and job description for each member of your practice staff and any incentives for significant performance such as bonuses or potential ownership privileges.

Operations

Discuss the major business functions of your office, and describe how the work will get done. Note any services that are "special" for a practice that deals with your target population. For instance, your specialty area may be women's health care and your practice provides the services that are typically expected for this type of practice. However, you may also provide a special service such as bone density scanning, which is not typically offered in the area. This specialty service should be highlighted in the business plan. This could be the reason that your practice may be more effective in soliciting and retaining patients than the competition.

Financial Plan

In this section of the business plan you should discuss projected income, balance sheets, the income or profit-and-loss statements, cash flow projections, and the break-even analysis. You should plan to show financial projections for 3 to 5 years.

Projected income statements should describe the amounts and types of costs associated with the practice and the receipts and profits on both a monthly and annual basis for each year of the plan. Balance sheets should summarize the assets and liabilities of the practice and should be prepared for the practice start-up interval, then semiannually during the first year of operation, and annually for the remainder of your financial plan. The profit-and-loss statement will discuss the costs to run the practice and income projections. The projected income minus the practice costs will enable you to infer proposed profits. Cash-flow projections describe the management of the practice funds. These projections should be annually for the time period discussed in the financial plan and monthly for the first year of the plan. The break-even analysis identifies the amount of cash that will cover all practice costs. In the financial plan, describe how you would reduce the break-even point if practice receipts fall short.

The financial plan should include all information that will assist potential lenders in understanding your revenue calculations. These projections will be as important as the assumptions on which they are based.

Repayment Projections

When preparing your financial plan, be sure to specifically discuss how and when the borrowed funds will be repaid. Discuss the sources that will provide the funds for repayment, as well as any collateral you propose to use to guarantee the loan. Most individual investors typically prefer short to intermediate loans with repayment of the loan within a 5-year period. Commercial lending institutions frequently consider longer term loans and lines of credit.

DETERMINE FINANCING OPTIONS

Setting up a health-care practice involves many anticipated and established costs regardless of the target population or practice use. The most common source of start-up capital is personal funds or an investment in the business by family or friends. Personal loans are another alternative for attaining funds to use in setting up a practice. Equity in a residence is frequently used as collateral to obtain personal bank loans or establish lines of credit with a financial institution. Personal loans are generally easier to obtain through a bank than a business loan unless the business has a history of being profitable. Bankers may look at the hard assets of the practice, such as equipment, as collateral for a business loan. Criteria for securing a business loan vary among lenders, as does the emphasis they place on particular factors such as hard asset collateral, profitability, or years in business.

The Small Business Administration (SBA) offers many financial programs for the small business owner. The SBA frequently funds federally specified projects and objectives. Frequently the SBA will guarantee up to 90% of a bank loan for a small business rather than make a direct loan to the business. The amount of the loan that the SBA will guarantee depends on the business equity. This guaranteed loan protects the lender in case of default by the business owner and is made available to small businesses unable to secure funding from conventional lenders. Information about SBA programs and requirements for participation can be obtained from their Web site at www.sba.gov/financing.

State and local government agencies are other sources of assistance for the small business owner. These agencies have a vested interest in enhancing the economic well-being of the community, and many offer various services to the entrepreneur. Information about programs offered by government agencies can be obtained by contacting the local chamber of commerce or state and city government offices.

Foundations frequently provide grants to businesses that focus on a specific area or related project and are another good source of funding. Geographical limitations are not often imposed on foundation funding.

DEVELOP FEES, REIMBURSEMENT, AND BILLING PROCEDURES

Establishing Fees

In the managed care world in which we practice, fees for health-care services are usually set by MCOs. The usual, customary, and reasonable fees of indemnity insurers are largely being replaced by a contracted fee schedule of the MCO. The APN can charge anything he or she wants; however, the MCO will reimburse only up to the maximum contractual allowance determined by its fee schedule. Is it worth the time and effort to develop a fee schedule?

Definitely develop a reasonable fee for your services. In developing this fee, you will have to consider a multitude of factors, including the work performed, clinical skills required, time spent with a patient, practice expenses (e.g., rent, staff salaries and benefits, supplies, utilities, insurance, etc.), and risk involved in treating the patient, as well as indirect care such as making referrals to other health-care professionals and reviewing and evaluating laboratory and x-ray results. Ultimately, your fees should reflect what you believe your services are worth. They should not vary according to the type of insurance plan a patient carries or an MCO's maximal allowable fees.

In determining reasonable fees, the practitioner can review the annual Medicare rules and regulations published in the end of the year edition of the *Federal Register.* This edition lists all current procedure terminology (CPT) codes and their CMS-determined resource-based relative value scale (RBRVS). The more complicated a patient visit or a procedure, the greater the RBRVS attributed to the service.

Establish the relative cost of a visit and compare the RBRVS for appropriate CPT codes and then set your fees accordingly. Another yardstick for measurement of your fee schedule is the MCO allowance for the service. If your fee is less than that approved by the MCO, your fee is unreasonably low. Finally, consider your comfort in charging this fee to the self-pay patient. If you feel it is a reasonable cost for your services and you are not consistently writing off a percentage of the fee, it most likely is a reasonable fee.

Reimbursement

A 2006 U.S. Census Bureau report states that approximately 46.9 million consumers do not have health-care insurance (U.S. Census Bureau, 2007). Many of these consumers will seek out services on a self-pay basis. Approximately 15% of your patient caseload will be self-pay patients who are not covered by a health-care insurer (Boehler & Hansel, 2006) or who go out of plan because of the service you provide or the convenience of your service. Many patients will pay the fee for service in a walk-in, fast-track, health-care center, for example, because of the convenient location or extended hours. The best opportunity you have to collect a fee for service is while the patient is still in your office. Set up and publicize your policy that payment is expected at the time of service. Initial paperwork given to the patient on the first visit should include a financial policy that explains your payment expectations, any financial arrangements available, and your policy on filing insurance claims. Consider the acceptance of credit cards for payment of your fee for service. This provides a convenient method for your patient to pay your bill in full and transfers the risk of nonpayment to the credit card company. Most banks will process credit card transactions for a fee, and many credit card companies will electronically transfer funds to your bank for immediate access to the money.

Reimbursement from third-party payers varies according to the type of provider and usually requires specified billing forms with illness and procedure coding. Medicare and Medicaid insurers, as well as many indemnity insurers and MCOs, require the CMS 1500 insurance form to submit a claim for payment. The coding required on the claim forms refers to nationally accepted, standard billing and coding systems. The most commonly used are the American Medical Association's CPT codes, the International Classification of Disease, 9th Revision, Clinical Modification (ICD-9-CM), and CMS's Healthcare Common Procedure Coding System (HCPCS) for durable medical equipment, medical supplies, and drugs. Indemnity insurers are the traditional insurance companies who usually have no relationship with the health-care provider other than paying the bill for service for a covered patient. These insurers typically require an annual deductible paid by the patient, and then they pay 80% of the health-care provider's bill with the remaining 20% being the responsibility of the patient. Be aware that these insurers pay "usual and customary reimbursement" (UCR), which is rarely equal to the fee you charge for your service. The patient is responsible for any charges not covered by their insurance in addition to the 20% copay.

MCOs contract with health-care providers for patient services. Contracts may set specified fees for services provided to the patient or may be based on a monthly capitated fee, regardless of patient use. In either case, the health-care provider cannot bill the patient for the difference between the contracted or capitated fee and the provider's regular fee for service. The exception is patient copayment requirements for each MCO plan. Copayments may be different for each plan and are based on many factors, including the family's annual income level, the frequency of multiple encounters with the practitioner, or the nature of the health-care problem.

To contract with MCOs, the APN must apply and be accepted to each individual MCO provider panel.

Billing

There is a variety of medical management software that will automatically submit insurance claim forms. However, monitoring the claims submitted and tracking the date and amount of payments received requires an organized system. Controlling reimbursement will ensure the success and continuation of your practice. A billing protocol such as that shown in **Box 24-4** will allow you to track the timeliness of insurance payments and the number of insurance reductions and denials.

PURCHASE EQUIPMENT AND SELECT SUPPLIERS

Weigh the pros and cons of leasing versus buying equipment. Keep in mind that although leasing does not require the large up-front outlay, it does entail monthly payments with interest. Vendors typically have varied leasing options with opportunities to purchase the equipment at a lower price at

BOX 24-4
Billing Protocol

- File claims daily or at least twice per week.
- Check all claims for accuracy and completeness before submission.
- Develop a "claims pending" report and revise and print it daily. Most insurers guarantee payment within 30 days of filing an accurate and complete claim.
- After 30 days, call all insurance companies about unpaid claims and make a notation.
- Refile the claim if it has not been received by the insurer.
- Develop and print an "aged accounts" analysis for each insurance company to track payment patterns longer than 30 days.
- Contact the plan administrator of habitually poor payers and request an explanation. This could be a sign of a financially troubled insurance plan.
- Periodically review the explanation of benefits (EOB) sent by the insurers that explains reductions or denials of claims.
- Contact the insurer to discuss reductions or denials of claims, and revise and refile the claim if appropriate.

the end of the lease. Look at the total cash investment requirements for practice start-up, the capital you have available, current equipment costs, and interest rates on loans versus equipment leasing.

A phone system is the communication system of your practice. Choose a system that will meet your needs and one that has expansion capabilities for the future. Besides front office phone lines, consider phone lines for the examination rooms and your office, as well as dedicated lines for the computer modem and the facsimile machine. Typically, six lines are the minimum needed in a health-care practice, with costs for a basic system in the $3,000 range. Other phone costs you might incur include Yellow Pages listing and an after-hours answering service.

A computer system is another essential need for your office. Consider the number of computers needed for the medical biller and front office staff and the need for laptops for the providers to access patient files, document clinical encounters, formulate treatment plans, and prepare referral and consultation reports. Many health-care offices have multiple computers connected to form a local area network (LAN). This allows multiple staff members to access and share patient files, printers, hard disk drives, and CD-ROMS. A computer consultant will be able to recommend and install a system that will meet your practice needs.

Practice management software focuses on two basic areas for health-care practices. The medical care areas have a patient-driven management focus. They typically include copies of all front office forms, have the ability to generate insurance claims, assist in patient scheduling, bill insurance companies, and have a complete electronic charting and clinical documentation system. The management focus is profit based and provides managerial and cost accounting information to maximize time and profits. Items contained in this section include the general ledger, accounts payable and receivable, monthly and annual financial reports and ratios, capitation disbursements and utilization rates, and the detection and tracking of trends for each patient encounter.

CTS (Computer Training Services) *Guide to Medical Practice Management Software* is a software evaluation program that reviews and analyzes the strengths and weakness of the leading medical management systems available in the marketplace. CTS has been publishing managed care software selection tools since 1983 and enables the practitioner to make an educated choice of a management system that best fits his or her individual needs. Information about this software can be obtained at www.ctsguides.com. Before purchasing any medical management system, contact several vendors and request a demonstration of their products. It is also wise to obtain references and contact local practices that use a particular system and ask about ease of use and satisfaction with the system.

Durable equipment, such as office furniture, examination tables, electrocardiogram machines, and so on, can be obtained from vendors such as durable equipment companies and medical supply companies. Investigate the purchase of secondhand medical equipment through brokers or through advertising in nursing and medical journals. Occasionally you may find office and medical equipment for sale due to the retirement or death of a practitioner or the downsizing of a health-care facility. If you purchase equipment through a vendor, be sure to compare costs by obtaining quotations on equipment, warranties, and services offered. Be sure to include "hidden" costs, such as termination fees, if leasing; federal, state, and local taxes, if applicable; shipping and installation charges; postwarranty maintenance charges; and interest costs for installment purchases.

The purchase of disposable medical supplies and periodic reordering of supplies is another financial consideration. Establish an organized purchasing system by centralizing the ordering process. Consider assigning one person in the practice to be responsible for tracking and ordering supplies. The designated person will be the one to talk to sales representatives and will become familiar with suppliers and prices to comparison shop for the best-quality supplies at the cheapest price. Centralized ordering will enable the purchaser to ascertain the quantity of supplies used per month, which will assist in the development of an inventory process. This will decrease unnecessary inventory, prevent running out of needed supplies, and avert higher prices due to "emergency" ordering.

HIRING AND MANAGEMENT OF PERSONNEL

APNs who open an independent practice and hire employees must have a working knowledge of the laws and statutes regulating a health-care practice, as well as a working knowledge of how to develop internal guidelines for hiring and managing personnel. Human resource management incorporates all the federal, state, and local laws and regulations that must be complied with by the health-care practice. These laws govern how employees must be treated and paid, and they protect the rights of the employees in the workplace. The components of human resource management include the following:

1. *Administration:* Activities include developing and updating employee handbooks, guides and regulations, and posters; developing procedures for recruiting, hiring, review, discipline, and termination; and having labor law expertise or a consultant.
2. *Labor and liability issues:* Knowledge of and compliance with a multitude of government regulations such as the Civil Rights Act of 1964 and the Equal Employment Opportunity Commission (EEOC), Federal Age Discrimination in Employment Act (ADEA), Americans with Disabilities Act (ADA), and the Fair Labor Standards Act (FLSA). These laws deal with wrongful termination, unemployment, discrimination, sexual harassment, and employee rights. The practitioner additionally must deal with immigration regulations and other government rules such as personnel recording keeping (W4, I-9, etc.).
3. *Payroll information and processing:* Knowledge and management of activities that include employer tax administration, record keeping, reporting, payroll calculations and deductions, paycheck imprinting and distribution, W2 and W4 and quarterly reports, unemployment administration, management reports, and time-off use and accruals.

4. *Workers' compensation:* Knowledge of state law requirements and purchase of insurance from a qualified carrier, state insurance fund, or becoming self-insured according to state law regulations. Activities include claims filings, management and administration, fraud investigation and defense, audits and loss control, communication with injured employees, and return-to-work procedures.
5. *Safety:* The Occupational Safety and Health Administration (OSHA) regulations require that employees have a workplace safe from recognized hazards. Employer activities include the establishment and implementation of an illness and injury prevention program that includes general and specific safety training and required protective equipment.
6. *Benefits:* Knowledge and compliance of mandatory benefits that include overtime pay, unemployment insurance, and work breaks. Development and management of optional benefits such as health insurance, pension plans, vacation time, sick time, personal time off, continuing or advanced education credits, travel, bonuses, and so on.

There are many government regulations and time-consuming human resource responsibilities that must be dealt with before you open your practice. Some practitioners hire an experienced office manager and rely on outside service providers such as a payroll service, insurance agent, and bookkeeper, as well as the expertise of an accountant and lawyer on retainer. This still leaves the responsibility of developing the employee handbook and job descriptions, and advertising, interviewing, hiring, training, and evaluating personnel to the APN or a designee.

An innovative alternative to in-house human resource management is to outsource this responsibility to a professional employer organization (PEO). The PEO specializes in labor management and cost control and handles all of the human resource issues while the APN maintains functional control of the employees. The PEO becomes the "employer of record" for your workplace employees, and by combining your employees with the employees of many other practices, the PEO is able to offer the employees better benefits such as health insurance, retirement plans, credit unions, and so on. As the owner, the APN benefits because the PEO has relieved the APN of the liability of compliance and administration of mandated government regulations and payroll administration and management. The PEO has no financial interest or ownership in the practice and only deals with employee issues. An example of a company that is a PEO is Medical Management Consultants, Inc., which can be accessed at www.mmchr.com.

DEVELOP AN ORGANIZED DOCUMENTATION AND QUALITY ASSURANCE PROCESS

Documentation

Organizing documentation for a health-care practice will facilitate the smooth flow of business activity. In addition to the front office forms such as patient intake forms, patient rights forms, and release of information forms, the APN must develop and organize the medical record, patient educational materials, and patient authorization forms such as the "informed consent to treat" forms. One of the most important documents of an APN practice is the medical record. A well-documented, legible, and structured medical record will facilitate claims processing and may serve as a legal document to substantiate patient care. The medical record is confidential and can only be released to third parties with patient consent. Frequently the consent to treatment includes a "release of records" statement allowing records to be sent to third-party payers, if requested. Key elements of an effective medical record are as follows:

1. *Organizing format:* All medical records should be uniform, with separate sections for patient information, annual screening list, problem list, medication list, test results, consultations, daily

encounter or progress notes, and other forms necessary for your particular practice. Information contained in these sections must be adequately secured and in chronological order. All coding on the charts, such as allergies or chronic health problems, must be uniform, and the interpretation of the coding must be well known to all personnel.

2. *Timeliness:* Medical notations must be written at the time of the patient encounter. Always include the date and time of the patient contact in the progress notes. If notes are dictated, this should be at the time of the patient encounter and must be proofread and signed by the health-care provider, preferably before it is entered into the medical record.
3. *Accurate records:* Record all information using a concise and accurate format. Many APNs use a SOAP format to concisely record the patient's subjective **s**tatements and the provider's **o**bjective findings, **a**ssessment, and **p**lan of care. Handwritten progress notes must be legible to prevent misinterpretations and clinical errors.
4. *Corrections:* Alteration of a medical record is unlawful. If an error has been made, draw a single line through the entry and add the correct information. Be sure to include the date, time, and your signature next to the correction or in the margin of the record. An addendum is also acceptable and can be added at the end of the record with a cross-reference to the original note. The date and time of the addendum are noted and signed by the author.
5. *Telephone conversations:* Document all patient calls in the record with time, date, nature of the conversation, actions taken, and signature of the provider. Calls or conversations with family should also be included in the progress notes with the date, time, nature of the conversation, and provider signature. If calls were placed for consultations, appointments, or equipment rentals for the patient, this should also be recorded in the progress notes, dated, and signed.
6. *Treatment plan and instructions:* Record your plan of treatment for your patient including important instructions, educational information given verbally or in writing, and warnings about interactions or complications that may occur. A well-written and organized medical record will be your first line of defense against a malpractice claim and will facilitate accurate and timely claims processing.

Quality Assurance

MCOs, insurers, and the public are increasingly asking health-care providers to demonstrate the value and improve the quality of their services. If outcomes management (OM) and performance improvement (PI) processes are put into place when the practice opens, then data collection about the quantity, quality, and cost-effectiveness of the practice will be built into the foundation of the practice. OM is the process by which you measure, track, modify, and achieve the best clinical outcomes (quality), while incurring the fewest overall costs such as economic, intellectual, technical, and time spent (cost-effectiveness). PI involves the measurement, evaluation, and improvement in the quality of the services of the practice and the patient care received, through a systematic and collaborative examination of the practice's entire operation (quality and quantity).

The initial step of OM is to determine what outcomes are to be measured (e.g., up-to-date immunization status of children under age 6) or what change in functional status will be noted (e.g., maintain fasting blood sugar lower than 130 for the diabetic patient). Outcome measurements vary between what is valued by the patient and what provides information to the health-care provider to improve care and reduce cost. The diabetic patient values a good quality of life free from complications of diabetes mellitus, such as decreased vision, peripheral neuropathy, fatigue, and polyuria. The health-care provider values 100% immunization coverage of the pediatric patients to prevent unnecessary illness and complications that could lead to serious injury and costly health care. Both of these examples represent appropriate areas to monitor outcomes of patient care.

In addition to monitoring clinical outcomes measuring the effects of treatment and the functional status of patients receiving treatment, other areas to monitor include patient satisfaction and financial and economic factors. Patient satisfaction evaluates the patient's satisfaction with the services provided by the practice staff and the health-care provider. Although not an indicator of the clinical quality of the provider, it does measure the provider quality. A review of the literature suggests that patient satisfaction highly correlates to clinical outcomes. A patient who feels respected by the staff and informed, educated, and considerately treated by the health-care provider is more apt to follow a treatment regimen and return for follow-up care.

To maintain cost-effectiveness while offering quality services, financial and economic factors must be evaluated. Measuring the cost of resources consumed to produce a clinical outcome will evaluate these factors. Patients diagnosed with diabetes mellitus frequently require large amounts of time to educate them about the disease and possible complications, treatment plan, and medications. Measuring the time the health provider spends to maintain the health of these patients and the costs involved might justify the purchase of additional patient education materials or hiring a registered nurse (RN) who is also a diabetic educator.

PI integrates the concepts of outcomes management by evaluating the data received from the patient and the provider and using the findings to improve patient care and practice services. The benefits of PI include continuous monitoring of health-care delivery, effective use and cost containment, and the development of practice guidelines for your health-care practice. Performance improvement processes should permeate all facets of the practice to ensure high-quality health care at the lowest cost.

Primary accrediting bodies in health care and third-party payers are increasingly using and requiring outcomes management data from providers to accredit or evaluate their performance. Insurance companies use this information to evaluate the retention of practitioners on their provider panels, as well as to sell services to employers. Health-care providers are increasingly subject to clinical and economic profiling by MCO plans, insurance companies, and consumer groups.

The National Committee for Quality Assurance (NCQA) has included in its health plan employer data and information set (HEDIS) the monitoring of additional quality criteria such as access to and availability of care, health plan stability, use of selected services, patient orientation, and translation services, to name a few. The NCQA is the primary accrediting body of MCOs and health maintenance organizations and is a major organization looking after consumer interests and rating health plans and providers. Annually, the NCQA requests that all managed care plans submit information about themselves and publishes a report card titled "Quality Compass," which rates the health plans. This document is sold to medical plans, employers, and various other health-care consultants. For information about this report or to obtain a copy of this document, visit the NCQA Web site at www.ncqa.org.

Performance standards will become increasingly more important in the years to come as health-care providers are asked to document the value and improve the quality of their services. Strategies for complying with performance criteria must be a top priority for health-care practices. Delegating responsibility for continuous quality improvement monitoring and implementing tracking systems for compliance will greatly improve the use of performance standards for the practice. Revising practice services based on data from the performance standards and rewarding staff and providers for compliance and high scores will improve the practice's entire operation and increase the value and reputation of the practice.

DEVELOPING POLICIES AND PROCEDURES

Practice policies, procedures, and protocols should be written in great detail and should be part of every employee's orientation. Employees are expected to know these guidelines to ensure the smooth functioning of the practice. Additionally, important procedures and protocols should also be outlined in this manual such as a protocol for handling a medical emergency, a policy on confidentiality or annual equipment maintenance, and a procedure for handling patient complaints or termination of the professional relationship. Because this manual is essential to providing organized, high-quality services, each employee should sign a written acknowledgement that the practice manual has been read, and this form should become part of the employee's personnel record.

Specific office policies, procedures, and protocols that should be developed are listed in **Box 24-5.** Responsibility for the initial development of the practice policy manual should be the APN's. However, updates and maintenance of this manual can be delegated to the office manager or another employee after the manual is established.

DEVELOP MARKETING STRATEGIES

Marketing can take many forms from word of mouth to high-priced television appearances. These external marketing strategies are tangible ways of reaching your target population to advertise the

BOX 24-5
Necessary Policies, Procedures, and Protocols

- Communicating practice fees
- Office collection procedures
- Billing policies and follow-up
- Release of records procedure
- Registering a patient
- Source of patient referral log
- Setting up the patient record
- Completing the superbill
- Scheduling patient appointments
- Closing and reconciling daily cash collections and disbursements
- Cleaning laboratory equipment
- Performing an electrocardiogram
- Scheduling a laboratory test
- Handling test results and consultation reports
- Referring patients for consultation
- Arranging services for patient care
- Protocols for purchasing equipment and supplies
- Equipment maintenance policy
- Handling a medical emergency protocol
- Confidentiality policy
- Protocol for handling patient complaints
- Procedure for termination of patient care

location of your practice and the services you provide. There are also internal strategies that you can employ to retain your patient base and increase your patient loyalty. For example, the internal strategies of competence and concern can be expressed through efficiency and friendliness of the staff and health-care provider.

A marketing budget should be an essential part of your start-up operational budget. Marketing is your practice's form of communication to the target population. This is how you inform patients about your location and what you can do to help them maintain their health or resolve a health problem. Marketing is not an optional expense.

A marketing plan helps you to organize your activities and prevents "lost opportunities" to showcase your practice or high-cost, "emergency" printing of practice brochures or appointment cards. Opportunities to showcase your practice can be found in many areas. Contact your local chamber of commerce to see if there is a "Welcome Wagon" service for new residents in your town and inquire about including your practice brochure for distribution to these consumers. Join community organizations to become known in your area and volunteer to offer free seminars on health-care topics. Inquire about membership in local speakers bureaus in your community or through professional organizations such as the state nurses association or the state board of nursing. Offer to participate in community and organizational health fairs and screenings that are being planned in your area. Repetition is the name of the game. Your name, location, and services need to be repeated many times before they are remembered. Before opening your practice, be sure to order stationery, appointment cards, brochures, and announcement cards with your practice name, address, and telephone number engraved. Also order an inscribed stamp to imprint the name, address, and phone number of your practice on educational materials or any other forms of information that may be distributed to patients in your office or potential patients at speaking engagements and health fairs. Develop and submit articles that highlight health topics to local newspapers and community bulletins, being sure to briefly describe who you are, where you are located, and what services your offer. Before opening your doors, submit practice announcements to local media services such as cable television bulletin boards, community radio programs, local newspapers, and community bulletins, brochures, and calendars.

Don't underestimate the power of the Internet and social media networking. Patients search for health-care providers on the Internet using Google, and with over 88 billion Google searches per month, search engine optimization is a necessity (Jackson, Schneider, & Baum, 2011).

Developing a Web site to advertise key information about your practice is essential. Getting that Web site seen by consumers requires a strategy to reach the top of a search engine list. Two such strategies are repetition of key words in the title and beginning of any article and the frequency and repetition of these key words throughout the Web site, article, or advertisement (Maley & Baum, 2010). Additional social media networking includes advertising via YouTube, a professional page on Facebook for your business, and even having a following on your blog on Twitter. With 35-to 55-year-olds being the fastest growing segment on Facebook with an average daily use of 20 minutes, you will quickly build up an online community for your professional page. Twitter helps you build a community of people interested in what you have to say. Twitter reaches 800 million search queries each day and searches have increased by 33% in the last year (Schneider, Jackson, & Baum, 2010). These 21st century marketing tools will become a mainstay of your marketing plan.

Last, be sure to educate your staff about your credentials and what services you offer. Your staff is marketing your practice every time they answer questions or speak to a potential patient. Be sure they know about your education, experience, and specialty training, as well as what services you offer.

REFERENCES

Boehler, A., & Hansel, J. (2006). *Innovative strategies for self-pay segmentation.* Retrieved August 22, 2012, from www.hfma.org/hfm.

Brassard, A., & Smolenski, M. (2011). Removing barriers to advanced practice registered nurse care: Hospital privileges. *AARP Public Policy Institute Insight on Issues, 55.* Retrieved October 7, 2011, from http://assets.aarp.org/rgcenter/ppi/health-care/insight55.pdf.

Brown, D. J. (2007). Consumer perspectives on nurse practitioners and independent practice. *Journal of the American Academy of Nurse Practitioners, 19*(10). 523–529.

Carzoli, R., Martinez-Cruz, M., Cuevas, L., Murphy, S., & Chui, T. (1994). Comparison of neonatal nurse practitioners, physician assistants, and residents in the neonatal intensive care unit. *Archives of Pediatric and Adolescent Medicine, 148*(12), 1271–1276.

Cronenwett, L., Dracup, K., Grey, M., McCauley, L., Meleis, A., & Salmon, M. (2011). The doctor of nursing practice: A national workforce perspective. *Nursing Outlook, 59*(1), 9–17.

Fain, J., Asselin, M., & McCurry, M. (2008). The DNP . . . Why now? *Nursing Management, 39*(7), 34–37.

Jackson, R., Schneider, A., & Baum, N. (2011). Social media networking: YouTube and search engine optimization. *Journal of Medical Practice Management, 26*(4), 254–257.

King, E. S. (2008). A 10-year review of four academic nurse-managed centers: Challenges and survival strategies. *Journal of Professional Nursing, 24*(1), 14–20.

Kocher, R., Emanuel, E., & DeParle, N. (2010). The Affordable Care Act and the future of clinical medicine: The opportunities and challenges. *Annals of Internal Medicine, 153*(8), 536–539.

Maley, C., & Baum, N. (2010). Getting to the top of Google: Search engine optimization. *Journal of Medical Practice Management, 25*(5), 301–303.

Meleis, A. I., & Dracup, K. (2005). The case against the DNP: History, timing, substance, and marginalization. *Online Journal of Issues in Nursing, 10*(3).

Mirvis, D. (1999). The behavior of physicians. In J. Johnson & A. Kilpatrick (Eds.), *Handbook of health administration* (pp. 439–460). Boston: Marcel Dekker.

Mundinger, M., Kane, R., Lentz, E., Totten, A. M., Tsai, W. Y., Cleary, P. D., et al. (2000). Primary care outcomes in patients treated by nurse practitioners or physicians: A randomized trial. *Journal of the American Medical Association, 283*(1), 59–68.

Newhouse, R., et al. (2011, Sept-Oct). Advanced practice nurse outcomes 1990–2008: A systematic review. *Nursing Economic$, 29*(5). Retrieved August 22, 2012, from https://www.nursingeconomics.net/ce/2013/article3001021.pdf.

Office of Technology Assessment. (1986). *Nurse practitioners, physician assistants, and certified nurse-midwives: A policy analysis.* Washington, DC: Author.

Pearson, L. (2007). The Pearson report. *American Journal of Nurse Practitioners, 11*(2), 10–101.

Pearson, L. (2011). The Pearson report. *National Overview of Nurse Practitioner Legislation and Healthcare Issues.* Retrieved October 4, 2011, from http://www.pearsonreport.com.

Schneider, A., Jackson, R., & Baum, N. (2010). Social media networking: Facebook and Twitter. *Journal of Medical Practice Management, 26*(3), 156–157.

Spitzer, W., Sackett, D., Sibley, J., Roberts, R. S., Gent, M., et al. (1974). The Burlington randomized trial of the nurse practitioner. *New England Journal of Medicine, 290*(5), 251–256.

U.S. Census Bureau. (2007). *Income, poverty, and health insurance coverage in the United States: 2006.* Retrieved April 2008 from www.census.gov/prod/2007pubs/p60-233.pdf.

Vincent, D., MacKay, T., Pohl, J., Hirth, R., & Oakley, D. (1999). A tale of two nursing centers: A cautionary study of profitability. *Nursing Economics, 17*(3), 257–262.

25

The Advanced Practice Nurse as Employee or Independent Contractor: Legal and Contractual Considerations

Kathleen M. Gialanella

INTRODUCTION

Advanced practice nurses (APNs) need to be clear about whether they are practicing as employees or as independent contractors. The difference between an employee and an independent contractor is a legal one based on common law or statutory definitions (Internal Revenue Service [IRS], 2011a). In general, if the individual or entity for whom the APN performs services controls what the APN does and when and how he or she does it, the APN is an employee. If, however, the individual or entity oversees only the result of the APN's work and not the manner or method in which the work is done, the APN may be considered an independent contractor (IRS, 2011b). The distinction between the two has significant legal, tax, and financial implications. This chapter explores these implications and includes a discussion of the various contractual issues that apply to employment and independent contractor agreements. Pertinent case law is discussed as well.

EMPLOYEE OR INDEPENDENT CONTRACTOR: WHAT DIFFERENCE DOES IT MAKE?

An APN's status as an employee or independent contractor is a significant factor when considering issues pertaining to professional liability and other legal, tax, financial, and contractual situations.

Professional Liability Considerations

With regard to liability exposure, employees alleged to have engaged in negligence or malpractice will likely find a safe harbor in the doctrine of *respondeat superior*. This doctrine holds that an employer is responsible for the acts of its employee. Thus, if an employee is acting within the scope of his or her employment and is sued for negligent treatment of a patient, the employer is vicariously liable for the damages sustained by the patient. Although this doctrine is not an absolute bar to suing an employed APN individually, it does give the employee a level of protection that is unavailable to APNs who function as independent contractors. An in-depth discussion of these considerations and the liability insurance implications can be found in Chapter 27.

Financial and Tax Implications

APNs who practice as employees receive paychecks that have monies withheld by the employer. The monies that are withheld include state and federal income tax payments, payments to Social Security and Medicare, and unemployment and disability taxes. In addition, the employer is responsible for paying its share of any Social Security, Medicare, and unemployment and disability taxes due on that employee's wages. The employer is responsible for forwarding any amounts withheld from the employee's paycheck, as well as its share of such payments, to the government. The employer must also issue a Form W-2 statement to each of its employees showing the total amount of taxes that were withheld from the employee's pay during the previous year.

Employees may deduct unreimbursed business expenses (e.g., dues for professional organizations, subscriptions to professional journals, required continuing education, and premiums for professional liability insurance) on their tax returns, but only if the deductions are itemized and the unreimbursed expenses exceed 2% of the employee's adjusted gross income (AGI). For example, if an employed APN had an AGI of $100,000 in 2011, the APN could deduct unreimbursed employee expenses that exceeded $2,000 (2% of AGI). If the APN spent $3,500 that year on professional dues, subscriptions, continuing education, and liability insurance, the APN can deduct only $1,500—the amount that exceeds 2% of the APN's AGI.

If the APN practices as an independent contractor, the organizations to whom he or she provides services must issue a Form 1099-MISC showing the total amount of money it paid to the APN during the previous year. Unlike the employee, the independent contractor is responsible for paying his or her income and self-employment taxes. The organization is not required to withhold any taxes or make any Social Security or Medicare payments that an employer of an APN would be required to make. The savings in time and money that independent contractor arrangements present to the organization make it an attractive alternative.

If the APN is an independent contractor, his or her business expenses are reported annually on the income tax return. Unlike the unreimbursed business expense threshold of 2% of AGI that an employee must meet before being allowed to take a deduction, business expenses incurred by an independent contractor do not have to amount to any specific percentage of AGI to be deducted. Thus, in the example previously given, the APN would be able to deduct the full expenses incurred of $3,500.

The APN must keep other trade-offs in mind when contemplating employment versus an independent contractor arrangement. Employers often provide certain benefits to their employees (e.g., health insurance, pension plans, and paid personal time off for holidays, vacations, illnesses). These benefits are not made available to independent contractors. Some organizations prefer to offer an independent contractor arrangement to an APN to avoid the cost of providing such benefits. If an APN wants or needs these kinds of benefits, an independent contractor arrangement is not advisable.

Factors Used to Determine Status

Because the liability, financial, and tax implications of one's work status can be significant, it is important for APNs to understand the factors that are considered to determine whether an APN is an employee or an independent contractor. A determination is based on the facts. The Internal Revenue Service (IRS, 2011b) considers common law and looks at the degree of control asserted by the organization versus the degree of independence maintained by the worker. To determine whether an APN is an employee or an independent contractor from a federal tax perspective, the IRS would evaluate behavioral and financial controls and the type of relationship that exists between the APN and the organization for which the APN provides services.

Questions the IRS would pose to evaluate the status of the arrangement include the following:

- What instructions does the organization give to the APN? If the organization instructs the APN about when and where to work, the equipment and supplies to be used, who will assist the APN, and what work must be performed (or even how the results are to be achieved by the APN), these are factors that indicate the APN is employed by the organization.
- Does the organization educate and train the APN to perform services in accordance with certain policies and procedures, or does the APN have his or her own protocols for providing services? The former arrangement points to an employer–employee relationship. The latter would indicate the APN is an independent contractor.
- Does the APN have significant fixed unreimbursed business expenses (e.g., office rent, telephone and computer services, professional dues, and support staff to pay) in connection with providing services to the organization? If so, this generally indicates that the APN is an independent contractor.
- Does the APN advertise and are his or her services available to more than one organization or to individuals? If so, the APN is likely to be considered an independent contractor.
- How is the APN paid? Does the APN receive a set amount of pay over a certain period of time and receive benefits from the organization or is the APN's compensation based on a flat fee without the provision of benefits? The former arrangement indicates an employment situation, whereas the latter arrangement would suggest the APN is an independent contractor.
- Does the APN realize a profit or take a loss? If so, it indicates the APN is an independent contractor.
- What type of relationship exists between the organization and the APN? Is it for an indefinite period or will it end on completion of a particular project? Is there a written contract that describes the type of relationship that exists? (For example, if the contract is called an "employment agreement," the employer–employee relationship is obvious because it is specifically stated within the agreement.) Does the APN receive benefits such as health insurance, a retirement plan, and paid time off? If so, it indicates the APN is an employee.

State taxing authorities make similar inquiries for state tax purposes. The factors relied on by these taxing authorities can differ from the IRS and vary from state to state. Some states are more stringent than the IRS and other states when classifying workers as employees versus independent contractors. Thus, it is important for an APN to be familiar with the federal bases used to distinguish between employee and independent contractor arrangements, as well as the bases used by the states in which the APN practices. APNs should seek out sound legal and accounting advice to address these issues.

Failure to properly classify the work status of an APN can be costly to the APN if he or she is treated as an independent contractor but is, in fact, an employee. A case filed by individuals who had been classified as independent contractors rather than employees at Microsoft illustrates this. *Vizcaino v. Microsoft Corporation* (1997) arose out of a tax audit of Microsoft conducted by the IRS. The audit concluded that a number of individuals classified as independent contractors needed to be reclassified as employees, and the requisite taxes paid. The IRS concluded that the individuals were employees because Microsoft controlled the manner and way in which the individuals performed their services for the company. Microsoft ended up paying the required taxes and overtime that resulted from the reclassification, and it reclassified some of the individuals as permanent employees. Eight of these reclassified individuals demanded that they receive all of the employment benefits they did not receive during the time they were considered independent contractors, including participation in Microsoft's employee stock purchase plan. Microsoft refused to issue these benefits, so the individuals sued the company. The Ninth Circuit Court of Appeals in *Vizcaino* ordered Microsoft to provide employment benefits to its employees for the periods of time that those individuals had been erroneously classified as independent contractors. The financial impact on the company was significant, as were the financial gains realized by the reclassified workers. Although the workers in *Vizcaino* were not health-care providers, the findings and results of that case would apply equally in the health-care industry.

The Advanced Practice Nurse as Employee

Employees working without a contract guaranteeing a specific position for a definite time at a designated pay rate are referred to as employees "at will." In the past, this kind of employment arrangement allowed employers to terminate any at-will employee for any reason or for no reason. Although the general rule that an employee can be hired or fired for any reason or no reason continues to exist, there now are many exceptions in place. These exceptions include public policy concerns, antidiscrimination laws, and whistleblower statutes. Thus, employers no longer enjoy the unbridled latitude the general rule of law previously afforded them.

Although the absence of job security continues to be an issue for at-will employees, federal and state statutes have been enacted and judicial decisions have been made to ensure that employers treat employees more fairly, regardless of the employee's status as a contract or at-will employee.

One of the key limitations on an employer's ability to terminate an employee at will is called the "public policy" exception. It is a judicially mandated exception that permits a terminated at-will employee to pursue a wrongful termination claim against the employer in cases in which the employee has a reasonable basis to believe he or she was terminated in violation of a clear mandate of public policy. *Kirk v. Mercy Hospital Tri-County* (1993) is an example of such a case. Pauline Kirk worked as a registered nurse (RN) at the hospital until she was terminated. She was an at-will employee who reportedly told a family member that the death of one of the patients for whom she cared was hastened by the actions of the physician. She offered to assist the family with obtaining a copy of the patient's medical record. When hospital officials learned of Ms. Kirk's actions, she was terminated. Ms. Kirk filed a lawsuit claiming wrongful termination by the hospital. The case was dismissed by the trial court, but Ms. Kirk filed an appeal with the Missouri Court of Appeals. That court reversed the decision of the trial court and sent the case back for hearing. It agreed that Ms. Kirk had a right to pursue her wrongful termination lawsuit because of her claim that she was terminated for reporting serious misconduct that could constitute a violation of the law. The Court of Appeals recognized that Ms. Kirk's actions warranted protection under the public policy exception.

A more recent whistleblower case that gained national attention involved two Texas nurses employed by Winkler County Memorial Hospital. The nurses were concerned about the incompetent practice of a physician who was treating patients at the hospital. They reported their concerns to hospital administration and then reported the physician to the Texas Medical Board when the hospital failed to act. The hospital fired the nurses, who were also criminally prosecuted. They were improperly charged with releasing official hospital information to the medical board. The charges against one nurse were dropped and the other nurse was acquitted of wrongdoing at trial (Murray, 2011). The nurses then sued the hospital, the physician, and others based on a number of claims, including wrongful termination, and recovered $750,000.

APNs practicing as employees have the opportunity, like Kirk and the two Texas nurses, to pursue wrongful termination causes of action if they believe that adverse employment action was taken against them in violation of public policy. Many states and the federal government have adopted strong whistleblower statutes that enhance the common law public policy protections available to employees. Some of those laws have specific protections for health-care professionals. An example of such a statute is the New Jersey Conscientious Employee Protection Act (1986, as amended 1989, 1997, and 2005). It specifically prohibits employers from taking retaliatory action against health-care professionals, such as APNs, who disclose information about employers who provide improper patient care.

Other statutory protections include a variety of antidiscrimination laws. There are a number of federal laws, and many states have their own laws as well, that protect workers from discrimination based on race, sex, ethnicity, religion, and disability. The most recent antidiscrimination statute to be enacted by the federal government is the Genetic Information Non-Discrimination Act of 2008. It protects individuals in the workplace from discrimination based on their genetic information.

Employees are afforded additional protections under federal and state laws that provide benefits for unemployment, injuries on the job, the need for family and medical leave, and continuation of health-care benefits. APNs who work as employees should be aware of their many rights under these laws.

Some APNs may have written employment contracts that provide them with additional rights. Contractual issues are discussed in greater detail later in this chapter.

The Advanced Practice Nurse as Independent Contractor

An APN who is an independent contractor has a contract, which may be verbal, written, or implied, with another party to provide specific services. The contract does not stipulate a level of behavioral and financial controls over the APN that would be associated with an employer–employee relationship. If an APN is working as an independent contractor, he or she is not entitled to benefits that the organization provides to its employees. The APN also would not be able to obtain unemployment compensation, workers' compensation, or family and medical leave protections through that organization if the need arose. This is because the legal relationship is not an employment relationship. Of equal concern is the impact potential professional liability claims would have on the APN who is an independent contractor. For example, an APN who is not employed by the hospital, but has privileges there, would be individually responsible for his or her negligent acts that occur in the hospital.

The case of *Hansen v. Caring Professionals, Inc.* (1997) is illustrative. Although it does not involve an APN, it does involve a nurse and the issues presented in the case also would apply to APNs who work as independent contractors. The case examines whether the nurse, who was retained by Caring Professionals to provide temporary nursing services to a local hospital, was an employee or independent contractor of that agency. The distinction was fundamental in determining whether or not the agency could be held liable for the alleged negligent acts of the nurse. Mr. Hansen, the plaintiff in the case, claimed that a malpractice occurred when a central venous catheter that had been inserted into his wife's jugular vein became dislodged. It was alleged that air entered the intravenous line and created an embolus that caused Mr. Hansen's wife to sustain severe brain damage and total disability.

Eileen Fajardo-Furlin, RN, was named as a defendant in the case because she cared for Mrs. Hansen while she was in the hospital. Furlin was working at the hospital on temporary assignment through Caring Professionals. Caring Professionals also was named as a defendant. The patient's husband sought to hold Caring Professionals responsible for the alleged negligence of Furlin. Caring Professionals sought to be removed from the case, asserting that there was no employee–employer relationship, but rather an independent contractor relationship, thereby absolving Caring Professionals from any liability for Furlin's actions. The trial court agreed and dismissed Caring Professionals from the case. An appeal followed, but the appellate court agreed with the trial court. Caring Professionals succeeded in getting removed from the case because Furlin was an independent contractor. Furlin remained in the lawsuit as an individual defendant. This case illustrates how the type of working relationship an APN has with an organization could have a significant impact on the outcome of a negligence or malpractice case. This case also illustrates the importance of having individual professional liability insurance. Nurse Furlin, as the only remaining defendant in the case, would be responsible for the cost of her legal fees and any judgment or settlement unless she had carried her own malpractice policy.

CONTRACT ISSUES FOR APN EMPLOYEES AND INDEPENDENT CONTRACTORS

APNs should have a basic understanding of contract law. It is often advisable and sometimes a requirement for APNs to have written agreements in place to address certain work and practice issues. The remainder of this chapter introduces the APN to these types of considerations.

Types of Contracts

Contracts are promises or sets of promises that outline the rights and responsibilities of the parties. They are legally binding, and if valid, they can be enforced. When one or more parties fails to perform in accordance with articulated rights and responsibilities, that failure is termed a *breach*. When a breach occurs, remedies outlined in the agreement or contract are available to the nonbreaching party. In addition, when an agreement-related dispute is tried in the civil justice system or the subject of binding arbitration, the nonbreaching party can obtain damages if a breach is found to have occurred.

Contracts are usually categorized by the way in which they are formed. They can be express contracts, implied contracts, or quasi-contracts. Express contracts are promises or sets of promises to which the parties agree either verbally or in writing. Implied contracts are promises or sets of promises that are derived from the conduct of the parties to the contract. Quasi-contracts are not considered contracts *per se*, but they are used by courts in some jurisdictions to allow one or more parties to the quasi-contract to avoid unjust enrichment at the expense of the other party or parties. This is known as *equitable relief.*

Some contracts, whether express or implied, are considered invalid for various reasons. An invalid contract will not be enforced by the courts. An example of an unenforceable contract is one that is illegal because fulfilling its terms would be considered a crime. For instance, if an APN enters into a contract which provides that he or she would receive financial incentives for referring patients to a health-care facility, this would be an antikickback violation. Taking kickbacks for patient referrals is a crime and a court would not enforce such a contract. The contract is considered to have been void at its inception. Some contracts can be considered voidable. For example, if one of the parties to the contract is a minor or has a level of mental illness or dementia that prevented him or her from understanding the terms of the contract, the contract is considered voidable by that party. Unenforceable contracts are those that may be valid but not enforced because of some defense that may be asserted by one or more parties to the contract. An example would be if a party were tricked into signing the contract or entered into the contract by mistake.

For any contract to be enforced, the parties must have reached a "meeting of the minds" about its terms. When the parties have reached a meeting of the minds, the result is called *mutual assent.* Mutual assent is achieved when one party makes an offer and the other party unequivocally accepts the offer.

In addition to offer and acceptance, there must be an exchange of consideration for the contract to be valid. For example, an APN can enter into an employment contract with a physician practice. The consideration received by the APN is monetary compensation. The consideration received by the physician practice is the services that the APN provides to the practice.

Contracts can be unilateral or bilateral. A unilateral contract is one in which there is no opportunity for negotiation. An example of such a contract is a professional liability insurance policy. The insurance company promises to defend an APN in a malpractice case pursuant to the terms of the insurance policy in exchange for the payment of premiums by the APN. The terms of the policy (contract) are not negotiated. Once the APN pays the premium, the policy becomes effective. A bilateral contract is one in which the parties negotiate the terms. APNs often negotiate the terms of their employment contracts to obtain compensation and benefits that are acceptable to them.

Common Contractual Terms Included in Written Agreements

Agreements can be struck with a handshake or with the stroke of a pen. Agreements struck with a handshake, although honorable, may prove to be frustrating, unworkable, and largely unenforceable because many of the issues that normally are addressed in written agreements are not addressed in verbal agreements. In addition, it is much easier to prove the terms of an agreement that has been reduced to writing. Written agreements can help the parties avoid the misunderstandings that may arise with implied or verbal contracts. Thus, it is recommended that APNs who enter into employment and independent contractor agreements do so in writing whenever possible.

Written agreements can be brief, limited to just a few pages, or they can be lengthy, detailed documents. The length and terms of the agreement depend on the specific arrangements contemplated by the parties, as well as their needs and preferences. Regardless of the length of an agreement, there are certain terms that routinely are included in employment and independent contractor agreements for APNs. Among them are the scope of the contract; its effective date; the relationship and responsibilities of the parties; confidentiality; conflict of interest; compensation; indemnification and subrogation; dispute resolution; term, renewal, and termination; remedies for breach; notices; modification and assignment of the agreement; severability; conflict of laws; legal authority; force majeure; covenant not to compete; and signatures. Each of these provisions will be discussed.

Scope

The section of a written agreement addressing scope recites the activities governed by the agreement. In this section the services provided by the APN are identified. The services may be stated broadly, or they may be listed individually. A broadly written scope statement for an APN might state that he or she agrees to render services that are consistent with the scope of practice articulated in his or her state's nurse practice act and in accordance with all applicable national practice standards, such as the American Nurses Association's (ANA's) *Nursing: Scope and Standards of Practice* (2010). A more specific scope statement might identify the APN's specific job responsibilities and list the individual services to be provided. In either event, it is important to verify that the services contemplated by the agreement fit within the APN's scope of practice as defined by the state.

Effective Date

The section of a contract addressing the effective date will specify the date on which the agreement begins. It is also the date against which time frames identified in the agreement may be measured. For example, if the effective date of the agreement is July 1, 2011, and the APN is required to provide a certain report to the other party every 90 days, the first report is due on October 1, 2011.

Relationship of the Parties

In the relationship of the parties section of the contract the APN is identified as either an independent contractor or an employee. If the APN is going to be considered an independent contractor, it is important to keep that status in mind as other contractual provisions are written. Classifying an individual as an independent contractor but prescribing when, where, and how services will be performed may subject an organization to having that independent contractor reclassified as an employee. As previously discussed, this could expose an organization to liability for unpaid taxes and employment benefits, as well as governmental penalties.

In situations in which an APN is going to function in an independent contractor role, the contract should specifically state that the APN is not eligible for paid sick leave or vacation time, health insurance, retirement plans, and other benefits extended to the organization's employees. An employee contract, on the other hand, should specifically include all of the benefits to which the APN is entitled.

Responsibilities of the Parties

Once the relationship of the parties has been established, the responsibilities of each party can be more easily identified. Like other provisions, this section may be brief, or quite lengthy, comprehensively listing what the expectations are of each party. In situations in which an APN is going to work as an independent contractor, it is imperative that the APN maintain the decision-making ability with regard to the manner and means by which services will be provided to patients. In addition, the APN should contemplate adding a provision that he or she be consulted about any existing and future clinical practice guidelines the organization may have or consider and be permitted to provide appropriate changes, if necessary, before implementation.

Should an APN be identified as an independent contractor in the agreement and then be required to operate in a controlled manner proscribed by the other party, it is likely that the APN will be considered an employee, not an independent contractor. If, on the other hand, the agreement being executed is an employment contract, it is reasonable to identify when, where, and how the APN is to function.

Typically, APNs practicing as independent contractors have the responsibility to ensure that they are and remain properly credentialed, that they have adequate liability insurance, and that they perform contractual services in a manner that complies with professional practice and ethical standards, as well as all applicable local, state, and federal regulations, statutes, and case law. However, APNs might consider including a contractual requirement that the organization with whom they are contracting assist with the credentialing and recredentialing process for area hospitals, managed care organizations, third-party payers, and regulatory agencies. In addition, APNs, whether practicing as employees or independent contractors, may be asked to promptly disclose any disciplinary actions taken against them. If a contract contains this type of provision it is imperative that the APN understand his or her obligation to report and act promptly when the need arises. Otherwise, the failure to report may be an event identified in the agreement that would permit immediate termination of the APN.

Usually, the organization with whom the APN is contracting requires the APN's assistance and cooperation with the collection of data to confirm the APN's competency and proper credentialing. Required data may include confirmation of educational preparation, specialty certifications, licensure, prior employment, status of existing and past practice privileges, liability insurance, malpractice claims, criminal background information, membership in professional associations, and compliance with the Drug Enforcement Administration. In addition, APNs practicing as independent contractors may be asked to provide information regarding the types of client populations previously served, charges per encounter, visits per hour, visit frequency, incidence of diagnostic procedure use, admission and readmission rates, complication and mortality rates, outcomes, accessibility and availability history, appointment waiting times, and after-hours coverage history.

The responsibilities of APNs are delineated in written agreements and organizations with whom they contract should have their responsibilities delineated in the agreement as well. In that regard, it is the organization's responsibility to execute contracts that are consistent with the organizational bylaws. The APN may explicitly require that the organizational bylaws be incorporated into the agreement by reference and that he or she be provided the most current edition of the bylaws. The APN may also negotiate involvement on the bylaws committees or other organizational committees or panels.

It is also the organization's responsibility to have sound corporate compliance programs in place and to provide the APN with the information he or she needs to provide the agreed-to services. These and other organizational responsibilities can be stated broadly or can be delineated specifically and in detail with set deadlines and penalties for failure to meet those deadlines.

Confidentiality

The confidentiality section of a contract usually deals with information and documents that the parties wish to protect as confidential. The responsibilities of the parties with regard to this information and these documents is also outlined. Some confidentiality provisions simply state that confidential, proprietary, and trade secret information shall not be disclosed to third parties, without describing what information is considered to be confidential, proprietary, or a trade secret. If there are questions about what specific information is protected, it is prudent to clarify this so that potential breaches of confidentiality are minimized.

With regard to the privacy and confidentiality of protected health information, many contracts now address the requirements of the Privacy Rule and Security Rule adopted by the federal government in 2003 and 2005, respectively. These rules are commonly referred to by health-care providers as "HIPAA"—an acronym for the Health Insurance Portability and Accountability Act of 1996. The protections under HIPAA recently were expanded with the passage of the Health Information Technology for Economic and Clinical Health (HITECH) Act of 2009 and the subsequent adoption of additional federal rules. These laws enhance the privacy and security protections of the electronic health records that have become prevalent in today's health-care delivery systems. APNs must be fully familiar with the requirements that apply to them under these laws, as well as the HIPAA and HITECH Act policies and procedures of the organizations with whom they contract.

Conflict of Interest

Conflict of interest provisions are contained in written agreements in an effort to ensure that both parties are acting in the best interests of each other and promoting the mutual success of the relationship. Potentially conflicting loyalties can be problematic and should be avoided. Typically, conflict of interest provisions require the party who becomes aware of a potential conflict to promptly disclose it to the other party. When these provisions are included in an APN's written agreement, it is important for the APN to act in a manner that avoids potential conflicts and is not contrary to the contractual requirements, such as always acting in the best interest of the patients and not in the best interest of any other third party. For instance, an APN's prescribing habits ought to reflect what medication is most effective for the patient, not an interest or investment the APN has in a specific drug or drug company.

Compensation

Compensation provisions in written agreements delineate the payment that will be rendered once agreed-to services are provided. The sum may be listed as a total amount of money that will be paid over the course of the contract, or it may be listed as an incremental amount, paid according to established benchmarks. Caps may be identified that limit the total amount of money that will be paid, as well as any bonus payments. With regard to bonus payments, it is important to decide whether bonus payments will be based on profit that is generated from the services provided by the APN, the productivity of the APN, the quality of care given by the APN, or some combination thereof. Not only does the APN need to decide whether or not bonus payments are going to be incorporated into the written agreement, a great deal of attention needs to be paid to the formula used to calculate bonus payments. It is important to be sure the formulas used are reasonable, are regularly audited, and do not benefit one party more than the other. Care should be taken to avoid financial incentives that may be viewed as kickbacks or otherwise illegal.

In addition, health-care organizations, plans, and practice groups will likely include a statement conveying that it is the responsibility of the APN practicing as an independent contractor to pay all taxes associated with contracted services.

APNs executing written agreements need to consider adding specific dates on which payments will be made. When those payments are not forthcoming, a late fee can be imposed so long as it is included in the agreement. Additionally, when the compensation for the APN is based on billing receipts, the APN should be provided with ongoing documentation tracking the billing process and reimbursement levels from each payer, including secondary sources and previously denied claims. Time frames within which claims will be processed should be set, and penalties for failure to meet those time frames should be negotiated.

Indemnification and Subrogation

Indemnification and subrogation issues are typically addressed in written agreements. Indemnification is a promise between the parties to hold each party harmless for the wrongdoing of the other party. For example, an APN may enter into a contract with a physician practice as an independent contractor. The contract will contain language that says the APN is responsible for his or her own wrongdoings. If a malpractice occurs for which the APN is solely responsible, it is the APN who must bear the loss associated with that claim. The APN must indemnify the physician practice. The contract will also contain language that requires the APN to carry his or her own insurance coverage. It is important to ensure that an indemnification provision is reciprocal so that both parties are extended the same level of protection. The APN should be indemnified by the physician practice if someone other than the APN is responsible for a malpractice or other type of claim.

Subrogation, on the other hand, permits the substitution of one party for another. In health-care matters, the doctrine of subrogation has been used by health-care facilities to recover from the APN the monetary losses sustained after the health-care organization is found liable for the negligence or malpractice of the APN or other individual to whom the APN delegated any aspect of care or treatment. Like indemnification, a subrogation provision will likely be included in certain contracts. If it is, the APN should be sure the provision is reciprocal so that both parties to the contract have a right to subrogation.

Dispute Resolution

Dispute resolution provisions describe the process to be used when the parties disagree about any aspect of the contract. Usually, this provision states that both parties will use their best efforts to promptly resolve all disagreements. In situations in which the disagreement cannot be resolved, there may be a requirement for the parties to submit the dispute to mediation or arbitration as alternative dispute resolution mechanisms. The parties to the contract may negotiate terms that require either binding or nonbinding dispute resolution. If there is binding arbitration, for example, the parties to the contract are waiving their rights to file a lawsuit in the event one of the parties is dissatisfied with the arbitrator's decision. If the parties agree to a nonbinding dispute resolution process, it is important to state that the process must be concluded before filing a cause of action in court.

Term, Renewal, and Termination

Term, renewal, and termination provisions in written agreements specify the length of the contract, usually in months or years, and the process to be used to renew and terminate the agreement. Renewal clauses typically require one or both parties to notify the other party within a certain period of time of their intention to renew the contract. Some written agreements approach the issue differently by providing for automatic renewal for a specific period if one party does not notify the other of its intent to *not* renew the agreement.

Termination provisions in written agreements usually require the terminating party to notify the other party within a specific period, usually 60 or 90 days, of that party's intent to terminate the agreement. Agreements may be terminated with or without cause, and severance payment may or may not be incorporated into the agreement. "Termination without cause" provisions permit the APN to be terminated for any reason or no reason, so long as the termination is not unlawful. Sometimes courts consider "termination without cause" provisions in written agreements to be insufficient or unenforceable, thereby permitting the terminated party to pursue a wrongful termination in violation of public policy. This is especially true if the terminated party is characterized as a whistle-blower who reported an allegedly illegal practice and was subsequently notified of the termination of the agreement.

If a "termination without cause" provision is going to be included in the written agreement, it needs to be reciprocal, permitting the APN to terminate the agreement for any reason or no reason within a comparable period. APNs, like other parties to written agreements, need to be sure that their decision to terminate an agreement is lawful.

Not only may agreements be terminated without cause, they may be terminated with cause. An event giving rise to termination with cause usually results in the immediate dissolution of the contract. Terminations for cause are typically limited to instances in which the APN commits a crime, breaches his or her fiduciary duty to the organization, is disciplined by his or her professional board, or acts in a manner that potentially compromises the standing of the organization in the community. These provisions may also be stated more broadly by permitting "for cause" termination with any illegal occurrence. Like termination without cause provisions, termination of the agreement "for cause" may be exercised by an APN, so long as an identifiable "for cause" event has occurred and the agreement permits termination. It is, therefore, important to ensure that termination clauses are reciprocal and that the APN articulates the occurrence of those events that would permit the APN to terminate the agreement, as well as the financial consequences for each party if the agreement is terminated.

Remedies for Breach

Written agreements usually identify the remedy or consequence of breaching or failing to perform under the terms of the agreement. In an attempt to limit the circumstances that can give rise to a breach, and to establish the amount of money to be paid because of a breach (known as liquidated damages), one party may attempt to define the specific circumstances that would create a breach of contract. An example would be one party's failure to provide the other party with proof of insurance. In situations in which a specific definition of breach is acceptable to the APN, it is important to ensure that the limited definition is reciprocal and that each party be given a reasonable opportunity to "cure" the breach.

Notices

The notices clause in written agreements identifies the individuals who are to receive notice from the other party. The clause contains specific contact information for each of the individuals listed. The provision also outlines the process, such as certified mail, to be used when notifying the other party of any occurrence requiring notification, such as a decision to renew the contract for an additional term. It is important that the notification information be current so that the proper individuals are apprised of any communication between the parties to the agreement.

Modification

Modification provisions in written agreements permit the parties to modify the terms of the agreement without having to execute a new contract. For multiyear contracts, modification clauses are important because they permit an APN to renegotiate the compensation package or any other aspect of the agreement on an annual or other agreed-to basis. Any specific term of the contract may be modified so long as the modification provision states that the contract may be modified at any time and as long as both parties agree to the modification. Modifications invariably must be in writing and signed by all parties to the contract. Sometimes modification provisions will specify only certain components of the agreement that can be modified. Before executing an agreement, it is important for the APN to understand which terms of the agreement are subject to modification and, if necessary, negotiate for the right to modify additional terms before signing. Typically, modifications that occur during the term of the contract accompany the agreement in written form and are attached to the agreement as addendums.

Assignment

Assignment provisions in written agreements either permit or prohibit the assignment of the contract from one of the parties to another individual or entity. When assignment is permitted, one party may pass a contract on to a third party. That third party then assumes the responsibility for performing in accordance with the terms of the contract. On the other hand, when assignment is prohibited, the agreement cannot be sold or transferred to another party. Often, if an APN is contracting with an entity, the entity will want the ability to assign the contract to another entity or subcontractor (such as a hospital or group practice) but will be unwilling to allow an APN to assign the contact to another APN.

Severability

Severability clauses help to keep uncontested and enforceable provisions of the written agreement in effect. Sometimes one specific provision of an agreement is disputed and deemed unenforceable. The severability clause permits the rest of the contract to remain in full force.

Conflict of Laws

The conflict of laws clause in a written agreement identifies the jurisdiction within which the agreement was executed and the jurisdiction that governs contractual disputes that may arise. It is important for APNs to know which jurisdictions apply. For example, if an APN is contracting with a health-care facility that is owned by a company located in another state, the APN may be subject to that other state's laws if a dispute arises. Sometimes this clause will require the APN to seek relief in the other state's court system rather than the court system of the state where the APN is located. These types of provisions can make it quite difficult for the APN to obtain remedies if there is a breach of the contract.

Legal Authority

The legal authority section of a written agreement states that the parties to the agreement have the authority to enter into the arrangement. This provision ensures that only the individuals with the authority to bind the parties are participating in the negotiation and execution of the written agreement.

Force Majeure

The *force majeure* clause of a written agreement ensures that the contract will not be considered to be breached in situations in which an "act of God" prohibits one party from performing in accordance with the terms of the agreement. "Acts of God" include natural disasters such as floods, earthquakes, tornados, and hurricanes, as well as human disasters such as wars, terrorist acts, and riots. A *force majeure* clause has the effect of putting the performance requirements of the contract on hold until performance can be reasonably resumed.

Covenant Not to Compete

Covenants not to compete limit an APN's ability to enter into other ventures that would compete with the "interests" of the organization, plan, or practice group with whom he or she is contracting. Typically, covenants not to compete are time limited and may contain geographical limitations. That is, an APN may be prohibited from entering into other ventures that directly or indirectly compete with the other party for a certain period of time, such as 2 years after the contract terminates. The prohibition also may be limited to a certain geographical radius, such as a 10-mile radius from the location of the other party. This type of limitation is meant to protect the organization or practice group from direct competition by the APN, who could otherwise open a practice in the same general location and take business from the other party.

When a covenant not to compete is included in an independent contractor or employment agreement, it is important for the APN to know what organizations or entities the other party considers to be within the scope of the covenant not to compete. It is also important to clarify what the other party means by the use of the word "interests," to limit the applicable period to as narrow a time frame as possible, to limit the geographical restraints, and, if possible, to include a specific sum of money that will be received by the APN for agreeing not to compete. Each state has laws that govern whether a restrictive covenant is enforceable or not, and the APN should keep in mind that these laws vary from state to state.

Also, in exchange for retaining this covenant in an agreement, an APN should give serious consideration to requiring the other party to execute an exclusive agreement that would not allow the other party to contract with other APNs. Alternatively, the APN might ask for the right of first refusal on all projects and referrals for which the APN is qualified. An example might be the closure of a pain management clinic due to lack of funding and termination of the APN who functioned as staff, with subsequent reopening of the same service on receiving new grant monies. On reopening, the pain management clinic would give the APN the right of first refusal for rehiring.

Signatures

The signatures section of a written agreement is the place where the parties sign and date the document. After the parties sign the agreement, it is considered to be executed. An agreement that is executed signifies that the parties have reached a meeting of the minds and that both parties intend to interact with each other in accordance with the terms of the contract.

Other Provisions to Consider Including in Written Agreements

Although most written agreements contain some combination of the provisions previously identified, there are contemporary issues that may need to be addressed by APNs as well. Those issues include the proprietary rights of the parties and incentives, as well as the frequency with which clinical practice guidelines and collaborative practice agreements will be negotiated.

Proprietary rights of the parties should be discussed by the parties considering entering into a contractual business relationship. It is important to clarify who owns all tangible and intangible property at the beginning of the business relationship so that issues regarding ownership interests can be explored and restrictions on use, if any, can be articulated. Tangible personal property might include equipment, supplies, or furnishings. Intangible property, on the other hand, includes things such as intellectual property and good will. In situations in which these issues have been addressed during the negotiation period, the parties are clear about what property they each own and the expectations regarding the use of that property during the term of the contract and once the agreement expires or is terminated.

With regard to incentives, it is important for APNs to avoid agreeing to participate in any incentive arrangement that is based on the denial or rationing of care or schemes to acquire new patients in which the APN knowingly receives inducements. Incentive arrangements that fit into this category include any limitations on the numbers of diagnostic tests that can be performed, admissions ordered, patients seen in clinic settings, or drugs prescribed within any specific period. Engaging in these kinds of activities subjects health-care professionals to fraud and abuse allegations and to breach of fiduciary duty causes of action. Health-care providers are experiencing the consequences associated with these problems. The Office of Inspector General–U.S. Department of Health and Human Services (OIG-HHS) reported that the federal government obtained $2.5 billion in health-care fraud judgments and settlements in 2010 for alleged kickbacks and false claims—a figure that does not include recovered state Medicaid funds (OIG-HHS, 2011). APNs should be careful to avoid contracts and activities that the government might view as fraudulent. Investigations are on the rise as the federal government actively seeks to recoup significant amounts of money to help fund national health-care reform under the Affordable Care Act of 2010. It may be appropriate, however, for APNs to consider including legal incentives that are based on the achievement of quality outcomes. Quality outcomes that might be used as incentives include, but are not limited to, patient satisfaction, length of stay, mortality, readmission rate, and adherence to recommended clinical regimens.

Avoiding Legal Pitfalls Associated with Written Agreements

Written agreements are executed in an effort to establish the ground rules the parties agree to follow. Sometimes, however, these agreements are the subject of litigation. Usually, in litigation arising out of a written agreement executed between two parties, one party alleges that the other has breached the contract. In other instances, one party may attempt to argue that the contract should be deemed illegal or that certain provisions of the contract should be disregarded.

In 1999, juries in two Florida cases awarded health-care professionals significant damages for breach of contract by the health-care organizations with which the professionals had been working. In the first case, a jury awarded $22.8 million to two oncologists, Jerome J. Spunberg and Bruce W. Phillips, who had their practice agreements wrongfully terminated by Columbia/JFK Medical Center in

Atlantis, Florida (*Spunberg v. Columbia/JFK Medical Center,* 1999). In the second case, a jury awarded Ho Chung Tu, a neonatologist, $2 million in damages after it determined that Mount Sinai Medical Center of Greater Miami breached its contract with the doctor by directing patients to other physicians (*Tu v. Mount Sinai Medical Center,* 1999).

Some agreements entered into by health-care professionals are not only unenforceable, but they are also considered illegal. When that occurs, health-care professionals or the organizations they contract with may be subject to civil and criminal sanctions. In 2010 OIG-HHS reached a settlement with Rush University Medical Center in Chicago, Illinois. The hospital agreed to pay a civil monetary penalty of $1.5 million for leasing office space to physicians at less than fair market value (OIG-HHS, 2011). These types of arrangements are considered to be kickbacks from the hospital for patient referrals from the physicians. Also in 2010 a Texas nurse was sentenced to prison for participating in a kickback scheme with a durable medical equipment (DME) company. The DME company paid the nurse 10% of the Medicare payments it received for each patient the nurse referred to it (OIG-HHS, 2011). APNs need to be vigilant and avoid these and other types of arrangements that may be characterized as kickbacks.

The case that follows is illustrative of some of the contractual terms previously discussed in this chapter, as well as some problems APNs may encounter in situations involving written agreements. *Washington County Memorial Hospital v. Sidebottom* (1999) involved a nurse practitioner (NP) who entered into an employment agreement with the hospital in 1993. The employment agreement contained a covenant *not to compete* during the term of the agreement and for 1 year following the termination of the agreement. The covenant applied to the geographical area within a 50-mile radius of the hospital. The NP could not "directly or indirectly engage in the practice of nursing [elsewhere] without the express direction or consent" of the hospital. In February 1994, the NP was still employed at the hospital and asked for permission to provide prenatal care elsewhere. The hospital was not providing prenatal care for its patients at the time and allowed the NP to provide the care elsewhere. However, the hospital reserved the right to rescind its permission if it offered prenatal services in the future.

The employment agreement terminated in 1996, and the NP and the hospital entered into a new employment agreement that had a term of 2 years. The second agreement contained the same covenant not to compete. It also provided for an additional 2-year term, unless either party provided written notice of termination at least 90 days before its expiration in 1998. The agreement also gave the parties the right to review the NP's compensation at set intervals.

During the course of the second employment agreement there were some discussions between the parties about increasing the NP's compensation. In January 1998, the hospital unilaterally gave the NP a 3% salary increase, which the NP considered to be unfair, although she did sign a modification to the agreement concerning the increase. The NP resigned a few months later and immediately began employment with a physician practice that was located within the 50-mile radius of the hospital. The hospital went to court and obtained an order prohibiting the NP from practicing within the 50-mile radius for 1 year from the effective date of her resignation.

The NP appealed and argued the court should not enforce the covenant "because there was no threat of significant patient loss" to the hospital. However, the appellate court found the geographical limitations and time frame of the covenant to be reasonable and protective of the hospital's patient base, which was the source of its revenue. The court noted that the hospital had helped the NP get established in the community by setting up two clinics, advertising her services, and providing her with the support necessary to maintain her practice.

The NP also argued that the hospital materially breached the employment agreement by unilaterally amending the contract with a salary increase without the NP's review or any negotiations. The appellate court rejected this argument as well and found the hospital had acted in good faith by giving the NP an increase equal to a cap it had imposed on salary increases at the time. Had the court agreed that the hospital breached the employment contract, the NP would *not* have been subject to the covenant not to compete. The covenant would have been unenforceable and the court would have allowed the NP to continue to practice within the geographical area excluded by the contract.

CONCLUSION

Traditionally, nurses have practiced as employees and not independent contractors. However, more and more APNs are embarking on private practice careers and pursuing entrepreneurial opportunities that require the protections of a written agreement. In addition, more and more APNs and their employers are entering into written contracts to define their rights and responsibilities. Because executing written agreements governing the working relationship between the APN and another party is becoming commonplace, it is important to understand the basic, foundational issues that need to be addressed in written agreements. This chapter has identified a number of those issues.

Although written agreements can provide APNs with great flexibility and autonomy, they can also result in the APN, rather than the health-care organization, being held liable for alleged acts of negligence. In addition, the terms included in written agreements may be the focus of litigation themselves. Cases discussed in this chapter demonstrate how some courts have addressed these issues. In light of the principles discussed in this chapter, it is important for APNs to ensure that agreements regarding their status as employee or independent contractor be memorialized in writing. In addition, these written agreements need to be carefully reviewed for compliance with federal and state laws and regulations and to ensure that the written agreement accurately reflects the mutual assent of the parties.

REFERENCES

American Nurses Association. (2010). *Nursing: Scope and standards of practice* (2nd ed.). Washington, DC: American Nurses Publishing.

Hansen v. Caring Professionals, Inc., No. 1-95-2346 (appeal from the Circuit Court of Cook County, February 20, 1997).

Internal Revenue Service. (2011a). *Publication 15.* Washington, DC: Department of the Treasury, Internal Revenue Service.

Internal Revenue Service. (2011b). *Publication 15-A.* Washington, DC: Department of the Treasury, Internal Revenue Service.

Kirk v. Mercy Hospital Tri-County, 851 S.W.2d 617 (Missouri 1993).

Murray, John S. (2011). What every nurse needs to know about whistle-blowing. *OR Nurse, 5*(4), 39–42.

New Jersey Conscientious Employee Protection Act. (1986, as amended 1989, 1997, and 2005).

OIG-HHS. (2011). *Health care fraud and abuse control program annual report for fiscal year 2010.* Retrieved November 27, 2011, from http://oig.hhs.gov/publications/docs/hcfac/hcfac/hcfacreport2010.pdf.

Spunberg v. Columbia/JFK Medical Center, Inc., No. CL-97-008937 (Florida 1999).

Tu v. Mount Sinai Medical Center of Greater Miami, Inc., No. 93-03552 (Florida 1999).

Vizcaino v. Microsoft Corporation, 120 F.3d 1006 (Ninth Circuit 1997).

Washington County Memorial Hospital v. Sidebottom, No. ED75301 (Circuit Court of Washington County, Missouri, 1999).

26

The Law, the Courts, and the Advanced Practice Nurse

David M. Keepnews
Kammie Monarch

INTRODUCTION

The focus of this chapter is to highlight several areas of the law that directly affect the role and practice of advanced practice nurses (APNs). It gives an overview of the sources of law in the United States; how each branch of government, especially the judicial branch, works; and discusses some specific areas of law that guide all APNs in their daily practices. We do not directly address issues related to negligence and malpractice—as important as those issues are—because they are addressed separately in another chapter.

THE BROAD CONTEXT FOR LAW

Sources of Law

The legal environment for nursing practice is derived from a number of sources, including *legislation* that governs and otherwise affects practice; *regulations* that implement; and the *decisions* of courts that interpret and enforce laws, including both legislation and regulation.

Legislation

Much of the legal context for advanced nursing practice originates in statutes—that is, in legislation that is passed in Congress and in state legislatures. Legislation defines the legal authority for practice, legal responsibilities of practitioners, many of the penalties for failing to live up to those legal responsibilities, and other critical aspects of practice, including reimbursement.

Different responsibilities fall to the state legislatures and to Congress. Congress votes on legislation that involves the use of federal funds, relates to issues that span across state boundaries, or affects commerce between states. For example, the Medicare program was created by federal legislation in 1965, and Medicare funding, financing, eligibility, coverage, and payment are all governed by federal law. State laws are still relevant—Medicare requires that services must be within a practitioner's scope of practice, which is determined by each state, in order for them to be eligible for payment—but Medicare is a federal program, and Congress and the federal government have the power to define and shape that program.

A large number of health-care issues are the responsibilities of the states. State legislatures define licensure requirements for health-care professionals, hospitals, and other health-care organizations. States also determine issues related to the scope of practice of APNs and other health-care professionals—these include major issues such the scope of APN prescriptive authority and whether APNs must practice in collaboration with physicians.

In theory, Congress passes laws that deal with national or federal issues, whereas most health-care issues are reserved for the states to address. In practice, this line has become harder to draw. For example, although states are responsible for regulating hospitals and other health-care organizations, such organizations must be in compliance with Medicare requirements, including Medicare conditions of participation (COPs), in order to participate in the Medicare and Medicaid programs—that is, to be eligible for payment by those programs. The states have traditionally been responsible for regulating health insurance, but Congress has determined that many insurance issues are areas of national concern. Accordingly, the Affordable Care Act (Public Laws 111-148 and 111-152)—the health reform law enacted in 2010—sets out a framework for state health insurance exchanges, mandates most employers to provide health insurance or pay a penalty, and mandates individuals not covered by their employer or a government health-care program to purchase insurance. Some have argued that this "individual mandate" exceeds Congress's powers—that this is a matter for states to decide. This issue has been litigated, with varying results, in federal court and, as of the time this chapter was written, is awaiting a decision by the U.S. Supreme Court.

Generally speaking, when Congress acts in a given area, it overrides states' actions in the same area—a doctrine known as *preemption.* For instance, the federal Employee Retirement Income Security Act of 1974 preempts any state laws regulating employee benefit plans, including employer-provided health insurance. This provision in the law has had the effect of exempting self-insured plans (in which employers bear their own insurance risk directly) from state regulation. It also has had the effect of preempting state courts' ability to try damage suits based on damages allegedly caused by the actions of an employer-provided health plan.

Federal legislation, the National Labor Relations Act, defines the rights of private sector employees to engage in collective bargaining and concerted activity related to wages, hours, and working conditions. If a state legislature were to pass its own law addressing the rights of private sector employees to form unions, those laws might be challenged based on being preempted by federal law.

In some instances, however, both Congress and the states may act—either because Congress explicitly allows the states to act or because Congress and the states address different aspects of the same issue. For example, the federal Occupational Safety and Health Act addresses health and safety issues of employees, but it allows states to pass more stringent laws and regulatory mechanisms to protect employees within the state. Both the Congress and many state legislatures have enacted antitrust laws, which address anticompetitive marketplace activity. Although Congress has strengthened and broadened federal laws on health-care fraud and abuse, including fraudulent and abusive activities directed against private health insurers, states also have laws that address health-care fraud and abuse.

Government Agency Rulemaking

The actions of federal and state government agencies have a critical role to play in health care, including the practice of APNs. The rules and regulations they issue have the force of law.

In the United States, government is divided into three branches: legislative, executive, and judicial. Under this scenario, the legislature passes laws, the executive branch implements them, and the judicial branch interprets them when controversies arise.

The executive branch is headed by a chief executive—either the president (at the federal level) or the governor (at the state level). It includes a number of different agencies that administer the day-to-day workings of the government; these are headed by officials who report to the president or governor and who (generally) are appointed by him or her. These agencies cover all areas of government. In health care, relevant agencies include the U.S. Department of Health and Human Services (DHHS) and agencies within it, such as the Centers for Medicare and Medicaid Services, the Food and Drug Administration, the Centers for Disease Control and Prevention, and the National Institutes of Health. But many other agencies have an impact on health care and health professionals in one way or another—the U.S. Department of Labor, the Department of Defense, the Department of Veterans Affairs, and others.

These agencies act based on the authority given to them through Congress (for federal agencies) or the state legislatures. A common explanation of these agencies' responsibilities is that they implement legislation. This description is not inaccurate, but it may be deceptively simple. "Implementation" may involve a range of activities, from simply operationalizing a clear legislative mandate, to filling in complex details in a legislatively developed program, to acting on its own initiative based on a long-standing, broad grant of legislative authority.

The following examples may help illustrate the differences between each of these types of executive agency action.

In one hypothetical state, following lobbying efforts by nursing organizations, the state legislature passes legislation authorizing APNs to prescribe drugs without physician supervision or mandatory collaboration. The relevant part of this legislation reads as follows:

1. An advanced practice nurse (APN) shall be authorized to write prescriptions for drugs, regardless of class of drug, provided that the APN:
   a. Is certified by a national accrediting body recognized by the National Commission on Certifying Agencies or the American Boards of Nursing Specialties; and
   b. Has successfully completed 100 hours of coursework in pharmacology offered by an accredited school of nursing, either as part of an educational program leading to preparation as an APN or subsequent to completing such program.
2. The board of nursing shall establish and maintain a mechanism for ensuring that APNs meet the above requirements before prescribing drugs.
3. The board of nursing shall maintain a list of APNs who are qualified to prescribe drugs and shall make this list available to the board of pharmacy.
4. A licensed pharmacist, upon being presented with a valid prescription written by an APN who is qualified to prescribe drugs, shall fill such prescription in the same manner as a prescription written by any other qualified prescriber.
5. Nothing in this section shall be construed as requiring physician supervision of APN prescriptions or prescribing practices.

To implement this change in the law, the state board of nursing (BON) and state board of pharmacy might then propose amendments to their regulations. The BON's regulations would include a process for tracking and verifying completion of required pharmacology coursework and for maintaining a list of APNs who are authorized to prescribe.

This is the simplest form of implementation—providing a mechanism to operationalize a clear legislative mandate. Imagine that the law was written a little differently and instead reads as follows:

An advanced practice nurse shall be authorized to prescribe drugs, provided that she or he has completed coursework in pharmacology, and in accordance with standards and mechanisms as determined by the board of nursing.

This law is much less precise. How much coursework do APNs need in order to prescribe? Where can they obtain it—must it be from a school of nursing, or can it be provided by another continuing education provider? What other standards should be included—should there be restrictions based on the APN's area of expertise or certification? Are pharmacists required to fill prescriptions written by APNs? What role (if any) will physicians have related to APN prescribing? These are all issues that are left to the government agency (in this case, the BON) to address when it proposes and issues regulations.

Why would a state legislature adopt a law that is so sparse on details? Perhaps it was the result of a compromise following a failure to reach consensus on the details among interest groups and legislators and an agreement to let those details be worked out in regulation. Or, as is often the case, perhaps legislators preferred to leave some of the important details to the government agency that is expected to have the requisite expertise to set appropriate standards, based on the belief that legislators lack the expertise (or time) to debate whether 75, 100, or 200 hours of pharmacology coursework is appropriate, but that the government agency charged with regulating nursing practice is in a better position to make such a determination.

This type of scenario—the legislature enacting legislation that leaves it to a government agency to determine major details—is fairly common. When Congress passed the Health Insurance Portability and Accountability Act (HIPAA) in 1996, it included requirements for safeguarding the privacy of health information. It was left to DHHS to develop and promulgate rules that spell out the mechanisms for implementing and enforcing standards for doing so. When Congress expanded the scope of Medicare reimbursement for APNs as part of the Balanced Budget Act (BBA) of 1997, it was up to DHHS (and, specifically, to the Health Care Financing Administration, now the Centers for Medicare and Medicaid Services [CMS]) to address important questions such as who would qualify for reimbursement and how statutory requirements that APNs work in collaboration with a physician would be implemented.

The Affordable Care Act (ACA) introduced several important new measures to expand access to health-care coverage, curb abusive practices by some insurers, and expand primary care and preventive services, among many others. Many of the provisions of the ACA require DHHS and in some cases other agencies, including the Department of Labor and the Internal Revenue Service, to issue implementing rules. These include rules addressing basic issues such as determining what is included in "essential health benefits" and what constitutes "preventive services."

Sometimes government agencies act under a broad scope of authority that has been granted to them in a specific area by Congress or a state legislature, rather than in response to a recent legislative mandate. A state health department may be granted the authority to establish licensing standards for hospitals, for instance. After initially establishing regulations containing standards for licensure, the agency may subsequently decide to revise those standards as part of its broad mandate to protect the public's health.

The Court System

What Courts Do

Courts administer justice by applying laws to controversies. Facts are determined, the law is applied to those facts, and a decision is rendered. Civil courts adjudicate controversies between individual parties or ascertain the enforcement and redress the rights of the parties. Parties in these matters are referred to as *plaintiffs* and *defendants.* Plaintiffs are the suing party, and defendants are the party defending the cause of action filed against them.

Criminal courts, on the other hand, are charged with administering criminal laws and determining penalties for wrongs against society. In some states, criminal and civil courts are separate, whereas in others a court of general jurisdiction exists.

Structure of the U.S. Court System: Federal and State

In the United States, there is a federal court system and each state has its own court system. In state-based civil proceedings, breach of contract, negligence, and malpractice causes of action are typically heard, as well as domestic relations, real estate, probate, and other state-specific matters. These cases may or may not be heard by a jury, but they are always overseen by judges.

In most states, the party losing the case at the trial court level has the opportunity to appeal the matter to an appellate court. States use different names for this level of court, but they all are considered intermediate appellate courts. Generally, these courts are referred to as *courts of appeals.* In these courts, the appealing party is referred to as the *appellant,* and the other party is the *appellee.* Cases coming before a court of appeals are not retried. Generally, appellate judges determine whether or not the trial was properly conducted and/or whether the right law was correctly applied. After reviewing the trial court record, the court of appeals may affirm, modify, reverse, or remand the judgment made at the trial court level. Affirming the trial court decision upholds the original determination made in the matter. Modifying the trial court decision changes the decision in some way. Reversing the decision of the trial court results in nullifying it. Remanding the decision results in the case being sent back to the trial court.

The losing party at the appellate court level may have the opportunity to appeal the matter to the state supreme court. Many state supreme courts have the discretion to determine which cases it will and will not hear. Cases raising federal constitutional issues may be appealed to the U.S. Supreme Court.

Unlike the varied nature of the state court systems, the federal court system is uniform. Every state is divided into federal districts. Some larger states such as California, New York, and Texas are each divided into four districts. In total, there are 94 federal district courts. These district courts are presided over by appointed federal district judges. Federal district courts hear both civil and criminal matters. Cases tried in federal district courts include those in which the United States is a party; disputes between states, between a state and a citizen of another state, between citizens of different states, and between a state or its citizens and a government abroad; disputes affecting foreign ambassadors; cases arising under federal law and the U.S. Constitution; and admiralty and maritime cases.

After a judge in a federal district court has rendered his or her decision, the losing party may appeal that decision to a federal court of appeal (often referred to as circuit courts). There are 13 such courts in the United States. The losing party at this level may request to appeal the decision to the U.S. Supreme Court.

The U.S. Supreme Court is located in Washington, D.C., and is composed of nine justices, one of whom serves as the chief justice. Supreme Court justices—like all federal judges—are nominated by the President of the United States and confirmed by the U.S. Senate.

The Role of Precedent

In making their decisions, courts look at how prior cases raising similar issues have been decided. Previously decided cases with similar facts or legal issues are called *precedents.* Courts will look to these prior decisions as guides to deciding current cases, by either following them or distinguishing a current case to explain why previous decisions do not apply.

SELECTED LEGAL ISSUES

Legal Scope of Practice Issues

State laws define the boundaries within which members of each health-care profession may practice. This is referred to as that profession's *scope of practice*. The scope of practice of APNs is generally found in each state's nurse practice act. Typically, scopes of practice for nurses, including APNs, are written broadly and do not delineate specific tasks.

State laws governing APN scope of practice vary considerably. Twelve states and the District of Columbia currently allow APNs to practice without any legal requirements for physician supervision or collaboration. Other states require varying degrees of involvement by physicians. State laws also vary in APN authority to prescribe medications—some require collaboration with a physician; some allow only some categories of APNs to prescribe; some impose restrictions in terms of types of medications that can be prescribed. New York State permits nurse practitioners (NPs) to prescribe only within their specialty area.

These varying restrictions on APN practice have been cited as a barrier to expanding access to health-care services. The Institute of Medicine (IOM) report on *The Future of Nursing* (Committee on the Robert Wood Johnson Foundation Initiative on the Future of Nursing, at the Institute of Medicine, 2010), included a recommendation to remove scope-of-practice barriers, declaring that "advanced practice registered nurses should be able to practice to the full extent of their education and training" (p. 278).

In 2008, the APRN Consensus Group and the National Council of State Boards of Nursing issued a *Consensus Model for APRN Regulation: Licensure, Accreditation, Certification and Education*. This document sets out a uniform model of APRN regulation with the intent that it be adopted by all U.S. states. The model has been endorsed by a wide range of nursing professional and specialty organizations.

Advanced Practice Nurses in the Courts

In 1936, for the first time, scope of practice issues between nurses and physicians were addressed in a published opinion. That case, *Chalmers-Francis v. Nelson* (1936), involved a nurse's administration of anesthesia over the objection of a physician and one of his associates. The physician asserted that administration of anesthesia by a nurse was a violation of the California Medical Practice Act and should be immediately stopped. The case was eventually heard by the California Supreme Court. In reviewing the matter, the Court concluded that anesthesia administration by nurses did not constitute diagnosing or prescribing within the state medical practice act.

In *Fein v. Permanente Medical Group* (1981), an NP was alleged to have been negligent when she assessed a patient with chest pain as having a muscle spasm rather than a myocardial infarction. At trial the patient was awarded almost $1 million in damages. The case, which presented a number of issues, was eventually appealed to the California Supreme Court. One of the issues raised was whether an NP's professional conduct should be judged according to a physician standard of care. The court found that an NP—not physician—standard of care should apply because the NP's scope of practice includes examining and diagnosing a patient, and that the activity engaged in by the NP was within her scope of practice even though that activity overlapped with activities engaged in by physicians.

In *Sermchief v. Gonzales* (1983), the Missouri Board of Registration for the Healing Arts threatened to charge two nurses with the unauthorized practice of medicine and to charge five physicians with aiding and abetting the unauthorized practice of medicine. These health professionals all practiced at a clinic in which the nurses performed family planning, obstetrics, and gynecology services using standing orders and protocols that were approved by physicians. In an attempt to resolve the issue, the health professionals asked for an injunction prohibiting the Board from taking action and to declare that their actions were lawful. The case eventually went to the Missouri Supreme Court, which ruled in favor of the nurses and physicians, affirming the ability of the nurses to practice as APNs. In reaching its decision, the court reviewed the state's definition of professional nursing and noted that the scope of practice for nurses had been expanded and that the nurses in this case were practicing in accordance with applicable laws. Because these nurses' conduct was consistent with the state nurse practice act, they were not engaging in the unauthorized practice of medicine.

Bellegre v. Board of Nurse Examiners was decided in 1985. In this case, physicians challenged the validity of rules promulgated by the Texas Board of Nurse Examiners concerning advanced nursing practice. The case went to the state appellate court, which ruled that the Texas BON had the statutory authority to make and issue rules pertaining to advanced practice nursing.

Planned Parenthood v. Vines (1989) was decided by a Court of Appeals in Indiana. In this case, a patient sued Planned Parenthood, alleging that an NP had inserted an intrauterine device (IUD). One of the issues addressed by the court was the standard of care required of the NP. After considering the matter, the court concluded that the NP was a specialist and should be held to the standard of care for a person with superior knowledge and skill, and thus must practice consistent with others with superior knowledge and skill. At trial, expert testimony asserted that the standard of care for inserting IUDs was the same for nurses and physicians. As a result, the NP was required to insert the IUD using the care and skill of others, including physicians, performing that same task.

Berdyck v. Shinde and HR Magruder Memorial Hospital was decided by the Ohio Supreme Court in 1993. In this case, the court ruled that the standard of care applicable to any other health-care professional was the same, regardless of the particular health-care professional performing that skill. Here, a nurse and physician were both accused of negligence with regard to recognizing the signs and symptoms of preeclampsia. One of the issues the justices dealt with on appeal was the duty of care owed to the patient. In rendering its decision to affirm the lower court's denial of the hospital's motion for summary judgment, the justices noted that the fact that a physician owes a particular duty of care to a patient does not mean that the nurse is exempt from owing that same duty of care. The court observed that the same act may be within the practice standards for both nurses and physicians, and that both groups of health-care professionals must embark on the completion of that act in a way that is consistent with their respective duties of care to their clients.

The Ohio Supreme Court's determination in the *Berdyck* case was reiterated in *Ali v. Community Health Care Plan, Inc.* (2002). The plaintiff sued a health maintenance organization (HMO) that employed a nurse-midwife. The plaintiff alleged that she was treated negligently during her pregnancy, thereby causing her to lose the baby. She had reported the development of a vaginal discharge to the HMO's nurse-midwife during a telephone conversation approximately 2 weeks after having an amniocentesis. She claimed the nurse-midwife failed to direct her to see a physician. The nurse-midwife countered that the character of the vaginal discharge reported by the patient was not indicative of a loss of amniotic fluid. The nurse-midwife's documentation supported her position. The case was tried and the judge instructed the jury to apply a certain standard of care: what a reasonable and prudent nurse-midwife practicing obstetrics and gynecology would have done under the same circumstances. The jury rendered a verdict in favor of the HMO. The plaintiff appealed and argued the trial judge should have directed the jury to apply a different standard: what a reasonable and prudent *professional* practicing obstetrics and gynecology would have done under the same circumstances. The plaintiff contended the nurse-midwife standard was a lower standard. The appellate court disagreed and determined that any professional practicing obstetrics and gynecology would be required to direct a patient to be seen if the patient reported signs and symptoms consistent with loss of amniotic fluid. The verdict rendered by the trial court was affirmed.

Spine Diagnostics Center of Baton Rouge Inc. v. Louisiana State Board of Nursing (2008) concerned a Louisiana State Board of Nursing Advisory Opinion, which concluded that interventional pain management falls within the scope of practice of certified registered nurse anesthetists (CRNAs). A trial court ruled that the Advisory Opinion constituted a regulation expanding the CRNA scope of practice into a new area. An appellate court affirmed, finding that interventional pain management is "solely the practice of medicine" and agreeing that the Advisory Opinion was a regulation that the BON had issued without providing notice and an opportunity to comment, as required by the state Administrative Procedures Act, and finding it invalid. The state supreme court declined to hear the case, allowing the appellate court ruling to stand.

In 2011, an Iowa court invalidated rules issued by the state board of nursing and department of public health, authorizing NPs to supervise fluoroscopy. Iowa physician groups argued that the rules were invalid because state law prohibits the expansion of nursing into medicine without official recognition by physicians. The court found that state law also required that the agencies first establish a curriculum, safety standards, and an examination before authorizing NPs to supervise fluoroscopy. Nursing organizations unsuccessfully argued that the law should be upheld (*Iowa Medical Society and Iowa Society of Anesthesiologists v. Iowa Board of Nursing and Iowa Department of Public Health*, 2011).

Professional Discipline

Boards of nursing govern the practice of nursing in every state. It is the responsibility of the BON to protect the public from conduct that poses a threat to the public health, safety, and welfare. Each state's nursing practice act and/or regulations set out specific grounds for professional discipline, but generally they include acts of unprofessional conduct, gross negligence, endangering patient safety, unethical conduct, and acting outside of one's scope of practice (Monarch, 2002).

In 1980 an APN was disciplined because he was found to have violated the nurse practice act in Florida. The case was *Hernicz v. State of Florida, Department of Professional Regulation.* Hernicz's license was suspended because he was alleged to have treated two patients without physician supervision. Disciplinary action was taken in this case because the state of Florida required APNs to work with a sponsoring physicians. In this case, the Florida Court of Appeals concluded that the disciplinary action taken was proper because the Florida Department of Professional Regulation presented credible and substantial evidence that the NP did not have a supervising physician when he treated two patients.

When an APN is accused of violating the state nurse practice act, he or she must be notified in the complaint of the specific alleged violations. A disciplinary action process will be held in accordance with the state's administrative procedures act (APA). It is the provisions of the APA that ensure that individual disciplinary action proceedings occur in a manner that respects the constitutional rights of the nurse. Of particular concern are the nurse's rights to due process. This requires that the nurse have a meaningful opportunity to respond to the complaint and to be meaningfully heard.

Following disciplinary proceedings, a BON will issue final agency orders. This document describes any disciplinary action that was taken, outlines the finding of facts, and outlines the conclusions of law that were relied on in rendering the decision. Disciplinary action may include issuing a reprimand, suspending the APN's license, or revoking it. Once a final agency order is issued by a BON, the matter is concluded, unless one of the parties elects to appeal the decision in court.

Courts will generally not substitute their own judgment for that of the board of nursing. However, there are instances in which a court reversed BON action. Typically, reversals occur when a court determines that the nurse's due process or other constitutional rights were violated, the board acted beyond its statutory authority, it failed to follow required procedures, committed an error of law, or made an arbitrary and capricious decision.

Hogan v. Mississippi Board of Nursing (1984) is an example of a case in which a BON decision involving an APN—in this case, a nurse anesthetist—was overturned by a court. Hogan was investigated by the Mississippi Board of Nursing for allegedly misappropriating narcotics from the hospital where she worked. The BON conducted a hearing, found her guilty, and her license was revoked. She appealed. The Mississippi Supreme Court found that the BON had applied the wrong standard of proof in determining that Hogan had misappropriated narcotics. Whereas charges of misconduct generally require the BON to prove the charge by a *preponderance of the evidence* (showing that it is more likely than not that the accused party committed the alleged acts), in this case the court ruled that charges leading to license revocation must meet a higher standard—*clear and convincing evidence*—but the BON failed to apply this standard in Hogan's case. The court thus directed the BON to restore Hogan's license.

FRAUD AND ABUSE

Responsibility and accountability are not new concepts for APNs or for any professional nurse. As APNs have broadened their roles in health care, areas of potential legal risk have grown. Many of the issues that were formerly of primary concern to other health-care professionals are now much more clearly relevant to APNs as well.

As Medicare providers, APNs are able to receive Medicare provider numbers (known as Unique Physician Identification Numbers, or UPINs) and to bill Medicare directly for covered services. APNs are recognized as providers by increasing numbers of group and private health plans as well. Recognition as providers has also brought an increased responsibility (and need) for APNs to understand the requirements for sound, legal billing practices.

Federal and state governments have sharpened their focus on fraudulent and abusive practices by all health-care providers. Government agencies have concentrated increasing resources on investigating and prosecuting fraud and abuse. As independently accountable professionals, it is in APNs' interests to understand what is expected of them as providers under Medicare, Medicaid, and other health-care programs and plans. In this as in most other areas of law, ignorance of the law does not excuse violations. The fact that a practice may use billing staff or an outside billing specialist does not mean that providers are not expected to know, and to be responsible for, claims and documentation submitted under their names and UPINs.

APNs need to have some familiarity with reimbursement laws and what they are expected to do to avoid violations. Some common examples of conduct that may be considered to violate fraud and abuse laws include billing for services that were not actually furnished to the patient, misrepresenting the patient's diagnosis (providing a false or more severe diagnosis to justify payment or increase the amount of payment), misrepresenting the services provided (billing for more complex or intense services than those that were actually furnished to the patient), misrepresenting the medical necessity of services provided, and billing for services under circumstances in which requirements for payment have not been met.

The federal government and many state governments have been stepping up investigation and enforcement activities related to fraud and abuse for several years. The Affordable Care Act increases federal sentencing guidelines for health-care fraud that involves more than $1 million in losses; increases coordination between CMS, the HHS Office of Inspector General (OIG), and the Department of Justice; and adds greater oversight of private insurance abuse. It expands resources devoted to fraud and abuse enforcement and sets the stage for possible further expansion of fraud and abuse laws.

Assessing Risk and Avoiding Fraud and Abuse

Whether in their own practices, in physician-based practices, or in hospital-based practices, APNs should be aware of programs in place to ensure compliance with applicable laws on billing for services. APNs should not assume that billing practices that have been in place for some time must be okay because "we have always done it this way." Enforcement agencies are generally concerned more with *patterns* of inappropriate, illegal billing practices over time than with isolated, accidental events.

The Health-Care Fraud Prevention and Enforcement Action Team (HEAT), a joint initiative of DHHS and the U.S. Department of Justice, includes a Provider Compliance Training Initiative to encourage compliance and to advise providers on how to avoid fraud and abuse. Several resources have been developed as part of this initiative, including instructional videos and podcasts. These can be accessed at http://oig.hhs.gov/compliance/provider-compliance-training/index.asp. In addition, the DHHS OIG Web site (http://www.oig.hhs.gov) includes advisory opinions and compliance guidance resources that can be readily accessed.

Billing, coding, and payment policy are complex. Most APNs are not experts in this area, but all should have a general understanding of coding, billing, and payment. In most instances, working with a billing specialist—either one employed by the practice or an external consultant—is highly advisable. However, each APN must have sufficient knowledge to work with these specialists to ensure their accuracy.

One specific area in which APNs (and the practices in which they work) must be careful is the area of "incident to" billing. Since its inception, Medicare Part B has paid not only for "physician services," but also for services and supplies furnished incident to the services of a physician (CMS, 2011). Among other things, this has allowed physician practices to bill for services provided by other staff—not just APNs, but also staff nurses, medical assistants, and other office personnel. For many years, this was the only way that services provided by APNs were covered under Medicare. As APNs won Medicare reimbursement for eligible services, more and more APNs have been billing Medicare directly for their services. However, many practices have chosen to continue billing APN services as incident to services. When an NP or a clinical nurse specialist (CNS) bills Medicare directly for services (under their own names and UPINs), Medicare pays for those services at 85% of what it would pay a physician. (Certified nurse-midwives' services are paid at 100% of the physician rate as of January 1, 2011.) Incident to services are billed under the physician's name and number, and are paid at 100% of the physician rate—in essence, they are treated as if the physician performed the service. Thus, many physician practices that employ APNs see a financial incentive in billing under incident to.

Incident to billing, however, comes with several requirements (CMS, 2011). The physician must initiate the patient's course of treatment and must provide subsequent services frequently enough to reflect the physician's continuing active participation in and management of the course of treatment. The services must be provided under direct physician supervision—the physician must be present in the office suite and immediately available to provide assistance and direction throughout the time the APN is providing services to the patient. The APN must be an employee, leased employee, or independent contractor of the physician, or of the entity that employs or contracts with the physician. (So, for example, the APN and physician may both be employees of the same clinic or health system.)

These requirements reflect the fact that incident to payment was not designed as a mechanism for paying independent providers of care, but rather as a way to reimburse physicians for services provided by office staff. Incident to billing long predates recognition of APNs as Medicare providers. Also, keep in mind that these conditions do not apply to APN services billed under the APN's name and UPIN.

The potential for incorrectly billing for services is increased when practices depend on incident to billing for services provided by APNs. Is there a physician on the premises and available at all times, or do APNs cover for physicians during hospital rounds, or at other times when no physician is in the office? Are there times when a new patient is seen by an APN? Are there times when an established patient is seen by an APN for a new health problem? If the practice complies with all of the conditions for incident to billing, are the details of such compliance adequately documented?

Notably, in addition to the restrictions and risks inherent in incident to billing for APN services, it also renders those services invisible—they are reflected in Medicare data as having been provided by the physician, not the APN.

ANTITRUST LAW

Antitrust is another area of the law that can have an important bearing on health professionals' practices. It is an area in which the courts have played a significant shaping role. Antitrust laws apply much more broadly than just to health care. The first federal antitrust statute, the Sherman Act, was passed by Congress in 1890, followed by the Clayton Act and the Federal Trade Commission Act, both in 1914. Congress's goals in enacting these statutes was to ensure free competition by countering business practices and transactions "which tended to restrict production, raise prices or otherwise control the market to the detriment of purchasers or consumers of goods and services" (*Apex Hosiery Co. v. Leader,* 1940). When competitors work together to restrain competition by others, they deprive consumers of the purported benefits of a free economic market—it removes incentives to lower prices and improve quality. Some activities that had been undertaken by large industries at the end of the 19th century—dividing up economic markets, agreeing on minimum prices, boycotting other competitors—were seen as inherently injurious to consumers. As part of a populist reaction to the "robber barons" in industries such as steel and oil, the antitrust laws were seen as an effort to reclaim the free enterprise system as the United States had previously known it. For instance, in describing the Sherman Act, the U.S. Supreme Court noted that this statute was "designed to be a comprehensive charter of economic liberty aimed at preserving free and unfettered competition as the rule of trade. It rests on the premise that the unrestrained interaction of competitive forces will yield the best allocation of our economic resources, the lowest prices, the highest quality, and the greatest material progress, while at the same time providing an environment conducive to the preservation of our democratic, political, and social institutions" (*Northern Pacific Railway Co. v. United States,* 1958).

The U.S. Department of Justice (DOJ) and the Federal Trade Commission (FTC) share federal enforcement responsibilities for these antitrust statutes; in addition, state attorneys general and private parties may also bring suit under these laws. Most states also have their own antitrust laws, generally with provisions parallel to the federal laws.

The antitrust laws are written broadly. The application of these laws has been shaped by decades of judicial interpretation. Some activities—price-fixing, group boycotts, and market allocation (dividing up markets among competitors)—are considered *per se* violations. This means that once it has been established that a competitor has engaged in one of these activities, the courts do not inquire as to its anticompetitive effects, such as whether and how it has harmed competition or injured consumers. Other activities are analyzed under a *rule of reason* approach. Under this approach, the court analyzes an alleged restraint on competition, weighing the procompetitive effects of an agreement against its anticompetitive effects (Marsh, 2010). This means that the court carefully examines the industry involved, the history and purpose of the restraint, the relevant market, and any special circumstances that exist in that market (*United States v. Topco Associates,* 1972). Meeting this standard is clearly a much more involved, costly, and time-consuming analysis than that required for activities that are considered *per se* violations.

Another example would be if a group of physicians organizes to disadvantage another group of health-care providers. In *Wilk v. American Medical Association* (1990), the American Medical Association (AMA) was found to have engaged in a boycott of chiropractors. The AMA's code of ethics had declared it unethical for physicians to associate with unscientific practitioners and later determined that chiropractic practice lacked a scientific basis. The effect of these determinations was a pronouncement that any physicians who referred patients to chiropractors, accepted referrals from chiropractors, or taught at a chiropractic school would be committing an ethical violation. A group of chiropractors sued the AMA, alleging that it was attempting to eliminate chiropractic care through an illegal boycott. The U.S. Court of Appeals for the Seventh Circuit eventually determined that this AMA policy (which had subsequently been changed) was, in fact, a *per se* violation of the Sherman Act.

For many years, the antitrust laws were considered by the courts to be inapplicable to the activities of most professionals. "Learned professions" such as law and medicine generally were considered sufficiently different from other businesses for concerns about anticompetitive conduct to be relevant. In 1975, in *Goldfarb v. Virginia State Bar,* the U.S. Supreme Court found setting minimum attorneys fees to be a Sherman Act violation, rejecting the defendant bar association's argument that they were exempt because the law is a learned profession. Subsequently, the U.S. Supreme Court made the application of the antitrust laws to medicine explicit in *Arizona v. Maricopa County Medical Society* (1982). In that case, local physicians had agreed on maximum fees that could be charged. This decision indicated that such acts were price fixing and effectively eliminated any belief that health care was outside the reach of antitrust laws.

In one of the few antitrust cases involving APNs, a group of CNMs brought suit against hospitals, a physician-owned insurance company, and several physicians. The CNMs charged that the defendants had engaged in concerted actions to prevent them from gaining hospital privileges, required physician supervision, and the ability for their collaborating physician to secure liability insurance. Their thriving practice was eventually forced to close. Eventually, the CNMs won settlements against some of the defendants, and the U.S. Court of Appeals for the Sixth Circuit ruled against the remainder of the defendants (*Nurse Midwifery Associates v. Hibbett,* 1990).

In *Oltz v. St. Peter's Community Hospital* (1994), the Ninth Circuit Court of Appeals examined a case brought by a nurse anesthetist whose contract with a hospital was cancelled after a competing group of anesthesiologists obtained an exclusive contract with the same hospital. The hospital, located in a rural community in Montana, provided 84% of the surgical services rendered in the area. The anesthesiologists did not want to compete with Oltz, who charged a lower rate for anesthesia and enjoyed a good relationship with local surgeons. After the hospital cancelled Oltz's contract, he was effectively put out of business and had to relocate to find suitable employment. Oltz sued the anesthesiologists and the hospital, and claimed their actions constituted a violation of the Sherman Act. On appeal from a trial court verdict awarding him no damages, the Ninth Circuit Court of Appeals ruled in his favor, finding that Oltz had presented ample evidence to support his claim that the hospital and physicians had conspired to eliminate him as a competitor.

Enforcement of the Antitrust Laws

Changes in health care have posed new challenges and concerns for health-care providers. In the 1990s, the DOJ and the FTC issued their *Statements of Antitrust Enforcement Policy in Health Care* (FTC & DOJ, 1996) to offer guidance on types of arrangements or combinations that would generally not be subject to antitrust enforcement. These statements represented an attempt by these two agencies to provide a degree of flexibility in antitrust enforcement in health care, particularly during a period of rapid transformation of the industry.

The Affordable Care Act established a Medicare Shared Savings program that encourages the formation of accountable care organizations (ACOs) involving combinations of health-care providers. In October 2011, the FTC and DOJ issued a joint "Statement of Antitrust Enforcement Policy Regarding Accountable Care Organizations Participating in the Medicare Shared Savings Program" to provide procedures for reviewing prospective ACOs.

Promoting Competition

Not all conduct that hinders competition constitutes antitrust violations. The FTC often provides analysis and advice on the potential impact on competition of proposed legislation and/or regulations. For example, in 2010, the staffs of the FTC's Office of Policy Planning, Bureau of Economics, and Bureau of Competition issued a letter advising that proposed Kentucky rules governing "limited service clinics" (such as retail clinics) would unjustifiably restrict the activities of health professionals practicing there, potentially hindering the ability of these clinics to compete with other types of clinics (DeSanti, Farrell, & Feinstein, 2010). The FTC may also initiate an administrative complaint when it believes that a practice is anticompetitive, as it did after investigating a North Carolina Board of Dental Examiners rule restricting the ability of non-dentists to provide tooth-whitening services (FTC, 2010).

In its report, the IOM Committee on the Future of Nursing took note of these and other opinions and actions by the FTC. As part of its recommendation to remove scope-of-practice barriers to allow advanced practice registered nurses to practice to the full extent of their education and training, the committee suggested that the FTC and the Antitrust Division of the DOJ "review existing and proposed state regulations concerning advanced practice registered nurses to identify those that have anticompetitive effects without contributing to the health and safety of the public. States with unduly restrictive regulations should be urged to amend them to allow advanced practice registered nurses to provide care to patients in all circumstances in which they are qualified to do so" (Committee on the Robert Wood Johnson Foundation Initiative on the Future of Nursing, at the Institute of Medicine, 2010, p. 279).

CONCLUSION

Laws, regulations, court decisions, and other arenas of public policy continue to affect health care and nursing. As important as it is for APNs to be aware of how the law affects them, it is also critical for them to play a role in shaping laws today and tomorrow. Organizations representing nursing and APNs have an important role to play in advocating for policies that can expand access to health care, including advanced practice nursing services. Nursing is key to achieving the goals of health reform—something that is recognized not just by nursing groups, but also by broader groups of health-care leaders, as demonstrated by the IOM report's recommendation that APNs should be able to practice to the full extent of their education and training. The opportunity is ripe for APNs—through increased advocacy and collaboration with a broad array of partners and allies—to shape the legal and regulatory environments to maximize their role in health care and expand consumers' access to their vitally needed services.

REFERENCES

Affordable Care Act, Public Laws 111-148 and 111-152 (2010).
Ali v. Community Health Care Plan, Inc., 801 A 2d 775 (Ct. 2002).
Apex Hosiery Co. v. Leader, 310 U.S. 469 (1940).

Arizona v. Maricopa County Medical Society, 457 U.S. 332 (1982).
Bellegre v. Board of Nurse Examiners, 685 SW 2d 431 (1985).
Berdyck v. Shinde and H.R. Magruder Memorial Hospital, 613 NE 2d 1014 (1993).
Centers for Medicare and Medicaid Services. (2011). *Medicare benefit policy manual Chapter 15—Covered medical and other health services.* Retrieved August 20, 2012, from https://www.cms.gov/manuals/Downloads/bp102c15.pdf.
Chalmers-Francis v. Nelson, 6 Cal. 2d 402 (1936).
Committee on the Robert Wood Johnson Foundation Initiative on the Future of Nursing, at the Institute of Medicine (2010). *The future of nursing: Leading change, advancing health.* Retrieved August 20, 2012, from http://www.iom.edu/Reports/2010/The-Future-of-Nursing-Leading-Change-Advancing-Health.aspx.
DeSanti, S. S., Farrell, J., & Feinstein, R. A. (2010). *Letter from FTC staff to Kentucky Cabinet for Health and Family Services* (January 28, 2010). Retrieved from, http://www.ftc.gov/os/2010/02/100202kycomment.pdf.
Employee Retirement Income Security Act. (1974). P.L. 93-406.
Federal Trade Commission Act. (1914). U.S.C. Sec 44–48.
Fein v. Permanente Medical Group, 121 Cal. App. 3d 135 (1981).
Federal Trade Commission. (2010). *Federal Trade Commission complaint charges conspiracy to thwart competition in teeth-whitening services: North Carolina dental board charged with improperly excluding non-dentists.* Retrieved August 20, 2012 from http://www.ftc.gov/opa/2010/06/ncdental.shtm.
Federal Trade Commission & U.S. Department of Justice. (1996). *Statements of antitrust enforcement policy in health care.* Retrieved August 20, 2012, from http://www.justice.gov/atr/public/guidelines/0000.htm.
Federal Trade Commission & U.S. Department of Justice. (2011). Statement of antitrust enforcement policy regarding accountable care organizations participating in the Medicare Shared Savings program. *Federal Register, 76*(209), 67026–67032.
Goldfarb v. Virginia State Bar, 421 U.S. 773 (1975).
Health Insurance Portability and Accountability Act. (1996). Public Law 104-191.
Hernicz v. State of Florida Department of Professional Regulation, 390 So. 2d 194 (1980).
Hogan v. Mississippi Board of Nursing, 457 So.2d 931 (1984).
Iowa Medical Society and Iowa Society of Anesthesiologists v. Iowa Board of Nursing and Iowa Department of Public Health. Iowa District Court for Polk County, CV 8252 (October 31, 2011). Retrieved August 20, 2012, from www.iowa.gov/nursing/images/pdf/ARNP%20Fluoroscopy%20Order.pdf.
Marsh, R. E. (2010). The health care industry and its medical care providers: Relationship of trust or antitrust? *DePaul Business and Commerce Law Journal, 8,* 251–273.
Monarch, K. (2002). *Nursing and the law: Trends and issues.* Washington, DC: American Nurses Publishing.
Northern Pacific Railway Co. v. United States, 356 U.S. 1, 4 (1958).
Nurse Midwifery Associates v. Hibbett, 918 F.2d 605 (1990).
Oltz v. St. Peter's Community Hospital, 19 F.3d 1312 (1994).
Planned Parenthood v. Vines, 543 NE 2d 654 (Indiana, 1989).
Sermchief v. Gonzales, 660 SW 2d 683 (Missouri, 1983).
Spine Diagnostics Center of Baton Rouge Inc. v. Louisiana State Board of Nursing CA 0813 (2008).
United States v. Topco Associates, 405 U.S. 596, 621 (1972).
Wilk v. American Medical Association, 895 F.2d 352 (1990).

27

Malpractice and the Advanced Practice Nurse

*Carolyn T. Torre**

INTRODUCTION

Professional liability insurance is essential for advanced practice nurses (APNs), who, because of their autonomy, exercise of independence in clinical decision making, provision of complex care, and prescription of medications, assume an increased risk of being sued for malpractice. The purpose of this chapter is to provide some basic information about the legal accountability of APNs, an overview of the current health-care practice climate and the process of litigation, the risks that affect being sued for malpractice, and those that affect liability insurance availability and cost. Finally, the chapter discusses steps APNs can take to minimize the risk of being sued for malpractice, including (a) maintaining current clinical skills and knowledge; (b) communicating clearly with patients regarding treatment options and ensuring informed consent; (c) documenting clear, supportable reasons for taking or not taking diagnostic and therapeutic actions, as well as recording the patient's response to interventions; (d) recognizing the timely need for consultation and referral; (e) nurturing the optimal professional and business relationships that are a part of advanced practice nursing; and (f) knowing and abiding by state and federal laws governing APN practice.

NURSING TRADITION AND THE PARADIGM SHIFT

Historically, nurses were perceived to be protected against malpractice liability because most were employed in hospitals (Shinn, 1998). As "charitable organizations," hospitals were generally exempt by statute or common law from malpractice liability. When charitable immunity statutes were eliminated and institutions began to insure against liability, nurses assumed that they were protected under the hospital's or facility's insurance policy by virtue of their employment relationship. Many nurses persist in this assumption, which, as Buppert (2008) points out, is unwise because institutions are primarily concerned about protecting their own interests and may choose not to vigorously defend particular nurses. Should these nurses not also have their own individual liability insurance, they can be at risk of financial ruin particularly if they decide to settle or are ultimately found guilty. Malpractice insurance is a hedge against such risk.

Current APN Practice and the Impact of Health-Care Reform

Approximately 32 million uninsured Americans are expected to obtain health-care insurance by 2019 as a result of the passage of the Patient Protection and Affordable Care Act (ACA) in March

*Earlier versions of this chapter were authored by Sharon Muran, Amy Muran Felton, and Marie Infante.

2010 (Kaiser Family Foundation, 2011). Separate elements in the ACA such as the ability of young adults to stay on their parents' insurance plans until age 26, nondeniability by insurance to children with preexisting conditions, and the reimbursement of preventive services (without a copay) for new Medicare recipients have already been implemented. This rise in the number of insured will be accompanied by the need for a substantial increase in the availability of primary care providers, and the utilization of APNs to meet this increased need is the logical solution.

The APN title in most states includes nurse practitioners, clinical nurse specialists, nurse anesthetists, and nurse-midwives. Determining which APNs are included when examining data related to malpractice rates is important because some advanced practice specialties are riskier than others, in particular, obstetrics and anesthesia. Advanced practice nursing programs have evolved to educate registered nurses at the master's and doctoral level in specialties designed to cover primary, specialty, and acute-care needs across the entire age spectrum. APNs work in a variety of practice settings including federally qualified health-care centers, private physicians' offices, nursing homes, correctional facilities, schools, college health centers, hospitals, and patient's homes, as teachers in schools of nursing, and as policy makers at the state and federal level in both governmental departments and nonprofit organizations. By 2009, 49.1% of physicians were in practices that employed nurse practitioners and certified nurse-midwives (Park, Cherry, & Decker, 2011).

Over the past years APN educators, policy makers, researchers, and practitioners have defined and tested standards of care. By September 2011, APNs in 16 states and the District of Columbia had achieved full practice independence by legislatively eliminating requirements for collaborative agreements and joint protocols with physicians from their APN statutes (Fairman, Rowe, Hassmiller, & Shalala, 2011). A white paper published by the New Jersey State Nurses Association in 2009 described the need to eliminate legislative, regulatory, and practice barriers for APNs in that state to make them maximally accessible as primary and specialty care providers (Torre, Joel, and Aughenbaugh, 2009). The comprehensive 2010 report on the future of nursing released by the Institute of Medicine (IOM), underscores the cost-effectiveness and high quality of care offered by APNs and argues that legislative, regulatory, and insurance barriers must fall for them to be able to practice to their full scope and educational preparation (IOM, 2010). A related article by the primary authors of the IOM report contends that APNs are integral to meeting the nation's primary care provider shortage and concluded that there are "no data to suggest that nurse practitioners in states that impose greater restrictions on their practice provide safer and better care than those in less restrictive states or that the role of physicians in less restrictive states has changed or deteriorated" (Fairman et al., 2011, p. 194). APNs are directly reimbursed by insurers at both the federal and state levels such as Medicare and Medicaid; by private insurance companies such as Blue Cross/Blue Shield, United Healthcare, and Oxford; and by many health maintenance organizations (HMOs) and managed care organization (MCOs), but outdated Medicare laws and company policies can and do impose significant restrictions on if, how, and at what level this reimbursement occurs.

With more APNs expected to be acting as the primary and specialty care providers of a growing number of insured, APNs can anticipate being subject to an increased risk of professional liability. Because the best defense is a good offense, APNs must actively and continuously engage in effective risk management strategies including ensuring that they have the consistent protection of malpractice insurance.

THE RISKS OF ADVANCED PRACTICE NURSING

There are at least three types of exposure that APNs should seek to avoid: (a) financial exposure in terms of judgments or settlements from a civil lawsuit, (b) licensure or certification actions by the relevant state agencies or private associations, and (c) civil or criminal sanctions and exclusion from participation in the federal health-care programs for fraud or abuse.

Civil Lawsuits

The first type of exposure is liability for professional malpractice. Malpractice is a type of professional negligence that results when the practitioner fails (by act or omission) to exercise the degree of skill and learning expected of a reasonably prudent, reputable member of the (APN) profession (Black, 1979). Negligence includes failure to follow up, failure to refer when necessary, failure to disclose essential information, and failure to give necessary care (Buppert, 2008). When the appropriate standard of care is not followed and results in harm to the patient, financial exposure to compensate the patient or the patient's family occurs. This exposure is the typical risk that most malpractice insurance policies cover.

Licensure or State Certification Exposures

There are other types of direct or indirect financial exposures that arise from breaking state statutes or regulations that control advanced practice. Substance abuse, fraud, unprofessional conduct, failure to fulfill requirements for continuing education, and failure to renew state licenses by deadlines or to have a written collaborative agreement or joint protocol with a physician where one is required are other examples of charges that can result in licensure sanctions or loss of APN certification by a state board of nursing (BON). These types of risks may or may not be covered by a professional liability insurance policy. The wise APN will comparison shop to locate the liability insurance that will cover the costs of defending against such licensure actions.

Federal Health Program Exclusion

Another type of legal risk is noncompliance with laws and regulations of the federal health-care programs that provide direct reimbursement for the services of APNs (Buppert, 2002, 2008; Infante, 2000). The penalties can be both criminal and civil. A conviction for fraud is referred by the courts to the state BON for appropriate action with respect to the license of the guilty nurse (Bureau of National Affairs, 2004). The most severe civil penalty for breaking these laws is exclusion from federal health-care programs based on the authority of the Secretary of the U.S. Department of Health and Human Services (DHHS) to ban practitioners from receiving payments from any federal health-care program when they have violated certain laws. These risks are generally not covered in a typical professional liability insurance policy. In addition, all providers (e.g., hospitals, HMOs, home health agencies, nursing homes, and others) and all other practitioners (e.g., physician, group practices, and others) who themselves participate in federal health-care programs are banned from hiring the excluded APN at risk of losing their own federal reimbursement. Therefore, program exclusion is a career-ending event for most individuals. It should be pointed out that in the period between September 1, 1990, and April 2, 2011, no advanced practice nurse-nurse practitioner, nurse anesthetist, nurse-midwife, or clinical nurse specialist has been reported to the National Practitioner Data Bank for exclusion from Medicaid or Medicare (NPDB, 2011a).

Although a thorough discussion of statutory and regulatory risks is beyond the scope of this chapter, APNs must know the laws that control their practice and their reimbursement, develop behaviors to ensure compliance with these laws, recognize the risks associated with noncompliance with these laws and regulations, and use risk prevention strategies to manage their professional practices and minimize those risks (Buppert, 2008; Infante, 2000). Increasing use of telemedicine, will, for example, require knowledge of state laws where the patient resides because in some states, such as New Jersey, the BON requires that a registered nurse (RN) or APN be licensed there to provide clinical care to a NJ resident, even remotely. One of the most important ways to keep up with current state and federal laws and regulations and other practice-and policy-related issues is to be an active member of your state nurses association, an affiliated APN group, and at least one national organization representing APNs. Doing so means you can participate in initiating policy changes that control APN practice, stay abreast of changes in state and federal laws affecting APN practice, and develop and sustain supportive relationships and communication networks with other APNs.

MALPRACTICE AND THE ADVANCED PRACTICE NURSE

How frequently are APNs sued for malpractice? There is no reliable way to gather information on the number of lawsuits filed on a national basis. There is also little to stop a patient from bringing a malpractice lawsuit regardless of the ultimate merits of the allegations against the practitioner. The fact is that that APNs are being sued more frequently, and that the cost of both malpractice payouts and average expenses related to defending claims have risen (CNA HealthPro, 2010; Miller, 2009). The most comprehensive source of reports on verdicts and settlements resulting from malpractice claims against health-care professionals is the National Practitioner Data Bank (NPDB) of the DHHS, Health Resources and Services Administration (HRSA). Data from NPDB shows that though reports of malpractice suits and settlements for all APN categories—nurse anesthetists, nurse-midwives, nurse practitioners, and clinical nurse specialists—have risen since 1990, they remain low in number compared to reports against physicians.

The National Practitioner Data Bank and Healthcare Integrity and Protection Data Bank

The NPDB was established by Congress in 1986 (NPDB, 2008). DHHS is responsible for implementing and maintaining this databank. The NPDB is intended to improve the quality of care by restricting the ability of incompetent practitioners to move from state to state without disclosure of previous malpractice payments or adverse actions.

In 1996, Congress created a second data repository, the Healthcare Integrity and Protection Data Bank (HIPDB), to combat fraud and abuse in health insurance and health-care delivery (HIPDB, 2008). The HIPDB collects, reports, and discloses information regarding licensure and certification actions, program exclusions, criminal convictions, and other adjudicated actions and decisions against both individual practitioners and institutional providers. Although there is some overlap between the NPDB and the HIPDB, only the NPDB reports malpractice judgments and settlements.

State licensure boards, hospitals, and other eligible entities access these databanks to assess an individual practitioner's (including APNs') responsibility for errors and professional misconduct when considering applications for state license, employment, staff privileges, or other affiliations.

The NPDB collects information on all malpractice payments made by insurance companies on behalf of individual health-care practitioners. Payments must be reported to the NPDB no matter how small the amount, whether or not the case is settled before filing suit, and whether or not the payment was the result of a confidential settlement. Reporting of malpractice payments is mandatory for all types of licensed health-care practitioners. The NPDB also collects information about adverse licensure or professional sanctions imposed on health-care practitioners. Reporting of adverse licensure actions, clinical privilege actions, and professional society actions is mandatory for all physicians and dentists in the United States. Adverse actions against APNs and other health-care practitioners may be voluntarily reported to the NPDB.

Trends in Malpractice Claims

The NPDB began collecting and analyzing data on malpractice claims in 1990 and issues annual cumulative reports of its findings. The most recent data are from the 2011 Summary Report, which reviews reports for all individual health-care providers (NPDB, 2011a). Before March 2002, the NPDB classified nurses into four categories: professional (registered) nurses (RNs), certified registered nurse anesthetists (CRNAs), certified nurse-midwives (CNMs), and nurse practitioners (NPs). A fifth category, advanced nurse practitioners, subsequently amended to clinical nurse specialist, was added in 2002. The 2011 summary report provides an opportunity to review the reports submitted for each category of APN over the period September 1, 1990, through April 2, 2011, by state. See **Table 27-1.** Comparing and contrasting both the number and rates for each of those APN categories, as well as comparing and contrasting them to the reports and rates for two other similar health-care professionals (physicians and physician assistants [PAs]), provides the following picture (NPBD, 2011a): nurse anesthetists have the highest number of reports over this 21-year period (1,461 reports out of an estimated 44,000 providers), but nurse-midwives have the highest rate of reports (830 out of an estimated 6,700 providers), calculated as 3% (nurse anesthetists) and 12% (nurse-midwives), respectively. Nurse practitioners have a total number of reports approaching that of nurse anesthetists (1,150) but a very low rate (0.6%) because of the total number of these providers (167,857).

(text continues on page 506)

TABLE 27-1

NPDB Summary of APNs Reported by State: 1990–2011

The following is a summary of reports submitted and accepted into the NPDB for those nursing specialties falling under the APN rubric: clinical nurse specialist, nurse anesthetist, nurse-midwife, and nurse practitioner. Since all states do not include nurse anesthetists and nurse-midwives under the title APN, the data are presented separately for each specialty. The data cover the period from September 1, 1990, through April 2, 2011. Professional categories that were not available for the entire time period are noted.

Data disclaimer: Reports of adverse clinical privileges and professional society membership actions against practitioners other than physicians and dentists (e.g., chiropractors, psychologists, podiatrists) are submitted voluntarily.

Clinical Nurse Specialist (Date Profession Code First Available for Use: September 9, 2002)

State	Medical Malpractice Reports	Licensure, Clinical Privileges, Medicare/ Medicaid	Professional Society Membership Exclusion Reports and Peer Review Organization Reports
AL	0	4	0
CA	0	1	0
CO	2	0	0
CT	1	0	0

Continued

TABLE 27-1

NPDB Summary of APNs Reported by State: 1990–2011—cont'd

State	Medical Malpractice Reports	Licensure, Clinical Privileges, Medicare/ Medicaid	Professional Society Membership Exclusion Reports and Peer Review Organization Reports
IN	1	0	0
KY	0	6	0
LA	0	1	0
MA	2	1	0
ND	0	1	0
NJ	1	0	0
OH	0	2	0
OK	0	1	0
OR	0	1	0
RI	2	0	0
SC	0	2	0
TX	1	1	0
UT	1	0	0
WA	1	0	0
WV	1	0	0
TOTAL	**13**	**21**	**0**
Nurse Anesthetist			
AK	7	1	0
AL	30	87	0
AR	20	1	0
AZ	15	2	0
CA	42	7	0
CO	20	1	0
CT	9	0	0
DC	3	0	0
DE	1	0	0
FL	132	8	0
GA	45	6	0
HI	3	0	0
IA	19	2	0
ID	16	3	0
IL	34	1	0
IN	6	1	0
KS	56	4	0
KY	25	7	0
LA	91	23	0
MA	15	11	0
MD	36	1	0
ME	6	2	0
MI	54	40	0

TABLE 27-1

NPDB Summary of APNs Reported by State: 1990–2011—cont'd

State	Medical Malpractice Reports	Licensure, Clinical Privileges, Medicare/ Medicaid	Professional Society Membership Exclusion Reports and Peer Review Organization Reports
MN	12	2	0
MO	45	2	0
MS	19	7	0
MT	7	1	0
NC	23	4	0
ND	4	4	0
NE	25	2	0
NH	8	2	0
NJ	26	1	0
NM	17	1	0
NV	8	0	0
NY	64	2	0
OH	64	7	0
OK	34	13	0
OR	9	4	0
PA	48	4	0
PR	2	0	0
RI	5	3	0
SC	15	25	0
SD	2	1	0
TN	63	13	0
TX	189	12	0
UT	10	5	0
VA	23	3	0
VT	1	0	0
WA	18	8	0
WI	18	2	0
WV	8	0	0
WY	6	1	0
TOTAL	**1,461**	**337**	**0**
Nurse-Midwife			
AK	2	0	0
AL	3	4	0
AZ	13	5	0
CA	40	1	0
CO	20	2	0
CT	14	3	0
DC	4	0	0
DE	4	0	0

Continued

TABLE 27-1

NPDB Summary of APNs Reported by State: 1990–2011—cont'd

State	Medical Malpractice Reports	Licensure, Clinical Privileges, Medicare/ Medicaid	Professional Society Membership Exclusion Reports and Peer Review Organization Reports
FL	126	5	0
GA	32	1	0
HI	2	0	0
IA	3	0	0
ID	1	0	0
IL	15	0	0
IN	2	0	0
KS	1	0	0
KY	12	1	0
LA	2	0	0
MA	47	2	0
MD	25	0	0
ME	3	0	0
MI	34	4	0
MN	9	2	0
MO	3	0	0
MS	1	0	0
MT	2	0	0
NC	9	1	0
ND	1	0	0
NE	1	0	0
NH	13	3	0
NJ	41	10	0
NM	21	3	0
NV	9	1	0
NY	113	10	0
OH	26	5	0
OK	8	1	0
OR	9	0	0
PA	91	15	0
RI	4	0	0
SC	9	4	0
TN	7	0	0
TX	9	1	0
UT	5	1	0
VA	12	0	0
VT	2	0	0
WA	11	6	0
WI	4	2	0
WV	5	1	0
TOTAL	**830**	**94**	**0**

TABLE 27-1

NPDB Summary of APNs Reported by State: 1990–2011—cont'd

State	Medical Malpractice Reports	Licensure, Clinical Privileges, Medicare/ Medicaid	Professional Society Membership Exclusion Reports and Peer Review Organization Reports
Nurse Practitioner			
AE (military)	1	1	0
AK	6	18	0
AL	3	188	0
AR	9	12	0
AZ	47	5	0
CA	81	16	0
CO	33	0	0
CT	4	32	0
DC	5	0	0
DE	3	0	0
FL	182	49	0
GA	19	4	0
GU	2	0	0
HI	1	2	0
IA	8	1	0
ID	9	7	0
IL	16	6	0
IN	11	1	0
KS	9	9	0
KY	13	16	0
LA	22	24	0
MA	62	2	0
MD	25	3	0
ME	6	3	0
MI	16	19	0
MN	8	1	0
MO	18	0	0
MS	22	15	0
MT	7	0	0
NC	2	29	0
ND	2	1	0
NE	3	0	0
NH	11	1	0
NJ	29	1	0
NM	22	2	0
NV	9	6	0
NY	91	36	0
OH	7	7	0
OK	12	73	0

Continued

TABLE 27-1

NPDB Summary of APNs Reported by State: 1990–2011—cont'd

State	Medical Malpractice Reports	Licensure, Clinical Privileges, Medicare/ Medicaid	Professional Society Membership Exclusion Reports and Peer Review Organization Reports
OR	30	27	0
PA	33	39	0
RI	8	6	0
SC	12	16	0
SD	4	6	0
TN	40	49	0
TX	80	5	0
UT	9	15	0
VA	25	59	0
WA	40	87	0
WI	3	1	0
WV	5	0	0
WY	5	1	0
TOTAL	**1,150**	**921**	**0**

Total APNs reported, 1990–2011: 1,150 (NPs) + 830 (CNMs) + 1,461 (NAs) + 13 (CNSs) = **Total:** 3,454 reported out of total APNs: 277,574 = **about 1%.**

*Number of reports, source: NBPD, 2011; rates determined using approximate total numbers of APNs based on figures obtained from the following sites, retrieved September 6, 2011:

Nurse anesthetists: http://www.aana.com/ataglance.aspx

Nurse-midwives: http://www.allnursingschools.com/nursing-careers/nurse-midwife/nurse-midwife-career

Nurse practitioners: http://www.statehealthfacts.org/comparemaptalbe.jsp?ind=773&cat=8

Clinical nurse specialists: http://www.nacns.org/html/cns-faqs1.php

Physicians: https://catalog.ama-assn.org/Catalog/product/product_detail.jsp?productId=prod1910039

Physician assistants: http://www.statehealthfacts.org/profileind.jsp?rgn=1&cat=8&ind=440

Clinical nurse specialists have an extremely low number of reports: only 13 over 21 years, out of a total of 69,017 providers (0.01%), perhaps reflecting that the CNS category was not separately reported before 2002 and, in addition, that the role, except for psychiatric CNSs, has been less likely to involve diagnostic decision making and medication management requiring prescription writing than other APN categories. In contrast to APNs, physicians (including DOs/DO interns/residents and MDs/MD interns/residents), who number approximately 985,000, experienced a total of 281,463 reports between 1990 and 2011, a rate of 28.5%. In the same period, PAs had 1,650 reports to the NPDB out of a total of 74,755 PA providers, a rate of 2%; this compares to the rate of the combined APN category reports: 3,454 out of approximately 277,574 APN providers, about 1% (NPDB, 2011a).

An assessment by Hooker, Nicolson, and Le (2009) of whether or not the utilization of PAs and APNs increases professional liability determined that the probability of making a malpractice payment during the period they examined was 12 times less than that of physicians for PAs and 24 times less than that of physicians for APNs. This same study described higher average malpractice payouts for APNs compared to PAs, even slightly higher than those for physicians. The reason for these variations may be found in an explanation provided by the NPDB (2011b, p. 30): that there are fewer claims made against nurses than physicians so one large payment for an APN negatively affects the mean. Note, in addition, that PAs are much less likely to be involved in the provision of obstetrical and anesthesia care than APNs and the highest claims payments made by all nurses in 2006 were related to obstetrics. A survey of Michigan certified nurse-midwives (Xiao, Lori, Siefert, Jacobson, & Ransom, 2008) confirms the professional liability exposure of these professionals, 15.5% of whom had a malpractice payment of more than $30,000 (the threshold at which reports are sent to NPDB) made on their behalf. Hooker and colleagues (2009) found that female clinicians of all clinical types paid higher malpractice payments than male clinicians and that with regard to APNs, female patients were involved in bringing significantly more suits than male patients.

What Are APNs Sued For?

As would be expected, the highest number of claims made for nurse anesthetists are related to the anesthesia care, and claims are made for CNMs in relation to obstetrics (NPDB, 2011b, p. 29). A 2009 analysis of malpractice claims data for nurse practitioners covered by the Nursing Service Organization over the period 1998–2008 determined that the "predominant allegations" for open and closed claims were related to diagnosis, treatment, and medication, in that order (CNA HealthPro, 2010). Patients who sustained long-term permanent injury involving paralysis or brain injury received the highest monetary awards, significantly higher than the survivors litigating claims of wrongful death although the most frequently cited injury was wrongful death. The injury that most often resulted in death in this study was infection/abscess/sepsis. Scope-of-practice-related allegations were rare but associated with the highest average payments made. Adult/geriatric, family, and pediatric/neonatal NP specialties had the highest number of claims, and the highest average amount paid was to the pediatric/neonatal specialty (CNA HealthPro, 2010). The fact that pediatric patients have a longer time to sue and are awarded higher damage awards when suits are successful because they have a longer predicted time to live with the pain, suffering, and expense of care related to injury is reflected in higher malpractice rates for APNs providing obstetrical, neonatal, and pediatric care.

When the NPDB (2011a) data are examined based on reports of payments by state, it is apparent that the number of reports for APNs varies depending on the practice category. The highest number of reports made for nurse anesthetists between September 1990 and April 2011 was in Texas, followed by Florida; the highest number of reports for CNMs in the same time period was in Florida, followed by Pennsylvania; and the highest number of reports for NPs was in Florida, followed by New York (see Table 27-1). The number of payments in any given state is affected by the number of APNs and may represent a reflection of the professional opportunities in that state. The numbers are also a function of the specific provisions of the malpractice and evidence laws in each state.

There continues to be little in the scant claims experience or research to explain why APNs are sued so much less frequently than physicians. Pearson (2011) calculated the ratio of reports to NPDB for medical malpractice and Medicare/Medicaid exclusion per nurse practitioner in 2010 to be 1:160 compared to 1:4 for their physician colleagues. Although substantial evidence exists that many more medical errors are made than lawsuits filed, little is known about why malpractice claims are filed in some circumstances but not in others, regardless of the type of health-care provider (Schmidt, Heckert, & Mercer, 1992; Weiler et al., 1993). A 2011 study of physician malpractice risk according to specialty estimates that whereas 99% of physicians in the highest-risk specialties (neurosurgery, thoracic-cardiovascular surgery, and general surgery) and 75% of physicians in low-risk categories (psychiatry, pediatrics, and family practice) are likely to face a claim by age 65, 78% of all claims, annually, did not result in payments to claimants (Jena, Seabury, Lakdawalla, & Chandra, 2011).

Physicians see large numbers of patients on a daily basis in an effort to maximize the income stream for a practice; as a consequence, less time is spent with individual patients, which carries increased liability risk. Levinson and colleagues (1997) found that physicians with no claims made against them spent a longer time in an encounter. The Nursing Service Organization study of nurse practitioner claims data determined that NPs typically see 16 patients per day and that those with claims reports see more than 18 patients per day (CNA HealthPro, 2010). It makes sense that spending less time means communicating less with patients about their concerns and about their treatment, which is especially problematic when patients have complicated histories and complaints. A systematic review of 11 randomized clinical trials and 23 observational studies evaluating data on patient satisfaction, health status, cost, and/or process of care by Horrocks, Anderson, and Salisbury (2002) determined that nurse practitioner and physician outcomes were comparable but that patient satisfaction was highest among patients of nurse practitioners. This review also found that nurse practitioners offered more advice or information to patients, documented findings in greater detail, and had better communication skills than their physician colleagues; no differences were determined between nurse practitioners and physicians in the health status of their patients, in the number of prescriptions written, in return visits requested, or in referrals to other providers. A meta-analysis of the Cochrane database by Laurant and colleagues (2006) involving 16 studies evaluating primary care provided by nurses and APNs, in contrast to that of physicians, found that resource utilization and costs were equivalent for comparable care but that patients were more satisfied with the care of nurses. It has been suggested that a clinician is less likely to be sued when patients perceive genuine interest in them, when they believe their care to have been competent, and when careful documentation has been made of services provided (Lefevre, Water, & Budetti, 2002; Sloan & Hsieh, 1995; Wright, 2008). Buppert (2008, p. 261) emphasizes that good communication is essential because it leads to satisfied patients and "satisfied patients generally don't sue."

Malpractice Lawsuits and State Laws

Malpractice lawsuits, with rare exceptions, are filed in state court under state law rather than federal law. State laws pertaining to filing a malpractice claim vary widely and may make it easier or more difficult for patients to sue for malpractice and obtain a judgment or settlement. For example, differences in statute of limitations (the time from discovery of an injury to filing of a lawsuit), burdens of proof, caps on noneconomic damages (e.g., pain and suffering), attorneys' fees, and use of mandatory medical review panels or arbitration to resolve issues make a great difference in the frequency of malpractice lawsuits in a given state and the amount of a judgment or settlement.

Advanced Practice Nurses and Tort Reform

Often health-care professional stakeholders seek state or federal legislation to solve the problems of too many lawsuits and too little access to affordable insurance. Commonly referred to as *tort reform,* these proposed laws seek to make it more difficult or less profitable to file claims against health-care professionals. The intended results are (a) to create a more favorable market for malpractice insurance carriers to continue to provide coverage and (b) for health-care practitioners to continue to provide services. In every session of Congress there are legislative proposals and political calls for national tort reform at the federal level (Underwood, 2009). Although there are strong policy arguments to support Congress taking such action, malpractice litigation is a matter of state law and state legal practice. National tort reform, although repeatedly proposed, remains unlikely any time soon. Meaningful state tort reform laws have been passed in a number of states, and to keep up with the fluid nature of these changes, it is prudent to check state-by-state specifics regarding the current nature of medical liability legislation, which can be found at the National Conference of State Legislatures (NCSL) Web site (NCSL, 2011).

An extensive analysis by Mello (2006) of multiple studies examining the impact of state tort reforms on the malpractice crisis concludes that caps on noneconomic damages reduce the average size of malpractice awards by 20% to 30% and have a modest impact on malpractice insurance premium growth but that these caps have "disproportionately" negative effects on the most severely injured. Mello contends that state reforms such as changes to joint-and-several liability, statutes of limitations, or attorney contingency fees have not had the expected intent of changing the underlying elements of the malpractice crisis by reducing premiums, making malpractice insurance more readily available, or improving the financial health of insurance companies; that research fails to support the perception that overall physician supply has significantly decreased; or that there is a relationship between malpractice cost and physician supply. Mello agrees that the evidence indicates physicians do practice defensive medicine—ordering referrals, medications, and tests to protect themselves from liability—but says that the impact of these strategies is hard to measure.

Alternative and potentially more productive reforms may occur related to the increasing attention that the Congress, federal agencies, and The Joint Commission (TJC) is devoting to prevention of medical errors (Bovgjerg, Miller, & Shapiro, 2001; Clinton & Obama, 2006; Institute of Medicine, 2000; TJC, 2008).

Notwithstanding their historically low incidence of claims, APNs can expect to find themselves increasingly affected by situations that arise in a "hard" malpractice insurance market. The effects are escalating insurance premiums, coverage limitations, insurance company insolvencies, or decisions by carriers to stop covering medical malpractice altogether, limiting access to whatever liability insurance is available (America Association of Nurse Anesthetists [AANA], 2002a; American Society for Healthcare Risk Management, 2002; Silverman, 2004). As a result of prohibitive insurance costs or complete lack of insurance, some practitioners have taken drastic actions, including early retirement, closure of high-risk practices such as obstetrics, or relocation to a state where the claims experience is more reasonable and insurance is available (Freedman, 2002; Silverman, 2004). Because of the malpractice burden, Xiao and colleagues (2008) found that many Michigan CNMs moved from private practice to salaried employment (where the employer pays the medical malpractice premium); those who were independently covered or who were "going bare" were significantly less likely to provide obstetrical care. In another response, associations such as the American College of Nurse-Midwives (ACNM) and other professionals, including a number of physician groups, have formed their own insurance companies to ensure insurance access to their members in the periodic downturns of the insurance business.

Although the aggregate claims history for APNs may seem modest, a hard market for malpractice insurance affects APNs, as well as physicians and all licensed health-care practitioners. The best advice is for APNs to engage in a form of risk management called *risk prevention* and make every effort to reduce errors.

PRACTICE SETTINGS AND SPECIALTY PRACTICE RISKS

As an initial legal principle, each person is always individually accountable for his or her own torts (wrongs). As demonstrated by the NPDB statistics, APNs can and do get sued in their own right. Liability in all cases turns on whether the APN exercised due care under the circumstances. This conclusion is determined by examining the duty owed to the patient, the professional standards that apply to a reasonable APN practicing under similar circumstances, and the causal effect of any act or omission of the APN to the injury suffered by the patient. Whether anyone else, such as collaborating physicians, are accountable and can be sued for the harm caused by substandard acts or omissions of the APN depends on the relationship between the parties and on the facts and circumstances of the incident.

EMPLOYED ADVANCED PRACTICE NURSES

APNs such as NPs and clinical nurse specialists (CNSs) are employed by health-care systems, as well as by acute-care, extended care, and home care facilities, managed care organizations, and private physician practices. CNMs and nurse anesthetists may be employed either by acute-care institutions or by physician groups of obstetrician-gynecologists and anesthesiologists, respectively. As employees, APNs are presumed to be covered by the employer's malpractice program because under the concept of "vicarious liability" the employer is held responsible financially for harm caused to a patient by its employee. The Latin term for this principle of imputed responsibility is *respondeat superior.* It applies only in an employment situation because the employer effectively controls the manner in which the care is rendered (i.e., the employer has legal control over the actions taken by the employee that are within the scope of the employee's job description). When hospitals or health-care systems are sued, it is typically a result of errors or omissions committed by employees such as physicians, technicians, nurses, and APNs. From an economic perspective, employers have more assets to pay a settlement or a judgment and therefore are better able to bear the risk.

When an APN is in a true employment relationship, liability for negligence continues to flow through to the employer as a consequence of this traditional principle of tort law. The insurance rates charged to the employer reflect the risks associated with the entire pool of employees. However, this allocation of risk also provides the employer with the best opportunity to manage the risk through direct payment of claims. Many health-care employers are self-insured, meaning they personally "retain" risk or fund the settlement of claims to a given dollar ceiling. In effect, they are settling with their own money, thus avoiding the higher insurance premium costs. Self-insured employers are thus strongly motivated to keep claim settlements below their self-insured limit. To achieve this objective, it is common to agree to a settlement without disputing which of the named health-care employees were actually liable.

The danger to the employed APN is twofold. First, if named individually in a lawsuit, the APN can be found jointly and severally liable or liable for contributory negligence as an individual, not just an employee. If, under these circumstances, the APN relies only on the employer's malpractice insurance to cover the claim, the hospital defense counsel could decide to settle the case and leave the remaining liability to the APN individually. Second, an APN without individual malpractice insurance coverage is subject to the decisions of the one hospital lawyer, which may not be in the APN's best interest. Moreover, if the APN is at the mercy of the hospital insurer, a settlement of a suit on behalf of any named health-care practitioner must be reported to the NPDB as required by law. Such a settlement could be negotiated without knowledge or consent of the APN. With the APN's professional reputation and financial well-being at stake, the APN cannot afford to abdicate responsibility to an employer. It is advisable to carry sufficient amounts of individual malpractice insurance to maintain control and to avoid these types of conflicts (Buppert, 2008, 2011; CMF Group, 2002; Philipsen, 2008) With individual malpractice insurance coverage, the APN has separate counsel who is not conflicted by the interests of the hospital and can zealously represent the interests of the APN.

INDEPENDENT VS. COLLABORATIVE PRACTICE RISKS

The APN, subject to state nurse practice acts, is increasingly likely to become an independent practitioner who controls his or her own professional judgments and actions. With greater autonomy comes greater individual accountability for actions. In this type of practice arrangement the APN may deliver health-care services in any one or more of several settings, including traditional employer settings. Independent practice is usually accomplished through solo practice, group practice with other APNs, or business arrangements in which the APN and the health-care system, HMO, physician, or group practice structure their relationship as one of "independent contractor" or as a credentialed member of a hospital's medical staff with defined privileges.

As an independent contractor, the general rule is that no vicarious liability flows from the APN to the institution, physician, or other third party (Ingram, 1993). In real life, however, even when the APN is not the employee of the institution, or physician, a lawyer may still argue that the institution or physician is responsible because ostensibly the APN and the hospital or practice encourages patients to believe the nurse is employed by the institution. This type of ostensible agency theory is frequently argued in emergency room and anesthesia cases or whenever the lawyer wants to get to the (presumably) "deep pocket" of the hospital or the physician as a source of money for the patient. A plaintiff's lawyer will argue that responsibility is shared by all who were involved in the events leading to the claim of injury, including the institutional provider and any physician (or APN) involved in the care of the patient at the time under legal theories of joint and several or contributory liability (Buppert, 2008; Philipsen, 2009; Silverman, 2004).

Whether vicarious liability is imputed to the hospital, group practice, HMO, physician, or other party turns on the specific relationships and the degree of control exercised by one professional or party over the APN. A hospital, for example, is not held liable for the professional negligence of non-employed medical staff members regardless of whether they are physicians or APNs. Although courts take many factors into account, the final decision in any case depends on the facts and circumstances particular to that situation (Feld & Moses, 2009; Silverman, 2004). If physicians are, by law or policy, required to supervise APNs, then the degree to which they are held accountable for APN practice is greater than if they are in a collaborative relationship; in the latter case, "some neglect by the physician must be proven" (Buppert, 2008, p. 262). From a litigation perspective, this makes the ongoing effort of anesthesiologists to continue to supervise the practice of nurse anesthetists in states such as New Jersey puzzling. Nurse anesthetists provide 65% of all anesthesia care in the United States annually, are the sole providers in two-thirds of rural hospitals in the United States, and are the primary anesthesia providers for the military. A large study comparing the care of nurse anesthetists in 14 states (2 more, Colorado and California, have now joined them) that had opted out of the Medicare rule requiring anesthesiologist supervision to those of nurse anesthetists in states that have not opted out found no increase in risk to patient safety in the opt-out states (Dulisse & Cromwell, 2010). Multiple court decisions have concluded that surgeons, dentists, and health-care centers working with CRNAs do not accrue increased liability because they are *not in control of the CRNA* (AANA, 2002b). The 2009 Nursing Service Organization analysis of claims brought against CNA-insured nurses practitioners between 1998 and 2008 determined that nurse practitioners with claims were more likely than nurse practitioners without claims to say that their state regulations require direct physician supervision (CNA HealthPro, 2010).

Since APNs are significantly less likely than physicians to have claims payments made against them (Hooker et al, 2009; NPDB, 2011a; Pearson, 2011), it can be reasonably concluded that physicians should be more concerned about the litigation risk posed by their physician colleagues than their APN colleagues. Still, anecdotal reports of an increasing number claims made, for example, against obstetrician/gynecologists in New York and New Jersey who work with CNMs and NPs (Silverman, 2004), create anxiety for physicians about APN liability risk and result in some physicians refusing to sign collaborative agreements/joint protocols or demanding large payments because they fear automatic surcharges to or rises in their insurance rates (Torre, Joel, & Aughenbaugh, 2009). When, as happened to CNMs in New York and New Jersey in 2004, insurance rates doubled, physicians or hospitals may be less enthusiastic about hiring these providers, considering them too costly (Silverman, 2004).

Although many APNs work in what they would describe as collaborative practices with physician colleagues, legal parameters set by Board of Medical Examiners' Corporate Practice Rules in some states (for example, New Jersey) preclude physicians from being a corporate partner with (or an employee of) professionals of "lesser licensure," such as APNs, so most APNs are employees. Where APNs work in practice together and are required to have a joint protocol or collaborative agreement with a physician, they may contract with physicians as consultants. In a true collaborative practice, the APN is an independent practitioner and not an employee. This business arrangement is a prudent form of risk management for all parties because accountability rests with the individual provider. No one practitioner controls or is liable for the activities of another. This risk control strategy does not ensure an APN will not be sued, but it does appreciably diminish the chances of unprotected and unwarranted vicarious liability for all parties. Although it is true that the physician who employs an APN can be liable, like any employer, for the negligence of their employees under the theory of *respondeat superior*, if another type of business relationship exists between the physician and the nurse, there is no legal basis on which to impute liability automatically to the physician.

Removing the statutory and regulatory requirements for supervisory or collaborative agreements and joint protocols from all state statutes will make it clear that the responsibility for the totality of APN care resides solely with them and that should reduce real or perceived physician anxiety about increasing liability risk when sharing care with their APN colleagues.

MALPRACTICE INSURANCE AS A RISK MANAGEMENT TOOL

Liability for individual acts or judgments as a professional cannot be transferred, but financial responsibility for damage awards (indemnity) and legal (defense) fees incurred in arriving at damages may be transferred. The objective is to limit the financial effect should you cause or be accused of causing injury to another (Buppert, 2008; Shinn, 1998). Purchasing professional liability coverage involves thorough investigation and selection of insurance with a regular review of coverage to be sure it continues to meet practice risks. A suggested process includes the following steps:

- **Identify a carrier:** Professional liability carriers differ from one specialty to another. APN professional associations and their Web sites are a reliable source of information about insurers who can be expected to understand and have experience in representing advanced practice nurses. Practicing colleagues with coverage are another source of information. Choose a company with a sound financial reputation, preferably one with an A to A++ rating (A. M. Best & Co., 2002).
- **Select the type of coverage:** Although it seems to be increasingly difficult to find (and may be completely unavailable for CNMs and nurse anesthetists), Buppert (2008) encourages trying to purchase occurrence rather than a claims-made coverage because occurrence policies will cover the APN regardless of when the incident occurred and whether or not the policy is currently active; claims-made policies cover the APN only when the contract is currently active.

Additional tail-funding can (and should) be purchased to extend the period of coverage with a claims-made policy, but this will add to the cost of the insurance.

- **Select level of coverage:** Since so many cases occur where damage awards exceed $1 million, Buppert (2011, p. 17) counsels that nurse practitioners should purchase "as much insurance as you can get, and afford."
- **Understand the coverage limits:** For example, $1,000,000 each occurrence/$5,000,000 annual aggregate means the most paid for any one claim is $1,000,000 and the number of claims at that amount that can be paid in 1 year is five. Find out if legal costs are included in the policy. Are they included within the limits of liability or are they in addition to the limits? If they are not included, the APN would be responsible for these costs (CMF Group, 2002).
- **Determine policy settlement provisions:** Look only for an insurer who agrees to consult, will permit choice of counsel, and will not settle without written consent.
- **Understand costs of malpractice insurance:** Rates differ considerably for APN specialties and the cost burden of malpractice insurance therefore also varies by specialty. The average salary of a CNM in Michigan in 2011 was about $61,000, and malpractice rates for Michigan CNMs, determined in a 2006 survey, averaged $11,131 (ERI, 2011; Xiao et al., 2008). In contrast, the average salary for a New Jersey NP in 2011 was approximately $92,000 (*Advance for Nurse Practitioners,* 2011) whereas the average annual cost for full-time malpractice coverage for a New Jersey pediatric or family nurse practitioner (who, among NPs, pay the highest rates) was less than $1,400 (Marsh, 2011). Comparing costs of malpractice insurance for nurse practitioners in those states that have achieved full scope of practice independence to those in states that have not demonstrates no significant increases in rates for NPs in the independent states.
- **Know contractual obligations:** In addition to the duties the insurer has to you, there are limitations of which the APN needs to be aware. All policies have specific exclusions under which the insurance does not apply. All policies exclude criminal acts or events that are "against public policy." In general, the broader the coverage, the higher the premiums. Maintaining professional liability protection is a partnership. The insured also has obligations to the insurer that must be honored if professional risks are to be successfully managed. Truthfulness when applying for insurance, timely premium payments, and complying with the conditions of coverage as stated in the policy are essential. Key among all policy conditions is notification of the insurer as soon as possible if an adverse event occurs (Buppert, 2008; Coakley, 2010).

What Happens When a Lawsuit Is Filed

APNs justifiably dread the prospect of a lawsuit, which will impugn professional competency, create personal and family anxiety, and incur financial hardship. Education about an issue can reduce stress and promote informed decision making. The same approach applies here. Know what to do if the lawsuit appears. Patients bring lawsuits against nurses with the belief that the nurse, or the nurse's insurance company, can pay the damages that the patient alleges were caused by the nurse's negligence (Sloan & Hsieh, 1995). As a practical matter, the lawyer for the patient or the patient's family makes a case assessment before filing the lawsuit to determine whether the case has merit. For a malpractice lawyer who takes cases on a contingency basis (i.e., the lawyer is paid a percentage of any award, but only if the patient wins), the golden rule is to go after only the "live fish." In other words, malpractice lawyers only sue professionals, including doctors or nurses, who have the money or insurance to pay any judgment or settlement. To ensure there will be someone at the end of the lawsuit to pay an award, lawyers for patients frequently name any and all entities or individuals who could possibly have something to do with the claim of injury. When a suit is filed, an APN should anticipate the following:

- The APN is served with copy of the suit that includes the summons and complaint filed by the plaintiff (patient).
- The professional liability coverage must be activated by immediately by notifying the insurance agent or the insurance company verbally.
- The specifics of the claim and the date of notification are recorded. Any conversations must be thoroughly documented, including the next steps each party is to take.
- One copy of the summons is retained; one copy is sent to the insurance agent and one to the employer, if applicable.
- Anecdotal documentation is prepared (i.e., all that can be recalled about the incident: who, what, when, where, how, and why). If possible, the patient record should be consulted. Dates, times, and people involved should be noted.
- If employed, the APN is to notify the risk manager verbally and in writing, again documenting the interaction with risk management.
- The temptation to discuss the suit with others should be avoided. Discussions should be limited to the insurance agent, claims representative, attorney, and, if applicable, the employer's risk manager. Do not discuss the case with anyone related to the plaintiff, anyone who might be a witness for the plaintiff, or the news media.
- Do *not* assume any financial obligation or pay any money without the insurance company's consent. If this occurs, the APN cannot expect the costs to be covered by the liability policy (Shinn, 1998).

Insurer's Response

- Within 24 to 48 hours from the time of notification of the filing of a claim, the APN should be contacted by the insurer's claim representative whose skills have been matched with claim specifics to ensure the best-qualified person manages the claim.
- The insurer will have determined whether other providers covered by the insurer are being sued or have been sued by the same patient. If so, the insurer will determine whether there is any conflict in having one person manage the lawsuit for all the insured providers. The assignment of a single claims representative occurs when all the insured agreed with the carrier that no one is at fault or fault lies with someone not insured by the liability carrier.
- The claim representative interviews the APN by phone and explains what the insurance policy covers. In addition, the claim representative contacts any other carriers (e.g., the employer) that should or might be providing coverage for the APN (Shinn, 1998; Shinn & Curtin, 2001).

Legal Counsel

- Once coverage is confirmed, the APN is advised by the claim representative what law firm will be providing counsel. Attorneys are usually from local or regional firms who have negotiated fee arrangements to handle the insurer's claims and have medical malpractice experience related to the specific claim.
- The assigned lawyer interviews the APN. The objectives are for the lawyer to become more familiar with the case while the APN becomes comfortable with the lawyer. To facilitate this process the APN should ask for (a) the lawyer's credentials, (b) the number of cases of this type previously litigated, (c) the number of cases that have gone to trial, and (d) the outcomes.

- The APN should contact the claim representative immediately if he or she is dissatisfied with the assigned attorney and request that a change be made. Walker (2011) emphasizes that the APN's lawyer should be an expert in APN statutes and regulatory requirements, and fully understand APN scope of practice and the professional standards of APNs.
- Once the lawyer is agreed on, the APN should receive a written outline from the insurer's claim representative stating what law firm will provide defense, as well as any investigative firm that will be used, and an explanation of how the claim will be handled. Coverage issues should be described along with current status and detailed resolutions.
- The APN's counsel and the plaintiff's lawyer then engage in discovery (i.e., investigation of the facts of the claim). Written questions called *interrogatories* are served by both sides, followed by written responses and the appearance of the plaintiff, defendant, and witnesses at depositions where a court reporter will take their testimony under oath. In the end all information gathered is used to settle or ready the case for trial (Coakley, 2010; Shinn & Curtin, 2001).

Settlement

- Although each case should be evaluated on its merits, it is possible for settlements to be reached regardless of whether the APN has some fault or not. In the first instance, variables include some degree of fault, social climate, plaintiff socioeconomic factors, local statutes, previous jury verdicts for similar claims, the APN's ability to pay the claim, and the potential for a verdict in excess of the liability limits. Reasons for settlement even when the APN is not at fault include economics, medical records that do not support APN actions, impracticality of having the APN testify in his or her own defense, or the desire to avoid the unpredictability of a jury trial (Coakley, 2010; Shinn & Curtin, 2001).
- In the end the best rule for the APN is never to agree on a settlement until having had the opportunity to express personal opinions about the case, have them seriously considered, and conclude personally that a settlement is the best resolution of the matter (Coakley, 2010; Shinn & Curtin, 2001). Remember that a settlement will be reported to the National Practitioner Data Bank. This means it will be part of an APN's permanent professional record.

TRIAL

Risks Inherent in Witness Testimony

In a trial, the patient has the burden of proof. To be successful, evidence must be sufficient to meet the four elements of negligence: duty, breach of duty, causal connection, and damage. The plaintiff's attorney typically presents the case with as many types of witnesses as possible. Witnesses may include the patient, aggrieved family members, APN experts, medical experts, hospital employees, or economic experts. Each of these witnesses plays a different role in the plaintiff's case.

The patient allegedly injured by the APN is often the most powerful witness. If possible, the injured party describes firsthand what he or she thinks occurred, as well as the bad effect caused by the APN's actions or omissions. Family members are effective witnesses because they serve to personalize the patient, demonize the APN, evoke jury sympathies, and inflame jury passions.

The testimony of nursing and medical experts is crucial to a plaintiff's case because it provides a clinical perspective on the problems described by the patient and the patient's family members. The plaintiff's APN experts explain how the APN breached the standard of nursing care owed to the patient. They do so by pointing out problems found in the APN's own clinical records and other ways in which the care was allegedly substandard. They also challenge the adequacy of the APN's continuing education.

Medical experts testify about the nature and extent of the patient's injuries and describe the pain and suffering, disability, or additional health risks resulting from these injuries. In addition, the experts opine on the manner in which the APN's breach of the standard of care directly caused these injuries and point out any ways in which the APN and, often, the collaborating physician failed to comply with the applicable standard of care. Finally, they explain why the patient's injuries were *not* a natural and unavoidable result of the individual's medical condition, known risks associated with the procedure or treatment, the aging process, or a preexisting health problem.

It is not unusual to see experts attack the qualifications, training, and continuing education of the APN. Perhaps of greatest importance are their attempts to increase the opportunity to have the judge or jury assess punitive damages by linking a lack of qualifications to a wanton or reckless disregard for the welfare of the patient. Finding evidence in memos and e-mail files of shortcuts, failure to respond to telephone calls, or undue financial controls is usually not difficult. "Putting profits or self-interest before patients" is a common mantra of the plaintiff's argument.

Testimony of current and former colleagues and employees of a hospital on behalf of the plaintiff presents a danger to the APN because they will claim that the APN treated them badly, was unprofessional, unreliable, and consistently put his or her own self-interests ahead of patient care by consciously not responding when needed or simply not knowing the appropriate thing to do. Employee testimony is orchestrated to increase the APN's punitive damages exposure by showing a pattern of callous behavior toward both patients and employees.

In the trial process, the plaintiff's witnesses are questioned by the plaintiff's attorney and cross-examined by the APN's counsel. Once the plaintiff concludes, the APN's counsel has the opportunity to present witnesses to rebut the plaintiff's allegations. The APN may or may not testify, depending on the specifics of the suit (Myers & Fergusson, 1989).

Trials may end with the successful defense move for a directed verdict against the plaintiff. This means the APN's lawyer asserts and succeeds in arguing the plaintiff failed to meet the burden of proof or has not made a valid case for malpractice. If the trial is a bench trial, the judge rather than a jury decides on the verdict (Aiken, 2004). Most plaintiffs demand a jury trial. If the verdict is against the APN, the APN, counsel, and insurer determine the next steps (Shinn & Curtin, 2001). One option following an unacceptable verdict is to file an appeal to the next higher court (Buppert, 2008).

Risk Reduction Strategies

To avoid malpractice, Buppert (2011) recommends that APNs be wary of developing a patient-provider relationship (implicitly a duty to the patient) with colleagues, neighbors, family, and friends outside of a formal practice relationship; practice within established standards of care; be sensitive to the limits of education, expertise, and scope of practice; consult with and refer to other providers as early and often as necessary, especially if "the history and examinations suggest a deadly condition and it hasn't been ruled out or treated" (p. 17); carefully document so that clinical choices are clear and justifiable; find another work setting if the current one is not permitting safe practice; and purchase an individual occurrence malpractice insurance policy.

Strategies for limiting exposure to a significant malpractice case must focus on neutralizing the factors that are favorable to the plaintiff's case or on turning them to the APN's advantage. In the best of all circumstances, these interventions and practices are put into action to prevent a lawsuit from being filed in the first place and they are thoroughly documented to provide evidence of the APN's good faith in the event of litigation. Broadly, these actions are described as caring, communication, competence, and charting (Giessel & Palentino, 2006).

Caring and Communication: Fostering Positive Relationships With Patient and Family

APNs must manage expectations by providing the patient and family with a realistic depiction of care and treatment needed, as well as expected outcomes. This message should be reinforced consistently in clinical records and written materials, including educational materials and all one-on-one communications. If a significant gap exists between what is promised and the actual capacity to deliver care and services, there is a high risk that the patient and the family will be disappointed.

In addition, when discussing any aspect of care and services, particularly any aspect of informed consent, the APN should present the information in easy-to-understand lay person's terms that take into account the patient's condition and the limitations of treatment. Finally, the APN should explain issues typical to all patients in similar circumstances and encourage the patient and family to work with the APN to identify and prevent problems.

In the event of a poor outcome or adverse reaction, every effort must be made to disclose the events to the patient and family, respond to their concerns, ameliorate the patient's condition, and address either the professional conduct or system's failure that led to this outcome. Making apologies to patients and families for bad health-care outcomes is an emerging strategy; ethicists and liability experts increasingly argue that providers have a moral responsibility to admit medical error and that disclosure linked with offers of compensation may reduce total liability costs, notwithstanding the complexity of appropriately providing such an apology and the emotional impact of an apology on both patients and provider (Gallagher, Studdert, & Levinson, 2007; Kachalia, 2009). The good faith effort of this practice standard should be noted by APNs as it is now recognized and protected in many states (NCSL, 2007).

In these days of instant communication, maintaining an appropriate level of accessibility to both patients and institutions is a must. It is far better for patients to contact the APN directly at any time than for them to feel they must call an attorney or a government agency to report substandard care or medical errors. Work hard to avoid making a diagnosis and providing treatment by phone or email.

Office and hospital staff members should be encouraged to get to know the patients. Staff members who know their patients' names and individualized care needs and preferences make better caregivers and poorer litigation targets than staff members who do not take the time to develop such relationships. Emphasize this point to staff whenever possible. It seems too obvious to state, but everyone wants to be treated with dignity and recognition of their individuality. Positive relationships may be one of the primary reasons why people decide *not* to sue a health-care professional.

APNs must pay particular attention to the patient's medical history and understand the patient's underlying medical conditions and concurrent treatment and drug therapies to meet their medical needs. In a lawsuit it may be necessary for the APN to address medical progress by explaining how that patient's underlying medical conditions affected any negative outcome experienced by the patient. At the beginning of evaluation and treatment it is prudent, if not always practical, for the APN to obtain from the patient or a legal representative an authorization to release medical information from all other facilities where the patient has been treated and to obtain these materials and review them. This activity not only helps the APN to appreciate and understand the patient's full medical and behavioral picture, but also provides a wealth of information in the event of a subsequent lawsuit.

In turn, the patient's medical history is essential for determining the patient's prognosis, rehabilitation prospects, and medical risks; for developing and carrying out an effective care plan; for providing a context in which to evaluate the patient's progress; and for providing possible medical explanations for negative outcomes experienced by the patient while under the APN's care. Buppert (2008) urges APNs to be alert to high-risk patients characterized by multisystem failure, substance abuse, and cognitive and emotional challenges. She suggests that APNs refer early; carefully document care and failures to follow up; review medications at each visit and provide easily understood and clearly legible dosing instructions; where possible, involve guardians or family members when counseling or teaching patients with cognitive challenges to ensure patients understand their circumstances and have truly consented to treatment; and be aware that if a patient has sued another provider, the patient may seek to sue his or her current one as well.

Fostering Positive Staff Relationships

To cultivate office and hospital staff, the APN should acknowledge and respect them. To the extent possible, APNs should ensure that their own office staff are paid and treated as well as their counterparts at other offices. Acknowledging caring behavior early and often is important. Employees appreciate the opportunity to participate in decisions that affect their work environment. Feedback should always be encouraged on issues of importance to staff. Staff training not only is the key to improving the delivery of care but also may be presented as a benefit, particularly to employees of the hospitals and nursing home where the APN practices. It helps to have employees and staff members improve their business, administrative, and clinical skills. In many ways the APN depends on them for carrying out orders. In addition, staff who are not health-care professionals but filling positions such as receptionist, appointment secretary, or business administrator may be the first and most frequent individuals with whom a patient interacts; it is essential that patients perceive these key people to be accessible and interested in addressing their needs speedily, competently, and courteously. In support of positive conduct, all training efforts by the staff should be encouraged and rewarded.

Fostering Positive Relationships With Physicians and Other Professional Colleagues

Maintaining open lines of communication with collaborating and attending physicians, with other health-care providers in the community, and with facility nursing and medical staff is also essential to minimizing the risks of future lawsuits. As for the legal relationship with the collaborating physician, the APN must be informed about the requirements, if any, under the state nurse practice acts for advanced practice nursing and follow them.

APNs must also manage the business relationships between themselves and their physician colleagues and institutions. It is essential to review all written agreements and institutional credentialing procedures and bylaws to be sure they do not create the impression of an employee relationship or impute vicarious liability on the physician or the institution unless that is what both parties intend. Requirements for unnecessary controls, such as supervision or practice restrictions, should be addressed because, as described previously, they could actually increase rather than decrease exposure to legal liability for both the physician and the institution.

APNs should keep collaborating physicians informed of developments in the practice or the care of a specific patient that might create the risk of a lawsuit. The physician-APN team should confer and decide whether changes in care are indicated and whether both need to more closely monitor care delivery systems and identify potential areas of concern. APNs should seek the collaborating physician's help in resolving any concerns about a patient's course of treatment.

Maintaining Competence

APNs are required by both state law and national certification requirements to complete a specified number of continuing nursing education contact hours in their specialty for recertification and it is essential that they keep ready files to document this education should they be audited by either state boards of nursing or national certification bodies. To provide evidence-based care, APNs must reach out to seek the clinical, procedural, and legal information that will guide "best practice" for their patients. Ready accessibility to online learning options make keeping up easier, and utilization of handheld electronic tools means information can be uploaded, viewed, and used nearly immediately.

Documenting Care

Keeping detailed records of care provided is time consuming and often onerous, but it is imperative for liability risk reduction. Electronic medical records systems, although complicated and often expensive to implement, help accurately share patient information between providers, increase legibility, and may make the process of record-keeping less labor intensive; however, they are only as accurate and complete as the information entered into them. When quotations from patients (who have declined care or been noncompliant with treatment, for example) will help make clear actions the provider has taken, be sure they are included in the record and keep them objective. Include summaries of phone conversations and email messages that contribute to understanding patients' concerns and providers' suggested next steps. If a patient misses an appointment, record that. Document informed consent. Never alter a record, as written (Giessel & Palentino, 2006; Miller, 2009).

CONCLUSION

Although APNs are sued for malpractice relatively infrequently, it is an experience to be strenuously avoided. Thoughtfully reviewing liability risk reduction strategies before beginning practice and repeatedly reminding oneself of them thereafter can help achieve this goal: know and follow state and federal laws governing APN practice; know institutional policies and abide by them; maintain clinical competency and expertise through ongoing continuing education; warmly engage patients and families in their own care using clear communication; document care carefully, preferably using an electronic medical record; follow evidenced-based practice guidelines; understand the limits of your knowledge and expertise; consult often and refer in a timely and appropriate manner; foster positive relationships with staff and professional colleagues; and purchase, and keep current, the most comprehensive malpractice insurance policy that is available for your specialty and within your budget.

REFERENCES

Advance for Nurse Practitioners. (2011, August). 2010 nurse practitioner salaries by state. *Advance for Nurse Practitioners,* p. 5.

Aiken, T. D. (2004). *Legal, ethical and political issues in nursing* (2nd. ed.). Philadelphia: F.A. Davis.

A. M. Best & Company. (2002). *Rating insurers.* Retrieved July 2, 2008, from www.ambest.com/ratings/about.asp.

American Association of Nurse Anesthetists. (2002a). *CRNA malpractice update.* Retrieved July 3, 2008, from www.aana.com/insurance/insur042302.asp.

American Association of Nurse Anesthetists. (2002b). *Legal issues in nurse anesthesia practice.* Retrieved July 3, 2008, from www.aana.com/crna/prof/legal.asp.

American Society for Healthcare Risk Management. (2002). Perspectives on the state of the insurance market and answers to health care risk managers' million-dollar questions. *Monograph of the American Society for Healthcare Risk Management.* Retrieved July 2, 2008, from www.hospitalconnect.com/ashrm/resources/files/monograph.pdf.

Black, H. (Ed.). (1979). *Black's law dictionary* (7th ed.). St. Paul, MN: West.

Bovgjerg, R. R., Miller, R. H., & Shapiro, D. W. (2001). Paths to reducing medical injury: Professional liability vs. patient safety. *Journal of Law, Medicine and Ethics, 29*(3-4), 369-380.

Buppert, C. J. (2002). Steering clear of Medicare fraud. *NSO Risk Advisor, 11,* 1–2. Retrieved July 2, 2008, from www.nso.com/newsletters/newsletters.php#archives.

Buppert, C. J. (2008). *Nurse practitioner's business practice and legal guide* (3rd ed.). Sudbury, MA: Jones & Bartlett.

Buppert, C. J. (2011). Three frequently asked questions about malpractice insurance. *Journal for Nurse Practitioners, 7*(1), 16–17.

Bureau of National Affairs. (2004). Nurse-anesthetist sentenced to probation, restitution for fraudulent health care billing. *BNA Health Fraud Report, 6*(4), 424.

Clinton, H. R., & Obama, B. (2006). Making patient safety the centerpiece of liability reform. *New England Journal of Medicine, 354,* 2205–2208.

CMF Group. (2002). *Don't make mistakes when buying your malpractice insurance.* Retrieved July 2, 2008, from www.npjobs.com/malpractice/buying.mistakes.shtml.

CNA HealthPro. (2010). *Understanding nurse practitioner liability: CNA HealthPro nurse practitioner claims analysis 1998–2008.* Retrieved October 2, 2011, from http://www.nso.com/pdfs/db/Nurse_Practitioner_Claim_Study_02-12-10.pdf?fileName=Nurse_Practitioner_Claim_Study_02-12-10.pdf&folder=pdfs/db&isLiveStr=Y.

Coakley, C. (2010, June 14).What if I'm sued: here's what to expect from a malpractice suit. *Advance for NPs and PAs.* Retrieved September 23, 2011, from http://nurse-practitioners-and-physician-assistants.advanceweb.com/Features/Articles/What-If-Im-Sued.aspx.

Dulisse, B., & Cromwell, J. (2010). No harm found when nurse anesthetists work without supervision by physicians. *Health Affairs, 29*(8), 1469–1475.

ERI. (2011). *CNM salaries.* Salary Expert. ERI Economic Research Institute. Retrieved September 28, 2011, from http://www.salaryexpert.com/index.cfm?fuseaction=Browse.CNM-salary-data-details&PositionId=111296.

Fairman, J. A., Rowe, J. W., Hassmiller, S., & Shalala, D. E. (2011). Broadening the scope of nursing practice. *New England Journal of Medicine, 364*(3), 193–195.

Feld, A. D., & Moses, R. E. (2009). Most doctors win: What to do if you are sued for medical malpractice. *American Journal of Gastroenterology, 104,* 1346–1351.

Freedman, M. (2002, May 24). The tort mess. *Forbes,* 90–98.

Gallagher, T. H., Studdert, D., & Levinson, W. (2007). Disclosing harmful medical errors to patients. *New England Journal of Medicine, 356,* 2713–2719.

Giessel, C., & Palentino, J. (2006). Malpractice and risk management: A look at current issues and practices. *Medscape Nurses, 8*(2). Retrieved September 4, 2011, from http://www.medscape.com/viewarticle/543977_2.

Healthcare Integrity and Protection Data Bank. (2008, May). *Fact sheet.* Washington, DC: Author. Retrieved July 2, 2008, from www.npdb-hipdb.hrsa.gov/pubs/.

Hooker, R. S., Nicholson, J. G., & Le, T. (2009). Does the employment of physician assistants and nurse practitioners increase liability? *Journal of Medical Licensure and Discipline, 95*(2), 6–16.

Horrocks, S., Anderson, E., & Salisbury, C. (2002). Systematic review of whether nurse practitioners working in primary care can provide equivalent care to doctors. *British Medical Journal, 324,* 819–823.

Infante, M. C. (2000). Legally speaking: Malpractice may not be your biggest risk. *RN, 63*(6), 67–71.

Ingram, J. D. (1993). Liability of medical institutions for the negligence of independent contractors practicing on their premises. *Journal of Contemporary Health Law and Policy, 10,* 221–231.

Institute of Medicine. (2000). *To err is human: Building a safer health system.* Bethesda, MD: National Academy of Sciences.

Institute of Medicine. (2010, October 5). *The future of nursing: Leading change, advancing health.* Washington, DC: National Academies Press.

Jena, A. B., Seabury, S., Lakdawalla, D., & Chandra, A. (2011). Malpractice risk according to physician specialty. *New England Journal of Medicine, 365,* 629–636.

Kachalia, A. (2009, January). Disclosure of medical error. *Perspectives on Safety in Morbidity and Mortality Rounds on the Web.* Agency for Healthcare Research and Quality. Retrieved September 26, 2011, from http://www.webmm.ahrq.gov/perspective.aspx?perspectiveID=70.

Kaiser Family Foundation. (2011). Summary of coverage provisions in the Patient Protection and Affordable Care Act. *Focus on Health Reform.* Retrieved October 2, 2011, from http://www.kff.org/healthreform/upload/8023-R.pdf.

Laurant, M., Reeves, D., Hermens, R., Braspenning, J., Grol, R., & Sibbald, B. (2006). Substitution of doctors by nurses in primary care. *Cochrane Database of Systematic Reviews,* Issue 1.

Lefevre, F. V., Water, T. M., & Budetti, P. P. (2002). A survey of physician training programs in risk management and communication skills for malpractice prevention. *Journal of Law, Medicine and Ethics, 28*(3), 258–266.

Levinson W., Roter, D. L., Mullooly, J. P., Dull, V. T., & Frankel, R. M. (1997). Physician-patient communication. The relationship with malpractice claims among primary care physicians and surgeons. *Journal of the American Medical Association, 277,* 553–559.

Marsh. (2011). *Malpractice rates for employed nurse practitioner in NJ.* Retrieved October 2, 2011, from https://proliability.marshpm.com/ahc/prol/?APPLICATION=PROL&professionCode=NURSE&associationAbbreviation=ANA.

Mello, M. M. (2006). *Medical malpractice: Impact of the crisis and effect of state tort reforms.* Robert Wood Johnson Foundation Synthesis Project. Project No. 10. Retrieved September 25, 2011, from http://www.rwjf.org/files/research/15168.medmalpracticeimpact.report.pdf.

Miller, K. P. (2009). Malpractice trends: Viewing the data and avoiding the hot seat of litigation. *Journal of Nurse Practitioners, 5,* 662–665.

Myers, K., & Fergusson, P. S. (1989). *Nurses at risk.* Des Moines, IA: HealthPro & Kirke Van-Orsdel.

National Conference of State Legislatures. (2007). *Medical malpractice tort reform: 2006 state introduced legislation.* Retrieved July 2, 2008, from www.ncsl.org/standcomm/sclaw/medmalrefrom06.htm.

National Conference of State Legislatures. (2011, August 15). *Medical liability/medical malpractice laws.* Retrieved September 27, 2011, from http://www.ncsl.org/?tabid=18516.

National Practitioner Data Bank. (2008). *Fact sheets.* Washington, DC. Retrieved June 26, 2008, from www.npdb-hipdb.hrsa.org.

National Practitioner Data Bank. (2011a). *NPDB reports on individuals. 2011 summary report.* Washington, DC. Retrieved September 6, 2011, from http://www.npdb-hipdb.hrsa.gov/resources/reports/NPDBSumRpt.pdf.

National Practitioner Data Bank. (2011b). *2006 annual report.* Washington, DC. Retrieved December 29, 2011, from http://www.npdb-hipdb.hrsa.gov/resources/reports/2006NPDBAnnualReport.pdf.

Park, M., Cherry, D., & Decker, S. L. (2011). Nurse practitioners, certified nurse midwives and physician assistants in physician offices. National Center for Health Statistics: *NCHS Data Brief.* No. 69, August 2011.

Pearson, L. (2012, April). The Pearson report. *American Journal for Nurse Practitioners.* Retrieved May 1, 2012, from http://www.pearsonreport.com/.

Philipsen, N. C. (2009). Resolving conflict: A primer for nurse practitioners on alternatives to litigation. *Journal for Nurse Practitioners, 4*(10), 766–772.

Schmidt, W. C., Heckert, D. A., & Mercer, A. A. (1992). Factors associated with medical malpractice: Results from a pilot study. *Journal of Contemporary Health Law and Policy, 7,* 157–182.

Shinn, L. J. (Ed.). (1998). *Taking control: A guide to risk management.* Chicago: Kirke Van-Orsdel, Inc. & Chicago Insurance Company.

Shinn, L. J., & Curtin, L. L. (2001). What to do if you are sued. *Nurse Risk Management Series,* Article 3, pp. 1–7. American Nurses Association. Retrieved September 23, 2011, from http://www.nursingworld.org/mods/archive/mod310/cerm103.htm.

Silverman, J. (2004, June 15). Premiums doubled since last year: Nurse-midwives feel sting of rising premiums, lawsuits; professional collaboration increases ob. gyns' litigation exposure, vulnerability. *OB/GYN News.* Retrieved July 2, 2008, from www.imng.com/titles/OBGYN/index.html.

Sloan, F. A., & Hsieh, R. (1995). Injury, liability and the decision to file a medical malpractice claim. *Law and Society Review, 29,* 413–438.

The Joint Commission. (2008). *2008 patient safety goals.* Retrieved July 2, 2008, from www.jointcommission.org/PatientSafety/NationalPatientSafetyGoals.

Torre, C., Joel, L., & Aughenbaugh, A. (2009). Maximizing access to health care in New Jersey: The case for APNs: A white paper. *New Jersey Nurse,* April 2009.

Underwood, A. (2009). Would tort reform lower costs? *NYTimes.com,* August 31, 2009.

Walker, R. (2011). Elements of negligence and malpractice. *Nurse Practitioner, 36*(5), 9–11.

Weiler, P., Hiatt, H. H., Newhouse, J. P., Johnson, W. G., Brennen, T. A., & Leape, L. I. (1993). *A measure of malpractice: Medical injury, malpractice litigation and patient compensation.* Cambridge: Harvard University.

Wright, W. (2008). Preventing malpractice. Lecture presented at NJSNA/FNAP APN Professional Education Day, Atlantic City, New Jersey, April 2, 2008.

Xiao, X., Lori, J. R., Siefert, K. A., Jacobson, P. D., & Ransom, S. B. (2008). Malpractice liability burden in midwifery: A survey of Michigan certified nurse-midwives. *Journal of Midwifery and Women's Health, 53*(1), 19–27.

28 Ethics and the Advanced Practice Nurse

Gladys L. Husted
James H. Husted
Carrie Scotto

Experience and knowledge alone do not ensure the development of ethical practice. Rubin (2009) described the structure of a type of nursing practice that restricts the development of clinical knowledge and ethical judgment even in experienced nurses. Elements of this restrictive practice include stereotyping patients; failure to recognize qualitative distinctions in physical, mental, or contextual circumstances; failure to accept responsibility for professional decisions; and lack of a sense of agency. This type of practice impedes the progression of nursing practice beyond the novice level.

Benner's (2001) novice-to-expert theory of nursing practice development allows for the newly practicing registered nurse (RN) to begin at the novice level. However, models for advanced practice require expert nursing practice and do not allow for novice practice (Walsh & Bernhard, 2011). Based on the *Essentials of Doctoral Education for Advanced Practice Nursing* (American Association of Colleges of Nursing, 2006), advanced nursing practice education must move the nurse beyond the novice level. Advanced nursing practice education ought to provide opportunities to achieve essential and specialty competencies of advanced practice. In addition, opportunities for feedback and reflection necessary for synthesis and broader learning must be included to bring the advanced practice nurse (APN) beyond the level of knowledge and practice acquired in baccalaureate education. Therefore, the theoretical foundation of advance practice education must be based on models that include self-reflection and intellectual dialogue in addition to knowledge and skill acquisition (Fawcett, Newman, & McAllister, 2004).

The symphonological model, as will be demonstrated, ensures that practitioners will begin with patient-centered, holistic assessment including the contexts of knowledge, situation, and awareness. The consideration of the bioethical standards to direct practice within the patient's circumstances will facilitate the type of reflection that will preserve a nursing model rather than a medical model for practice, thereby enhancing the lives of their patients and of themselves, albeit in different respects.

THE VALUE OF COMMUNICATION

One day two nurses in a jungle village passed under a coconut tree. As they passed, a coconut fell from the tree to the ground. An argument arose between them as to who had a right to possession of the coconut. Finally, they decided to do what seemed the only fair and ethical thing to do. They *would split the coconut in half and each nurse would take one half of the coconut. They shook hands and each prepared to go on her* way.* — *(Husted & Husted, 2008a, p 41.)*

Nurses (and everyone else) sometimes make unfortunate decisions without ever realizing it and without learning anything from it (Tuckett, 1999). This is especially likely to occur when we do not engage ourselves in a process of discursive thought.

Fortunately, before the nurses parted, a colleague passed them. She was an APN whose years of well-examined experience had developed in her the habit of seeking out reasons and relevance. When she asked them what they were going to do with the coconut, each was surprised by the answer of the other. One wanted the shells to use as cups for holding water and was not interested in the meat of the coconut. The other only wanted the meat and had no interest in the shells. As a result of the APN's intervention, one nurse now has twice as much coconut meat as she would have had otherwise and the other nurse has two cups instead of one.

Responsible ethical decision making and action in health care is somewhat like the division of coconuts. It requires awareness and understanding of the context in which the decision is to be made. All health-care professionals should assume the responsibility of seeking out what ought to be done and *why* it ought to be done. None of the contemporary ethical systems, as we will discuss, consistently recommends attention to these distinctions. "APNs are frequently at the forefront of advocating for patients seeking primary and/or specialty care and must be knowledgeable about the nature of ethical dilemmas and skilled in making ethical decisions" (Kalb & O'Conner, 2007, p. 197).

Nursing is not only concerned with patients in crisis; it is about patients in temporarily unpleasant conditions. Ethics is not only about difficult dilemmas; it is also about everyday occurrences. "Although ethical issues in health care receive much publicity, attention is rarely given to the non-dramatic, everyday ethics of health care" (Smith, 2005, p. 32). If an APN faces a choice between following present convenience and the welfare of her patient, she should recognize that an ethical responsibility is at play here. And, hopefully, she will choose her patient's welfare.

A practice-based ethical system, understandably, attends to practice. The welfare of her patient is the focus of a nurse whose ethical practice is mature and advanced.

PRACTICE-BASED BIOETHICS

For bioethics, one disability defines and sets apart every patient regardless of the nature of his affliction. This is the loss of agency—the power of an individual person to initiate and sustain action, the power to act on his purposes. . . . To achieve this purpose [returning agency to the patient], symphonology interweaves professional (therapeutic) practice and ethical interaction. — *(Husted & Husted, 2008b, p. 104.)*

The purpose of symphonology is to return the patient to a state of agency, where he can be his own agent to the extent possible in the context. A practice-based, symphonological (*symphonology* from *symphonia,* a Greek word meaning agreement) approach to ethical interaction is an approach from professional responsibility. Symphonology defines ethics as a system of standards to motivate,

*We use the pronoun "she" for the nurse or any health-care professional and "he" for the patient. This convention is for the reader's ease of understanding and to keep understanding in context. The singular is preferred to the plural or indeterminate because professionals and patients are individuals, and a practice-based ethic is, and ought to be, an individualistic ethic.

determine, and justify actions directed to the pursuit of vital and fundamental goals.† Ethics is not convenience; it is not etiquette, and it is not that which brings on a state of self-satisfaction. Symphonology is a *practice-based bioethic* derived from, and appropriate to, the self-determination of a patient, the purposes of a health-care setting, and the role of a health-care professional.

Practice-based bioethics aims to relate professionals and patients internally (to bring them into the same ethical context), to make human values its focus, and to make the health-care setting maximally purposeful.

Practice-based bioethics is based on interactions between a professional and a patient who relate themselves through agreement and understanding. When a nurse strengthens a patient's confidence in his recovery or supports him in dealing with a morbid prognosis, she is nursing within a practice-based ethical system.

The measure of success for a practice-based bioethic is a patient's vital objective that he shall regain or retain his power to initiate and sustain actions. An ethic that is not skillfully exercised and harmoniously interwoven with practice cannot justifiably be the ethic of a health-care professional. It is the "ethic" of a nurse who is merely "going through the motions."

The nurses who passed the coconut tree made a valuable discovery. The best action to take depends on the nature of the context, the motivations of the persons involved, and what it is possible to do in this context. The best professional actions depend precisely on the same realities—and on respect for individual rights. These produce relevant, appropriate, and justifiable ethical actions.

RIGHTS

Rights (a singular term denoting a single, noncomplex agreement) is the product of an implicit agreement among rational beings made and held by virtue of their rationality, not to obtain actions or the product or conditions of action from one another, except through voluntary consent, objectively gained. It is freedom from aggression—an agreement not to aggress (Husted & Husted, 2008a, p. 22). See **Table 28-1.**

†All definitions, unless otherwise stipulated, are taken from the text by Husted and Husted, 2008a.

TABLE 28-1

Individual Rights

Individual rights	The state of nonaggression that results from this implicit agreement.
Among rational beings	Beings who can think, a capacity of all humans.
Made and held by virtue of their rationality	Made because of their rationality and the fact that, being rational, they can see the advantage to it.
Not to obtain actions	For example, by coercion.
Nor the product of actions	By taking over a person's life.
Or conditions of actions	By changing the circumstances of the person's life for the worse.
Except through voluntary consent	One is not coerced—the agreement establishes the terms of interaction.
Objectively gained	One is not deluded or deceived, but is fully informed.

Adapted from the digital supplement for educators accompanying G. L. Husted & J. H. Husted. (2008a). *Ethical decision making in nursing and health care: The symphonological approach* (4th ed.). New York: Springer.

In any society to the extent people recognize and are faithful to this agreement, its members respect and enjoy human rights. When this is lacking, they do not. "When ethical agents live and interact together, the benefit of the rights agreement is so great and so obvious, the detriment of not having this agreement is so manifestly ruinous, that the agreement literally 'goes without saying'" (Husted & Husted, 2008a, p. 23).

Ethical practice does not allow a professional to violate the rights of a patient. A dedication to human values is internal to the ethical nature of the health-care setting. This presupposes respect for the rights of patients.

The practice of nursing, ideally, goes beyond respect for rights. However, a professional, practice-based ethic must *begin* with the recognition of a patient's rights. Through this recognition, a nurse provides a bridge between a patient's present condition and situation and the realization of the values her profession promises.

The reality of individual rights is not complex. It is present whenever two or more people are together. Each has a right not to be aggressed against by the other. Rights surround every human interaction, however insignificant. Rights are a reality so familiar and all encompassing that, in normal circumstances, it is the last thing with which one has to be concerned.

The rights agreement is the ethical foundation for all explicit agreements. It is the already preestablished implicit agreement that explicit agreements will be made without deception and will be honored.

The rights agreement structures and defines *human* interaction and the pursuit of human values. The recognition of rights produces interaction according to the standard of reciprocity—a voluntary process of give and take, without force or deception, and without interference with the other person's pursuit of values.

ADVANCED PRACTICE AND A PRACTICE-BASED BIOETHIC

Rapid advances in technology make many demands on the character, education, and abilities of the advanced practice nurse. The emphasis on scientific developments throughout the past several centuries has caused ethics to take a quantitative rather than a qualitative approach. Science has sought to separate itself from concerns about human values and values systems. — (Callahan & Mannino, 1998, p. 282.)

Whenever the need for an ethical decision arises in the health-care setting (and this is daily), it is confined within a specific, radically limited, yet complex context. The more complex the context, the more valuable are the ethical attitudes of a nurse who makes decisions that are based on this context—a nurse who makes practice-based decisions.

All of a nurse's experience that is relevant to her ethical competence is, ultimately, experience with individuals. The health-care setting is defined by the nature and purposes of human beings. A practice-based ethic is defined by the same realities. Each follows and enhances the other.

There is no such thing as skillful nursing without skillful ethical analysis. Ethical reasoning and clinical judgment share a common process, and both serve to teach and inform the other. The importance, therefore, of attention to clinical practice, regardless of how far removed an APN is from the clinical setting, cannot be overemphasized (Solomon et al., 1994). A person does not graduate from nursing school or enter a nursing graduate program already skilled in bioethical decision-making. Just as clinical expertise requires experience and attention, so does ethical expertise.

THE CONTEMPORARY ETHICAL THEORIES

If professional nursing practice is to be shaped by bioethical concerns, the ethic of nursing, of necessity, must be derived from, and relevant to, the profession and its practice. Attention to the context and careful thought and analysis are the essence of any competence, including advanced practice competence. Contemporary ethical theories do not lend themselves to the health-care professions or to ethically defensible decisions in health-care practice. None of the dominant ethical theories could be discovered in, or derived from, the profession of nursing. None can be made relevant to nursing practice.

> *Skillful ethical comportment will deteriorate to a merely competent level if we apply norms and principles to complex practical situations where we have the potential for skillful recognition of patterns. . . . Strategies of adjudication and the search for certitude through the application of norms and principles, though comforting, do not produce skillful ethical comportment.* — *(Benner, Tanner, & Chesla, 1996, pp. 276–277.)*

Yet, this is exactly what the contemporary ethical theories demand. See **Table 28-2.**

> *Things are seldom what they seem. Skim milk masquerades as cream; Highlowes pass as patent leather; Jackdows strut in peacock' feathers.* — *(H.M.S. Pinafore, Gilbert & Sullivan, 1885.)*

A young woman or man entering the profession has every reason to believe that the purposes of nursing are shaped by the deepest and most vital human concerns—those concerns that are related to the life, health, and well-being of those who are sick and disabled. Unfortunately for nursing students, the contemporary ethical theories being taught are not *relevantly* related to these purposes.

The dominant ethical theories of today being taught to nurses are deontology, utilitarianism, and cultural or social relativism. The result always involves an element of emotivism.

Deontology is the theory that actions in conformance with formal rules of conduct are obligatory regardless of their results (Angeles, 1992). Deontology requires a nurse to attend to out-of-context duties. Intention is the overriding ethical concern while *consequences* are viewed as irrelevant. The individual motivations and character-structures of a patient are secondary, or more often, *unrelated* to the ethics of nursing practice.

TABLE 28-2

Contemporary Ethical Systems

Systems	Defining Characteristic	View on Consequences
Deontology	Following the rule.	Not important.
Utilitarianism	Doing the greatest good for the greatest number.	Consequences to the greatest number.
Social or cultural relativism	Beliefs of a particular society, culture, or religion are paramount.	Social mores do not relate to individual consequences.
Emotivism	If I feel it is right, it is right.	The individual determines consequences for self; consequences to others are irrelevant.

There is nothing inherent in the practice of nursing that implies that in a dispute between the requirements of a patient's welfare and the demands of deontology, a nurse ought to choose deontology. Van Hooft (1990) states, "The idea that we are following rules when we act morally is a tired hangover from the days when the lives of people were controlled by religious and secular absolute rulers who accorded no respect or independence to ordinary people" (p. 211). "Deontology is entirely concerned with an agent's actions. It is unconcerned with consequences. It is also indifferent to the agent's intentions, except his intention to do his duty" (Husted & Husted, 2008a, p. 211).

Utilitarianism is the theory that one should act so as to promote the greatest happiness (pleasure) of the greatest number of people (Angeles, 1992). Utilitarianism requires a nurse to pay attention to consequences, but consequences to a larger number than one patient. It is impossible for a nurse to give her concern to the largest number possible, and at the same time, provide optimum care for her individual patients. Only optimum care—the best care a professional is capable of—is ethical care. There is no such thing as indifferent ethical care.

There is nothing in nursing as a profession that justifies the idea that, once a nurse has accepted a patient, she ought never to abandon concern for her patient in favor of pursuing the greatest good for the greatest number. The profession of nursing is incompatible with such a demand. Utilitarianism is a theory in which the end is said to justify the means (Gibson, 1993). It would, all too often, make the patient a means, and the desires of the patient's family or the nurse's outlook on life, for example, an end. The purposes of individual patients, and not the whims of a greater number, are the reason for being of professional nursing. Nothing in the principle of utility (i.e., the greatest good for the greatest number) establishes the principle of individual justice (Sarikonda-Woitas & Robinson, 2002).

Social or cultural relativism is the theory that what is ethical and what is unethical is determined by the customs, beliefs, and practices of a society or a culture (Angeles, 1992). There is nothing in the purposes or traditions of nursing to suggest that, in a clash between the requirements of a patient's welfare and the demands of one's society or culture, a nurse should choose the sentiments of the society or culture. This would turn a nurse's attention onto the views of a society or culture and away from her patient. Relativism undermines professional practice and the well-being of patients. A patient's culture may be important, but it can be of no greater importance than the importance given to it by a patient. "Culture provides a set of perspectives about how the group interprets its life and what happens to it, including sickness and death. However, culture is not a discrete trait descriptive of all individuals in it. Rather, culture should be understood as having a dynamic nature" (Kim, 2005, p. 164).

Barnes and Boyle (1995) observe that: "Unfortunately, the emphasis on shared patterns has rather rigidly defined nursing's perceptions of people from specific cultures and has not allowed for personal variations [of individual persons] within a given culture" (p. 414). Communication between patients and cultures is, at best, a figure of speech. Cultures, as such, have no tongues, no ears, and no ability to evaluate an individual's values and circumstances. Only individuals have this (Kikuchi, 1996).

> *While cultural factors are a valuable blueprint to caring for a patient, there can be no justification for failing to allow for the patient's personal evaluation of the beliefs of her culture to serve as the standards of culturally congruent care. Otherwise one is caring for the culture and not the patient, and the concept of "care" will have been subjected to a radical change in meaning. — (Zoucha & Husted, 2000, p. 326.)*

A flawed definition of a human being is more virulent than a plague.

Emotivism is the doctrine that holds that feelings or emotions are forms of ethical knowledge. The doctrine states that every ethical judgment and decision is simply a disguised description of a person's feelings (Angeles, 1992). The irrelevance of the contemporary ethical systems inevitably leads ethical agents to depend on emotions, rather than objective awareness.

There is nothing in the nature of nursing to suggest that, in a clash between the requirements of her patient's welfare and the demands of her present emotional state, a nurse should guide her actions by her feelings—quite the contrary. Emotivism turns a nurse's attention into herself and away from her patient. It replaces her professional responsibility with an obsession onto her ever-changing emotional moods. It makes ethical interaction between a professional and her patient entirely illusory.

"Knowledge" of all these theories is gained by cultural osmosis and expressed in largely unverbalized feelings. None of these theories produces a concern for the person in one's care. Close attention to the appropriate context, and careful analysis based on the nature and purposes of nursing, is what defines nursing.

A Rational Form of Bioethical Decision Making

The intrinsic ethic of a profession is structured by a process of discovering facts, causes, and motives. The contemporary theories demand that a nurse evade her objective, contextual awareness, and the discovery and recognition of immediately given facts relevant to her patient's individual situation. The theories project discovery and recognition away from a patient's values onto her first emotional responses, or onto the sentiments, opinions, and desires of others. For a practice-based ethic, an answer to a dilemma that a nurse and patient share is one that is independent of out-of-context beliefs and attitudes. Ideas based on one or more of these theories strengthen views such as the following:

- Ethics constitutes from issues—euthanasia, harvesting organs from anencephalic infants, research on the incompetent, cloning, medical use of marijuana, and so on.
- Unanalyzed and largely irrelevant individual or cultural opinions are ethical facts.
- Ethical action, in certain circumstances is important, but the circumstances requiring ethical action are unimportant.
- What is true or false in any circumstance is true or false in every similar circumstance.
- Rights are alienable. I would not let you decide for me, but I will decide for you.
- It is the role of a professional to make ethical decisions for her patients, but these roles are not reversible.

MORAL COURAGE/MORAL DISTRESS

Nurses are obligated to practice in a way that seeks benefit and avoids harm for the patient. Accordingly, the practice of nursing must be moral. Due to economic, political, and social influences the APN role has expanded and evolved to include more direct and autonomous practice. This progression has brought an increase in responsibility for APNs that demands not only expert practice, but also an increased understanding and commitment to ethical practice (Benner, Tanner, & Chesla, 2009; Buerhaus, 2011). To meet this demand, APNs must possess strong moral courage.

Moral courage is the ability to do what is right or moral despite elements that would influence a person to act in another way (Lachman, 2011). It is the resolute commitment to ethical principles despite threat or risk (Murray, 2011). Ethical competence is essential for moral courage and consists of the ability to analyze and respond to moral problems uninhibited by routine, emotional, or dogmatic tenets (Lachman, 2011). Thus, moral courage precludes moral elitism and allows no claims of ethical superiority. The patient within the context is the basis for decision making and action.

Moral courage develops as a result of repeated experiences that move the practitioner beyond competent practice to one in which there is persistent integration of ethical principles (Miller, 2005; Murray, 2011). Threats to moral courage arise as individuals may face risks such as loss of employment, professional reputation, future advancement, or other negative outcomes. This can lead to moral distress. Moral distress results when the nurse knows the ethical action best suited for the patient in context, but is unable to act because of such considerations as inadequate staffing, institutional requirements, health policy constraints, or cost containment (Repenshek, 2007).

> *The relationship between moral courage and moral distress is not straightforward. It is tempting to say that if nurses have sufficient moral courage they need not experience moral distress. . . . However, given that organizations are not always supportive and do not always react appropriately, but rather may act defensively to concerns about standards of care raised by conscientious practitioners, even the most morally courageous staff may fear to speak up. — (Gallagher, 2010, para. 15.)*

"As nurses advance into leadership positions, the complexity of the decisions they need to make increases, as does the potential for moral distress" (Edmonson, 2010). Unfortunately, "nurse educators . . . have tended to focus [when teaching ethics] simply on the ethical principles . . . [not] on their work environment [as] an ethical context" (Corley, 2002, p. 637). Although moral courage is not sufficient to avoid moral distress (Gallagher, 2010), the practice of APNs, based on the symphonological ethical model, dealing with individuals within the context of their professional practice, will support and advance moral courage. Each experience will be a patient-centered, ethical event. In addition, it will enable APNs to be able to justify their decisions and actions. The accumulation of these events will prepare the APN with a strong foundation that will promote ethically driven patient care (Sekerka & Bagozzi, 2007).

THE IMPORTANCE OF CONTEXT

Ethics is concerned with the good of the individual. The good of an individual can only be discovered in a context. A professional ethic assumes that a professional's strength of character is appropriate to produce the flourishing of her patients. So do her patients (Guido, 2006). "Ethics provides structure for placing conduct into action" (Guido, 2010, p. 3). This is basic and the defining end of a professional ethic.

A professional ethic aims at a single end—the end that is the reason for being of the profession. This reason for being establishes and structures the APN's professional context. It relates an APN and a patient internally within this context.

Gastmans (1998) states, "The nurse functions both as a professional and as a human being within a variety of contexts. These contexts influence directly or indirectly the way in which the nurse performs caring tasks" (p. 126).

When a nurse, as an ethical agent, learns how to identify the various parts of an ethical context and their interrelations, she has developed a significant practical skill. When she is able to understand the individual human values that make each context what it is, she has developed an advanced practice competency. The ancient Greek philosophers described this ability as "practical wisdom." The great Chinese thinkers (whose benign influence in the West, although largely unacknowledged, was enormous) called it the *Way*—acting in harmony with the nature of things.

"Context is complex and comprehensive, dynamic, and interactive. Despite how tempting and how much easier it is to resort to the general, the abstract, and the theoretical, any form of bioethics that does not put moral [ethical] problems in their myriad contexts is, in many senses of the word, unreal" (Hoffmaster, 2006, p. 40).

There are three elements of every context that guide objective awareness and action. See **Table 28-3.** First is the *context of the situation.* This context is comprised of the interwoven aspects of a situation that are fundamental to understanding the situation and to acting effectively in it. These are the facts that are necessary to act on to bring about a desirable result.

The second is the *context of knowledge.* This is the agent's understanding of the aspects of the situation that are necessary to an understanding of the situation and to acting effectively in it. In other words, this is the knowledge one has of how to deal with these facts most effectively. These resources of knowledge enable a nurse to identify and interweave the two sides of the context into a coherent plan of action.

The third is the *context of awareness.* This is a bridge between the agent's present awareness of the relevant aspects of the situation and of her present knowledge. An agent's context of awareness includes her awareness of those aspects of the situation that invite action. Every decision that an agent makes, if she acts in (or according to) the context, must be made according to:

- Her knowledge.
- That which is appropriate to the situation.
- Her present awareness of what she knows, and of what is relevant in the situation (Husted & Husted, 2008a, p. 89; also see Table 28-3).

A person's context is the interweaving of these three elements, which provides the resources for making a justifiable decision. Reigle (1996) states, "Knowledge of facts is insufficient if not tempered with the contextual features of each case. Only after the unique conditions of the case are considered can an ethically acceptable solution be identified" (p. 275).

Everything relevant to a context is contained within the context. A multitude of factors that surround that context are irrelevant. These are the factors that play no part in the nature of the dilemma. They neither cause the dilemma nor can they help to resolve it. The resources of the context are resources because they provide *relevant* criteria for ethical decision making.

Here is a simple example: A nurse discovers that a patient is allergic to a certain medicine and acts accordingly. The fact that he is allergic is one part of the context of the situation. Her discovery of this fact, made by virtue of her past experience and her present thinking processes, becomes one part of her context of knowledge. Her purpose is to protect him. This is made possible by her context of awareness.

A context always forms itself around a purpose. One discovers a change to be made or a goal to be achieved and sets about to learn how, in the circumstances, this is to be done. The key to this is to be able to know the difference between the relevant and the irrelevant. The relevant is any factor in the context that will enable a profession to bring about a change in the context and facilitate the achievement of a purpose. The irrelevant is that which does neither. That which threatens to frustrate the purpose is the inappropriate.

TABLE 28-3

The Three Elements of the Context

Of the situation	The interwoven aspects of the situation that are fundamental to understanding and to acting effectively in it
Of knowledge	The relevant knowledge that a health-care professional brings to the situation
Of awareness	The bridge between an agent's present awareness of the relevant aspects of the situation and of her present knowledge

Wurzbach (1999) states that although persons seek certainty in their decisions, "ethical certainty can provide [unwarranted] comfort for the ethical decision maker . . . and stifle dialogue and in-depth discussion of the [situation]" (p. 287). All the certainty that one has in any given context is the certainty that the context allows. One can have contextual and contingent certainty but never final and immutable certainty.

The Levels of a Context

There are a number of levels to every context. The first level is the split second, immediate present—the sensory level of awareness. Observations are taken of all the objective factors comprising the situation at any given moment taken in isolation from one another but without the awareness of their vital influence and relationship. This is the level of the contemporary ethical systems.

The second level is brought into being by a cognitive level of awareness. This level is provided by one's grasp of the nature and relationship of the objective factors as they exist in the present. This is the level of a nurse whose overriding concern is the well-being of her patient.

The third level is produced by foresight. Foresight provides the awareness of relationships, events, and causal sequences as they have evolved out of the past into the present and how they are relevant to the future. This is, or ought to be, an APN's bioethic.

The higher the level of a context and the more an APN relates herself internally to the context, the more appropriate her decisions and the more effective her actions will be. A nurse is "the agent of a patient doing for a patient what he would do for himself if he were able" (Husted & Husted, 2008a, p. 21). Her patient is the center of the context. She is acting internally to the context when the values and motivations that produce decisions and actions on her part are her patient's values and motivations. Values and motivations that are not her patient's, but demanded by the contemporary ethical theories, are external and irrelevant, and often inappropriate, to the context. They produce externally related, out-of-context actions, and very often, tragic examples of injustice.

That which is relevant to a practice-based professional ethic is not a matter of tradition or social convention. In the health-care setting, ethical decisions and actions begin with a grasp of those things that are crucially important in the life of a human individual. An APN is a human individual and is capable of understanding and dealing with this.

THE FLOURISHING OF AN APN

Decision-making is that which most characterizes advanced practice. . . . Underlying decision-making are clinical judgments, scholarly inquiry, and leadership. . . . The work of the advanced practice nurse is practice, the product is patient care; therefore, leadership in the advanced practice role supports the scientific process by:

- *Interpreting the context of practice*
- *Demonstrating influences on care*
- *Leading changes in practice* — *(Erickson & Sheehy, 1998, p. 244.)*

That ethical decision-making skills are part of the core competencies of all APNs is a basic tenet and central to the definition of advanced nursing practice (Reigle, 1996). Ideally, the ethical aspects of her practice will have developed along with the clinical aspects.

A practice-based ethic aims to relate professionals and patients internally, to bring them into the same ethical context, to make human values its purpose, and to make the health-care setting maximally purposeful and mutually intelligible. An APN can master the art and science of ethical decision making and interacting with what is important in her patient's life. In doing so, she increases her patient's well-being, strengthens the profession of nursing, keeps the practice of nursing contextually intelligible, and establishes for herself the conditions of pride in herself and her profession.

Only by following the definition of her profession can a nurse make her profession intelligible to her patient and to herself. Being the agent of her patient defines her profession. She takes actions for a patient—a person who has been formed by a lifetime of unique experiences and unique reactions to these experiences. In doing this, she develops pride in herself and in her practice. To allow a relatively helpless but competent person to decide for himself is the highpoint of a nurse's pride in her profession and her self-esteem.

She takes actions that a patient cannot take for himself. Yet, although she takes these actions, they are his actions. In coming under her care, he does not give up his right to self-determination—his right to think, decide, and act for himself. He is in a health-care setting to gain the power of expressing himself in action. He is there so that health-care professionals can take the actions that he would take if he were able. These are actions that he has lost the power—but not the *right*—to take.

Every action of an APN is an interaction, whether the action is a cause that results in an immediate effect or a cause whose intended effect occurs farther on down a chain of causal sequences. All cooperation requires interaction.

The noblest action a nurse can take, without which no justifiable action is possible, is her act of accepting her patient as a human being as real as she is. Without this, the context is unintelligible and no real interaction is possible. For the APN, "the importance of developing skills of critical thinking, self-exploration, and the ability to sift through contextually relevant elements of ethical situations" (Doane, Pauly, Brown, & McPherson, 2004) cannot be overlooked.

THE NURSE/PATIENT AGREEMENT

Interaction requires intelligibility. Interaction is not possible unless all parties to the interaction know what they are doing, why they are doing it, and what they intend to accomplish. All of this requires a prior agreement. An agreement is a shared state of awareness on the basis of which interaction occurs (Husted & Husted, 2008a).

A nurse agrees that, for a time, she will be part of a patient's world. Her skills make her a vital part. Decisions can be made and actions can be taken based on an ethical agreement between a professional and her patient. The nature of these decisions and actions is limited by the terms of their agreement. Non–practice-based ethical theories demand that in her ethical decisions and actions she abandon her patient and his world. Her patient is protected by nothing. He cannot rely on his nurse's dedication. To a greater or lesser extent, his rights and human dignity—his very reality—have been dispensed with.

An APN has the resources for appropriately meeting the demands of the context. An effective health-care setting encourages her in discernment and discovery. Hardt (2001) states: "The . . . [APN] cannot practice successfully in an environment that does not foster context-driven decision making. If [caring nurses] . . . are not able to apply the knowledge they have gained from patients, related to their patient's preferences, then the patient's context is not honored" (p. 45).

A professional, through her open declaration that she is a professional, takes on various obligations as part of the nurse–patient agreement. Through these obligations a patient can rightfully expect the nurse to act ethically and conscientiously within the context. These obligations and these expectations are an integral part of the agreement between a nurse and her patient (Husted & Husted, 2008c).

If a patient's context is not honored, the APN's agreement, in whatever form it takes, is not honored. If the APN–patient agreement is not honored, then the professional is not practicing a profession, but a sham.

Professional practice is sufficient to establish a health-care professional–patient agreement. One human recognizes another. "Seeing each as human, diverse, equal, and worthy were all part of the view of the meaning of human dignity" (Kalb & O'Conner, 2007, p. 200). They recognize the human values that are the basis of their interaction and the attitudes appropriate to guiding these interactions. Because of this, the agreement between them can be formed spontaneously and on an implicit level—the level implied by their relationship. Under the circumstances, the human nature of each guides their awareness, the forming of an implicit agreement to interact, and their interaction. Even with an incompetent, comatose, or very young patient, the nurse's responsibility remains the same. There is a professional agreement in place. She does not have an explicit agreement with this patient. But she does have an implicit, professional agreement.

Even APNs, who are not practicing in the arena of direct patient care, still have the nurse–patient agreement in place. Educator, administrator, and researcher are ultimately responsible for patients and their well-being. The role of the educator is for the benefit of the patient. There is a teacher–student–patient agreement. A nurse administrator is ultimately responsible for patients and their well-being. There is an administrator–staff–patient agreement. A researcher must have the well-being of her subjects uppermost in mind, and thus there is a researcher–subject agreement. The research cannot come before the welfare of persons. Research for the welfare of persons ought not to come before the welfare of persons.

THE AGREEMENT ONE HAS WITH ONESELF

Socrates, the first systematic ethicist of the Western world (470–399 BC), is known to have observed that the unexamined life is not worth living.

> *Every nurse, [every APN], ought to examine her life, at least to the point at which she comes to an agreement with herself that she will be a nurse. To the extent that a nurse has not made this agreement with herself—a commitment to be a nurse—she resembles a patient more than she resembles what she would be if she were a nurse.* — *(Husted & Husted, 2008a, p. 48.)*

A nurse who directs her long-term actions guided by her awareness of what is needed for her to keep that agreement embraces her profession. A nurse who is inspired by it, and who is dedicated to it, is far less likely to experience burnout. She experiences joy in taking action . . . and pride and confidence in acting as she does.

> *A nurse [who] tries to avoid taking those long-term actions that constitute her professional life breaks the agreement she made with herself to be a professional. She becomes indifferent. She undermines herself as a professional and as a person. If she has replaced her confidence and pride with indifference, she has done this because she abandoned herself when she abandoned her profession.*
>
> *If one is a nurse and is likely to continue to be a nurse, one ought to take the actions [nursing] calls for. At worst, this will make life far less boring. At best, it may restore her to the confident expectations and the pride that she began with at the beginning of her career.*
>
> *Dedication to what one professes—acting on that which one affirms and believes—is sometimes difficult to do. Adversities and frustrations arise. And these attack one's desire and one's sense of self.* — *(Husted & Husted, 1999, p. 17.)*

Overcoming adversities through dedication produces pride in oneself as a professional. A patient could not reasonably ask for more and should not find less. He needs a rational agent to do for him what he would do for himself simply because his well-being depends on acting on the basis of reason.

THE ADVANCED PRACTICE NURSE AND THE ETHICAL AGREEMENT

To the extent that an APN acts without regard for her patient's needs and values, she assumes that his decisions and actions have no ethical standing. To the extent that an APN acts for a patient—according to his rational motivations—she shares her patient's rightful authority over himself. His rightful authority over himself is absolute.

Many agreements require detailed, explicit discussion. For obvious reasons, the agreement between an APN, or any nurse and patient, cannot require this. A nurse's interventions, quite often, must begin immediately. What will be discovered during the course of treatment is unpredictable.

An implicit agreement can be formed immediately. This is made possible by the fact that the role of nurse and patient are firmly settled in rational human expectations. Reflection on herself and on her needs gives a nurse a clear idea of a patient's needs and values. Although it is not possible for any person to know fully and completely the lived reality of another, it is the nature of human understanding to draw on common experiences and images to form agreements.

BIOETHICAL STANDARDS

The bioethical standards (autonomy, freedom, objectivity, self-assertion, beneficence, and fidelity) signify properties inherent in the nature of every human person. See **Table 28-4.** They are the innate and defining properties of a human life. As guidelines they prevent "contradictions," actions or interactions that conflict with a patient's power to act—his agency.

There are certain individualized characteristics that every patient brings into the health-care setting and retains by right. Any human characteristic—any virtue—that is necessary to his successful interaction, first as a human and then as a patient, is a resource that cannot, in any way, be justifiably violated.

It greatly increases an APN's efficiency if she understands the functions of these characteristics to exercise and to interact with them. The bioethical standards signify these characteristics. They are the resources without which any interpersonal agreement or interaction would be impossible, without which a patient's recovery would be inconceivable, and without which a nurse could not function. These are the characteristics of a nurse and patient:

- **Autonomy**—The individual uniqueness of each patient. This uniqueness is the structure of his individual nature, the liaison of his character structures.

His autonomy is structured by the way he uses his mind, the decisions he has formed, his view of his life, his purposes, and the powers and disabilities of his agency. His autonomy includes his power

TABLE 28-4

The Bioethical Standards

Autonomy	Uniqueness, independence, and ethical equality
Freedom	Right to direct the course of one's life
Objectivity	Ability to deal with the reality of one's situation
Self-assertion	Right to control of one's time and effort
Beneficence	Right to judge benefit and harm for one's self
Fidelity	Faithfulness to the terms of an agreement

of reason and his animal nature. As a consequence of his rational animal nature, his ethical equality with all other rational agents is established.

Primarily, however, autonomy refers to a person's uniqueness. No two people develop identically. There is no alternative to a human person being unique. Therefore, his uniqueness is a person's innate right. It is a nurse's guidepost to her professional actions.

There is no possibility of one's sustaining the excellence of the person he is, unless he sustains who he is. Thus, autonomy is a basic virtue.

- **Freedom**—Self-directedness. An agent's capacity, and consequent right, to take independent, long-term actions based on his own evaluation of his present situation.

It is the responsibility of a nurse to enable a patient to exercise his freedom. The ability to foresee, plan, and act effectively in his future is a value to, and an excellence of, any human being as a human being.

- **Objectivity**—The ability to focus one's attention onto an objective context.

Objectivity is a person's need and right to achieve and sustain his exercise of objective awareness. This standard calls for a nurse to sustain this in her patient and in herself.

To the extent one fails to exercise objectivity, he cannot act to enhance his life. The complete absence of this would destroy the ability to sustain his life. Objectivity is a necessary element of human excellence.

- **Self-assertion**—The power and right of an agent to control his time and effort.

This power produces each person's self-ownership. It establishes the right of an individual to be free of undesired or undesirable interaction; the right to initiate individual actions. On a nurse's part, it is her actions in nurturing and sustaining this power.

No human excellence would be possible without the power to control one's time and effort. This is a basic virtue and a value.

- **Beneficence**—The natural inclination of a person to act to achieve that which is beneficial and to avoid that which is harmful. This implies rational self-interest as the basis of the nurse–patient interaction.

A nurse's actions assist this effort. This standard establishes the right of a patient (or professional acting as the agent of a patient) to act for his benefit. It is the self-interest processes that define life. Rushton (1992) points out that as nurses we have an obligation to ourselves as well as to our patients and others. This is in keeping with rational self-interest as discussed by Husted and Husted (2008a). And following on this, "respect for one's own dignity . . . [is] a prerequisite to respecting the dignity of patients, colleagues, and others" (Gallagher, 2004, p. 220).

It is established by the necessity he faces to act, insofar as possible, to acquire the benefits he desires and the needs his life requires.

The ability to achieve benefits is what makes life worth living. The ability to avoid harms is a correlate of this.

- **Fidelity**—Adherence to the terms of an agreement. More generally, an individual's faithfulness to his autonomy. And, finally, fidelity to the context.

For a nurse, fidelity is a commitment to the obligations she has accepted as part of her professional role—her professional role being a significant part of her autonomy.

The dedication to continue on courses of action that are appropriate to enhancing life and well-being—this is fidelity. This is essential to human excellence. It is a most desirable virtue.

A nurse ought to recognize these virtues, not as obstacles to be overcome, but as character resources to be nurtured. She ought to recognize these virtues as her own. A person's life would be a woebegone affair without them. See **Figure 28-1.**

THE NECESSITY OF THE AGREEMENT

Every APN is at least implicitly aware of a patient's possession of these virtues. She cannot escape awareness of them. Without these virtues, their agreement would not be possible. Without agreement, their interaction would not be possible. If their interaction is not possible, professional actions are not possible. If the virtues are violated, the nurse–patient agreement cannot be sustained. If the

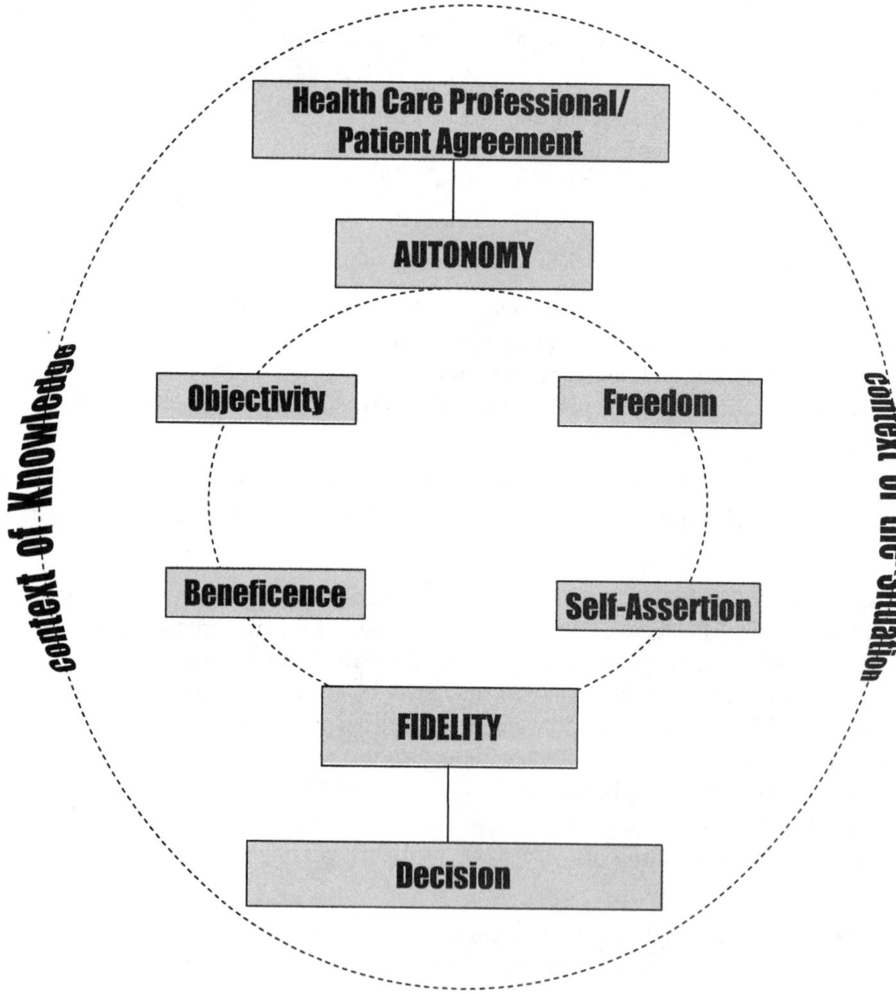

FIGURE 28-1 Husteds' symphonological bioethical decision-making guide. *(Source: J. H. Husted & G. L. Husted. (2008a.) Ethical decision making in nursing and health care: The symphonological approach (4th ed.). New York: Springer. Used with permission of Springer Publishing Company.)*

agreement is not sustained, interaction, properly so called, is impossible. If interaction is not possible, the practice of a profession is not possible. This is the source of the importance of the bioethical standards to professional practice. Their irreplaceable importance arises in the very first moment.

The Virtues of an Advanced Practice Nurse

Here we are using virtue in its original Greek and Chinese sense: the excellence of a person in performing his role as a person. Thus, the virtue of a farmer is to farm well, of a tailor is to make excellent clothing, and of a nurse is to nurse well. The virtue of every human being is to *live* well, to sustain and enhance his life. Thus, virtue is the excellence of a human being in being human.

Aristotle states, "Now fine and just actions . . . admit of much variety and fluctuation of opinion, so that they may be thought to exist only by convention, and not by nature" (as cited in McKeon, 1941, p. 936). However, fine and just actions follow from characteristics that are fundamental aspects of human nature and the virtues of a human person.

The standard of autonomy includes the inescapable fact (that is too often evaded) that every member of the human species—every rational animal—derives his ethical dignity from his nature as a member of the human species. This produces the fundamental ethical reality. Every ethical agent is the ethical equal of every other. No ethical agent can rightfully aggress against another for the benefit of that second ethical agent (Mill, 1988). Infidelity to, and aggression against, another can never arise from the virtues.

An APN is much more able to take direction from her patient's *autonomy*—his uniqueness—because she is not as engrossed in her own uniqueness as she would be if she were relatively new to the profession. If she is new to the profession, she is more focused on herself because she is, quite rightly, unsure of the requirements and techniques of her profession.

An APN is much more capable of allowing and fostering the *freedom* of her patient because she, herself, has mastered the skills that an advanced beginner must still acquire. Therefore, she is free to act within her patient's entire context. Every APN has taken independent and long-term actions to become an APN. Now she can assist her patient to take the independent and long-term actions that will restore him to a state of agency. Here, her experience is her best teacher.

An APN has a much greater ability to observe a context and to form *objective,* meaningful patterns of action because her body of knowledge is greater. She has had to exercise objective awareness to acquire the skills of an APN.

An APN has been able to gain more control over her time and effort because she can now sort out the relevant and the irrelevant aspects of her profession. She can focus on her patient's individual and vital needs. An APN is aware of a person's *self-assertion*—the right to control his own time and effort. In becoming an APN, she has exercised this right. An advanced beginner may be aware of this but may be unable to act on it.

An APN has exercised a greater than average *beneficence* (rational self-interest) toward herself in achieving the benefit of becoming an APN. She has also made herself better able to assist her patient in pursuing his values. She sees the patient as the beneficiary of her actions and has, hopefully, automatized this in her practice. This is the ethical foundation of her practice.

An APN has had the opportunity to develop a personal and professional integrity to the point that she understands that fidelity to her patient is *fidelity to herself,* to her professional practice, and to her life. As a nurse, she does not see this fidelity as separate from herself.

Because an APN does not have to think solely about the technical aspects of her professional practice, she is free to see the agreement as reciprocal (given the differences in their roles) and necessary.

An APN's knowledge is comprehensive and elaborately organized so that information storage and retrieval is easy. Her clinical knowledge is linked into networks of concepts and relationships, which are then compiled into a higher order knowledge structure that links intricate mental networks into a scheme of relationships and interaction.

Through experience, an APN has become capable of discovering much that a less experienced nurse is incapable of discovering. Progress in an APN's development will move through, and be structured by, her experience to the extent that she has capitalized on her experience. Retaining her experience of ethical situations will increase her context of knowledge. It will enable her to structure and integrate it. As her context of knowledge becomes greater, the context of every situation can become clearer to her. If she deliberates about the meanings of her experiences, this produces a relationship between her context of knowledge, the context of each individual situation that leads to an increase in her professional skill, and her context of awareness. This is also true of her ethical skill generally.

The big picture, and its meaningful details, will become evident through an increase in her knowledge and its attendant power to increase her awareness of present facts and future conditions. The increased acuity of her awareness will form an ever-greater body of knowledge with its power to clarify and sharpen her awareness of her patient's context. This is the source of her ethical competence.

This process of an APN's discovery and learning can never be complete. Learning that makes further learning seem impossible or unimportant has destroyed itself as a biological instrument in human life. The nature of every new situation must be learned. It can only be learned through contextual analysis of each situation. By its nature and its function in human life, learning can never be complete.

Ethical efficiency requires that every situation be approached without one's mind being enclosed in a handful of out-of-context-assumptions. Out-of-context truths work *against* ethical judgment.

Even the knowledge that character and motivations are produced by the dynamic complex of relationships among one's virtues (the bioethical standards) is a dead-end to practice if knowledge stops there. This knowledge of the bioethical standards is not sufficient to ethical decision making. It is not knowledge of self-sufficient rules. Through analysis, the bioethical standards are simply sufficient to guide the awareness that they can produce practice-based resolutions to every *individual* dilemma. *The standards must always be applied in the context.*

If there is any reason why nursing diagnosis and treatment is centered on her patient, there is no reason why her ethical decisions and actions should not be. Each serves the same values. To be faithful to the context, an APN cannot turn her back on anything in the context, most especially on her patient. If her patient cannot "call out" to her, then nothing in the context can.

A context-based model actualizes the concept of treating persons as individuals, and therefore, selecting individualized interactions based on a unique patient's needs and circumstances. It is a nurse's awareness of the patient's perceptions of his situation that assists her in understanding her patient's needs and desires. Symphonological theory is not just another compilation of traditional cultural platitudes. Symphonology presents a method of helping the nurse determine what is practical and justifiable regarding those aspects of her practice. Further, the theory of Symphonology recognizes that the context guides what is possible and desirable in the agreement (Scotto, 2008).

ABOUT CASE STUDY ANALYSIS

When ethically analyzing a case study, a difficulty arises in that, in practice, one would request more information—more pieces of data, answers to a greater number of questions—but the nurse can only work with what she has. And so, in a case study, the dilemma must occur entirely within the given context. Now consider the case presented in **Box 28-1.**

BOX 28-1
Case Study

Lois Ott, a 58-year-old, is suffering from end-stage renal disease. She can no longer do anything that gives her pleasure, and she is exhausted all the time. She has decided to forego dialysis and let the disease take its course. She has given this decision careful thought. Her family disagrees with her decision and has tried to talk her out of it. They are even thinking about trying to have her declared incompetent on the basis that the toxins in her blood system are making her thought process erratic. Roger, a family nurse practitioner, has been seeing Lois in the dialysis clinic for years. Lois has discussed her plans with Roger. Her family has tried to elicit Roger's help in getting her declared incompetent.

With the dialysis, Lois could probably live another 6 to 9 months. In supporting Lois, Roger can argue as follows:

Lois has had a lifetime of experiences. She has made a lifetime of choices and decisions and formed her life and *herself* according to her experiences and choices. If we, as professionals, have a right to ignore this, then her rights in the health-care system are displaced by habit and force. What we have become through our experiences and choices does not entitle us to erase the person that Lois is and treat her as one object among other objects in the health-care system. There is nothing in this situation that would, objectively, justify our stripping Lois of the right to determine her own life. On the surface, it seems that Lois's family is acting in her place and trying to think and decide with her. However, what Lois needs most is help in convincing her family that they are abandoning her and leaving her all alone in the experience of dying. Lois should not be all alone.

The course of action that Lois has chosen will injure no one and violate no one's rights. If we join her family in making her the instrument of what they desire, we will be harming her and violating her rights. However we go about the business of violating Lois's rights, we cannot make our actions right. We cannot make our actions appropriate and justifiable. It is not appropriate that Lois spend another 6 or 9 months alone, abandoned by the health-care system and her family and suffering during this time.

If we take control of her life and actions, her life will not belong to her. It will belong to us. We will act as though she is not the one living her life. We would not be content for someone else to choose the level of suffering we should endure and the way we should end our life. By the same token, *we* should not choose for *her.*

Lois has expressed her individual desires. Many people would not desire this, but many would, and Lois does. If, in every difficult decision, we were determined that those who disagree with us must accept our perspective, we would simply be acting as terrorists. These arguments can be offered in support of Lois. No comparable arguments can be made against Lois's position.

We made an agreement with Lois that we would act as her agent. Now we are entertaining the justifiability of breaking that agreement. This will make us unfaithful to Lois and unfaithful to our profession. There is no logical way we can justify this.

Notice that in analyzing this case we did not once use the term *ethics* nor did we name the bioethical standards. Nonetheless, our process was one of ethical decision making from a practice-based perspective. In a more complex case, analysis through each standard would be desirable to arrive at the most appropriate decision within the context. (For examples of more complex cases in which analysis is done through bioethical standards, see Husted & Husted [2008a]).

In a study done by Irwin (2004), when patients had an ethical decision to make, it was found that in talking about the decision and in trying to reach a conclusion, patients used all the bioethical standards (albeit not the words) in arriving at their conclusions.

As we have demonstrated through the contemporary ethical theories, ethics means different things to different people. By concentrating on decision making and speaking in human terms, terms that everyone can understand, you can probably avoid the chaos that results when, for instance, the head of a societal expectation bumps into the head of a scheme for the greatest good for the greatest number. Or either bumps into the head of an irreconcilable rule.

MUSINGS

Each patient entering the health-care system hopes to derive some benefit. He hopes to regain his competence to perform his normal functions and to live his life as he chooses. He wishes to enter again into the pursuit of his happiness. At the very least, he expects to come out better able to live than when he went into the health-care system. Each of the bioethical standards is appropriate to these purposes:

1. The *standard of autonomy* enables a patient to maintain his way of understanding himself and his world. (In a psychiatric setting, objectivity often replaces autonomy as a goal. Objectivity—an awareness of the facts of the external world—is a necessary precondition of autonomy. An autonomous being is autonomous in his relation to the external world.)

Sara is a timorous 82-year-old lady. Roseanne, her nurse practitioner, relates to her in a manner that implies that it is all right to be a timorous 82-year-old lady. When Sara leaves the health-care setting she will have a sense of her autonomy as strong as, or stronger than, when she entered.

2. The *standard of freedom* supports a patient's right to function as an independent being. It is the freedom to make the ethical decisions that affect his life.

Billy is a curious 6-year-old boy. Jane, his pediatric nurse practitioner, talks to him. She explains things to him. She asks his opinion. She allows him to make appropriate choices. Billy leaves the hospital as independent and self-confident as he was when he entered, or more so. In relation to his sense of freedom, Billy's hospital stay has had a positive effect.

3. The *standard of objectivity* is a patient's ability to function as a reasoning being.

To do this, he must have access to the understanding of his situation.

Jeff has been put on a low-salt, low-fat diet. Robert, his nurse practitioner, takes the time to explain to Jeff why he ought to stay on the diet. He motivates Jeff to stay on his diet by appealing to his understanding (his reason). He makes Jeff an active participant in his plan of care. He does not depend only on a passive emotional motivation that, in a few weeks, will probably fade away.

As Oscar Wilde (1989), tongue in cheek, remarks: "The only difference between a caprice and a life-long passion is that the caprice lasts a little longer" (p. 27).

4. The *standard of self-assertion* demands recognition of a patient's self-ownership. Leah is careful not to do anything that would interfere with her patient's control of his time and effort.

Ronnie is a 7-year-old child who is dying. He comes to the clinic every week for a transfusion. One day he says to Leah, his pediatric nurse practitioner, "I don't want this anymore." Leah explains what will happen if he does not get the transfusion. Ronnie says that he knows and he still does not want the transfusion. Leah gets the parents, physician, and other consultants together and tells Ronnie's story. Ronnie takes control of his life with Leah's help. — (Woods, 1999.)

5. The *standard of beneficence* protects a patient's reasonable expectation that he will derive some benefit from the health-care system. It is also recognition of a person's right *not* to be harmed.

A patient is dying of metastatic cancer. His family believes that he is going to recover and has made him a full code, despite the evidence of his suffering. He has expressed not wanting to live while he was conscious. He is now semiconscious and cannot make his wants known. The only thing he has to look forward to is avoidance of suffering. Barbara, his nurse, arranges to discuss the situation with the family. If she is unsuccessful, she will request an ethics consult.

6. The *standard of fidelity*—faithfulness to the nurse–patient agreement—is to establish assurance that purpose of action is not abandoned.

A child has wet the bed. He begs his nurse not to tell his parents. She promises that she will not. Fidelity establishes a predictable universe for the nurse and for her patient.

The agreement, with the bioethical standards as preconditions, is designed to enable a patient to bring his virtues into a biomedical setting, retain them while he is there, and have them intact when he leaves.

Bioethical analysis and interaction guided by the standards is not possible, in any objective sense, apart from the patient's purposes and attitudes. A patient is passive. His entire ethical purpose is to recover his agency, to act, to once again take charge of his life. The best thing that can happen to him is to encounter a nurse whose purpose is the same.

Through her progress as a nurse, an APN has, if only potentially, come to a greater understanding and experience of herself, of who she is, and, hopefully, she has come to appreciate the importance of this. Through her experience, she has come to understand the difference in the uniqueness in individuals and has gained a clearer insight into the meaning of this to an individual's progress toward a better life.

Through her experience, she has developed a greater than average skill at pursuing long-term goals guided by her objective awareness and an understanding of the importance and joy of this. Because of this, she is able to lead her patient down a version of the same path she has taken.

REFERENCES

American Association of Colleges of Nursing. (2006). *The essentials of doctoral education for advanced practiced nursing.* Washington, DC: Author.

Angeles, P. (1992). *Dictionary of philosophy.* New York: Harper Collins.

Barnes, D. M., & Boyle, J. S. (1995). *Transcultural concepts in nursing case* (2nd ed.). Philadelphia: Lippincott.

Benner, P. (2001). *From novice to expert: Excellence and power in nursing practice* (2nd ed.). Menlo-Park, CA: Addison Wesley.

Benner, P., Tanner, C. A., & Chesla, C. A. (1996). *Expertise in nursing practice.* New York: Springer.

Benner, P., Tanner, C., & Chesla, C. (2009). Entering the field: Advanced beginner practice. In P. Benner, C. Tanner, & C. Chesla (Eds.), *Expertise in nursing practice: Caring, clinical judgment, and ethics* (2nd ed., pp. 25–60). New York: Springer.

Buerhaus, P. (2011). Have nurse practitioners reached a tipping point? Interview of a panel of NP thought leaders. *Nursing Economics, 28*(5), 346–349.

Callahan, L., & Mannino, M. J. (1998). Legal aspect of advanced nursing practice. In C. M. Sheehy & M. C. McCarthy (Eds.), *Advanced practice nursing* (pp. 281–302). Philadelphia: F.A. Davis.

Corley, M. C. (2002). Nurse moral distress: A proposed theory and research agenda. *Nursing Ethics, 9,* 636–650.

Doane, G., Pauly, B., Brown, H., and McPherson, G. (2004). Exploring the heart of ethical nursing practice: implications for ethics education. *Nursing Ethics,* 11(3):240–53.

Erickson, R., & Sheehy, C. M. (1998). Clinical research in the advanced practice role. In C. M. Sheehy & M. C. McCarthy (Eds.), *Advanced practice nursing* (pp. 241–263). Philadelphia: F.A. Davis.

Fawcett, J., Newman, D., & McAllister, M. (2004). Advanced practice nursing and conceptual models of nursing. *Nursing Science Quarterly, 17*(2), 135–138.

Gallagher, A. (2004). Dignity and respect for dignity—two key health professional values: Implications for nursing practice. *Nursing Ethics, 11,* 587–599.

Gallagher, A. (2010). Moral distress and moral courage in everyday nursing practice. *OJIN: The Online Journal of Issues in Nursing, 16*(2).

Gastmans, C. (1998). Challenges to nursing values in a changing nursing environment. *Nursing Ethics, 5*(3), 236–245.

Gibson, C. H. (1993). Underpinnings of ethical reasoning in nursing. *Journal of Advanced Nursing, 18*(12), 2003–2007.

Gilbert, W. S., & Sullivan, A. (1885). *The mikado.* Retrieved June 9, 2007, from http://math.boisestate.edu/ gas/mikado/webopera/operhome.html.

Guido, G. W. (2006). *Legal and ethical issues in nursing* (4th ed.). Upper Saddle River, NJ: Prentice Hall.

Guido, G. W. (2010). *Legal and ethical issues in nursing* (5th ed.). Upper Saddle River, NJ: Prentice Hall.

Hardt, M. (2001). Core then care: The nurse leader's role in "caring." *Nursing Administration Quarterly, 25*(3), 37–45.

Hoffmaster, B. (2006). "Real" ethics for "real" boys: Context and narrative. *American Journal of Bioethics, 4*(1), 40–41.

Husted, J. H., & Husted, G. L. (1999). Agreement: The origin of ethical action. *Critical Care Nursing, 22*(3), 12–18.

Husted, J. H., & Husted, G. L. (2008a). *Bioethical decision making in nursing and health care: The symphonological approach* (4th ed.). New York: Springer.

Husted, G. L., & Husted, J. H. (2008b). The ethical experience of caring for vulnerable populations: The symphonological approach. In M. de Chesnay (Ed.), *Caring for the vulnerable: Perspectives in nursing theory, practice, and research* (2nd ed., pp. 103–113). Boston: Jones & Bartlett.

Husted, G. L., & Husted, J. H. (2008c). The nurse as ethical shield: The symphonological approach. *Perioperative Advanced Practice Nurse, 3,* 175–182.

Irwin, M. (2004). Application of symphonology theory in patient decision-making: Triangulation of quantitative and qualitative methods. Ph.D. dissertation, School of Nursing, Duquesne University.

Kalb, K. A., & O'Conner, S. (2007). Ethics education in advanced practice nursing: Respect for human dignity. *Nursing Education Perspectives,* 196–202.

Kikuchi, J. F. (1996). Multicultural ethics in nursing education: A potential threat to responsible practice. *Journal of Professional Nursing, 12*(3), 159–165.

Kim, S. H. (2005). Confucian bioethics and cross-cultural considerations in health care decision making. *Journal of Nursing Law, 10*(3), 161–166.

Lachman, V. (2011). Strategies necessary for moral courage. *OJIN: The Online Journal of Issues in Nursing, 15*(3).

McKeon, R. (Ed.). (1941). *The basic works of Aristotle.* New York: Random House.

Mill, J. S. (1988). *On liberty.* New York: Penguin. (Original work published 1819.)

Miller, R. (2005). *Moral courage: Definition and development.* Washington, DC: Ethics Resource Center.

Murray, J. (2011). Moral courage in health care. *OJIN: The Online Journal of Issues in Nursing, 15*(3).

Reigle, J. (1996). Ethical-decision making skills. In A. B. Hamric, J. A. Spross, & C. M Hanson (Eds.), *Advanced nursing practice: An integrative approach* (3rd ed., pp. 273–295). Philadelphia: Saunders.

Repenshek, M. (2007). Moral distress: Inability to act or discomfort with moral subjectivity? *Nursing Ethics, 16*(6), 734–742.

Rubin, J. (2009). Impediments to the development of clinical knowledge and ethical judgment in critical care nursing. In P. Benner, C. Tanner, & C. Chesla (Eds.), *Expertise in nursing practice: Caring, clinical judgment, and ethics* (2nd ed., pp. 171–199). New York: Springer.

Rushton, C. H. (1992). Caregiver suffering in critical care nursing. *Heart and Lung, 21,* 303–306.

Sarikonda-Woitas, C., & Robinson, J. (2002). Ethical health care policy: Nursing's voice in allocation. *Nursing Administration Quarterly, 26*(4), 72–80.

Scotto, C. (2008). Symphonological bioethical theory. In A. M. Romey & M. R. Alligold (Eds.), *Nursing theorists and their work* (7th ed.). St. Louis: Mosby.

Sekerka, L., & Bagozzi, R. (2007). Moral courage in the workplace: Moving to and from the desire and decision to act. *Business Ethics: A European Review, 16*(2), 132–149.

Smith, K. V. (2005). Ethical issues related to health care: The older adult's perspective. *Journal of Gerontological Nursing, 31*(2), 32–39.

Solomon, M. Z., Jennings, B., Guilfoy, V., Jackson, R., O'Donnell, L. Wolf, S. M., et al. (1994). Toward an expanded vision of clinical ethics education: From individual to the institution. *Kennedy Institute of Ethics Journal, 1*(3), 225–245.

Tuckett, A. (1999). Nursing practice: Compassionate deception and the good Samaritan. *Nursing Ethics, 6*(5), 383–389.

Van Hooft, S. (1990). Moral education for nursing decisions. *Journal of Advanced Nursing, 15*(2), 210–215.

Walsh, M., & Bernhard, L. (2011). Selected theories and models for advanced practice nursing. In J. Stanley (Ed.), *Advanced practice nursing: Emphasizing common roles,* (5th ed., pp. 89–114). Philadelphia: F.A. Davis.

Wilde, O. (1989). *The complete works of Oscar Wilde.* New York: Harper & Row.

Woods, M. (1999). A nursing ethic: The moral voice of experienced nurses. *Nursing Ethics, 6*(5), 423–433.

Wurzbach, M. E. (1999). Acute care nurses' experiences of moral certainty. *Advanced Nursing, 30*(2), 287–293.

Zoucha, R., & Husted, G. L. (2000). The ethical dimensions of delivering culturally congruent nursing and health care. *Issues in Mental Health Nursing, 1*(3), 325–340.

Index

Note: Page numbers followed by "f" indicate figures, those followed by "t" indicate tables, and those followed by "b" indicate boxes

A

B

C

O

Q

R

S

T

U

V

W

Y